Essential Respiratory Medicine

Essential Respiratory Medicine

Shanthi Paramothayan
Consultant Respiratory Physician
UK

WILEY Blackwell

Registered Office(s)
John Wiley & Sons, Inc., 111 River Street, Hoboken, NJ 07030, USA
John Wiley & Sons Ltd, The Atrium, Southern Gate, Chichester, West Sussex, PO19 8SQ, UK

Editorial Office
9600 Garsington Road, Oxford, OX4 2DQ, UK

For details of our global editorial offices, customer services, and more information about Wiley products visit us at www.wiley.com.

Wiley also publishes its books in a variety of electronic formats and by print-on-demand. Some content that appears in standard print versions of this book may not be available in other formats.

Library of Congress Cataloging-in-Publication Data

Names: Paramothayan, Shanthi, author.
Title: Essential respiratory medicine / Shanthi Paramothayan.
Description: Hoboken, NJ : Wiley Blackwell, 2019. | Includes bibliographical references and index. |
Identifiers: LCCN 2018024800 (print) | LCCN 2018024971 (ebook) | ISBN 9781118618325 (Adobe PDF) | ISBN 9781118618318 (ePub) | ISBN 9781118618349 (pbk.)
Subjects: | MESH: Lung Diseases
Classification: LCC RC756 (ebook) | LCC RC756 (print) | NLM WF 600 | DDC 616.2/4–dc23
LC record available at https://lccn.loc.gov/2018024800

Cover Design: Wiley
Cover Image: © SCIEPRO/SCIENCE PHOTO LIBRARY/Getty Images

Set in 10/12pt Adobe Garamond by SPi Global, Pondicherry, India
Printed and bound in Singapore by Markono Print Media Pte Ltd

10 9 8 7 6 5 4 3 2 1

This textbook is dedicated to the memory of my aunt and teacher
Miss Sushila Balamani Navaratnasingam

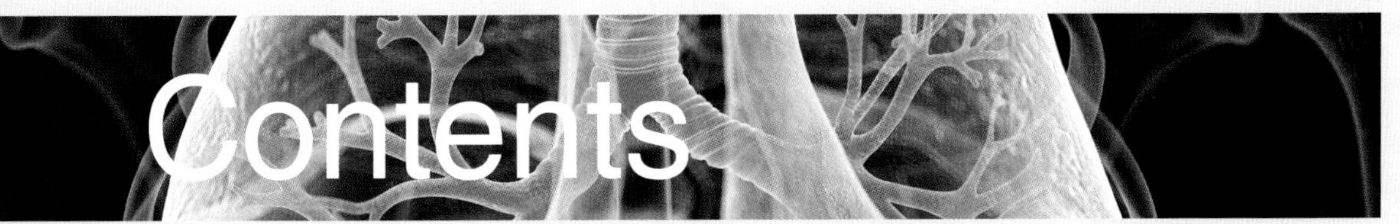

Contents

About the author

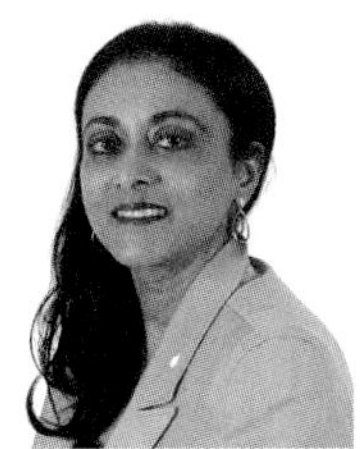

This textbook is written by Dr. Shanthi Paramothayan, a Consultant Respiratory Physician with 17 years of clinical experience in the NHS. As an Honorary Senior Lecturer for 15 years, the author has significant experience in teaching, assessing and examining undergraduates, foundation doctors, core medical trainees and respiratory registrars. She is a Fellow of the Royal College of Physicians, Fellow of the American College of Chest Physicians, and a Fellow of the Higher Education Academy. She has been a member of the Education and Training Committee of the British Thoracic Society, a member of the Question Writing Committee for the specialist respiratory examinations, a member of the MRCP 1 Board and a PACES examiner for the Royal College of Physicians. She has been a Foundation Training Programme Director, Director of Medical Education, Associate Medical Director for Education and Associate Foundation Quality Dean, Health Education South London.

Acknowledgements

I would like to thank the following people for their invaluable help with the writing of this textbook. Consultant Radiologists, Alaa WitWit, Konstantinos Stefanidis, Chandani Thorning, and Valmai Cook were crucial as they sourced many of the radiology images for the book. Alaa WitWit and Konstantinos Stefanidis also read and checked the accuracy of the radiology section of Chapter 4. The Librarians, Potenza Atiogbe, Marisa Martinez Ortiz, and Yin Ping Leung checked the references to ensure that they were all correct and in the right style. They also provided me with encouragement and support.

I am grateful to Tina Matthews, Rukma Doshi and Michael Lapsley, Consultant Histopathologists, and to David Cook, Biomedical Scientist, for providing the histopathology images. Saeed Usman, Consultant Ophthalmologist, provided the image of anterior uveitis.

I would like to thank John Clark, Consultant Microbiologist, for reading and recommending changes and additions to Chapter 8.

I would like to thank Carol Tan, Consultant Thoracic Surgeon, Jaishree Bhosle, Consultant Medical Oncologist, and Fiona MacDonald, Consultant Clinical Oncologist, for reviewing the relevant parts of Chapter 9 and recommending appropriate changes and additions.

I am grateful to Ginny Quirke, Siva Ratnatheepan, Vicky Taylor, and Rajiv Madula for reading chapters and making suggestions and corrections.

Ian Ellerington, Yvonne Welbeck-Pitfield and David Farrow from the Medical Illustration Department at Epsom and St. Helier University Hospitals NHS Trust were responsible for the clinical photographs and the videos for the supplementary material. My special thanks to Sophie Mitchinson, James Hambley, Rajiv Madula, Helen Parnell, Katherine Bintley, Patricia Lowe, Ella Sultan, Jennifer Swaby, Lucy Stratford, and Amy Grierson for willingly appearing in the photographs and videos of the supplementary material.

My thanks to Ahalya Sahadevan, Rajapillai Ahilan, Arjunan Ahilan, and Sanjeevan Ahilan for their support with IT, medical drawings, and comments on Chapter 1.

About the companion website

This book is accompanied by a companion website:

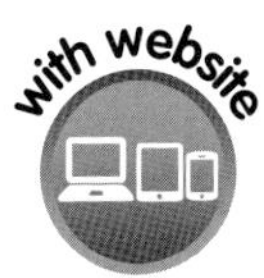

www.wiley.com/go/paramothayan/essential_respiratory_medicine

The website includes:
- Image bank
- Videos of patient examination
- Example respiratory sounds
- Multiple-choice questions

Scan this QR code to visit the companion website:

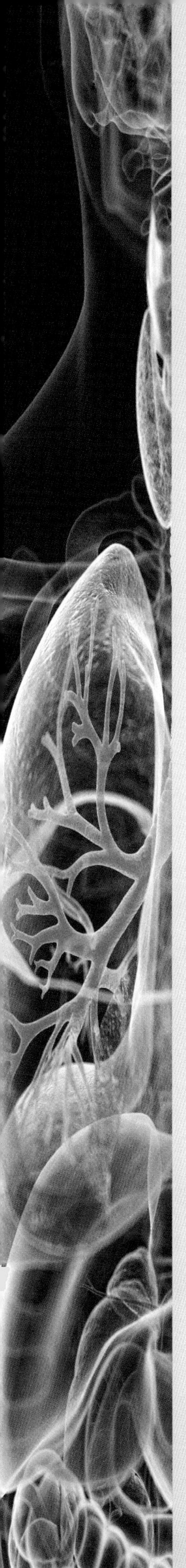

CHAPTER 1

Introduction to respiratory medicine

Essential Respiratory Medicine, First Edition. Shanthi Paramothayan.

Companion website: www.wiley.com/go/paramothayan/essential_respiratory_medicine

The respiratory system is essential for gas exchange in a multicellular organism. The lungs are also important as a defence against infectious microorganisms. Worldwide, diseases of the respiratory system cause significant morbidity and mortality; this includes infectious diseases, malignancies, allergic diseases, autoimmune disorders, and occupational diseases. Diseases of other parts of the body, for example, rheumatological and renal conditions, often affect the lungs.

Respiratory diseases can present acutely with severe, life-threatening breathlessness, for example, when someone develops a pulmonary embolus or a pneumothorax, or more insidiously with a steady decline in lung function over time, as occurs in chronic obstructive pulmonary disease or parenchymal lung diseases. In the United Kingdom (UK), respiratory diseases account for one-third of acute admissions to hospitals and for more than a quarter of all deaths in hospitals. Respiratory tract infections are the commonest conditions seen in General Practice.

In the last half a century there has been a decline in the prevalence of certain diseases, such as pneumoconioses, and other occupational lung diseases because of the recognition of the harm caused by exposure to certain agents at work. The introduction of masks, better ventilation, and other safety measures at work, together with appropriate legislation, has been the key to this success.

In the next few decades it is likely that asbestos-associated diseases (asbestosis and mesothelioma) will reduce in incidence and prevalence in the UK because of the prohibition of the use of asbestos. Asbestos, however, is still used in several developing countries. The recognition that air pollution is responsible for respiratory diseases will, hopefully, lead to cleaner air, especially in urban areas.

However, there has been an increase in the prevalence of allergic asthma, and there are various hypotheses to explain this increase. *Mycobacterium tuberculosis* has still not been eradicated, resulting in millions of deaths across the globe. Tuberculosis, also called 'phthism', 'consumption', or the 'white plague', was found in the spines of Egyptian mummies dating back to 3200–2400 BCE and is associated with poverty and deprivation.

Respiratory diseases are managed jointly by respiratory physicians, specialist nurses, physiotherapists, and occupational therapists in a multi-disciplinary way. Other specialists, including radiologists, pathologists, oncologists, thoracic surgeons, palliative care physicians, intensivists, and physiologists (for example, lung function technicians) are also essential in the management of patients with respiratory diseases. Patients who are acutely ill are managed in hospital, often on specialist respiratory wards, sometimes in single rooms if infectious, and in the Intensive Care Unit if respiratory support is required.

There has been increasing understanding of the physiology of the respiratory system and the pathophysiology of respiratory diseases in the last few centuries. Table 1.1 summarises some of the key developments in respiratory medicine.

About the book

Respiratory diseases are common, and this textbook offers a practical guide to those who care for patients with respiratory diseases. This textbook is aimed at medical students studying for their MBBS examination and postgraduate doctors of all grades, especially those studying for postgraduate examinations, including the MRCP examination. This book will also be useful for non-respiratory doctors, specialist nurses, physiotherapists, occupational therapists, pharmacists, respiratory physiologists, and physicians associates.

This text covers the entire respiratory curriculum and contains information that is useful and relevant to everyday clinical practice, with a focus on clinical presentation and management. Essential basic anatomy, physiology, pharmacology, and pathology are introduced to help understand the clinical presentation. A structured approach is taken to explain how to construct a sensible differential diagnosis of common respiratory conditions. There is a clear explanation of the common diagnostic tests required to make a diagnosis, including the interpretation of lung function tests. The mechanism of action of drugs commonly prescribed to treat respiratory diseases is discussed, with a description of their common side effects and interaction with other medications. The evidence-based management of common conditions is discussed with reference to the current British Thoracic Society (BTS) and National Institute for Health and Care Excellence (NICE) guidelines. Common pitfalls in diagnosis and management are highlighted.

Table 1.1 Brief history of respiratory medicine.

Year	Development	Scientist
Greece, 460–370 BCE	Beginning of modern medicine	Hippocrates
Greece, 304–250 BCE	Some understanding of the physiology of the lung	Erisistratus
Greece, 129–165 BCE	Anatomy of trachea, larynx, and lungs understood Believed air had substance vital for life	Galen
Egypt, 1210–1288	Some understanding of pulmonary circulation	Ibne Nafis
Italy, 1500	Understood anatomy and physiology of lungs Determined sub-atmospheric pressures inflated lungs	Leonardo da Vinci
Belgium, 1543	Tracheostomy used for ventilation	Andreas Vesalius
UK, 1700	Constructed first air pump for physiological research	Robert Hooke
France, 1778	Discovered role of oxygen	Antoine Lavoisier
France, 1816	Invention of stethoscope	René Laennec
Scotland, 1832	Invention of negative pressure tank-type ventilator	John Dalziel
Germany, 1882	Tuberculosis bacterium discovered	Robert Koch
Germany, 1895	First chest X-ray	Wilhelm Rötgen
UK, 1928	First non-invasive ventilation	Drinker-Shaw
USA, 1963	First human lung transplant	James Hardy
UK, 1972	First computed tomography scan	Godfrey Hounsfield

The book contains several boxes, tables, and algorithms set out in a clear, and concise way. It also contains several good quality colour photographs, and radiological and histological images to support the information in the text.

There are multiple choice questions which can be used by the reader to check their understanding, with a clear explanation of the correct answer. There is also a list of references for suggested further reading.

Supplementary material includes videos demonstrating how to take a history and conduct a clinical examination (http://www.wiley.com/go/Paramothayan/Essential_Respiratory_Medicine). There are also videos showing how to carry out common tests, such as peak flow, spirometry, the skin prick test, the Mantoux test, the shuttle test, and how to fit a patient for a sleep study.

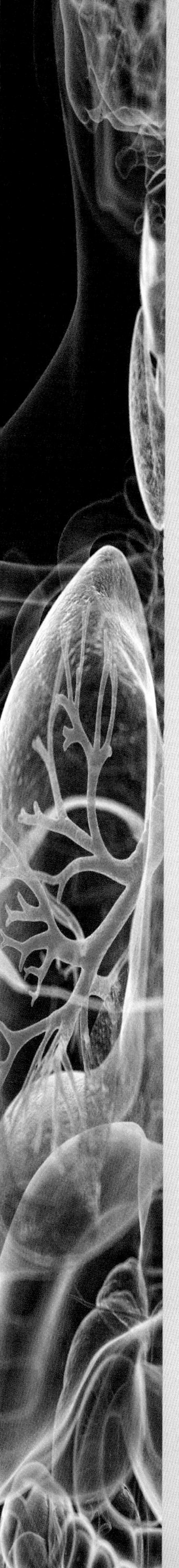

CHAPTER 2

Embryology, anatomy, and physiology of the lung

Learning objectives

- To gain a basic understanding of the development of the lung
- To be aware of the common developmental lung abnormalities
- To understand the anatomy of the respiratory system which is relevant to clinical practice
- To be aware of the structure and function of the diaphragm
- To understand the muscles of respiration
- To understand how mechanical ventilation occurs
- To gain knowledge of the structure of the bronchial tree and the alveoli
- To gain knowledge of the blood supply, nerve supply, and lymphatics of the respiratory system
- To understand the physiology of the respiratory system which is relevant to clinical practice
- To gain some understanding of the control of breathing
- To gain knowledge of the receptors in the lungs
- To appreciate the function of the central and peripheral chemoreceptors
- To understand how oxygen is transported in the blood from the lungs to tissues
- To understand how carbon dioxide is transported in the blood from tissues to the lungs
- To understand the importance of carbon dioxide in the acid-base balance of the body
- To understand the causes of physiological shunts
- To understand the causes of ventilation-perfusion mismatch
- To have some understanding of the defence mechanisms of the lungs

Essential Respiratory Medicine, First Edition. Shanthi Paramothayan.

Companion website: www.wiley.com/go/paramothayan/essential_respiratory_medicine

Abbreviations

ASD	atrial septal defect
CA	carbonic anhydrase
CO_2	carbon dioxide
COPD	chronic obstructive pulmonary disease
CSF	cerebrospinal fluid
FRC	functional residual capacity
H^+	hydrogen ion
H_2CO_3	carbonic acid
HB	haemoglobin
HCO_3^-	bicarbonate ion
MCE	mucociliary escalator
NANC	non-noradrenergic, non-cholinergic
NO	nitric oxide
O_2	oxygen
O_3	ozone
PCD	primary ciliary dyskinesia
PCO_2	partial pressure of carbon dioxide
PO_2	partial pressure of oxygen
R	respiratory quotient
SO_2	sulphur dioxide
VSD	ventricular septal defect

Introduction

The respiratory system's main role is to provide oxygen (O_2) that is required for glycolysis, and the removal of the waste product of respiration, carbon dioxide (CO_2). This involves two separate processes: (1) mechanical ventilation whereby air is moved into and out of the lungs, and (2) gas exchange across the alveolar-capillary membrane.

The respiratory system also has an important role in acid-base balance, the defence against airborne pathogens, and in phonation, which is essential for audible speech. The conversion of angiotensin 1 to angiotensin 11 occurs in the lungs as does the deactivation of bradykinin, serotonin, and various drugs, including propranolol.

The lungs act as a reservoir of 500 ml blood and therefore participate in heat exchange. The lungs filter and lyse microemboli from the veins, preventing them from reaching the systemic circulation.

Development of the respiratory system

The lungs are not required for respiration *in utero*, but start working as soon as the baby is born and is independent from its mother. The development of the lungs starts in week three of the embryonic period (3–16 weeks), continues through the foetal period (16–38 weeks), beyond birth, and into childhood. During intrauterine life, the lungs are an important source of amniotic fluid, producing around 15 ml kg^{-1} of body weight, which flows out via the trachea or is swallowed.

Development of the lungs

During the embryonic period, the structures of the respiratory system are formed: the trachea, bronchial tree, blood vessels, nerves, lymphatics, and the structures of the thoracic cage (Figure 2.1). In the latter part of the second trimester and during the third trimester, there is functional development, with lung maturation and the production of surfactant. Five phases of structural lung development are recognised. In the embryonic phase (3–16 weeks), at approximately 28 days after conception, lung development begins with the formation of the sulcus laryngotrachealis in the lower part of the pharynx. At 30 days, a bud, called the true lung primordium, forms from the lower part of the foregut, but remains in communication with it. The oesophagotracheal ridges then fuse to form the oesophagotracheal septum, which divides the oesophagus from the trachea. Failure of the formation of this septum occurs in 1 : 3000 births and results in the formation of a trachea-oesophageal fistula.

The diaphragm develops in the third week after fertilisation, with transverse and longitudinal folding. The septum transversum is the primitive central tendon and forms in the cervical region and migrates downwards, therefore the innervation is from the phrenic nerve that originates from the cervical spinal cord.

Failure of one of the pleuroperitoneal membranes to close results in a congenital diaphragmatic hernia which occurs in 1 : 2000 births. It occurs more commonly on the left side and results in the intestinal contents moving up into the left hemithorax, compromising lung development resulting in lung hypoplasia. Surgical repair carries a high mortality.

Normal lung development depends on the interaction between the epithelium and the mesenchymal tissue which lies beneath it. During the pseudoglandular period of the embryonic phase (5–16 weeks), there is an asymmetrical subdivision

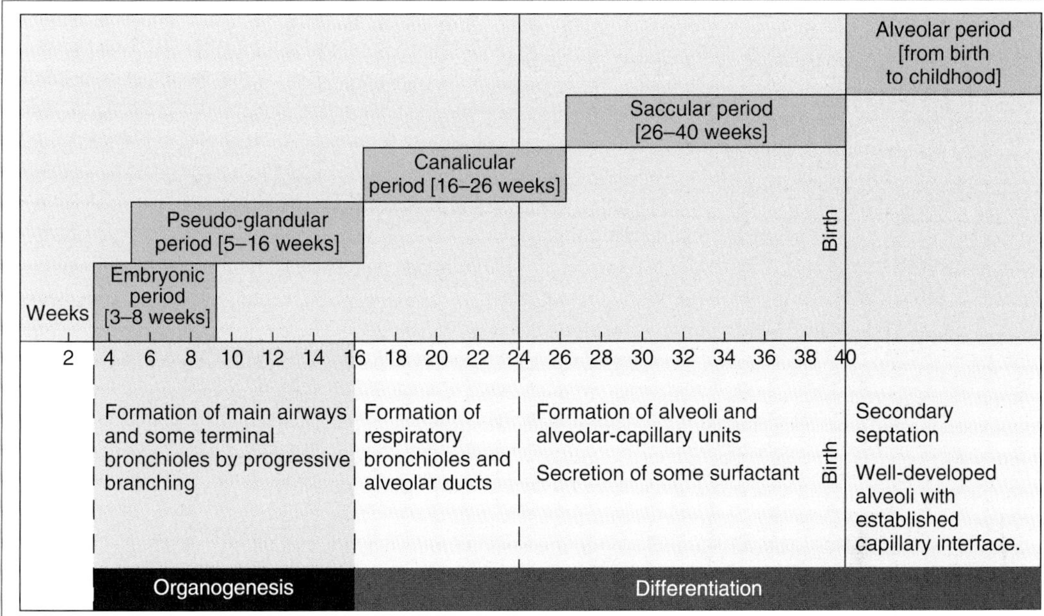

Figure 2.1 Stages of lung development.

of the lung primordium into the two buds which will form the main bronchi. The smaller left main bronchus is directed more acutely away from the trachea while the larger right main bronchus leads more directly from the trachea. The two main bronchi subdivide unequally, giving rise to three lobes on the right and two lobes on the left.

Progressive branching during the embryonic phase results in the formation of the first 16 generations of the conducting airways, composed of the trachea, bronchi, bronchioles, and terminal bronchioles. Differentiation of the epithelium derived from the endoderm, with formation of cilia in the proximal airways, occurs at 13 weeks and is controlled by the mesenchyme beneath it. This ciliated epithelium lines the entire conducting airway system and is important in host defence. In primary ciliary dyskinesia (PCD), the ciliary structure is abnormal, and the consequences are significant, as discussed in Chapter 12. The innervation of the lungs is derived from the ectoderm while the vascular structures, smooth muscle, cartilage, and connective tissue are derived from the mesoderm.

During the canalicular period (16–26 weeks), there is further branching of the bronchial tree, with the terminal bronchioles dividing into the respiratory bronchioles (generations 20–22), which further subdivide into the alveolar ducts (generations 20–22) and finally the alveolar sacs (generation 23). Generations 17–23 are called the respiratory zones and will be responsible for gas exchange. Once the alveolar sacs have been formed, further growth occurs by elongation and widening of the airways.

Type 1 pneumocytes, the main cells of the alveolus, are formed with very thin membranes. There is vascularization, with establishment of the capillary network very close to the type 1 pneumocytes in preparation for the gas exchange. Type 2 pneumocytes, which contain lamellar (or inclusion) bodies, also develop and will eventually synthesise and store surfactant.

At the end of the embryonic period (16 weeks), the pulmonary vessels have developed. The pulmonary circulatory system is smaller than the systemic circulatory system and is formed out of the sixth pharyngeal arch artery and a vessel plexus which originates from the aortic sac. The true sixth aortic arch is only then formed after vessels from the dorsal arch grow into this plexus and there is a connection between the truncus pulmonalis and the dorsal aorta.

During the terminal sac period of foetal development (26–38 weeks), there is further differentiation of the type 1 and type 2 pneumocytes, with progressive thinning of the alveolar walls which will facilitate gas exchange.

At full gestation, there are approximately 20×10^6 alveoli, often called 'primitive saccules', which mature during the neonatal period and connect to other alveoli through the pores of Kuhn. The pulmonary arterial network gradually develops a muscle layer during childhood and the capillary network extends and becomes entwined between two alveoli. The lungs continue to develop after birth until the age of 8, with the formation of a total of 300×10^6 mature alveoli.

As the alveoli in the foetus contain fluid and not air, the oxygen tension is low, resulting in pulmonary vasoconstriction and diversion of blood across the ductus arteriosus into the systemic circulation. After the first breath is taken, oxygen enters the alveoli, resulting in an increase in oxygen tension and increased blood flow to the alveoli. Nitric oxide (NO), a potent vasodilator, is secreted by the respiratory epithelium which results in significant vasodilation of the pulmonary blood vessels.

Surfactant is composed of a hydrophilic macromolecular complex of phosphatidylcholine (lecithin), phosphatidylglycerol and hydrophobic surface proteins B and C which project into the alveolar gas and float on the surface of the lining fluid. Surfactant decreases surface tension within the alveoli, preventing the collapse of the alveoli during exhalation. In the absence of surfactant, the alveolus would be unstable and would collapse at the end of each breath. During the latter part of gestation, surfactant production and secretion gradually increase. At 36 weeks of gestation there is sufficient surfactant so that spontaneous breathing can occur and the foetus is viable.

Prematurity carries a high mortality and a significant risk of neonatal respiratory distress syndrome. Corticotrophin stimulates the synthesis of the fibroblast pneumocyte factor from the foetal lung fibroblasts which stimulates surfactant production in type 2 cells. Corticosteroids given antenatally to premature babies will promote lung maturity. Exogenous surfactant can also improve the survival of the premature baby.

Amniotic fluid, originating in the foetal lungs and kidneys, is required for normal lung development. During foetal breathing movements, when the upper airways' resistance is decreased, diaphragmatic movements help maintain lung liquid volume. Oligohydramnios, called Potter's syndrome, occurs when there is a decreased volume of amniotic fluid, resulting in lung hypoplasia and renal agenesis. Other causes of lung hypoplasia include congenital diaphragmatic hernia, musculoskeletal abnormalities of the thorax which restrict the full expansion of the thoracic cage, and space-occupying lesions of the thorax.

The respiratory tract

The **upper respiratory tract** comprises of the nose, the paranasal sinuses, the epiglottis, pharynx, and larynx (Figure 2.2). The larynx is important in speech. During swallowing, the epiglottis closes the larynx which leads to the trachea, preventing food from entering the respiratory tract. Failure of this process will lead to aspiration of food contents into the lungs.

The **lower respiratory tract** begins at the trachea, which corresponds to the lower edge of the cricoid cartilage, at the level of the sixth cervical vertebra. The lower respiratory tract is enclosed within the thoracic cavity which is composed of the sternum anteriorly, the vertebral column posteriorly, the mediastinum, the diaphragm, which divides the thorax from the abdomen, and the ribs with their intercostal spaces (Figure 2.3, Figure 2.4). The bony sternum is divided into the manubrium, the body, and the xiphisternum, which is cartilaginous until late adulthood. The manubrium is joined to the cartilages of the first and second ribs at the level of T3 and T4, and to the body by the manubriosternal joint which lies at T4 and is called the angle of Louis or the sternal angle. This is an important landmark in surface anatomy. The body of the sternum joins the second to seventh ribs at the level of T5–T8.

The vertebrosternal, or true ribs, are the first to seventh ribs, and are connected to the sternum by their costal cartilages. Inflammation of the costochondral junction (costochondritis) results in 'pleuritic' chest pain which is worse on breathing, movement, and palpation. The eighth, ninth, and tenth ribs are called the vertebrochondral, or false ribs, and are joined to the cartilages of the ribs above. The eleventh and twelfth ribs are called floating or vertebral ribs.

Each rib is composed of a head and a shaft. The head is attached to the body and transverse process of the adjacent vertebra, the intervertebral disc, and the vertebra above (Figure 2.5). The shaft curves forward to join the sternum. The joints between the ribs and vertebra act like a hinge, causing the ribs to move during inspiration.

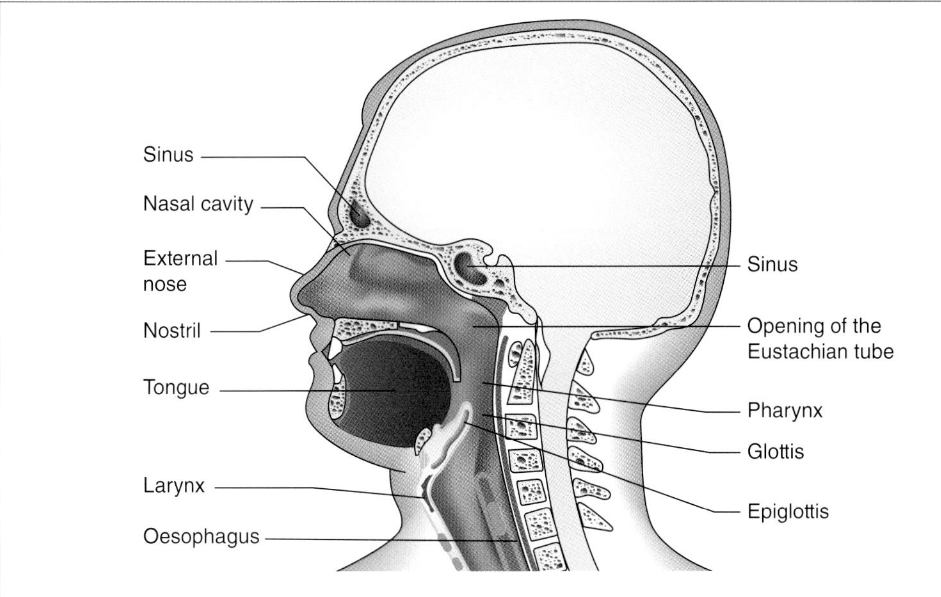

Figure 2.2 The upper respiratory tract.

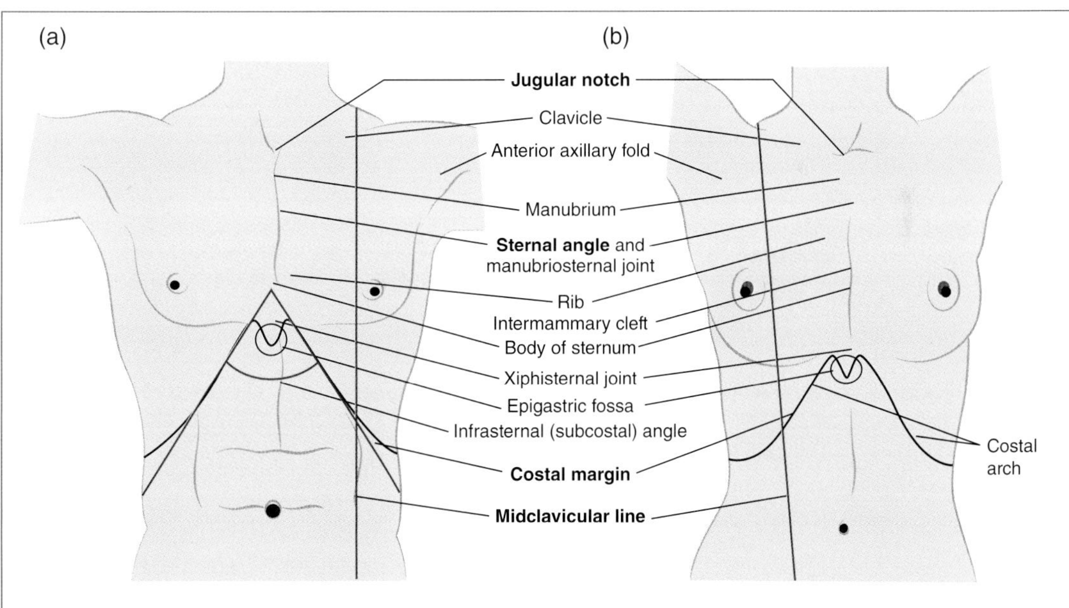

Figure 2.3 Surface anatomy of the thorax.

The rib cage protects the heart, lungs, and great vessels from damage. Trauma to the chest wall can result in fracture of the shaft of the ribs at the angle of the rib. Multiple rib fractures can result in a 'flail' segment which can cause significant difficulty with inspiration. The clavicles protect the first and second ribs which are less likely to fracture than the other ribs.

One in 200 people have a cervical rib which is attached to the transverse process of C7. A cervical rib can press on the brachial plexus and cause neurological symptoms, including paraesthesia of the arms and hands. Pressure on the subclavian artery can cause vascular symptoms.

The intercostal spaces between the ribs contain external and internal intercostal muscles (Figure 2.6).

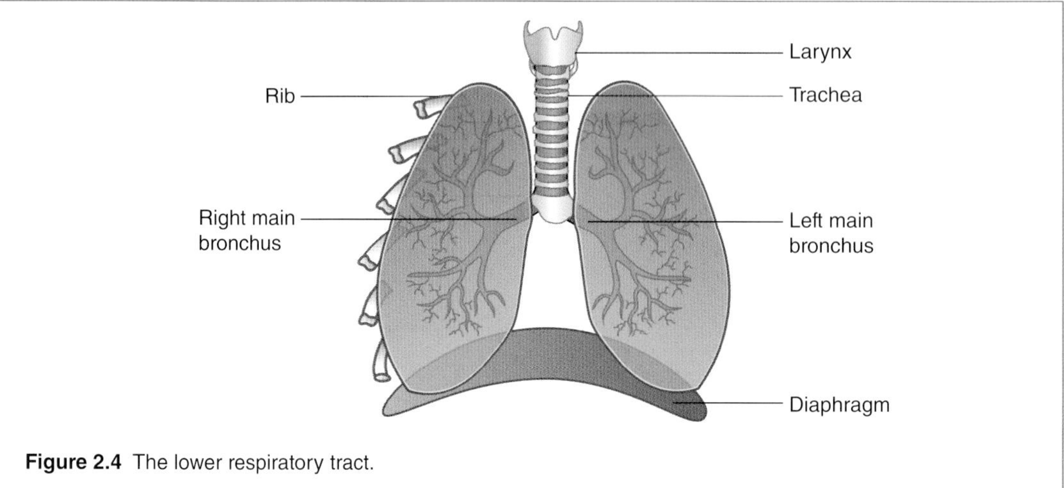

Figure 2.4 The lower respiratory tract.

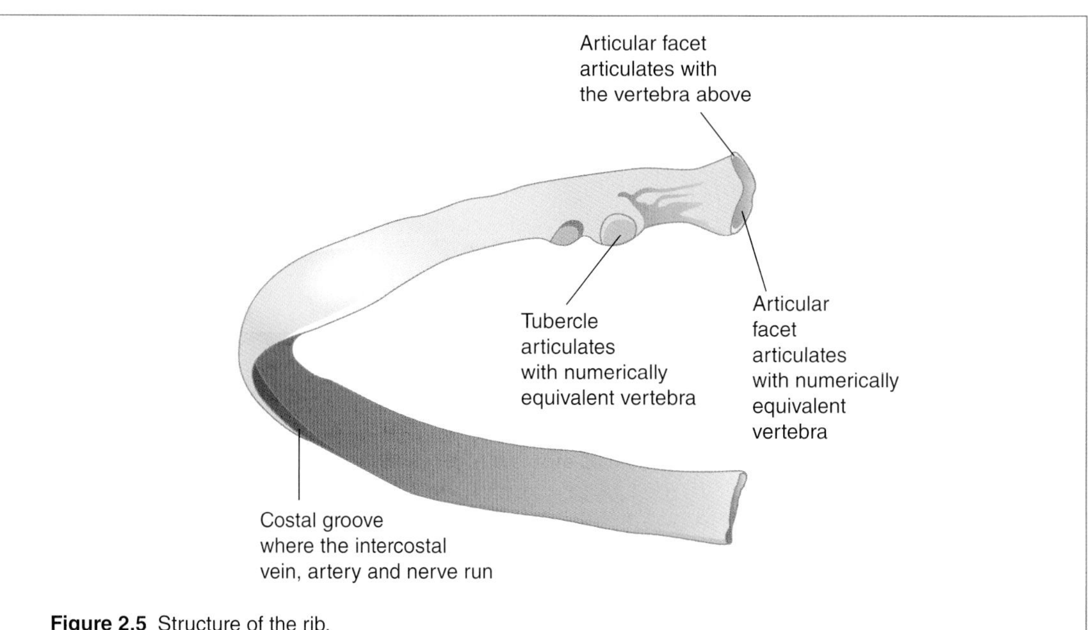

Figure 2.5 Structure of the rib.

The fibres of the external intercostal muscles pass downwards and forwards between the ribs, while the fibres of the internal intercostal muscles pass downwards and backwards. There is also an incomplete innermost intercostal layer. The intercostal muscles are innervated by the intercostal nerves, which are the anterior primary rami of thoracic nerves. The intercostal veins, arteries and nerves lie in grooves on the under-surface of the corresponding ribs, with the vein above, the artery in the middle and the nerve below. It is important, therefore, to avoid the underside of the rib when carrying out pleural procedures, but to insert the needle or drain just above the rib into the pleural space.

The **diaphragm**, which means 'partition' in Greek, has a central tendon which is attached to the pericardium, and thick skeletal muscle on either side, which separates the thoracic and abdominal cavities. It is the most important muscle of inspiration. Several key structures traverse the diaphragm between the abdomen and thorax. The sternal part of the diaphragm consists of two strips of muscle that arises from the posterior surface of the xiphisternum. The costal part comprises of six

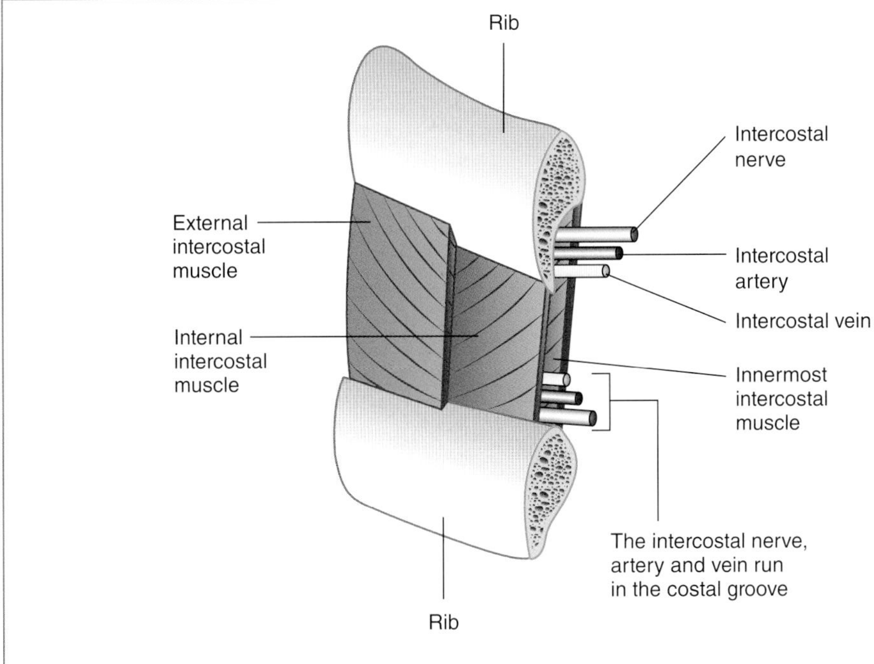

Figure 2.6 The ribs and intercostal space.

muscular strips that originate from the seventh–twelfth ribs and their costal cartilages. The vertebral part of the diaphragm originates from the crura and the arcuate ligaments on both sides. The muscular right crus arises from the bodies and intervertebral discs of the three lumbar vertebrae, and the left crus arises from the bodies and intervertebral discs of the upper two lumbar vertebrae. The medial and lateral arcuate ligaments are thickenings of the fascia overlying the psoas major and the quadratus lumborum respectively.

The inferior vena cava and right phrenic nerve pass through the diaphragm at T8, the oesophagus, branches of the left gastric artery, the gastric vein, and both vagi pass through at T10, and the aorta, thoracic duct, and zygos vein pass behind the diaphragm between the left and right crus at T12 (Figure 2.7). The sympathetic trunk passes through the diaphragm under the medial lumbocostal arch, and branches of the internal thoracic artery and lymphatics pass through the foramina of Morgagni.

The phrenic nerves (C3, C4, and C5) supply motor and sensory innervation to the diaphragm. Pain from irritation of the diaphragm is referred to the corresponding dermatome for C4 at the shoulder. Irritation to the phrenic nerve can cause intractable hiccoughs. The lower intercostal (T5–T11) and subcostal (T12) nerves supply sensory fibres to the peripheral diaphragm. Damage to the phrenic nerve, for example, by a tumour, will result in a unilateral diaphragmatic palsy, as discussed in Chapter 9.

The blood supply to the diaphragm is from the pericardiophrenic, musculophrenic, lower internal intercostal and inferior phrenic arteries. The superior and inferior phrenic veins drain blood from the diaphragm into the brachiocephalic vein, the azygos vein, the inferior vena cava, and the left suprarenal vein.

Muscles of respiration and mechanical ventilation

The inspiratory muscles are the diaphragm, and the intercostal and the scalene muscles. When they contract to expand the thoracic cavity, there is a decrease in intrapleural and alveolar pressure which creates a pressure gradient between the alveoli and the mouth, resulting in air entering the lungs. Elastic recoil of the lungs and the chest wall results in expiration, which is a passive process, not requiring any muscular activity. Forced expiration, for example, coughing, will require contraction of the abdominal muscles which push the diaphragm upwards.

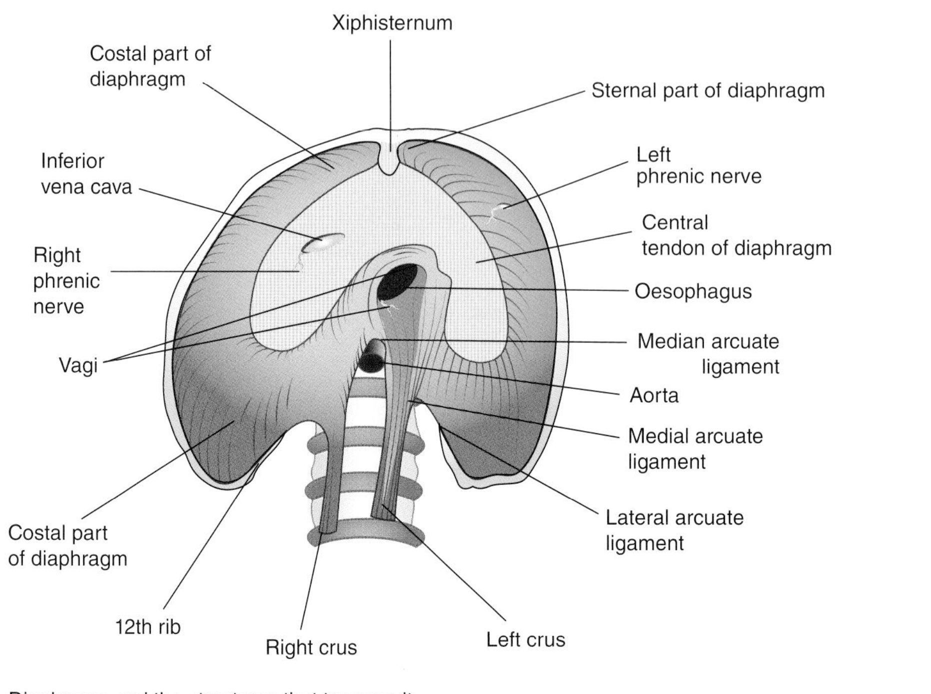

Figure 2.7 Diaphragm and the structures that traverse it.

Inspiration is an active process. The domed diaphragm is the main muscle of inspiration and is positioned high in the thorax at the end of expiration. During quiet breathing, the diaphragm contracts and moves down by 1.5 cm, pushing the abdominal contents down. This increases the intra-abdominal pressure and pushes the abdominal wall and the lower ribs outwards and downwards. During deep breathing, the diaphragm contracts harder and can move by as much as 6–7 cm.

During quiet breathing, the first rib remains almost motionless and the intercostal muscles elevate and evert the other ribs. The intercostal muscles support the intercostal spaces preventing them from being sucked in during inspiration. The scalene muscles, which insert into the first two ribs, are also active in normal inspiration. Movement of the upper ribs upwards pushes the sternum forward (the pump action), increasing the anterior–posterior diameter of the chest, and as the sloping lower ribs rise, they move out (the bucket handle action), and the transverse diameter of the chest wall increases. At the beginning of inspiration, the inspiratory muscles contract to overcome the impedance offered by the lungs and chest wall. The volume of the thoracic cavity can increase from 1.5 l up to 8 l with deep inspiration.

Diaphragmatic paralysis results in paradoxical movement: as the intercostal muscles contract and the ribs move, the diaphragm is sucked into the chest due to a fall in intrathoracic pressure. In a high cervical cord transection, all the respiratory muscles are paralysed, but when the damage is below the phrenic nerve roots, breathing continues via the diaphragm alone. In infants, the movement of the horizontal ribs cannot increase the volume of the chest, and breathing is reliant on diaphragmatic contraction alone; this is called abdominal breathing. As the infant grows, the ribs become more oblique and contribute to thoracic inspiration.

When the rate of ventilation or the resistance to breathing increases, the scalene muscles, sternocleidomastoids, and serratus anterior, which are called the accessory inspiratory muscles, are recruited to help inspiration. Splinting of the arms, for example, by grasping the edge of the table, will result in contraction of the pectoralis major muscle which will expand the chest further. When ventilation exceeds 40 l min^{-1}, there is activation of the expiratory muscles, especially the abdominal muscles, the rectus abdominis, the external and internal

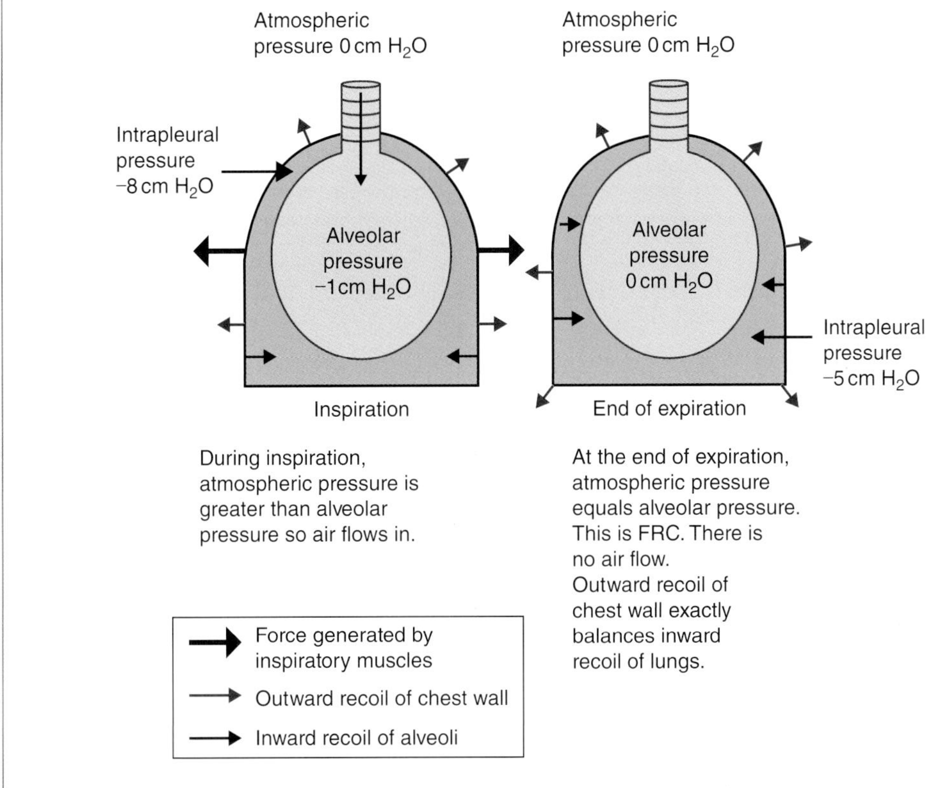

Figure 2.8 Relationship between elastic recoil and functional residual capacity.

oblique, which speed up recoil of the diaphragm by raising intra-abdominal pressure.

At functional residual capacity (FRC), the respiratory muscles are relaxed, and the outward recoil of the chest wall exactly balances the inward recoil of the lungs which creates a negative pressure in the space between them (Figure 2.8).

In lung fibrosis, the lungs are stiff (decreased lung compliance) and have increased elastic recoil, so the FRC is smaller. In emphysema, the FRC increases due to loss of alveolar tissue, loss of elastic recoil, increase in lung compliance, and air trapping. This leads to the development of a barrel chest. Mouth breathing, as adopted by patients with chronic obstructive pulmonary disease (COPD), decreases the FRC, enabling these patients to inspire.

Dynamic and static lung volumes and their measurements are discussed in detail in Chapter 4. The normal breath is called the tidal volume and is about 500 ml at rest, which is 10% of the vital capacity. At a normal respiratory rate of 15 breaths min^{-1}, the minute ventilation, which is the volume of air entering the lungs each minute is 7500 ml min^{-1} (500 × 15). Alveolar ventilation is the actual volume taking part in gas exchange every minute. As the dead space is 150 ml, alveolar ventilation is 5250 ml min^{-1} (7500-2250 ml/min).

The main resistance to airflow occurs in the upper respiratory tract, especially the nose, pharynx, and the large airways. The intrapleural pressure can be indirectly assessed from oesophageal pressure using a small pressure transducer. During inspiration, the chest wall expands and the intrapleural pressure falls. This increases the pressure gradient between the intrapleural space and the alveoli, stretching the lungs. The alveoli expand, and alveolar pressure falls, creating a pressure gradient between the mouth and the alveoli, causing air to flow into the lungs. During expiration, both intrapleural pressure and alveolar pressure rise. In quiet breathing, the intrapleural pressure remains negative for the whole respiratory cycle, whereas alveolar pressure is negative during inspiration and positive during expiration. Alveolar pressure is always higher than intrapleural pressure because of

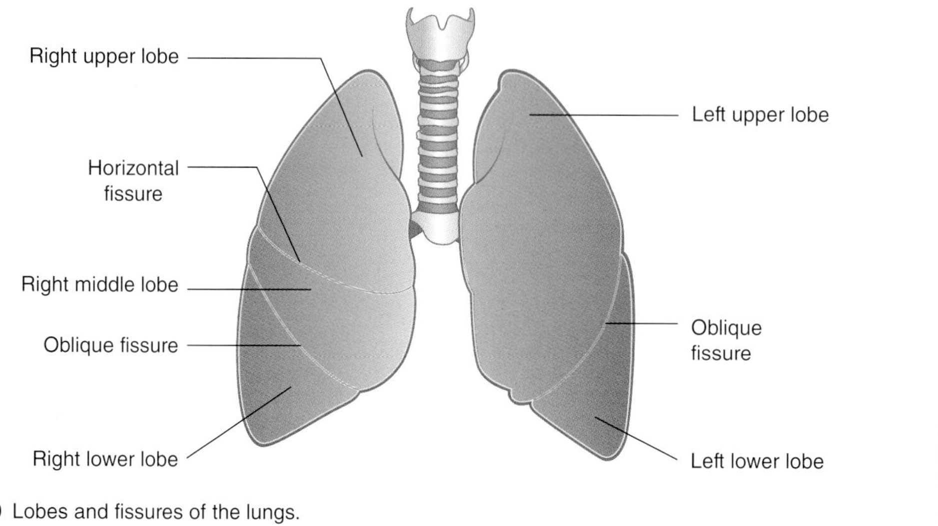

Figure 2.9 Lobes and fissures of the lungs.

the recoil of the lungs. It is zero at the end of both inspiration and expiration, and airflow ceases momentarily. When ventilation is increased, the changes in intrapleural pressure and alveolar pressure are greater, and in expiration intrapleural pressure may rise above atmospheric pressure. In forced expiration, such as coughing or sneezing, intrapleural pressure may rise to +8 kPa or more.

Structure of the lungs

The right lung has three lobes and the left lung has two lobes (Figure 2.9). The heart lies close to the left lung which has a cardiac notch. The conducting airways comprise of the trachea which bifurcates at the carina (T4/T5) into the two main bronchi which divide into smaller bronchi, eventually leading to the terminal bronchioles. The bifurcation of the trachea corresponds on the surface anatomy (see Figure 2.3) to the sternal angle or angle of Louis.

The trachea is a semi-rigid structure which leads from the oropharynx into the thoracic cavity. The trachea and main bronchi have U-shaped cartilage linked posteriorly by smooth muscle. The anterior and lateral walls of the trachea are supported by rings of cartilage, but the posterior wall does not have any cartilage and is therefore collapsible. Diseases of the cartilage, such as tracheobronchomalacia, can affect the entire tracheobronchial tree.

The right main bronchus is wider, shorter, and more vertical than the left main bronchus, so inhaled material is more likely to enter the right main bronchus. The left main bronchus is longer and leaves the carina at a more abrupt angle. The right lung is divided by the horizontal and oblique fissures into the upper, middle, and lower lobes. The left lung is divided into the upper and lower lobes by the oblique fissure. The vessels, nerves, and lymphatics enter the lungs on their medial surfaces at the hilum. Each lobe is divided into several wedge-shaped bronchopulmonary segments with their apices at the hilum and bases at the lung surface. Each bronchopulmonary segment has a bronchus, artery, and vein (Figure 2.10).

Each lung is lined by visceral pleura which is continuous with the parietal pleura, lining the chest wall, diaphragm, pericardium, and mediastinum. In health, the space between the parietal and visceral layer is very small with a few millilitres of pleural fluid. The right and left pleural cavities are separate and each extends as the costodiaphragmatic recess below the lungs. The parietal pleura is segmentally innervated by intercostal nerves and by the phrenic nerve (C3, C4, and C5), so pain from pleural inflammation is often referred to the chest wall or shoulder tip. The visceral pleura lacks sensory innervation.

The main bronchi divide into the three main lobar bronchi on the right (upper, middle, and lower) and into two lobar bronchi on the left (upper and lower). These lobar bronchi divide further into segmental bronchi (generations 3 and 4) which continue to divide further into 22

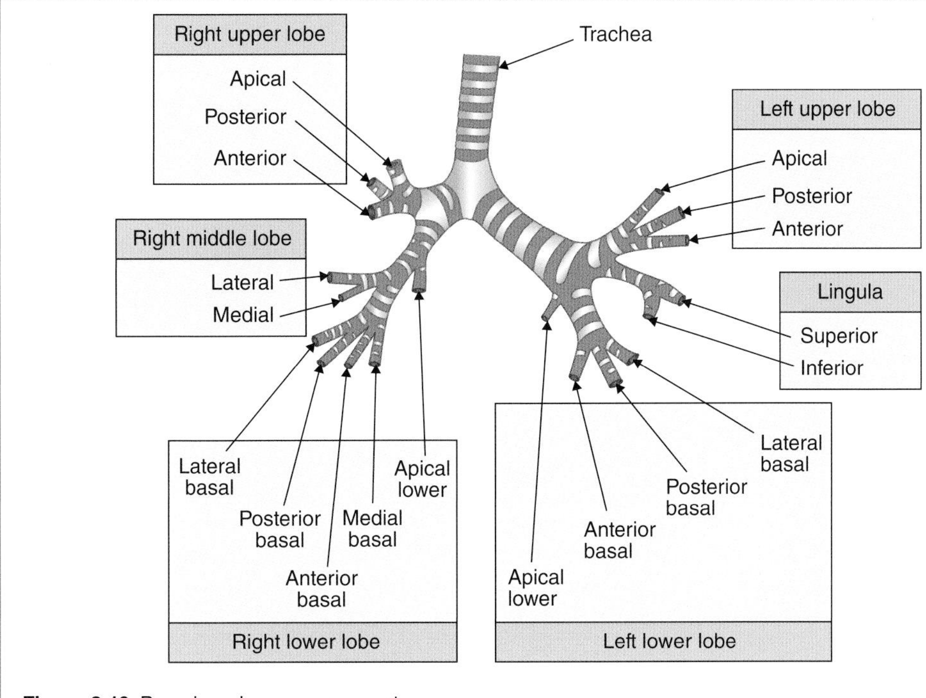

Figure 2.10 Bronchopulmonary segments.

generations, each successive generation approximately doubling in number. Generations 5–11 are small bronchi, the smallest measuring 1 mm in diameter. The lobar, segmental, and small bronchi are supported by irregular plates of cartilage, with bronchial smooth muscle forming overlapping helical bands. The muscle coat becomes more complex distally as the cartilaginous plate becomes more fragmentary and contributes 20% to the thickness of the walls in the distal airways.

The conducting airways from the trachea to the respiratory bronchioles are lined with ciliated columnar epithelial cells which become flatter through successive generations. The cilia beat synchronously, with a whip-like action, and waves of contraction pass in an organised fashion from cell to cell so that material trapped in the sticky mucus layer above the cilia is moved upwards and swallowed. The mucociliary escalator (MCE) is an important part of the lungs' defences. The larger bronchi have acinar mucus-secreting glands in the submucosa. These and goblet cells secrete mucus and become hypertrophied in chronic bronchitis. The function of the conducting airways is the filtration and humidification of air. Beyond this, there is a gradual transition from conduction to gas exchange.

Bronchioles, which start at generation 12, have no cartilage in their walls and are embedded in lung tissue and kept open by the tethering force of elastic recoil. Terminal bronchioles (generation 16) lead to respiratory bronchioles (generations 17–19), which represent the transition zone between the conducting airways and the gas-exchange part, containing ciliated and non-ciliated cells, and a well-marked muscle layer in their walls. The respiratory bronchioles lead to alveolar ducts and finally to the alveolar sacs (generation 23) which are entirely composed of blind-ending alveoli. The elastic tissue in the parenchyma enables the lungs to stretch when inflated and recoil during expiration.

An adult male has approximately 300 million alveoli. These are irregular polyhedrons measuring 0.1–0.2 mm in diameter. The number of alveoli depends on the height of the individual, and the size of the alveolus depends on the volume of air in the lungs. The acinus is the unit of respiratory function distal to the terminal bronchioles, comprising of the respiratory bronchioles, the alveolar ducts, and the alveoli. Many acinar together form a pulmonary lobule, which is separated by septae. The connections between these units lead to structural interdependence, which prevents the collapse

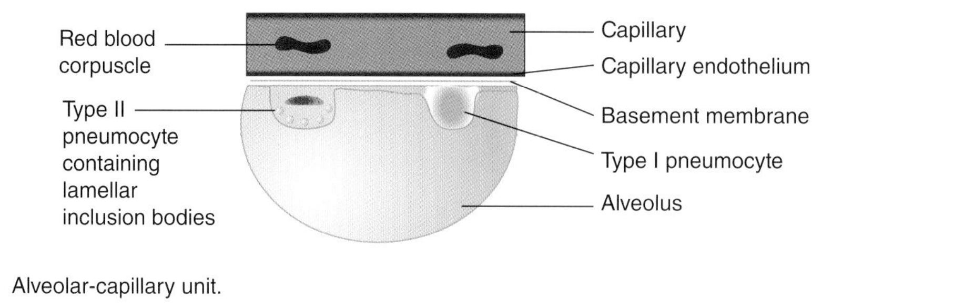

Figure 2.11 Alveolar-capillary unit.

of an individual unit, which is kept open by the expansion of the surrounding acinar.

Alveoli are lined by a thin layer of unciliated, squamous epithelial cells, of which there are two types. Type 1 pneumocytes have flattened processes that extend to cover most of the internal surfaces of the alveoli and do not contain any organelles. Type 1 pneumocytes rest on the basement membrane and interface closely with the capillary membrane, forming the alveolar-capillary unit where gas exchange occurs (Figure 2.11). This membrane is less than 0.4 μm, facilitating the easy movement of gases from the alveoli to the capillaries. The interstitial space contains pulmonary capillaries, elastin, and collagen fibres. This interface is affected in pulmonary fibrosis and pulmonary oedema.

Type 2 pneumocytes are less numerous, make up only a small proportion of the alveolar surface area, and are found at the junction between alveoli. They are round, have large nuclei, microvilli, and lamellar (inclusion) bodies which store and secrete surfactant, which reduces surface tension in the alveolar fluid as discussed later. Surfactant also plays a part in lung immunity.

Club cells (bronchiolar exocrine cells) are non-ciliated cells found in the epithelium of the bronchioles close to their junction with alveoli. They have microvilli and contain a lot of smooth endoplasmic reticulum which contains Cytochrome-P450. They secrete glycosaminoglycans, which are similar in composition to surfactants, into the alveolar space, which prevents alveolar collapse. They also secrete tryptase and uteroglobin. They may act as stem cells, multiplying and differentiating into ciliated epithelial cells. The club cells are the origin of bronchioalveolar carcinoma of the lungs (see Chapter 9).

The conducting airways, with a volume of 150 ml, form the anatomical dead space as they do not participate in gas exchange. The role of the conducting airways is to humidify, warm, and filter the air. Any alveoli that do not participate in gas exchange contribute to the dead space.

Blood supply of the lungs

The lungs and associated structures receive their blood supply from both the systemic and the pulmonary circulations. The pulmonary circulation has a pulmonary vascular resistance of 1/6th of the systemic circulation. The right ventricle, which needs only to generate a mean pulmonary artery pressure of 15–20 mmHg to pump blood through the lungs, is less muscular than the left ventricle.

The main pulmonary trunk arises from the right ventricle and divides into the right and left pulmonary arteries, the landmark for this division being on the left of the sternal angle. These two large pulmonary arteries divide progressively into smaller branches, with the eventual formation of capillaries which run alongside the bronchial tree and carry deoxygenated blood from the entire body to the respiratory bronchioles, alveolar ducts, and ultimately the alveolar sacs. This dense capillary network in the alveolar walls provides an extensive surface area for gas exchange, and is very close to the alveolar surface, so that the distance that O_2 needs to diffuse is less than 0.5 μm. The capillary network offers little resistance to blood flow; the capillaries are easily opened as the blood supply increases. The average transit time for a red blood cell to travel through the pulmonary circulation is 0.75 seconds, and during this time it can traverse several alveoli. The oxygenated blood drains into the left atrium through four peripheral pulmonary veins which arise in each lobe of the lung, although the right upper and middle lobe veins unite.

The pulmonary arteries are thinner and are more elastic than the systemic arteries. They transmit deoxygenated blood away from the heart to the lungs at a pressure of 20–30 mmHg. The right pulmonary artery is longer and wider than the left pulmonary artery, passes inferior to the arch of the aorta, and enters the left hilum of the lungs. It is connected to the arch of the aorta by the ligamentum arteriosum which is the fibrous remnant of the ductus arteriosus which closes at birth.

Pulmonary vascular resistance, which determines blood flow, is controlled by neural and non-neural factors. Efferent fibres from parasympathetic, sympathetic, and non-adrenergic, non-cholinergic fibres act on the arterioles. Whereas systemic arterioles dilate in response to hypoxia, resulting in an increase in oxygen delivery, the pulmonary arterioles undergo vasoconstriction in the presence of hypoxia. This diverts blood away from the under-ventilated areas of the lungs to the well-ventilated areas. This will occur, for example, when there is consolidation or atelectasis in an area of the lung resulting in reduced ventilation. There is no autoregulation of blood flow in the lungs as occurs in the brain or the kidneys.

Blood flow is greater at the lung base compared to the apex, partly due to gravity. Ventilation is also greater at the base, but the difference in the perfusion gradient is greater than the ventilation gradient, so that in a normal lung the bases are effectively over-perfused and the apices over-ventilated.

The bronchial arteries carry less than 1% of the cardiac output, arise from the descending aorta and supply blood to the trachea and the entire conducting system, down to the terminal bronchioles, but do not participate in gas exchange. They also supply the pulmonary vessels, nerves, interstitium, and pleura. After supplying the conducting airways, the deoxygenated blood drains into radicles of the pulmonary vein and then into the left atrium, contributing 2–5% to the right-to-left physiological shunt. Chronic pulmonary inflammation, for example, due to recurrent infections as may occur in a patient with bronchiectasis, can result in hypertrophy of the bronchial arteries and can be a cause of major haemoptysis. This can be treated with therapeutic bronchial artery embolisation.

Nervous supply of the lungs

The lungs are innervated by sympathetic and parasympathetic nerves which combine to form a nerve plexus behind the hila. The vagi contain parasympathetic fibres to the heart, motor fibres to the larynx and pharynx, and sensory secretomotor efferent nerves to the bronchial mucosa which are responsible for the cough reflex. The vagi also contain non-cholinergic fibres. The right recurrent laryngeal nerve arises as the vagus crosses anterior to the subclavian artery, hooks around that vessel and ascends between the trachea and oesophagus. The left recurrent laryngeal nerve arises as the vagus crosses the left side of the arch of the aorta, hooks around the inferior side of the arch to the left of the ligamentum arteriosum, and then ascends on the right side of the arch between the trachea and oesophagus. This nerve is liable to damage from tumours in the left lung which will result in hoarseness (see Chapter 9).

The sympathetic fibres arise from the second–fourth thoracic ganglia of the sympathetic trunk and enter the thorax anterior to the necks of the ribs. The thoracic part of each trunk has a dozen ganglia, the first of which is often found with the inferior cervical ganglion to form the stellate ganglia. Pre-ganglionic fibres from segments T1–T6 of the sympathetic chain supply the heart, coronary vessels and bronchial tree. The main visceral branches are the three splanchnic nerves. Pain fibres from the lungs and other thoracic structures travel to the spinal cord. The smooth muscle is supplied by a few sympathetic, noradrenergic fibres, which do not significantly affect smooth muscle tone. The smooth muscle contains β_{-2} adrenergic receptors which cause relaxation when stimulated by circulating adrenaline.

Lymphatics of the lungs

Lymph drains via superficial and deep lymphatic plexuses. The deep lymphatic plexus originates from between the alveoli and travels alongside the bronchopulmonary bundle to bronchopulmonary nodes at the hilum, then to the tracheobronchial nodes at the bifurcation of the trachea, which drains into the tracheal or paratracheal nodes. The superficial lymphatic plexus is subpleural. The visceral nodes drain the lungs, pleura and mediastinum. Mediastinal nodes in the superior mediastinum receive lymphatics from the thymus, pericardium, and heart. The efferents of the tracheal and mediastinal nodes form a bronchomediastinal trunk on each side of the trachea. Some lymph from the lower lobe drains to the posterior mediastinal nodes which drain directly into the thoracic duct.

The thoracic duct extends from the abdomen to the neck where it drains into the right and left brachiocephalic veins. Lymphatics have valves to prevent backflow. The total flow of lymph from the lungs is 0.5 ml min^{-1}. The lymph nodes may become enlarged in lung malignancies, infections, for example, *Mycobacterium tuberculosis* infection, and granulomatous conditions, such as sarcoidosis.

Control of breathing

Central control

The control of breathing is complex and conducted through inspiratory and expiratory neurones in the pons and lower medulla. The ventrolateral medulla contains a column of neurones called the **ventral respiratory group** which extends from the lateral reticular nucleus to the nucleus ambiguous. This is divided into four groups: (1) the caudal group which contains both inspiratory and expiratory neurones; (2) the rostral group which controls the functions of the larynx and pharynx; (3) the pre-Botzinger complex which contains inspiratory neurones (often called the Central Pattern Generator); and (4) the Botzinger complex which contains expiratory neurones. The respiratory rhythm begins with these associated groups of neurones generating regular bursts of activity lasting a few seconds, which stimulate the diaphragm and external intercostals to initiate inspiration. The antagonistic expiratory neurones then fire for a few seconds to cease inspiration and to initiate expiration. This interaction between inspiratory and expiratory neurones results in spontaneous ventilation or eupnoea.

The medulla also contains the **dorsal respiratory group** which lies close to the **nucleus tractus solitarium** and contains inspiratory neurones. These neurones receive input from the higher centres, including the cortex and hypothalamus via cranial nerves IX and X to modulate the response of the ventral respiratory group (Figure 2.12). The respiratory rhythm can be altered in response to smell, temperature, and emotion. The neurones of the dorsal respiratory group also receive feedback from central and peripheral chemoreceptors. Feedback from the stretch receptors in the lungs via the vagi is important in ceasing inspiration as lung volume increases. Voluntary control of breathing is mediated by motor nerves from the cortex contained in the pyramidal tracts which bypass the dorsal respiratory centre and directly stimulate the muscles of respiration.

Congenital central hypoventilation syndrome, called Ondine's curse, is a rare cause of fatal apnoea during sleep due to the failure of the autonomic control of respiration. Trauma to the brain can also result in a similar presentation.

Lung receptors and reflexes

There are various receptors throughout the conducting airways and alveoli which respond to irritants, stretch, inflammation, oedema, and position. These receive and send signals through the vagi.

Slow-adapting stretch receptors are located within the smooth muscle of the bronchial walls and fire with the continuing stimulation caused by distension of the lungs. The efferent nerves from the stretch receptors ascend via the vagi and result in shorter and shallower inspiration, delaying the next cycle of inspiration.

Irritant receptors are found between the epithelial cells in the bronchial smooth muscle throughout the airways and are stimulated by smoke, dust, and noxious gases, such as SO_2, O_3, and by histamine. These rapid-adapting receptors receive a parasympathetic bronchoconstrictor nerve supply of myelinated fibres from the vagi, which act via acetylcholine and muscarinic type 3 receptors. Stimulation of the irritant receptors in the smaller airways results in the deep sighs which occur periodically at rest and which prevent the lungs from collapsing. The receptors in the trachea are responsible for the powerful cough reflex, which expels particles and is an important part of the lung's defence system. Stimulation of these receptors also causes reflex constriction of the larynx and bronchi.

Juxtapulmonary (J) receptors, which are located on the alveolar and bronchial walls close to the capillaries, are stimulated by pulmonary congestion, pulmonary oedema, microemboli, and inflammatory mediators, such as histamine. Their afferents are small unmyelinated C-fibres or myelinated

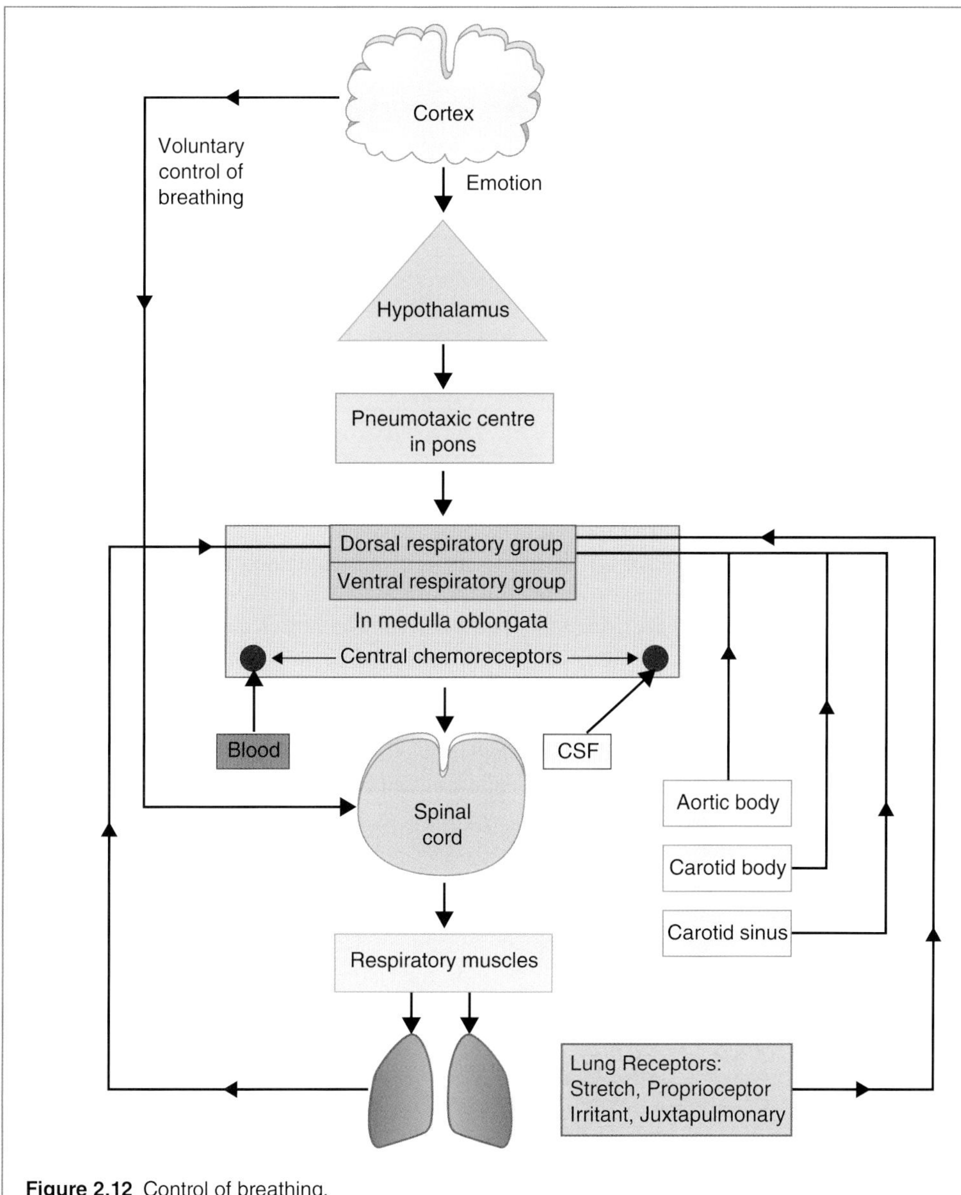

Figure 2.12 Control of breathing.

nerves in the vagi. Activation of the J receptors results in depression of somatic and visceral activity, with apnoea, rapid shallow breathing, a fall in heart rate, a fall in blood pressure, laryngeal constriction, and relaxation of skeletal muscles.

Proprioreceptors are found in the Golgi tendon organs, muscle spindles, and joints of the respiratory muscles, but not the diaphragm, and the afferents lead to the spinal cord via dorsal roots. These proprioreceptors are stimulated by shortening and load in respiratory muscles and are important during exercise.

Chemoreceptors

Chemical control of ventilation is mediated via **central chemoreceptors** which detect arterial partial pressure of carbon dioxide (PCO_2) and pH, and **peripheral chemoreceptors** which detect PCO_2, pH, and partial pressure of oxygen (PO_2) and feedback to the neurones in the dorsal respiratory group.

The central chemoreceptors lie near the venterolateral surface of the medulla, near the exit of cranial nerves IX and X. A tight, endothelial layer forms the blood-brain barrier which separates the cerebrospinal fluid (CSF) from blood and is impermeable to charged molecules such as hydrogen ions (H^+) and bicarbonate ions ($HCO3^-$), but permeable to CO_2, which can easily cross the barrier. The pH of CSF is therefore determined by arterial PCO_2 and CSF $HCO3^-$, and not affected directly by changes in blood pH. CSF contains little protein, so its buffering capacity is low. Therefore, a small change in the PCO_2 will result in a large change in the pH in CSF. The neurones of the central chemoreceptors are therefore very sensitive to CO_2 and an increase in PCO_2 in the CSF will result in an increase in minute ventilation in a linear fashion. These central chemoreceptors are therefore less sensitive to H^+ than they are to CO_2. The central chemoreceptors are responsible for about 80% of the response to CO_2. The response time is 20 seconds as CO_2 needs to diffuse across the blood-brain barrier. The central chemoreceptors do not respond to a drop in PO_2 (hypoxia).

An increase in alveolar PCO_2 above the normal value of 5.3 kPa results in a linear increase in minute ventilation (litres ventilated/minute) by about 15–25 l min^{-1} for each kPa rise in PCO_2. There is considerable variation between individuals. Athletes and patients with chronic respiratory disease often have a reduced response to PCO_2. If PCO_2 increases above 10 kPa, ventilation decreases due to direct suppression of the central neurones. Metabolic acidosis shifts the CO_2-ventilation response curve to the left whereas a metabolic alkalosis shifts it to the right.

There is little increase in ventilation until the PO_2 falls below 8 kPa (60 mmHg). The effect of reducing PO_2 is potentiated if the PCO_2 rises, so there is a synergistic relationship between the effects of PO_2 and PCO_2.

The peripheral chemoreceptors lie within the carotid and aortic bodies, both of which receive high blood flow relative to their size and respond within seconds to small changes in PCO_2, pH, and PO_2 by increasing the rate of firing, which will result in an increase in ventilation, especially if the PO_2 drops below 8 kPa. The carotid body is a 2 mg structure located at the bifurcation of the common carotid artery, just above the carotid sinus and contains type 1 glomus cells and type 2 sheath cells. The glomus cells contain dense granules of neurotransmitters and the sheath cells protect and support the glomus cells. The carotid body is innervated by the carotid sinus nerve, which leads to the glossopharyngeal nerve and responds to an increase in PCO_2 or H^+ and a decrease in PO_2 by increasing ventilation. The aortic bodies are distributed around the aortic arch, are innervated by the vagi, and they too respond to a drop in PO_2 and an increase in PCO_2 and H^+.

Adaptation of the chemoreceptors occurs in chronic respiratory disease and in those living at high altitude. When hypercapnia is prolonged, for example, in COPD, CSF pH gradually returns to normal with an adaptive and compensatory increase in $HCO3^-$ which is transported across the blood-brain barrier. The drive to breathe from the central chemoreceptor is consequently reduced, even though the PCO_2 is still high. There is also reduced sensitivity to further increases in PCO_2, so that a patient's ventilation is mainly controlled by the level of PO_2, which is called the hypoxic drive. If the hypoxic drive is suppressed by giving O_2 then this decreases ventilation. Therefore, in these patients, O_2 must be given cautiously, starting at a low level of 23–28%, with the lowest amount of inspired oxygen above 21% (room air) that is possible.

At high altitude, ventilation is stimulated by the low atmospheric PO_2 which results in hypocapnia and alkalosis and decreased ventilation. Over a few days of acclimatisation, the pH of CSF returns to normal due to $HCO3^-$ transport out of the CSF, even though the PCO_2 remains low, and consequently ventilation increases again. Over a longer period, blood pH returns to normal due to renal compensation.

Transport of oxygen

Oxygen is not very soluble in plasma and is therefore bound to haemoglobin (HB) to form oxyhaemoglobin and is transported from the lungs to all tissues. The oxygen capacity of haemoglobin is the amount of O_2 bound to HB, with each gram of HB combining with approximately 1.34 ml O_2. Therefore, in an individual with a normal HB of 150 g l^{-1}, blood will contain 200 ml l^{-1} O_2. Arterial blood has a PO_2 of approximately 13 kPa (100 mmHg) and

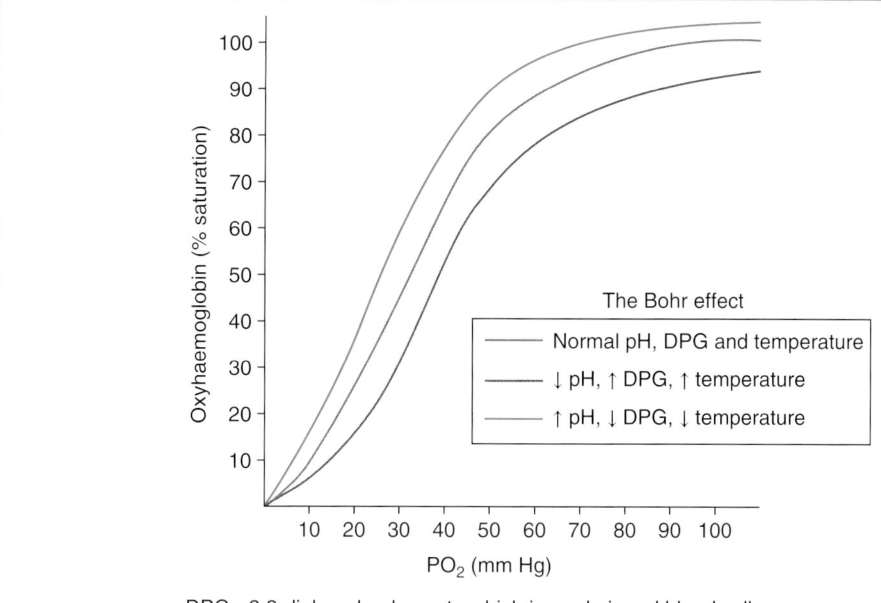

Figure 2.13 Oxygen-Haemoglobin Dissociation Curve and the Bohr Effect.

an O_2 saturation of 97%. The oxygen dissociation curve flattens at the higher levels of O_2 saturation, therefore hyperventilation and hypoventilation will cause little change in the arterial oxygen content. However, if the PO_2 drops below 8 kPa (60 mmHg), there will be a significant reduction in O_2 saturation and content.

The affinity of haemoglobin (HB) for O_2 depends on pH, PCO_2 and temperature and is called the **Bohr effect** (Figure 2.13). An increase in hydrogen ion (H^+) (a decrease in pH), an increase in PCO_2 and an increase in temperature, as occurs in metabolically active tissue, result in a shift of the oxygen dissociation curve to the right. A rise in the concentration of 2,3-diphosphoglycerate, caused by glycolysis in red cells, also results in a right shift. This results in the release of oxygen from HB to the tissues which require oxygen. Conversely, in the alveoli, the lower temperature, lower PCO_2, and higher pH result in a left shift of the dissociation curve and in an increased affinity of haemoglobin for O_2.

Transport of carbon dioxide

Carbon dioxide (CO_2) is 20 times more soluble in plasma than O_2 and 10% is carried dissolved in plasma. Some 60% of CO_2 is transported as bicarbonate ions. The relationship between pH, PCO_2 and HCO_3^- is described by the Henderson-Hasselbalch equation:

$$CO_2 + H_2O \leftrightarrow H_2CO_3 \leftrightarrow H^+ + HCO_3^-$$

with the enzyme carbonic anhydrase (CA) catalysing the left-hand side of the equation. This results in a high concentration of H^+ within the red blood cells as the membrane is impermeable to H^+. To maintain electrical neutrality, chloride ions diffuse into the red blood cells to replace bicarbonate, and this is called the chloride shift.

H^+ ions bind avidly to deoxygenated HB but not to oxygenated HB as it is more acidic. This contributes to the **Haldane effect** which states that for any given PCO_2, the CO_2 content of deoxygenated blood is greater than that of oxygenated blood. Therefore, when HB becomes deoxygenated, it can take up more CO_2 from respiring tissues. Conversely, oxygenation of HB in the lung assists the unloading of CO_2 from the blood so it can be expired (Figure 2.14). Some 30% of CO_2 is carried as carbaminohaemoglobin, formed by a combination of CO_2 with the terminal amino groups on proteins.

Ventilation is closely matched to the metabolic requirements of the body and can be estimated from the rate of CO_2 production (Figure 2.15). The respiratory gas exchange ratio or respiratory

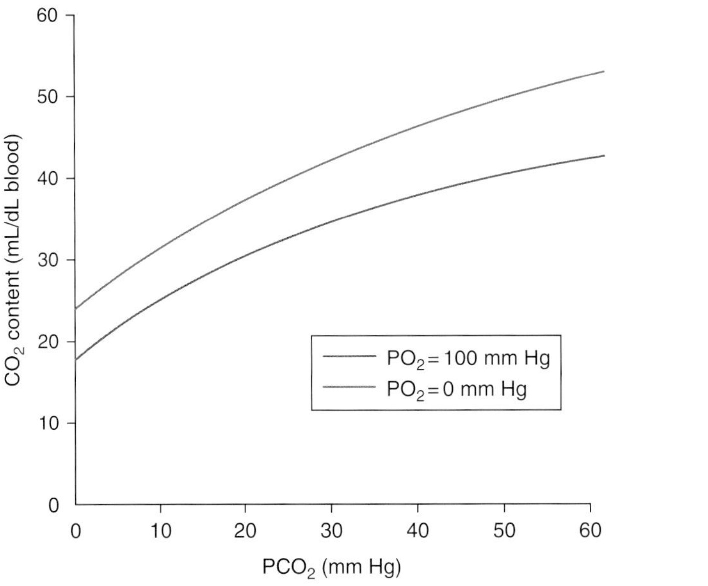

Figure 2.14 The CO_2 dissociation curve.

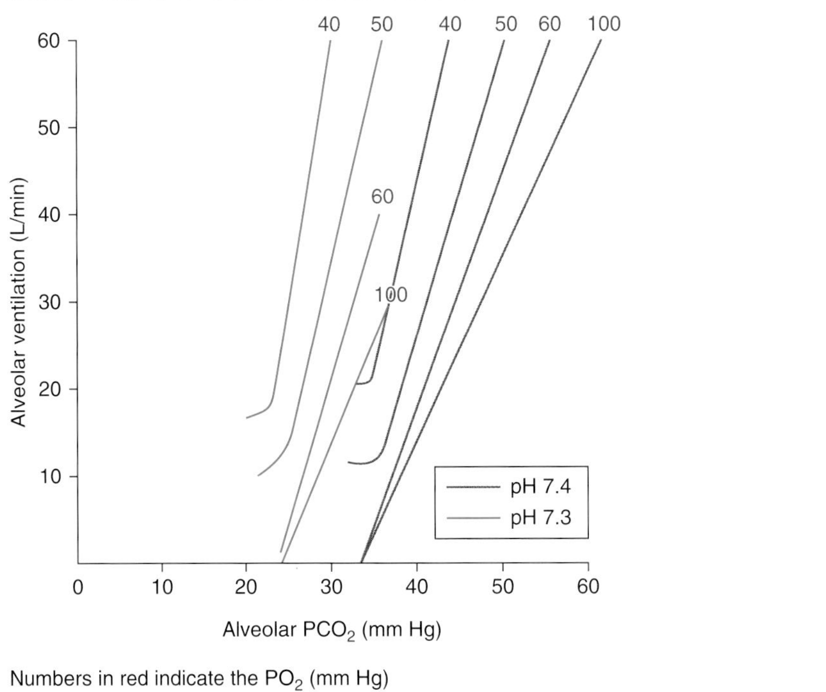

Figure 2.15 The effect of CO_2, pH, and O_2 on ventilation.

quotient (R) is the ratio of CO_2 production to O_2 consumption. Metabolising carbohydrates produces a volume of CO_2 equal to the volume of O_2 consumed, whereas metabolising fats and proteins produces a smaller volume of CO_2 than O_2 consumed. Therefore, for an average mixed diet, R = 0.8.

The acid-base balance

The pH of arterial blood is 7.4 with a H^+ concentration of 40 nmol l^{-1}. It is essential to maintain the pH between 7.35–7.45 (45–35 nmol l^{-1}) for enzyme function. The transport of CO_2 in blood is critical in acid-base regulation. Bicarbonate and deoxygenated HB are important buffers in blood, which bind and release H^+ according to the pH, thus limiting the change in pH that occurs when acid is added. One hundred times more acid equivalent is expired daily as CO_2 than the amount of acid excreted by the kidneys.

The concentration of bicarbonate in plasma is 24 mmol, the pCO_2 is 40 mmHg (5.3 kPa), and the pH is 7.4. If the ratio $[HCO_3^-]/[CO_2]$ remains constant at 20, then the pH will remain at 7.4.

Acute respiratory failure results in a decreased HCO_3^-/CO_2 ratio, and a decrease in pH resulting in respiratory acidosis. Hyperventilation results in an increase in HCO_3^-/CO_2 ratio and respiratory alkalosis. Chronic respiratory failure results in compensatory excretion of H^+ by the kidneys and reabsorption of HCO_3^- in the kidneys to maintain the pH within the normal range, which is called renal compensation.

The term metabolic acidosis is used when acid-base status is disturbed by changes in HCO_3^- rather than CO_2. A metabolic acidosis may be partially compensated for by an increase in ventilation and decrease in pCO_2. Base excess is the base deficit, which is a calculated value representing the amount of acid that would be needed to titrate the blood back to a pH of 7.4 at a pCO_2 of 5.3 kPa.

Ventilation-perfusion mismatch

Not all deoxygenated blood passes through the alveoli and participates in gas exchange. Some blood bypasses the alveolar capillary network for physiological reasons and this is called a **physiological shunt**. As already described, the bronchial arteries, which supply blood to the conducting airways, do not participate in gas exchange and the deoxygenated blood drains into the left atrium (Figure 2.16). Similarly, coronary venous blood, accounting for 2% of cardiac output, also drains into the left atrium. These physiological shunts result in a reduction in the partial pressure of oxygen in the left atrium.

Anatomical right-to-left shunts occur with congenital, cyanotic heart diseases, such as Tetralogy of Fallot, persistent truncus arteriosus, and transposition of the great vessels. Anatomical left-to-right shunts occur in atrial septal defect (ASD), ventricular septal defect (VSD), and patent ductus arteriosus. If the left-to-right shunts are not corrected, the individual will develop pulmonary hypertension, right ventricular hypertrophy, and the pressure in the right ventricle will exceed that in the left ventricle, resulting in a reversal of the shunt from left to right to right to left. This is called Eisenmenger's syndrome.

Lung defence

The upper respiratory system is open to the external environment. Infective pathogens, particles, dusts, pollen, and noxious substances can enter the body. There are several mechanisms to reduce the risk of pathogens reaching the alveoli. Nasal hairs will trap large particles and remove them. Sneezing will expel particles in the upper respiratory tract. The powerful cough reflex is essential in expelling irritants and large particles. In the lower respiratory tract, the MCE will remove particles trapped in the mucus by wafting the mucus upwards until it is swallowed.

Surfactant proteins have an important role in the immune function as do the enzymes lysozyme, tryptase, and cytochrome P450 secreted by the club cells. Invasion of the alveolar space by infective organisms will result in an acute inflammatory response with the recruitment of neutrophils which engulf particles. Lymphocytes will secrete antibodies to combat infections. Individuals with defective cilia, defective mucus, or immunodeficiency will develop severe, life-threatening bronchiectasis, as discussed in Chapter 12.

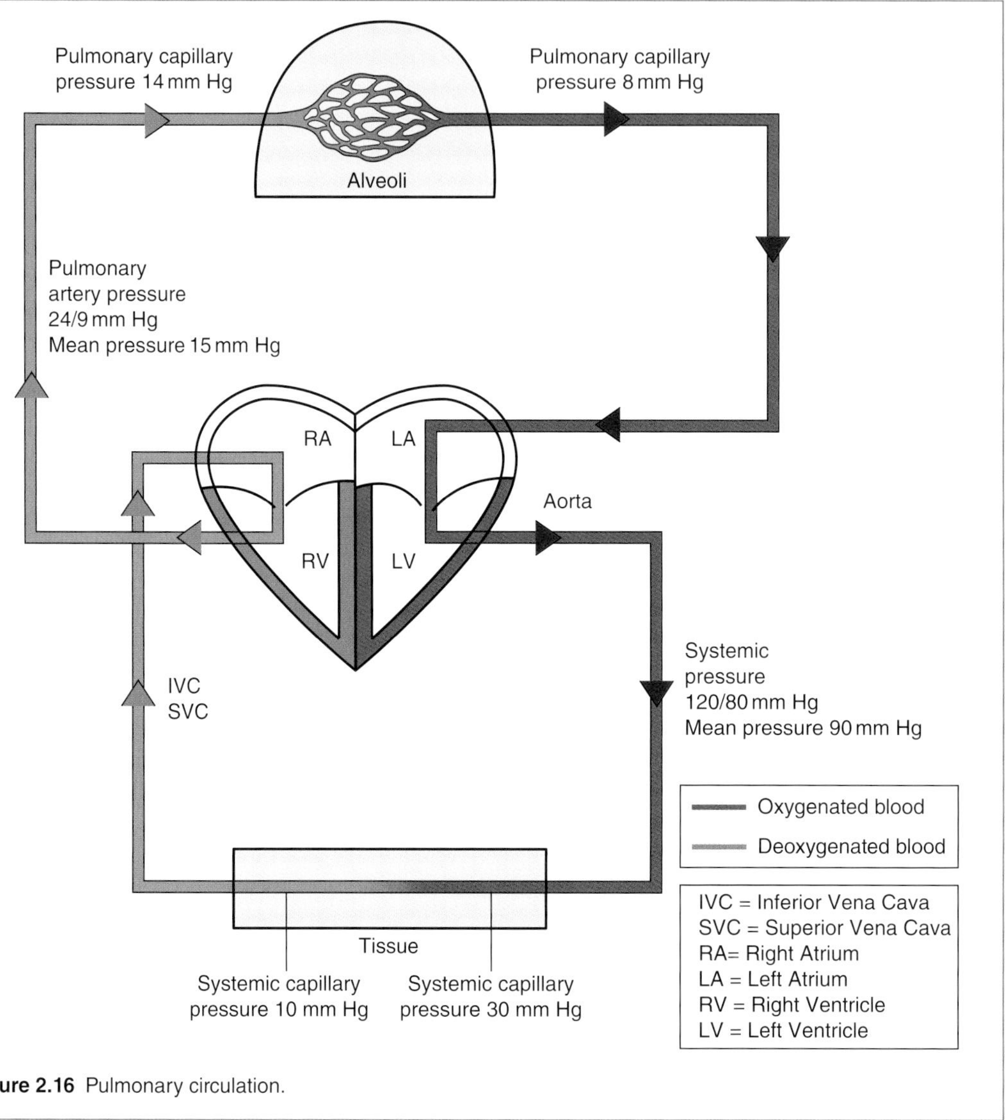

Figure 2.16 Pulmonary circulation.

SUMMARY OF LEARNING POINTS

- Development of the lung begins three weeks after fertilisation.
- The main structures of the respiratory system are formed at the end of the first trimester.
- The oesophagotracheal septum divides the trachea from the oesophagus.
- The lungs only reach full maturity at 36 weeks of gestation.
- The trachea divides into the two main bronchi and then a further 22 times, ending in the alveoli.
- The trachea down to the terminal bronchioles are the conducting zones which filter, warm, and humidify air.
- Generations 17–23 are the respiratory zones which are involved in gas exchange.
- The pulmonary circulation forms an extensive capillary network that is responsible for gas exchange in the alveoli.
- The bronchial arteries supply blood to the conducting airways, blood vessels, nerves, and pleura and do not participate in gas exchange.
- Bronchial arteries arise from the aorta and drain de-oxygenated blood into the left atrium, adding to the physiological shunt.
- The sympathetic, parasympathetic, and non-cholinergic, non-adrenergic nerves supply the lungs and associated structures.
- Lymphatic drainage of the lungs occurs along the superficial and deep plexuses.
- The thoracic duct drains into the right and left brachiocephalic veins.
- The diaphragm is a muscle with a central tendon that separates the abdomen from the thorax.
- The muscles of inspiration are the diaphragm and the intercostal muscles.
- Inspiration is an active process whereas expiration is passive.
- The control of breathing is from the respiratory centre in the medulla and the pons.
- The central chemoreceptors respond mainly to CO_2 and less to H^+ as the blood-brain barrier is impermeable to ions.
- The central chemoreceptors are not responsive to O_2.
- The peripheral chemoreceptors are in the carotid and aortic bodies and respond to CO_2, pH, and hypoxia with PO_2 below 8 kPa.
- There are stretch, J, and irritant receptors in the bronchial tree and lungs which respond to stimuli through the vagi.
- Oxygen is carried as oxyhaemoglobin as O_2 is not soluble in plasma.
- 60% of CO_2 is carried as carbonic acid, with 30% as carbaminohaemoglobin and 10% dissolved in plasma.
- The CO_2 and carbonic acid are responsible for the acid-base balance of the body and in maintaining the pH at 7.4.
- Anatomical right-to-left shunts occur in congenital heart defects.
- Anatomical left-to-right shunts occur in ASD, VSD, and patent ductus arteriosus.
- Lung defence mechanisms include: expelling of particles by sneezing and coughing, removal of foreign particles by MCE, surfactant proteins, enzymes, including tryptase and lysozyme, phagocytes which engulf organisms and the production of antibodies.

MULTIPLE CHOICE QUESTIONS

2.1 Failure of closure of the pleuroperitoneal membrane in development results in which condition?

A Diaphragmatic hernia
B Hyperplasia of the lungs
C Oligohydramnios
D Primary ciliary dyskinesia
E Tracheooesophageal fistula

Answer: A

Closure of the pleuroperitoneal membrane divides the thoracic and abdominal cavities. Failure of closure will result in a diaphragmatic hernia, with the abdominal contents being pushed into the thoracic cavity, causing lung hypoplasia and not lung hyperplasia. This occurs in 1 : 2000 births. Oligohydramnios occurs because of a decreased production of amniotic fluid and is also called Potter's syndrome. It will result in renal agenesis and lung hypoplasia. Primary ciliary dyskinesia occurs due to an abnormality of cilia. Failure of the oesophagotracheal septum, which occurs in 1 : 3000 births, results in a tracheooesophageal fistula.

2.2 Which of the following statements about the diaphragm are true?

A Blood supply to the diaphragm is from the vertebral arteries
B The aorta passes through the diaphragm at T10
C The inferior vena cava passes through at T8
D Damage to the spinal cord below the phrenic nerve roots results in complete cessation of breathing
E Diaphragmatic palsy causes increase in vital capacity when supine

Answer: C

The diaphragm receives blood from the pericardiophrenic, musculophrenic, inferior phrenic, and lower internal intercostal arteries. The aorta passes through the diaphragm at T12, together with the thoracic duct and zygos vein. Damage to the spinal cord below the phrenic nerve roots will enable diaphragmatic breathing to continue. Diaphragmatic palsy will result in a drop in vital capacity by 30% when supine due to pressure from the abdominal contents pushing upwards.

2.3 Which of the following statements about the lungs is true?

A Alveoli are lined with ciliated columnar epithelial cells
B Respiratory bronchioles contain no cartilage
C The trachea is held open by a complete ring of cartilage
D Type 1 pneumocytes synthesise and secrete surfactant
E Phrenic nerve innervates the visceral pleura

Answer: B

Alveoli are lined by type 1 and type 2 pneumocytes which are unciliated. The conducting airways are lined by ciliated columnar epithelium and contain cartilage but the respiratory bronchioles and alveolar ducts do not contain any cartilage, only smooth muscle arranged helically. The trachea has a U-shaped ring of cartilage, with smooth muscle at the posterior part, which makes it collapsible. Type 2 pneumocytes synthesise and secrete surfactant, necessary to prevent alveolar collapse. The phrenic nerves innervate the parietal pleura. The visceral pleura is not innervated.

2.4 Which of the following statements about the lungs is true?

A Blood supply to the conducting airways is from the pulmonary artery
B Blood vessels in the lungs vasodilate in response to hypoxia
C Deoxygenated blood from bronchial arteries drains into the left atrium
D Increase in PCO_2 shifts the oxygen dissociation curve to the right
E Hyperventilation will increase the arterial oxygen content

Answer: C

The bronchial arteries supply blood to the conducting airways and pleura and do not participate in the gas exchange. Pulmonary arterioles vasoconstrict as a response to hypoxia. Deoxygenated blood from the bronchial arteries and coronary venous blood drain into the left atrium, contributing to the physiological shunt. An increase in PCO_2 and a decrease in pH shift the oxygen dissociation curve to the left; this is called the Bohr effect and is important physiologically in releasing oxygen from haemoglobin in respiring tissues. As the oxygen arterial content is normally 95–98%, hyperventilation has no significant effect in increasing this.

2.5 Which of the following statements about CO_2 is true?

A Central chemoreceptors are sensitive to hydrogen ions
B CSF has good buffering capacity
C The majority of CO_2 is carried as carbaminohaemoglobin
D Carotid body responds only to hypoxia
E Acclimatisation at high altitude occurs due to renal compensation

Answer: E

Central chemoreceptors are more sensitive to CO_2 than H^+ as the blood-brain barrier is impermeable to ions. This means that the neurones in the medulla respond more quickly to respiratory acidosis (high PCO_2) than metabolic acidosis. There is very little protein in CSF, which therefore has little buffering capacity. Only 30% of CO_2 is carried combined to haemoglobin as carbaminohaemoglobin; 10% is carried dissolved in plasma. The majority is carried as carbonic acid. The carotid and aortic bodies respond to hypercapnia, to an increase in H^+ and to hypoxia, and the response is greatest if all three happen. Hypoxia becomes important only when PO_2 falls below 8 kPa. At high altitude, over time, there is renal compensation, with excretion of H+ and retention of bicarbonate ions which means that the pH returns to normal.

2.6 Which of these statements about ventilation is true?

A Anatomical dead space is 500 ml
B Alveolar ventilation is 5250 ml min^{-1} at rest
C Functional residual capacity is increased in emphysema due to increased lung compliance
D Lung compliance increases in fibrosis due to decreased elastic recoil
E Vital capacity at rest is 1000 ml

Answer: B

Alveolar ventilation takes into account the anatomical dead space of 150 ml. Vital capacity is only 500 ml during quiet breathing. FRC is decreased in emphysema due to decreased lung compliance caused by a reduction in alveolar tissue. In pulmonary fibrosis, lung compliance is decreased and elastic recoil increased, so the lungs are smaller.

2.7 Which of the following statements about alveoli is true?

A Alveoli contain irritant receptors which, when triggered, cause the cough reflex
B Adjacent alveoli are completely independent units that do not communicate
C Alveoli exhibit structural interdependence which prevents collapse
D The distance O_2 needs to diffuse from alveolus to capillary is 1 μm
E Surfactant allows greater flow of blood through the capillaries

Answer: C

Irritant receptors are found in the walls of the bronchi and not alveoli which contain J receptors which respond to pulmonary congestion. Alveolar units (pulmonary lobules) are connected to each other and prevent alveolar collapse by keeping neighbouring alveoli open. This is called structural interdependence. Oxygen diffuses 0.5 μm across the alveolar-capillary membrane in health. The role of surfactant is to reduce surface tension in the alveoli and prevent collapse.

2.8 Which of the following statements is true?

A Blood flow is greater at the apex compared to the base of the lung
B Hypertrophy of bronchial arteries commonly occurs in sarcoidosis
C Ligamentum arteriosus is the fibrous remnant of the ductus arteriosus
D The right recurrent laryngeal nerve is more likely to be damaged than the left recurrent laryngeal nerve
E The thoracic duct drains into the left atrium

Answer: C

Blood flow is greater at the lung bases (helped by gravity). Hypertrophy of the bronchial arteries occurs in bronchiectasis, aspergilloma, and lung cancers and is a cause of massive haemoptysis. The left recurrent laryngeal nerve has a longer and more tortuous route through the thorax and is more likely to be damaged or affected by bronchogenic carcinoma. The thoracic nerve drains into the left and right brachiocephalic veins. The pulmonary veins drain into the left atrium.

2.9 Anatomical right-to-left shunts occur in which of the following conditions?

A Atrial septal defect
B Patent ductus arteriosus
C Right ventricular hypertrophy
D Transposition of the great vessels
E Ventricular septal defect

Answer: D

Anatomical right-to-left shunts occur with congenital heart defects such as transposition of the great vessels and Tetralogy of Fallot. ASD, VSD and patent ductus arteriosus cause left-to-right shunts. Right ventricular hypertrophy does not cause a shunt.

2.10 Which of the following statements about the thoracic cage is true?

- **A** The cervical rib occurs in 1 : 2000 people
- **B** Floating ribs are the least likely to fracture of all the ribs
- **C** The intercostal vein, artery, and nerve run just above the rib
- **D** Vertebrochondral ribs are joined to the cartilages of the ribs above
- **E** The xiphisternum is composed of bone from early childhood

Answer: D

The cervical rib occurs in 1 : 2000 people and can cause paraesthesia and vascular symptoms. The first and second ribs are the least likely to fracture as they are protected by the clavicle. The intercostal vein, artery, and nerve run just below the ribs, so this area should be avoided. The xiphisternum remains cartilaginous until late adulthood. The vertebrochondral ribs (eighth, ninth, and tenth ribs) are joined to the cartilages of the ribs above.

FURTHER READING

Albert, R., Spiro, S., and Jett, J. (eds.) (1999). *Comprehensive Respiratory Medicine*. St Louis, MO: Mosby.

Bourke, S.J. and Burns, G.P. (2015). *Respiratory Medicine Lecture Notes*, 8e. Hoboken, NJ: Wiley-Blackwell.

Brewis, R.A.L. and White, F.E. (2003). Anatomy of the thorax. In: *Respiratory Medicine* (ed. G.J. Gibson, D.M. Geddes, et al.), 3–33. Edinburgh: Elsevier Science.

Colledge, N.R., Walker, B.R., and Ralston, S.H. (eds.) (2010). *Davidson's Principles and Practice of Medicine*, 21e. Edinburgh: Churchill Livingstone/Elsevier.

Harding, R. and Hooper, S.B. (1996). Regulation of lung expansion and lung growth before birth. *Journal of Applied Physiology* 81: 209–224.

Lumb, A.E. (2000). *TNunn's Applied Respiratory Physiology*, 5e. Oxford: Butterworth-Heinemann.

Moore, K. (2014). *Clinically Oriented Anatomy*, 7e, 306. Dordrecht: Walters Kluwer.

Ward, J.P.T., Ward, J., and Leach, R.M. (2010). *The Respiratory System at a Glanceh*, 3e. Chichester: Wiley-Blackwell.

West, J.B. (1987). *Pulmonary Pathophysiology: The Essentials*. Baltimore, MD: Williams and Wilkins.

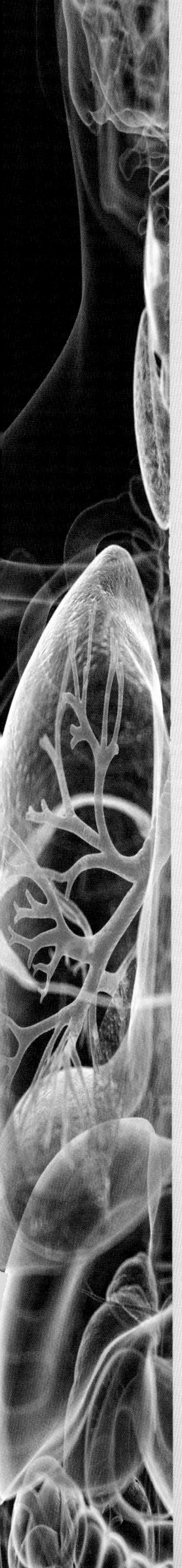

CHAPTER 3

Pharmacology of the lung

Learning objectives

- To understand how medications used to treat pulmonary disease are given
- To gain some understanding of the principles of drug deposition in the lungs
- To learn about the different devices used to deliver drugs to the lungs
- To learn about the medication used to treat obstructive airways disease
- To understand the pharmacology of short-acting and long-acting bronchodilators
- To understand the pharmacology of short-acting and long-acting anticholinergic drugs
- To learn about the benefits and side effects of inhaled and oral corticosteroids
- To learn how to prescribe long-term oxygen therapy
- To understand the role of selective and non-selective phosphodiesterase inhibitors
- To learn about the drugs given for acute asthma
- To gain some understanding of anti-immunoglobulin E therapy
- To appreciate the role of macrolides
- To understand the indication for systemic and topical adrenaline
- To gain some understanding of the drugs given for idiopathic pulmonary fibrosis
- To gain knowledge of pharmacotherapy for smoking cessation
- To gain some understanding of the types of drugs that damage the lungs

Essential Respiratory Medicine, First Edition. Shanthi Paramothayan.

Companion website: www.wiley.com/go/paramothayan/essential_respiratory_medicine

Abbreviations

ABG arterial blood gas
ABPA allergic bronchopulmonary aspergillosis
Ach acetylcholine
ARDS adult respiratory distress syndrome
BAL bronchoalveolar lavage
BTS British Thoracic Society
cAMP cyclic adenosine 3, 5, monophosphate
CAP community acquired pneumonia
CFC chlorofluorocarbon
COPD chronic obstructive pulmonary disease
CS corticosteroid
CT computed tomography
CXR chest X-ray
DPI dry powder inhaler
DPLD diffuse parenchymal lung disease
FGF fibroblast growth factor
FiO_2 inspired oxygen
FVC forced vital capacity
GCS glucocorticosteroid
HFA hydro-fluoroalkane
HPA hypothalamic pituitary axis
HSP-90 heat shock protein 90
ICS inhaled corticosteroid
IgE immunoglobin E
ILD interstitial lung disease
IPF idiopathic pulmonary fibrosis
kPA kilopascal
LABA long-acting β_2-agonist
LAMA long-acting muscarinic agonist
LTD4 leukotriene D4
LTOT long term oxygen therapy
MCE mucociliary escalator
MMAD mass median aerodynamic diameter
MRC Medical Research Council
mRNA messenger ribonucleic acid
NAC N-acetyl cysteine
NHS National Health Service
NIV non-invasive ventilation
NRT nicotine replacement therapy
NSIP non-specific interstitial pneumonia
OCS oral corticosteroid
OSAHS obstructive sleep apnoea/hypopnoea syndrome
PDGFR platelet derived growth factor receptor
pMDI pressurised metered dose inhaler
RAST radioallergosorbent test
SAA short-acting anticholinergics
SABA short-acting β_2-agonist
SAD seasonal affective disorder
SBOT short-burst oxygen therapy
SWSD shift worker sleep disorder
UK United Kingdom
VEGF vascular endothelial growth factor

Drugs and the lung

Diseases of the lung are treated with a variety of drugs. In this chapter, the mechanisms of action, side-effect profile, and interactions of the commonly used drugs are discussed. The clinical indications for the use of these drugs are described in more detail in the relevant chapters that follow. Obstructive airways disease is discussed in Chapter 6, diffuse parenchymal lung disease in Chapter 7, respiratory infections in Chapter 8, respiratory failure in Chapter 13, and sleep disorders in Chapter 14.

Principles of drug deposition in lungs

Inhaled therapy has been used for centuries: sulphurs and volatile aromatic substances, such as methyl and eucalyptus, have been used to relieve respiratory symptoms for many years. An inhaler or a nebuliser will deposit the drug directly into the lungs where it is absorbed and works rapidly. Systemic side effects from inhaled therapy are less than with oral or intravenous treatment.

All inhaler systems are relatively inefficient, with only 8–15% of the drug reaching the lung, no matter how good the inhaler technique is. Particle distribution within the lungs can be measured by radio-labelling the drug and using a gamma camera to quantify deposition. The factors that determine particle deposition in the lungs include the size of the particle, the inspiratory flow rate, and the distance the particle needs to travel, which is determined by the method of inhalation. Factors that favour distal particle sedimentation include small size and low flow rate.

An aerosol is a suspension of fine particles of varying sizes with a favourable surface-to-volume ratio, which allows a small dose to disperse widely over the airways and the alveolar surfaces (Figure 3.1). There is an optimal particle size which favours deposition. The mass median aerodynamic diameter (MMAD) of the aerosol is the diameter about which 50% of the total particle mass resides and this affects where most of the particles that enter the lung are deposited. Large particles of >6 μm in diameter are more likely

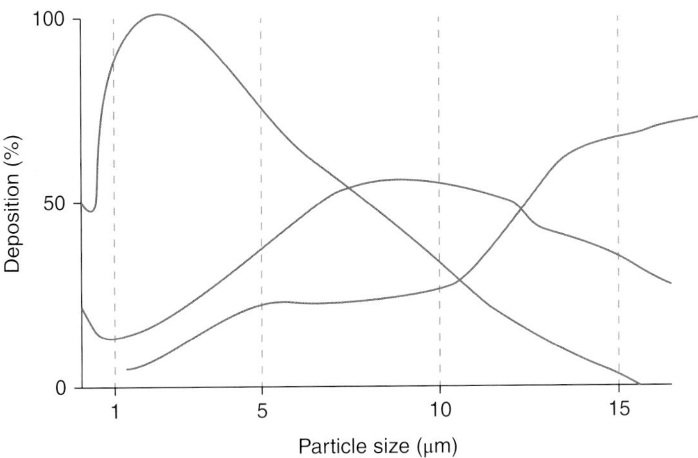

> 5 μm: Impaction – deposited into oropharynx and swallowed
1–5 μm: Sedimentation – optimal for delivery to the lower airways and parenchymal
< 0.8 μm: Likely to be exhaled by tidal breathing

Figure 3.1 Particle size and drug deposition.

to be deposited centrally, smaller particles <5 μm in diameter reach the smaller airways and those of 2–3 μm in diameter reach the alveoli. Particles which are even smaller than this may not settle and are expired. Drug deposition is enhanced by turbulent flow which predominates in these central passages, and particularly at airway bifurcations.

A faster inspiratory flow rate results in the particles being deposited more centrally because of inertial impaction. Slow inhalation with breath-holding results in the particles reaching the peripheral and distal bronchioles. Particles deposited in the conducting airways, which stretch from the larynx to the terminal bronchioles, will become trapped in the mucociliary escalator (MCE). In healthy individuals, the MCE clears the particles within 6–24 hours after deposition, but the clearance will be delayed in conditions such as bronchiectasis, where there is ciliary damage. Small particles in the alveoli are cleared very slowly via alveolar macrophages and lymphatics. The solubility of the drug also affects how quickly the drug is absorbed and cleared from the lungs.

Inhaler devices

The three main types of inhaler devices are pressurised metered dose inhalers (pMDI), dry powder inhalers (DPI), and soft mist inhalers (SMI) (Figure 3.2). Despite the differences in drug delivery to the lung with these various devices, no significant difference in bronchodilator effect has been found.

A **pressurised metered dose inhaler (pMDI)** can be used alone or with a spacer. It comprises of a canister, which can store up to 200 doses of the drug, and a plastic actuator. The drug in the small canister is either dissolved or suspended as crystals in a liquid propellant mixture of hydro-fluoroalkane (HFA) which has replaced the chlorofluorocarbon (CFC) which is detrimental to the ozone layer. A low concentration of surfactant prevents aggregation of the small particles and acts as a lubricant.

The patient should be instructed to shake the canister thoroughly, remove the cap, place the mouthpiece of the actuator between the lips, breathe out steadily, release the dose while taking a slow, deep breath in, hold the breath for a count to 10 and wait a minute before repeating. The use of the different inhalers and nebuliser is demonstrated in the supplementary video (www.wiley.com/go/ParamothayanEssential_Respiratory_Medicine)

The pMDI has several advantages: it is portable, relatively cheap, and small doses of the drug can be given. However, the elderly and young children can find it difficult to use as co-ordination is needed between actuation and inhalation. This can

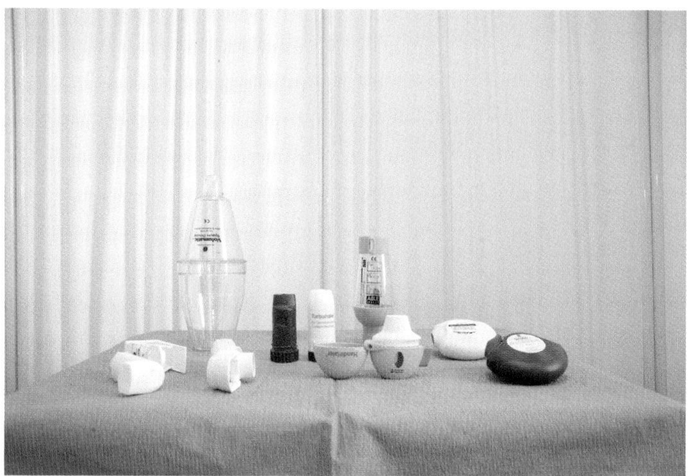

Figure 3.2 Several types of inhaler devices.

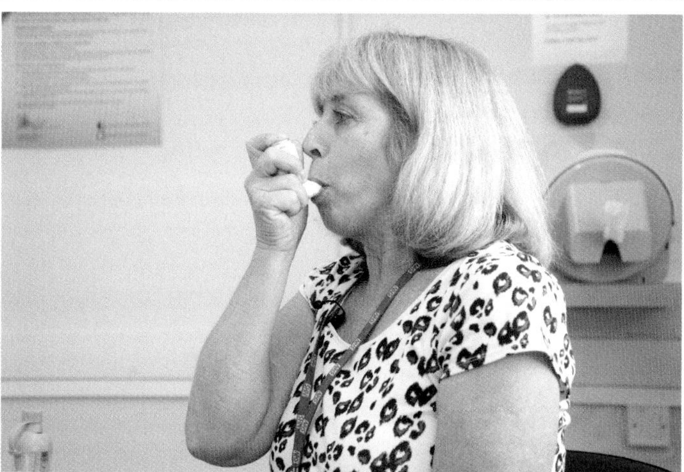

Figure 3.3 Individual using an MDI.

lead to poor compliance. Poor technique can result in deposition of the drug in the oropharynx rather than in the lungs. If inhaled corticosteroids (ICS) are being used, then oropharyngeal deposition can result in candidiasis and dysphonia. pMDI can be less effective in patients with significant airway obstruction as high inspiratory flow rates are required in this situation. It is generally recommended that the MDI is used with a spacer as this reduces oropharyngeal drug deposition and allows better penetration of the drug to the periphery of the lungs (Figure 3.3).

Dry powder inhalers (DPI) are breath-actuated devices that contain a desiccant which ensures that the powder is kept dry. Most adults and children prefer these as they require less co-ordination and are easier to use than a pMDI. The patient needs to be able to generate an inspiratory flow rate of at least $30\,l\,min^{-1}$ to ensure adequate drug deposition in the lungs and to reduce oropharyngeal deposition.

The **turbohaler** is the most commonly used DPI (Figure 3.4). It can hold 50–200 doses of the drug and a dose indicator gives a warning when only

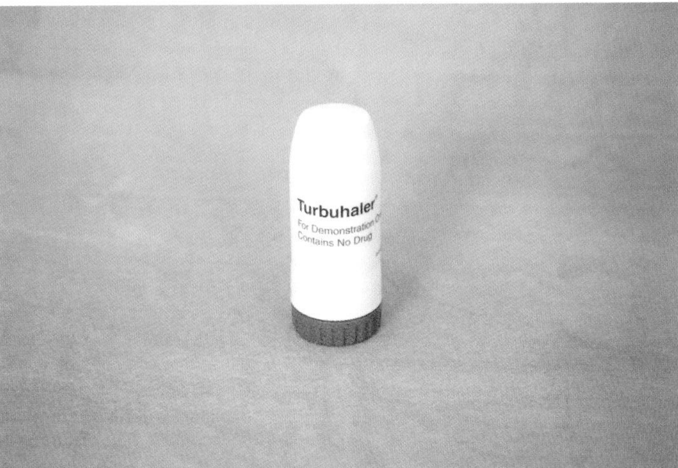

Figure 3.4 Turbohaler.

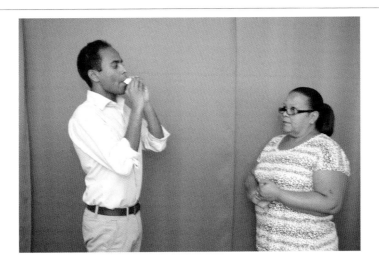

Figure 3.5 Patient using a turbohaler.

20 doses remain. Patients are often concerned because they may not feel any sensation in their oropharynx when they inhale (Figure 3.5). Other DPI devices include the spinhaler, rotahaler, discs, and blisters. These devices are similar in their efficacy.

A **spacer** device improves drug delivery and is recommended for use with all aerosol inhalers, including the pMDI. A large spacer with a one-way valve is called a volumatic device (Figure 3.6). This increases the distance from the actuator to the mouth and allows the particles time to evaporate and slow down before inhalation. This results in a larger proportion of the particles being deposited in the lungs and minimises oropharyngeal drug deposition, thus decreasing the incidence of oropharyngeal candidiasis. Patients should inhale from the spacer device as soon as possible after a single actuation because the drug aerosol is very short-lived. Tidal breathing is as effective as single breaths. The use of a large volume spacer is essential in young children and is an alternative to a nebuliser. The able spacer and aerochamber

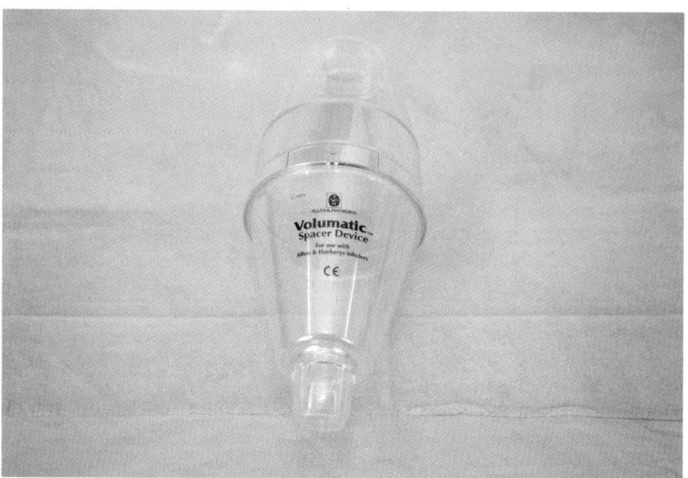

Figure 3.6 Volumatic device (spacer).

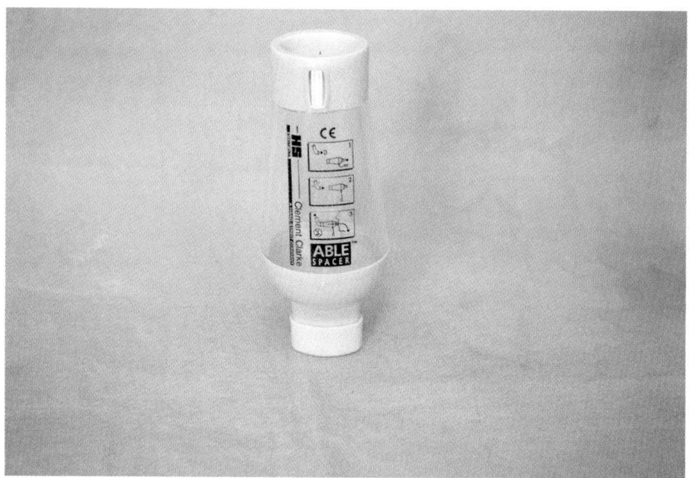

Figure 3.7 Aerochamber.

(Figure 3.7) are smaller volumatic devices which are more portable.

The spacer should be cleaned once a month by washing in mild detergent and allowed to dry in air without rinsing. The mouthpiece should be wiped clean of detergent before use. More frequent cleaning should be avoided as this can affect the electrostatic charge and drug delivery. Spacers should be replaced every 6–12 months.

Tube spacers are tube-like attachments to the pMDI with a much smaller interval volume than the large volume spacers. They too enable the aerosol to slow down before reaching the mouth.

Several studies have shown that in acute asthma, multiple doses of a bronchodilator given through a spacer have a similar bronchodilatory effect as if the drug is given through a nebuliser. However, a nebuliser has the advantage in that it can be used

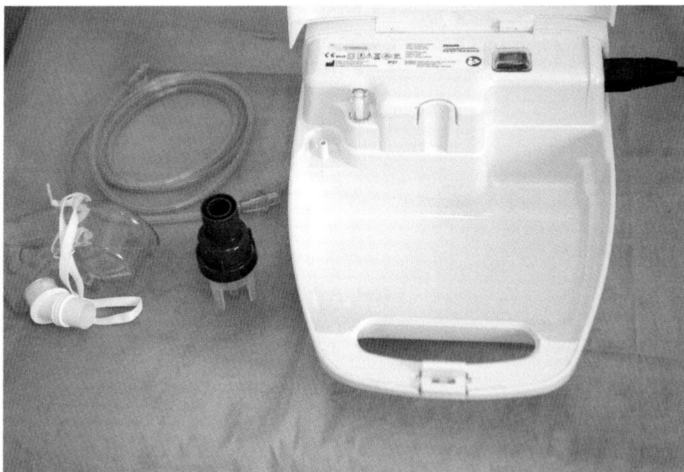

Figure 3.8 Portable nebuliser.

when the patient is very breathless and unable to make the inspiratory effort.

A **nebuliser** (Figure 3.8) can deliver a higher dose of drug to the airways than an inhaler. A solution containing the drug, usually 1 mg ml^{-1}, is turned into an aerosol for inhalation.

Nebulised short-acting β_2-agonists (SABA) and anticholinergic medication are used to treat patients with exacerbation of asthma or COPD. Nebulised SABA can also be used to assess airway reversibility in patients with asthma and COPD. Nebulised methacholine and histamine can be used to assess bronchial hyper-reactivity, and nebulised hypertonic saline can be used to induce sputum. Nebulised colomycin is used to treat pseudomonas aeruginosa infection associated with bronchiectasis and cystic fibrosis, and nebulised pentamidine can be used to treat pneumocystis jirovecii infection. Nebulised opiate can be given to relieve intractable breathlessness in the palliative care setting. There is no evidence for the use of nebulised steroids in exacerbations of asthma or chronic obstructive pulmonary disease (COPD).

Jet nebulisers are more widely used than ultrasonic nebulisers. The jet nebuliser requires an optimum gas flow rate of 6–8 l min^{-1}, which can be either piped air or oxygen. In patients who present with type 1 respiratory failure and require nebulised drugs, 6 l of oxygen should be used to drive the nebuliser. In patients who are at risk of type 2 respiratory failure, air should be used to drive the nebuliser. Supplemental oxygen can be given at the same time via a nasal cannula to maintain the oxygen saturation between 88% and 92%. Management of respiratory failure is discussed in Chapter 13.

Many different designs of nebuliser chambers are available which produce aerosols with particles of different sizes, depending on the design of the baffles in the chamber and the gas flow rate. They usually hold 4–6 ml of solution and have a flow rate of 6–8 l min^{-1}. Droplets with a MMAD of 1–5 µm are deposited in the conducting airways and are therefore suitable for treatment of asthma, whereas a particle size of 1–2 µm is needed for the alveolar deposition of pentamidine. Approximately 10% of a nebulised drug reaches the lungs, with most of the aerosol mist being wasted.

The ultrasonic nebuliser delivers large particles of 3–10 µm from high frequency (1–2 mHz) sound waves induced by the vibration of a piezoelectric crystal which, when focused on the surface of a liquid, creates a fountain of droplets. It has less clinical use than the jet nebuliser.

Oxygen

Long term oxygen therapy (LTOT) is indicated for patients with chronic type 1 respiratory failure with a resting $PaO_2 <= 7.3$ kPa or those with a resting $PaO_2 <= 8$ kPa with evidence of peripheral oedema, polycythaemia (haematocrit >55%) or pulmonary

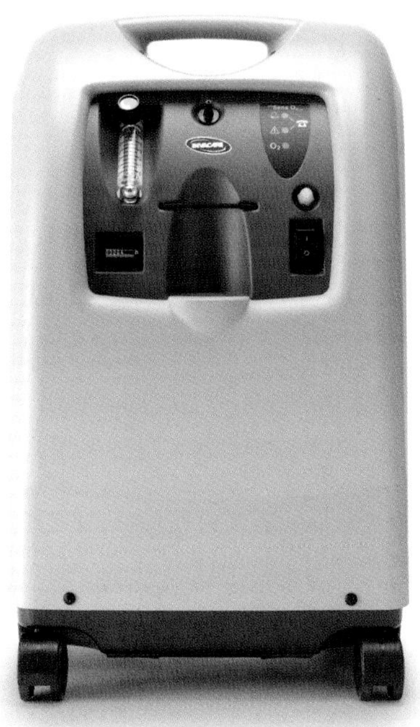

Figure 3.9 Oxygen cylinder. *Source: ABC of COPD, 3rd edition, Figure 11.7.*

hypertension. LTOT improves survival in patients with respiratory failure by reducing the risk of developing cor pulmonale. Controlled LTOT is indicated for patients with type 2 respiratory failure, but must be prescribed with care and closely monitored as there is a risk of CO_2 retention. The indications for oxygen therapy and principles of controlled oxygen are discussed in Chapter 13.

LTOT is given through a concentrator for those requiring oxygen for more than 15 h day^{-1}. The concentrator draws in air, filters out the nitrogen and concentrates the oxygen to reach 95% purity. The oxygen can be humidified to make it less drying to the nostrils (Figure 3.9). Other types of devices include oxygen reservoirs containing liquid oxygen or compressed oxygen. The percentage of inspired oxygen(FiO_2) required is determined by measuring the arterial blood gas (ABG) on air and then on oxygen. The concentrator can be pre-set to deliver the exact flow rate required. A back-up cylinder of oxygen is also supplied for use in an emergency, for example during a power cut, and can supply oxygen for several hours. If a flow rate of more than 5 l min^{-1} is needed, then more than one concentrator may be required.

Portable oxygen can be given for ambulant patients as bottled liquid oxygen which evaporates into the gas. Modern oxygen concentrators are light and portable and can be wheeled on a trolley. They have sufficient oxygen to last several hours and contain battery packs and electrical connections to charge them.

Oxygen can be prescribed for patients with intractable dyspnoea in the palliative care setting. There is little evidence that short-burst oxygen therapy (SBOT) is effective. Oxygen is flammable, so the patient and their family must be warned against the risks of smoking while on oxygen. Oxygen concentrators should be kept in a well-ventilated area, away from gas stoves and flames.

Inhaled drugs

Inhaled drugs are primarily used to treat obstructive airways diseases, such as asthma, COPD, and bronchiectasis. The evidence and indications for the use of these drugs are discussed in Chapter 6.

β_2-adrenoceptor agonists: the smooth muscle of the airways from the trachea to the terminal bronchioles has β_2-adrenoceptors. Direct stimulation of these receptors results in activation of adenylate cyclase and an increase in cyclic adenosine 3, 5 monophosphate (cAMP). The cAMP activates protein kinase A, which then phosphorylates several target proteins within the cell, resulting in the lowering of intracellular calcium concentration by the active removal of calcium from the cell into intracellular stores. Protein kinase A also inhibits phosphoinositide hydrolysis and myosin light chain kinase, resulting in the opening of the large-conductance calcium-activated potassium channels that repolarise the smooth muscle cell and stimulate the sequestration of calcium into intracellular stores. The overall effect is relaxation of the airway smooth muscle and bronchodilatation.

Short-acting β_2-agonists (SABAs) bind to the β_2-adrenoceptors and are effective bronchodilators with minimal side effects. β_2-agonists also have some anti-inflammatory properties: they inhibit mediator release from mast cells, thus reducing the development of bronchial mucosal oedema after exposure to mediators such as histamine and leukotrienes. SABAs also inhibit the release of inflammatory peptides, such as substance P, from sensory nerves which contributes to bronchodilatation. They increase the mucus secretion from the submucosal glands and ion transport across the airway epithelium, thus enhancing mucociliary clearance. However, these short-acting β_2-agonists do not have a significant inhibitory effect on the chronic inflammation of asthmatic airways.

Salbutamol and terbutaline are the safest and most effective SABAs used for treating asthma with rapid improvement in breathlessness and wheezing (see Chapter 6). Salbutamol can be given at a dose of 100 μg/metered inhalation via a pMDI alone or with a volumatic device and through a nebuliser, 2.5 or 5 mg as required. In severe acute asthma, intravenous salbutamol could be considered, although careful cardiac monitoring would be required. Oral preparations of salbutamol may be used by patients who cannot manage the inhaled route, for example, children and the elderly.

Terbutaline, also a SABA, is usually given via a turbohaler or nebulised at a dose of 5–10 mg, up to four times a day. It can also be given subcutaneously at a dose of 250–500 μg four times a day, or intravenously at a dose of 3–5 $\mu g\,ml^{-1}$, which equates to 90–300 $\mu g\,h^{-1}$ for 8–10 hours. Bambuterol, a long-acting oral preparation and pro-drug of terbutaline, may be of value in nocturnal asthma, but is rarely used.

The onset of bronchodilatation occurs within minutes after inhalation of a SABA and the effect is sustained for 4–6 hours. Patients with asthma and COPD are advised to carry SABAs to be used when they become breathless. Their use can protect against various challenges such as exercise, cold air, and allergens. β_2-agonists are more effective in relieving breathlessness in asthma than in COPD as there is more reversibility in asthma. Patients with asthma who are only on SABA and are using it many times a day for symptom control should receive additional treatment, as monotherapy in asthma is associated with an increased risk of death.

The main side effects of SABA, which are dose-related, occur due to stimulation of the β-adrenoceptors in the cardiac muscle and skeletal muscle, resulting in tachycardia (presenting with palpitations) and fine tremor, mainly of the hands. The selective β_2-agonists are associated with fewer side effects. Hypokalaemia can occur when β_2 agonists are given rapidly through a nebuliser, for example, in an acute exacerbation of asthma, because of the stimulation of potassium entry into skeletal muscle. The risk of hypokalaemia is increased when the patient is also being treated with theophylline, corticosteroids, and diuretics. β_2-agonists can also cause muscle cramps, headaches, paradoxical bronchospasm, urticarial angioedema, hypotension, and collapse. Tolerance can occur when the drug is given continuously due to down-regulation of the receptor. Theophylline, which can be used in acute asthma and COPD, can also cause tachycardia, so patients who are receiving both drugs should be carefully monitored.

Long-acting β_2-agonists (LABAs) have a slightly slower onset of action than SABAs but the bronchodilator effect is sustained for 12 hours; therefore, the drug should be taken twice a day. Salmeterol is a partial agonist which is given at a dose of 6 or 12 μg and acts within 20 minutes. Formoterol has a more rapid onset of action and is licensed for short-term symptom relief and for the prevention of exercise-induced bronchospasm.

LABAs should not be used for the relief of an asthma attack. It is recommended that formoterol and salmeterol are given in combination with ICS in asthma and COPD as these drugs act synergistically to improve symptoms, reduce exacerbations, reduce hospitalisation, and improve compliance. Preparations are available with different doses of each component so that patients can step the dose up or down as required. LABAs can rarely cause QT-interval prolongation, taste disturbance, nausea, dizziness, rash, and pruritus.

Short-acting anticholinergic (SAA) drugs are specific antagonists of muscarinic receptors and inhibit cholinergic nerve-induced bronchoconstriction, resulting in bronchodilatation. Normal airways have a resting vagal bronchomotor tone caused by tonic cholinergic nerve impulses which release acetylcholine (Ach) near the airway smooth muscle. Cholinergic reflex bronchoconstriction may be initiated by irritants, such as cold air and stress. This effect may be exaggerated in patients with COPD because of the fixed narrowing of the bronchi. Anticholinergic drugs, therefore, have a greater bronchodilator effect in COPD than in normal airways.

SAAs protect against the acute effects of irritants, such as sulphur dioxide, inert dusts, and cold air by blocking cholinergic bronchoconstriction. Anticholinergics are ineffective against antigen-induced or exercise-induced bronchoconstriction because they have no effect on mast cells and have no anti-inflammatory properties; they do not block the release of inflammatory mediators, such as histamine and leukotrienes.

Anticholinergics are less effective bronchodilators than β_2-agonists in acute asthma and offer less effective protection against various bronchial challenges, although their duration of action is significantly longer. Anticholinergics are slower in onset than β_2-agonists, reaching a peak only 1 hour after inhalation, with effects persisting for more than 6 hours. They may be more effective in older patients with asthma who may have an element of fixed airway obstruction. In the treatment of acute and chronic asthma, anticholinergic drugs, when combined with β_2-agonists, may have an additive effect.

Ipratropium bromide (atrovent) is a quaternary compound of atropine and a non-selective anticholinergic that blocks the muscarinic M3 receptors in the smooth muscle of the airways. Ipratropium bromide can be given by pMDI at a dose of 20–40 μg three or four times a day in patients with COPD where it has some bronchodilator effect as well as reducing the amount of mucus production, thereby improving chronic cough. It can also be given in the nebulised form at a dose of 250–500 μg four times a day for acute asthma or acute exacerbation of COPD. It is topically active and not significantly absorbed from the respiratory tract, so systemic side effects are minimal. The side effects, which are secondary to the muscarinic, anticholinergic actions, include dry mouth, blurred vision, and urinary retention.

Oxitropium bromide has a similar action to ipratropium bromide but is available in higher doses by inhalation. Its effects may be more prolonged so can be useful in some patients with nocturnal asthma.

Long-acting muscarinic agonist (LAMA) drugs cause bronchodilation, reduce bronchospasm and mucus production, and have a prolonged duration of action caused by slow dissociation from muscarinic receptors. They are licensed for use in COPD as first-line agents and have the advantage that they only need to be taken once a day. They are also indicated for patients with chronic asthma.

Tiotropium is given at a dose of 18 μg daily with a duration of action of 18–24 hours. Aclidinium bromide is also approved for use in COPD and is available as a dry powder. In trials, LAMAs have been shown to improve quality of life, reduce exacerbations and hospital admissions but with no evidence of a reduction in mortality. LAMAs can cause a dry mouth, blurred vision, closed-angle glaucoma, urinary retention, cardiac arrhythmias, taste disturbance, dizziness, and epistaxis, but systemic side effects are rare because little systemic absorption occurs.

Combinations of LABA, inhaled corticosteroid (ICS), and LAMA, improve compliance, maximise bronchodilation, improve symptoms, improve exercise capacity, improve quality of life, and reduce exacerbations in patients with COPD.

Corticosteroids (CS) are the most effective and most commonly used drugs for the treatment of lung disease apart from antibiotics. They are potent anti-inflammatory drugs which have a variety of different systemic effects. Glucocorticosteroid (GCS) receptors are found in most cells in the body. This receptor is bound to two molecules of heat shock protein 90 (HSP-90) and 1 molecule of immunophilin. Binding of GCS to the receptor dissociates the receptor from the HSP-90 and results in conformational changes of the receptor complex. The GCS-receptor complex (Figure 3.10) binds to the promoter-enhancer regions of target genes and up-regulates or down-regulates the gene and thereby the gene product through various pathways.

Oral corticosteroids (OCS) have a high oral bioavailability and are rapidly absorbed across the epithelial lining of the gastrointestinal tract by diffusion. OCS are used in the treatment of exacerbation of asthma, COPD, and diffuse parenchymal lung diseases (DPLD), usually at a dose of 0.5–1 $mg\,kg^{-1}\,day^{-1}$. OCS are also indicated for a variety of other conditions, such as sarcoidosis, allergic bronchopulmonary aspergillosis (ABPA), and vasculitis. Intravenous corticosteroids, such as methylprednisolone, are used to treat severe lung disease or when oral therapy is not possible, for example, when the patient cannot swallow or is vomiting.

Cortisone and prednisone are pro-drugs which require hydroxylation in the liver to the active compounds hydrocortisone and prednisolone. Prednisolone is more stable than cortisone, with twice the half-life and a much higher affinity for the glucocorticosteroid receptor. Dexamathasone is 25× times more potent than hydrocortisone (Box 3.1).

All the systemically available GCS are metabolised by the cytochrome P450 system in the liver. The systemic half-life varies from 1.9 hours for hydrocortisone to 4.4 hours for dexamethasone. Their clearance rates can be altered by severe liver

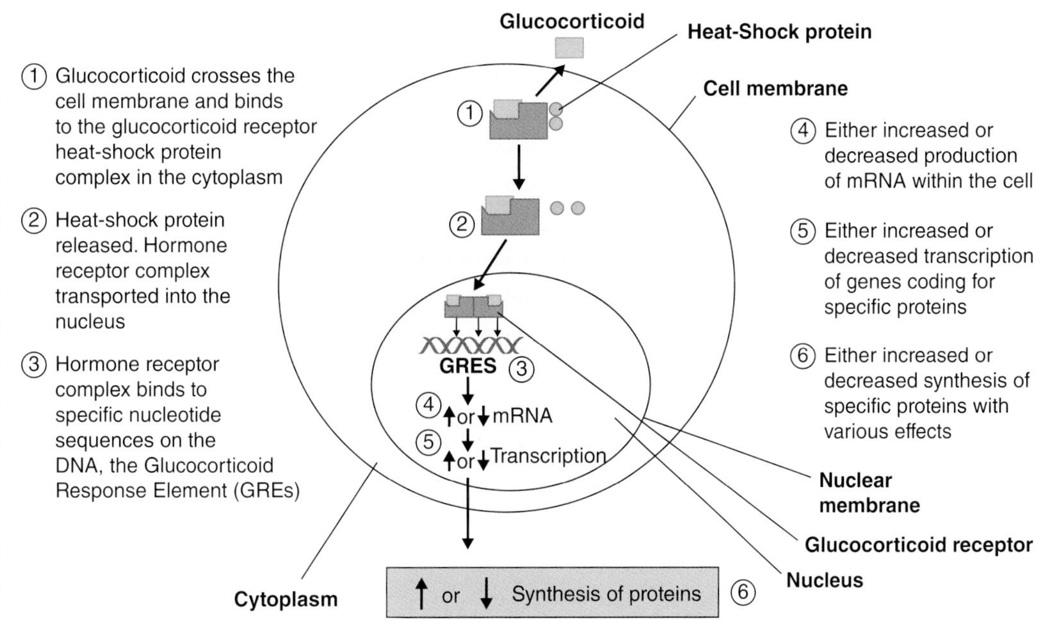
Glucocorticoid
Heat-Shock protein
Cell membrane
① Glucocorticoid crosses the cell membrane and binds to the glucocorticoid receptor heat-shock protein complex in the cytoplasm
② Heat-shock protein released. Hormone receptor complex transported into the nucleus
③ Hormone receptor complex binds to specific nucleotide sequences on the DNA, the Glucocorticoid Response Element (GREs)
④ Either increased or decreased production of mRNA within the cell
⑤ Either increased or decreased transcription of genes coding for specific proteins
⑥ Either increased or decreased synthesis of specific proteins with various effects
GRES ③
④ ↑or↓mRNA
⑤ ↑or↓Transcription
Nuclear membrane
Glucocorticoid receptor
Nucleus
Cytoplasm
↑ or ↓ Synthesis of proteins ⑥

Glucocorticoid receptor is a member of the nuclear hormone receptor super-family that includes receptors for steroid hormones, thyroid hormones, vitamin D and retinoids.

Figure 3.10 Glucocorticoid receptor complex and mechanism of action of corticosteroid.

Box 3.1 Comparison of systemic corticosteroids.

Drug	Equivalent glucocorticoid dose (mg)	Anti-inflammatory potency	Mineralo-corticoid potency	Biological half-life (hours)	HPA Axis suppression (mg)[2]
Hydrocortisone	20	1	1	8–12	20–30
Cortisone	25	0.8	0.8	8–12	25–35
Prednisolone	5	4	0.8	12–36	7.5
Methylprednisolone	4	5	0–0.5	12–36	7.5
Dexamethasone	0.75	30	0	36–54	1–1.5

disease, including liver cirrhosis. OCS can have significant systemic side effects, which are listed in Box 3.2.

Inhaled corticosteroids (ICS) are preferable to OCS for the treatment of obstructive airways diseases, such as asthma and COPD. The aim is to achieve the maximum anti-inflammatory effect in the lungs while minimising systemic absorption and unwanted side effects. A multicentre trial by the Medical Research Council (MRC) in 1956 first demonstrated improvement in acute asthma with ICS.

The commonly used ICS are beclomethasone, budesonide, and fluticasone which are lipophilic drugs and therefore effective when inhaled. They have a very high affinity for the GCS receptor, a hundred times greater than that of hydrocortisone. They also have a very efficient first-pass hepatic metabolism which results in an extremely low oral bioavailability. They are usually given combined with a LABA and given twice a day as this has been shown to improve symptom control, compliance, and better long term outcome.

The dose-response relationship for ICS is flat, so doubling the dose results in minimal benefit but with more side effects (Figure 3.11). It can take 6–8 weeks for ICS to achieve maximal clinical benefit and improvement in lung function. Airway hyper-responsiveness can continue to improve for up to 1–2 years.

Box 3.2 Side effects of oral corticosteroids.

Short term (days)	Medium term (weeks)	Long term (months)
Indigestion Skin bruising Insomnia Psychosis	Skin bruising Gastric ulcers Insomnia Psychosis	Posterior subcapsular cataracts Osteoporosis Growth retardation in children Weight gain Cushingoid appearance Adrenal suppression Hypertension Diabetes Avascular necrosis

Beclomethasone 17.21-dipropionate is biotransformed into its active metabolite beclomethasone mono-propionate in the liver but further metabolism of this is slower than that of budesonide and fluticasone. It is usually given at a dose of 200–2000 μg a day for asthma or COPD.

Budesonide has an oral bioavailability of 6–13%, with a high first-pass liver metabolism but minimal lung metabolism. After a single inhaled dose of 500 μg, the peak plasma levels are achieved within 30 minutes and the plasma half-life is two hours. Budesonide has a high binding affinity for the GCS receptor, ten times that of dexamethasone. Budesonide has a similar potency to beclomethasone.

Fluticasone is twice as potent as beclomethasone or budesonide and given at a dose of 25–250 μg twice a day (Figure 3.12). Fluticasone propionate has an oral bioavailability of <1%, which is the lowest available ICS. It has a rapid first-pass liver metabolism and poor absorption across the gut epithelium. Plasma half-life after intravenous administration varies from 3.7–14.4 hours. This is because it is very lipophilic and is retained in the lipid stores. Fluticasone has the highest binding affinity to the GCS receptor, 18 times that of dexamethasone.

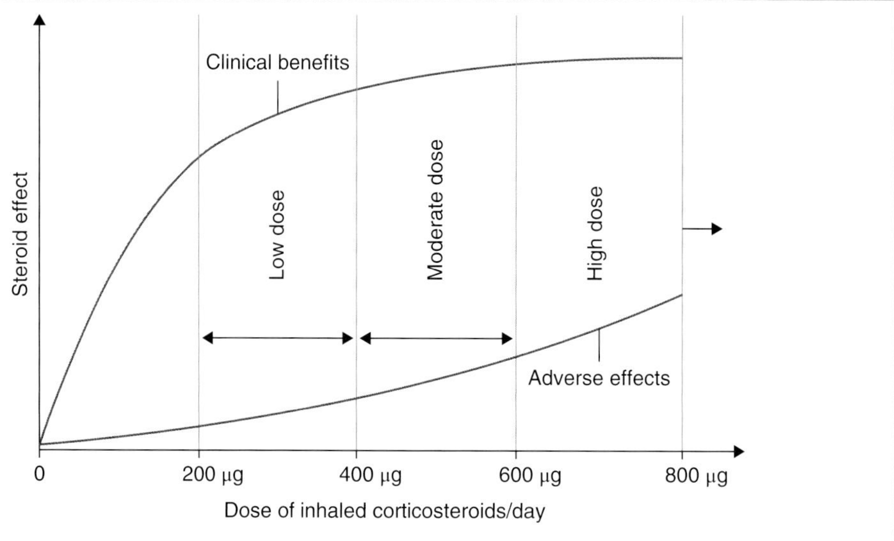

Figure 3.11 Dose response curve of inhaled corticosteroids.

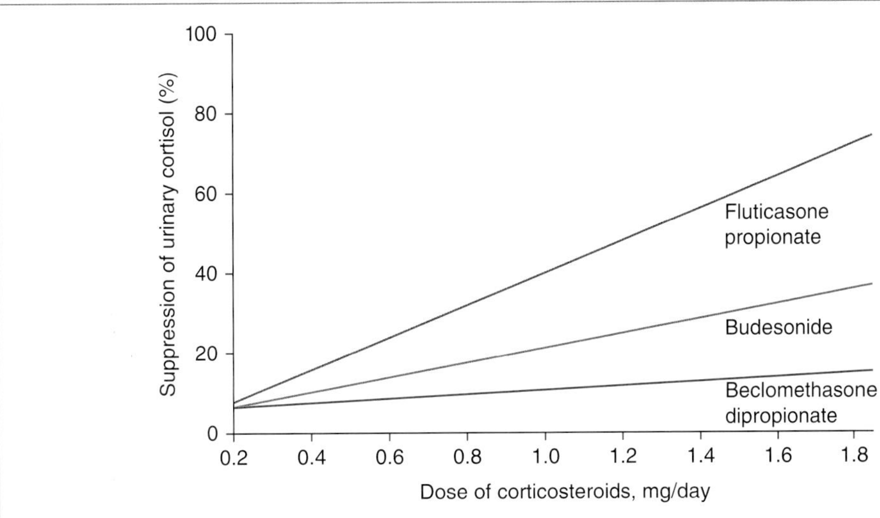

Figure 3.12 Potency of inhaled corticosteroids.

Local side effects of ICS include oral candidiasis and dysphonia, both secondary to oropharyngeal deposition. Clinically obvious oral candidiasis occurs in 5–10% of adult asthmatics and in 1% of children. However, oropharyngeal cultures for Candida species have been demonstrated in up to 45% of children and 70% of adults using ICS. The risk of candidiasis increases when antibiotics and ICS are taken concomitantly, and greatly reduced by using a large volume spacer and by mouth rinsing after use. Dysphonia occurs in up to 30% of those who use ICS and can be reduced by using a spacer.

Systemic side effects of ICS occur because of the absorption of the drug into the systemic circulation and are dose-related. There is little evidence of clinically relevant systemic side effects at doses $< 400\,\mu g\,day^{-1}$ of beclomethasone or budesonide in children and of $<1000\,\mu g\,day^{-1}$ in adults.

Normal doses of ICS have no clinically relevant effect on the hypothalamic pituitary adrenal (HPA) axis. With very high doses of ICS/nebulised CS, some adrenal suppression may occur. In children, there may be a reduction in growth velocity. ICS can affect bone metabolism but there is little evidence that they cause osteoporosis at the conventionally used doses and no evidence that they cause an increased risk of fractures. ICS can result in biochemical changes in bones, but overall height is unaffected. Skin bruising occurs as a dose-dependent side effect of ICS in 47% of patients, usually at daily doses of $>1000\,\mu g\,day^{-1}$. The incidence of skin bruising increases with age and duration of treatment.

Theophylline is indicated for the treatment of acute asthma, chronic asthma, and COPD. Caffeine, a methylxanthine with a small bronchodilator effect, was used to treat asthma in the early part of the twentieth century. Theophylline, also a methylxanthine, is a non-selective phosphodiesterase inhibitor which has minimal effect on bronchomotor tone in normal airways. It reverses bronchoconstriction in asthmatic patients by increasing intracellular cAMP concentration and by blocking the adenosine receptor, thereby reducing the bronchoconstriction that adenosine causes in asthmatic patients through activation of mast cells.

Theophylline has a smaller bronchodilator effect than β_2-agonists or ICS, but has an immunomodulatory role, reducing the number of T lymphocytes in the airways. Theophylline inhibits the late response to allergen challenge more effectively than the early response and inhibits the influx of eosinophils into the airways. Theophylline has an additive bronchodilator effect when used together with β_2-agonists, although this combination increases the risk of hypokalaemia and tachycardia.

Theophylline is used worldwide as a treatment for asthma. It is much cheaper than the current inhaled therapy and can be given orally. Although it is rapidly absorbed, it has a narrow therapeutic range because several factors affect plasma clearance. Many different formulations of slow release theophylline are available which differ in their pharmacokinetic profiles. It is usually given at a dose of 400 mg daily. While the aim is to achieve therapeutic drug levels of 10–20 $mg l^{-1}$, there is some evidence that plasma concentrations of 5–10 $mg l^{-1}$ may be effective, especially in combination with corticosteroids. Side effects occur with plasma levels over 20 $mg l^{-1}$ and include nausea in 10% of patients, and abdominal discomfort. Toxicity can result in tachyarrhythmias, and seizures, which are more common when the drug is given intravenously.

Theophylline is metabolised in the liver by the cytochrome P450 enzyme system and therefore interacts with many drugs that are also metabolised by this system. Drugs that are enzyme inducers, such as rifampicin and anticonvulsants, reduce the level of theophylline, as does excessive alcohol use. Drugs that are enzyme inhibitors, such as erythromycin or ciprofloxacin, increase the level of theophylline. Levels are also increased in heart failure, with viral infections, in those with liver cirrhosis, and in the elderly. Theophylline should be used with caution in patients with cardiac arrhythmias, severe hypertension, hyperthyroidism, epilepsy, and those at risk of hypokalaemia.

Aminophylline, the intravenous equivalent of theophylline, is a mixture of theophylline and ethylenediamine which is 20 times more soluble than theophylline alone. If the patient is not on oral theophylline, then a loading dose of 5 $mg kg^{-1}$ should be given (up to a maximum of 500 mg) followed by a slow infusion of 0.5 $mg kg^{-1} h^{-1}$ over at least 20 minutes for acute asthma and COPD. If intravenous aminophylline is given, a blood sample should be taken 4–6 hours after starting treatment. Plasma theophylline concentration should be measured five days after starting oral treatment and at least three days after any dose adjustment.

Roflumilast is a selective, long-acting phosphodiesterase-4 inhibitor, which is available as a tablet. It has been shown to reduce exacerbations in patients with severe COPD, especially when used in combination with LABA, for example, indacaterol or olodaterol. Side effects include diarrhoea, nausea, dizziness, and headaches.

Leukotriene antagonists are commonly used to treat allergic and exercise-induced asthma. Cysteinyl-leukotrienes (LTC4, LTD4, LTE4) are formed from arachidonic acid by the enzyme 5-lipo oxygenase. Leukotrienes stimulate the cys leukotriene 1 receptor, resulting in bronchoconstriction, activation and recruitment of eosinophils, microvascular leakage, and increased mucus production. Leukotriene D4 is the most potent of these. Elevated levels of leukotrienes are found in the bronchoalveolar lavage fluid and the urine of asthmatics.

Leukotriene 1 receptor antagonists block the effects of leukotrienes, causing bronchodilatation and reducing the eosinophilic response associated with inflammation. Leukotriene receptor antagonists are recommended for use in patients with mild to moderate asthma who are either unable to take ICS or who are not optimally controlled despite taking a combination of ICS and LABA. They are often used at Step 3 of the Asthma Management Plan. These drugs may benefit patients with asthma which is induced by exercise, allergens, cold air, and aspirin. Use of leukotriene inhibitors has been shown to reduce the need for short-acting bronchodilators. Leukotriene antagonists are given orally and generally well tolerated, with few side effects. There are differences in rates of absorption and metabolism between drugs in this class. Montelukast, 10 mg, can be given once a day whereas Zafirlukast, 20 mg, is given twice a day. Corticosteroids are not known to significantly inhibit the production of leukotrienes.

Magnesium sulfate is used to treat severe asthma. It is not entirely clear how it works, but it causes bronchodilation when given intravenously at a dose of 1.2–2 g over 20 minutes. A recent trial of intravenous or nebulised magnesium sulfate in adults with exacerbation of asthma found no benefit. However, a systematic review of randomised controlled trials found a reduction in hospital admissions in those with asthma exacerbations treated with magnesium sulfate and an improvement in lung function.

Sodium cromoglycate and nedocromil sodium belong to a group of drugs called the cromones and are licensed for use in asthma and rhinitis. Sodium cromoglycate is a derivative of khellin, an Egyptian herbal remedy that was found to protect against allergen challenge without a significant bronchodilator effect. Sodium cromoglycate stabilises the mast cell membrane, prevents degranulation, and inhibits the release of inflammatory mediators. Sodium cromoglycate is used in children as prophylaxis against the bronchoconstriction that can occur with exercise and cold weather. It has few significant side effects so is considered safe in children. Nedocromil sodium is structurally related and has very similar clinical effects.

Immunoglobulin E (IgE) levels are raised in patients with allergic asthma. IgE binds to receptors on mast cells and basophils, causing the release of inflammatory cytokines including histamine and cysteinyl-leukotrienes. IgE specific to allergens, such as house dust mite, can be measured by a radioallergosorbent (RAST) test. Anti-IgE therapy is used to treat allergic asthma.

Omalizumab (Xolair) is a recombinant IgG1 monoclonal antibody that binds to circulating IgE and prevents it from binding to the IgE receptor. The immune complexes formed by this process are then cleared by the liver. Omalizumab is indicated for patients with moderately severe or severe allergic asthma with IgE levels between 30 and 700 units ml^{-1} and who are not optimally controlled despite the use of LABA/ICS combined inhaled therapy and leukotriene inhibitor. Randomised controlled trials have demonstrated a reduction in exacerbations in patients treated with this drug and a reduction in steroid use. Omalizumab is given as a subcutaneous injection in hospital with close monitoring. Total IgE levels, which do not differentiate the free IgE from IgE complex to the drug, rise during treatment. The main concern about this treatment is anaphylaxis, which occurs in 1–2 in every 1000 patients, and can occur after any dose.

Mucolytic drugs are indicated in patients with COPD and bronchiectasis who are troubled by a regular productive cough which they find difficult to expectorate. The sputum of patients with COPD contains more glycoprotein which is more viscous and therefore difficult to expectorate. The retained secretions act as a culture medium and increase the frequency of infections. Thiol medications, such as N-acetyl cysteine (NAC) and erdosteine, contain free sulfhydryl groups which can split the glycoprotein bonds in mucus. They decrease the viscosity of the sputum within a few days of treatment and enhance mucociliary clearance. A Cochrane meta-analysis showed that NAC decreased the number of exacerbations in patients with COPD.

S-carboxymethylcysteine (carbocisteine) is also a mucoactive drug. Its structure and mechanism of action differs from that of NAC and erdosteine. Carbocisteine is well absorbed from the gastrointestinal tract, reaches peak serum concentrations within 2 hours, and has a plasma half-life of 1.5 hours. It penetrates lung tissues and makes bronchial secretions less viscous, thus aiding clearance. Carbocisteine has anti-inflammatory properties, scavenges free radicals *in vitro*, and may reduce the systemic inflammation associated with COPD. Alteration to the glycoprotein composition of the sputum may increase antibiotic penetration into bronchial secretions. There is some evidence that carbocisteine decreases cough sensitivity.

The clinical response to carbocisteine varies from one individual to another because of genetic polymorphism in the sulphoxidation capacity. NICE and British Thoracic Society (BTS) guidelines recommend the use of mucolytics in selected patients with COPD, particularly those troubled by chronic sputum production and frequent exacerbations. It is generally well tolerated. The main side effects are gastric ulcers and abdominal discomfort.

Adrenaline (epinephrine) is essential in the treatment of anaphylaxis, and 0.3–0.5 mg should be administered immediately as an intramuscular injection. This can be repeated at 10-minute intervals if required. Adrenaline works by preventing the release of mediators such as histamine and cysteinyl leukotrienes from mast cells, which cause bronchoconstriction and cardiovascular collapse. Side effects include anxiety, tachycardia, palpitations, pallor, and tremor. Rarely, adrenaline can result in angina, hypertension, myocardial infarction, and intracranial haemorrhage.

Topical adrenaline can be administered when there is bleeding after an endobronchial biopsy. The recommendations for the dose and amount which can be safely given vary in the different guidelines and there is no randomised trial evidence. The BTS Bronchoscopy guidelines recommend administering adrenaline, 1 : 10 000, through the bronchoscope onto the areas of bleeding while monitoring the heart rate and blood pressure. Many experts recommend giving this dose in 2 ml aliquots, not exceeding a dose of 0.6 mg.

Antibiotics are commonly used drugs for the treatment of bacterial infections. Inappropriate use of these has increased bacterial resistance to certain antibiotics. Antibiotics prescribed for respiratory tract infections, community acquired pneumonia, hospital acquired pneumonia, and *Mycobacterium tuberculosis* are discussed in Chapter 8.

Antituberculous drugs are given in combination and have many side effects. Compliance can be poor, especially as they must be taken for six months, so Directly Observed Therapy may be necessary. In addition, they interact with many other drugs through the cytochrome P450 enzyme system. Rifampicin in an enzyme inhibitor so can result in the elevation of plasma levels of several drugs, such as warfarin and anticonvulsants.

Macrolide antibiotics are used to treat many respiratory tract infections and community acquired pneumonia (CAP). Erythromycin is the original macrolide antibiotic but is poorly tolerated, with gastrointestinal side effects, prolonged QT interval, and elevated liver enzymes. Azithromycin and clarithromycin are derived from erythromycin after changes to the structure of the molecule. These newer drugs are more stable, have better oral bioavailability, are better tolerated, and have a broader spectrum of activity than erythromycin.

Macrolides bind to a subunit of bacterial ribosomes and inhibit protein synthesis. Clarithromycin and azithromycin are effective against *Streptococcus pneumoniae, Haemophilus influenzae, Moraxella catarrhalis*, and *Mycobacterium avium* complex. They are also used for their anti-inflammatory effects and in the prophylaxis of recurrent respiratory infections in patients with bronchiectasis, cystic fibrosis, and COPD.

As macrolides are metabolised by the cytochrome P450 system and are enzyme inducers, they interact with several drugs, including aminophylline, statins, warfarin, and anticonvulsants, and reduce the plasma level of these drugs. They should, therefore, be used with caution.

Modafanil is derived from adrafanil, a benzhydryl sulfinyl compound. Its exact mechanism of action is unknown, but it promotes alpha wave activity when awake and increases theta wave activity during sleep. It increases histamine levels in the hypothalamus and dopamine concentrations in the brain. Modafanil has been shown to increase wakefulness, alertness, concentration, and to improve mood.

It is licensed for use in narcolepsy, obstructive sleep apnoea/hypopnoea syndrome (OSAHS) and shift worker sleep disorder (SWSD). It can also be used for other hypersomnias, seasonal affective disorder (SAD), and fatigue secondary to chronic diseases. Case studies have suggested that it may benefit patients with type 2 respiratory failure who cannot tolerate non-invasive ventilation (NIV) or are unsuitable for NIV. Modafanil is given orally, either once or twice a day. It is a long-acting drug with a half-life of 15 hours. The main side effects include hypersensitivity reactions and psychiatric symptoms.

Doxapram is a respiratory stimulant which acts on the chemoreceptors in the carotid bodies and the respiratory centre in the medulla, increasing the respiratory rate. It can be used in patients with type 2 respiratory failure who cannot tolerate or are not suitable for NIV. It can also be used to treat respiratory depression secondary to opiate overdose in addition to naloxone. It is given intravenously but needs to be monitored carefully as it can cause arrhythmias and hypertension.

Pirfenidone is an anti-fibrotic drug which reduces fibroblast proliferation and the production of procollagens 1 and 11. It also has anti-inflammatory properties. It can be used in mild and moderately severe idiopathic pulmonary fibrosis (IPF) with forced vital capacity (FVC) of 50–80% predicted. It has been shown to reduce the decline in vital capacity and disease progression and may reduce mortality (see Chapter 7). Pirfenidone has many side effects, which include nausea and photosensitivity.

Nintedanib is an orally active tyrosine kinase inhibitor which targets vascular endothelial growth factor (VEGF), fibroblast growth factor (FGF), and platelet derived growth factor receptor (PDGFR). It inhibits angiogenesis but the exact mechanism of action in pulmonary fibrosis is not clear. It has been shown in trials to reduce the decline in FVC and time to exacerbation in patients with IPF. It can also be used with docetaxel as second-line treatment for non-small cell lung cancer.

Drugs prescribed for smoking cessation

Smoking is responsible for at least 5% of hospital admissions and is a preventable cause of ill health. Approximately 17% of adults in the UK smoke, but two-thirds of them have expressed a desire to quit. There is strong evidence that smoking cessation reduces morbidity and mortality, is cost-effective and should be emphasised to every patient at every encounter. All healthcare professionals, including pharmacists, should be encouraged to 'Ask, Advise, Assist and Arrange' to help smokers to quit.

Smoking cessation interventions are evidence-based and cost-effective. Repeated interventions and multiple attempts are often needed to permanently quit. A combination of behavioural support and pharmacological therapy increases the number of smokers who stop smoking. Counselling can be done one-to-one, in groups or via telephone, for example, the 'Quitline'. Some patients stop smoking after receiving psychotherapy, hypnotherapy, and acupuncture but these are not available on the NHS. There is evidence that banning cigarette smoking in public places has reduced the prevalence of smoking.

While brief advice from a doctor results in 2% of smokers stopping, the addition of medication increases this significantly. Drugs that are prescribed include nicotine replacement therapy (NRT), bupropion, and varenicline. NRT, given as patches, gums, lozenges, and sprays has been shown to double the chance of quitting in clinical trials. NRT reduces the symptoms of nicotine withdrawal, which includes irritability, restlessness, craving, anxiety, depression, and insomnia. NRT provides nicotine in a slower and safer way than cigarette smoke, without the tar and carbon monoxide. A transdermal nicotine patch should be applied daily, initially 21 mg day^{-1} for four weeks, reducing to 14 mg day^{-1} for two weeks and then 7 mg day^{-1} for two weeks. The onset of action is rather slow and therefore nicotine chewing gums, lozenges, inhalators, and nasal sprays can provide more rapid peak blood levels as the drug is absorbed directly through the buccal or nasal mucosa. Very few individuals become addicted to NRT. Weight gain is a common concern among smokers who want to quit, and this should be addressed in the counselling cessations.

Buproprion (Zyban) is an anti-depressant which works by increasing levels of dopamine and noradrenaline in the central nervous system. It has been found to double the rate of smoking cessation compared to placebo but is less effective than varenicline. A dose of 150 mg daily for three days, followed by 150 mg twice a day for 7–12 weeks, is given. There is evidence that a longer period of treatment may reduce relapse. It may be a good choice in those who are particularly concerned about weight gain and in those in whom varenicline is contra-indicated. The most worrying side effect of Buproprion is seizures which occurs in 0.1%, so it should be avoided in those with epilepsy or those with other risk factors for seizures. Buproprion can also cause insomnia, agitation, dry mouth, and headaches.

Varenicline (Champix) is a partial agonist which binds to the alpha-4 β-2 subunit of the nicotinic acetylcholinergic receptors in the brain. It blocks nicotine from binding to the receptor and, as a partial agonist, it reduces the symptoms of nicotine withdrawal. Varenicline is the most effective and cost-effective treatment for smoking cessation, with a rate of smoking cessation three times higher than with placebo. Several trials have found varenicline to be superior to buproprion or NRT. Varenicline is contra-indicated in individuals with a psychiatric history as it may predispose to suicidal ideation. It should also be used with caution in individuals with cardiovascular problems, particularly coronary artery disease and peripheral vascular disease.

E-cigarettes are available that deliver nicotine without the carcinogens in cigarette smoking. Vaping is now popular, and some studies have shown that this helps individuals from smoking cigarettes. The long term effects of vaping are not known, but many doctors feel that it is a safer option than smoking. Therefore, it could be considered when the patient is unable to stop smoking after trying all the other available measures.

Drugs that damage the lungs

A variety of drugs can damage the lung parenchyma, resulting in alveolitis, non-specific interstitial pneumonia (NSIP), pulmonary fibrosis, and adult respiratory distress syndrome (ARDS). As discussed in Chapter 7, a detailed history should be taken of all the medication the patient has taken in the recent past. If there is any indication that a drug may be implicated, then it should be stopped. The patient may need oxygen if hypoxic, and systemic glucocorticoids, for example, oral prednisolone 40–60 mg daily or intravenous methylprednisolone.

A chest X-ray (CXR) and a computed tomography (CT) thorax can show several different patterns, including alveolar opacities, interstitial or mixed opacities and focal nodular areas of consolidation. A bronchoalveolar lavage (BAL) may be required to rule out infection, malignancy, and pulmonary haemorrhage. A lung biopsy is rarely helpful once there is established fibrosis.

Box 3.3 Drugs causing diffuse parenchymal lung disease.

• Amiodarone	• Carmustine
• Methotrexate	• Chlorambucil
• Nitrofurantoin	• Naproxen
• Sulphonamides	• Flecanide
• Chemotherapy agents	• Statin

Box 3.3 lists some of the common agents. A more comprehensive list will be found at www.pneumotox.com

Chemotherapy drugs frequently result in pulmonary toxicity (Figure 3.13, Figure 3.14). Patients will present with cough and breathlessness, the differential diagnosis for which includes infection, pulmonary emboli, heart failure, and lung metastases. If the patient has had radiotherapy, then radiation damage will also be a possible cause (Figure 3.15). Parenchymal lung damage from drugs and radiation is discussed in Chapter 7.

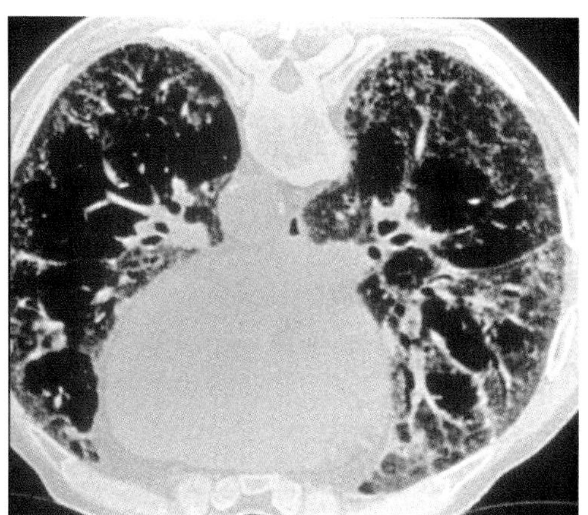
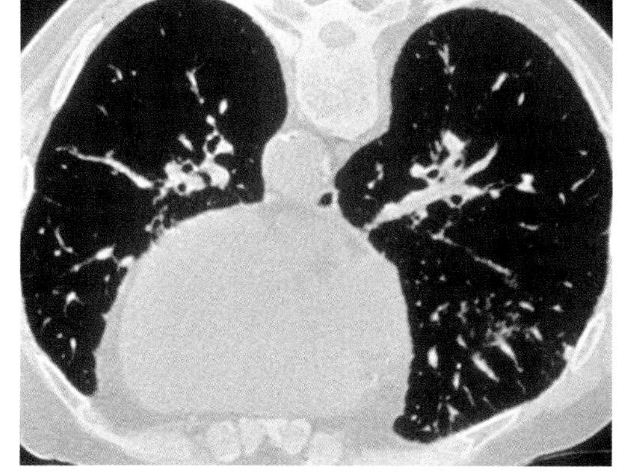

Figure 3.13 CT thorax showing nitrofurantoin toxicity.

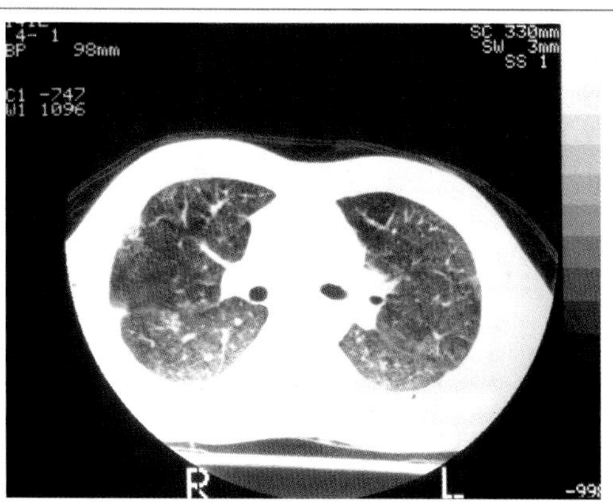

Figure 3.14 CT showing bleomycin toxicity.

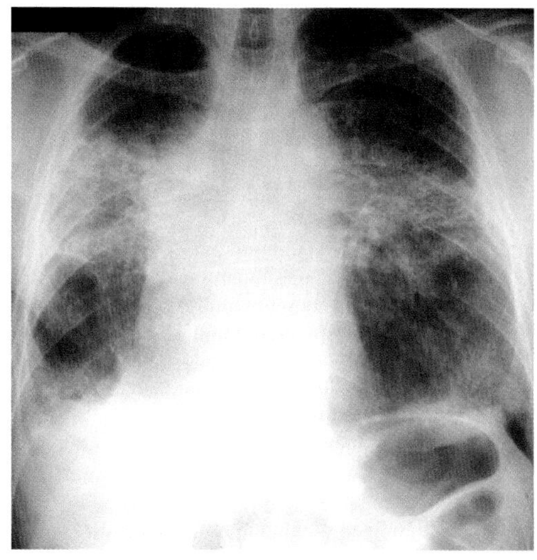

Figure 3.15 CXR showing radiation-induced fibrosis.

SUMMARY OF LEARNING POINTS

- Drug deposition in the lung is affected by the size of the particle, its solubility, the inspiratory flow rate, and the distance travelled.
- The inhaled route has many benefits over the systemic route.
- There are several devices for inhaling medication, but only 10% of the drug reaches the lungs.
- pMDI devices should be used with a volumatic device to improve drug deposition and reduce oropharyngeal deposition.
- Dry powder inhalers are easier to use but require an inspiratory flow rate of $30\,l\,min^{-1}$.
- Obstructive airways diseases are treated with a combination of SABA, LABA, SAA, and LAMA to optimise bronchodilation.
- ICS reduce chronic inflammation and bronchodilate the airways in asthma and COPD.
- ICS have fewer systemic side effects compared to OCS.
- Phosphodiesterase inhibitors have a role in the treatment of obstructive airways diseases.
- LTOT is indicated in patients with type 1 or type 2 respiratory failure with a $PaO_2 < 7.3\,kPa$ or 8 kPa and signs of cor pulmonale and polycythaemia.
- Magnesium sulfate is indicated in patients with acute asthma.
- Leukotriene antagonists are indicated in patients with allergic, exercise-induced, or aspirin-induced asthma.
- Anti IgE therapy (Omalizumab) can be given to patients with allergic asthma and raised IgE who are not optimally managed on other medication.
- Macrolides are antibiotics which have a wide spectrum of antibiotic and anti-inflammatory properties.
- Mucolytic drugs should be considered in patients with COPD and bronchiectasis who have chronic sputum production and frequent exacerbations.
- Intramuscular adrenaline at a dose of 0.3–0.5 mg should be given to patients presenting with anaphylaxis.
- Topical adrenaline (1 : 10000) can be given through the bronchoscope when bleeding occurs after an endobronchial biopsy.
- Doxapram is a respiratory stimulant that could be used in patients with type 2 respiratory failure who are unable to tolerate NIV.
- Modafanil increases histamine levels in the brain, promotes wakefulness, and is indicated for narcolepsy, OSAHS, shift worker sleep disorder, and seasonal affective disorder.
- Perfenidone and nintedanib are new drugs for the treatment of idiopathic pulmonary fibrosis.
- NRT, Buproprion, and varenicline are safe, effective, and cost-effective drugs prescribed for smoking cessation.
- A variety of drugs are toxic to the lungs and damage the lungs in several different ways.

MULTIPLE CHOICE QUESTIONS

3.1 Which of these factors does NOT influence the deposition of the drug in the airways?

A Inspiratory flow rate
B Size of the drug particle
C Turbulence of air flow
D Age of the patient
E Solubility of the drug

Answer: D

Drug deposition in the airways depends on the size of the particle, the inspiratory flow rate, the turbulence of the air flow, and the solubility of the drug. The age of the patient will only be relevant if they are unable to generate a sufficient inspiratory flow rate.

3.2 Which of the following statements about theophylline is true?

A Theophylline blocks the muscarinic cholinergic receptors in bronchial mucosa
B Theophylline blocks the movement of eosinophils into the lungs
C Theophylline causes significant bronchodilation in normal airways

D Theophylline is the most potent bronchodilator available
E Theophylline should be given intravenously as it is poorly absorbed from the gut

Answer: B

Theophylline, a methylxanthine, is a phosphodiesterase inhibitor. It does not affect the cholinergic receptor but does decrease the movement of eosinophils into the lungs. It is a weak bronchodilator compared to corticosteroids or β_2-agonists. It is well absorbed from the gastrointestinal tract and can be given orally.

3.3 Which of the following statements is true?

A Theophylline has no clinical benefit if the plasma level is less than $10\,mg\,l^{-1}$
B Macrolides will decrease the plasma concentration of theophylline
C The commonest side effects of theophylline are cardiac
D Intravenous aminophylline can be given safely if the patient is on oral theophylline
E Plasma theophylline concentration should be measured five days after starting oral treatment

Answer: E

There is some evidence that plasma theophylline level of $< 10\,mg\,l^{-1}$ may have some benefit when given with corticosteroids and or β-$_2$ agonists. Macrolides are enzyme inhibitors so they reduce the clearance of theophylline by the cytochrome P450 enzyme system, thus increasing the plasma theophylline concentration. The commonest side effects of theophylline are gastrointestinal. The plasma theophylline level should be measured in patients taking this drug before intravenous aminophylline is given. The plasma concentration should be measured five days after starting the medication.

3.4 Which of the following statements about leukotrienes and leukotriene receptor antagonists is true?

A Leukotriene E4 is the most potent leukotriene
B Increased levels of leukotriene are found in the urine of patients with asthma
C Leukotriene receptor antagonists increase eosinophilic infiltration of airways
D Leukotriene receptor antagonists have no benefit in patients with exercise-induced asthma
E Leukotriene receptor antagonists have no benefit if the patient is already on oral corticosteroids

Answer: B

Leukotriene D4 is the most potent of the leukotrienes, all of which are derived from arachidonic acid. Increased levels of leukotrienes are found in the urine and bronchoalveolar lavage of patients with asthma. Leukotriene receptor antagonists block the influx of eosinophils into the airways and so have an anti-inflammatory effect. They are therefore useful in the management of asthma induced by exercise, cold air, allergen, or aspirin. Corticosteroids have no effect on this pathway, so leukotriene receptor antagonists are indicated, even if the patient is already on steroids.

3.5 Which of the following statements about Omalizumab is true?

A Omalizumab is a monoclonal antibody that binds to circulating IgE
B Omalizumab is indicated only for patients with life-threatening asthma
C Omalizumab is available as an oral preparation
D Anaphylaxis occurs in 1% of patients treated with Omalizumab
E Anaphylaxis usually occurs after several treatments with Omalizumab

Answer: A

Omalizumab, a monoclonal antibody that binds to circulating IgE, can be used for patients with moderately severe asthma who are not optimally controlled on LABA and ICS. It is given as a subcutaneous injection. Anaphylaxis occurs in 0.1% of patients and can occur even after the first dose.

3.6 Which of the following statements about inhaled corticosteroids (ICS) is true?

A ICS cause adrenal suppression at a dose of 600 μg daily
B ICS increase the risk of osteoporosis and fractures at a dose of 800 μg daily

C ICS are hydrophilic drugs with a low affinity for the glucocorticoid receptor
D ICS have a flat dose-response curve so doubling the dose has minimal benefit but with increased side effects
E The effectiveness of ICS is reduced if given with LABA

Answer: D

ICS are not known to have significant systemic side effects at doses less than 1000 µg daily in adults. ICS are lipophilic drugs with a high affinity for the glucocorticosteroid receptor, ICS have a flat dose-response curve, therefore, it is better to add another drug, such as a LABA rather than double the dose. ICS and LABA are often given in combination and have a synergistic effect.

3.7 Which of the following statements about oral corticosteroids is true?
A Cortisone is an active compound and binds to the glucocorticoid receptor
B Prednisone is hydroxylated in the liver to prednisolone, the active compound
C Hydrocortisone is more potent than dexamethasone
D Corticosteroids are poorly absorbed from the gastrointestinal tract
E Glucocorticosteroid receptors are not found in lung tissue

Answer: B

Cortisone and prednisone are pro-drugs which are hydroxylated in the liver to the active drugs hydrocortisone and prednisolone. Dexamethasone is 25 times more potent than hydrocortisone. Corticosteroids are absorbed rapidly from the gastrointestinal tract, therefore are mostly given orally. Glucocorticosteroid receptors are found in most tissues in the body.

3.8 Which of the following statements about anticholinergic drugs is true?
A Anticholinergic drugs are effective against exercise-induced asthma
B Anticholinergic drugs have a greater bronchodilator effect than β_2-agonists
C Anticholinergic drugs block the release of histamine from mast cells
D Anticholinergic drugs are more effective in the airways of COPD patients than normal airways
E Short-acting anticholinergic drugs have a shorter duration of action than B_2-agonists

Answer: D

Anticholinergic drugs are not anti-inflammatory so do not affect histamine or leukotriene release. They are not effective against allergen-induced or exercise-induced bronchoconstriction. They are less effective bronchodilators than β_2-agonists but have a longer duration of activity, lasting 4–6 hours. They are more effective in COPD as the cholinergic bronchoconstrictor reflex is exaggerated in these patients due to chronic, fixed obstruction.

3.9 Which one of the following questions about macrolides is true?
A Azithromycin is never used to treat community acquired pneumonia
B Erythromycin can cause ototoxicity if given for more than two weeks
C Macrolides have anti-inflammatory properties
D Macrolide resistance occurs in less than 5% of the population
E Macrolides work by destroying the bacterial cell wall

Answer: C

Macrolides have anti-inflammatory properties although the exact mechanism is unknown. They inhibit protein synthesis in bacterial ribosomes but resistance is increasing and approaching 25%. Macrolides can be used to treat CAP, and ototoxicity is not a common side effect of macrolide treatment.

3.10 Which of the following statements about smoking cessation is true?
A Nicotine replacement therapy (NRT) is ineffective in patients who smoke more than 20 cigarettes a day
B NRT should not be given together with varenicline
C Buproprion blocks the nicotinic anticholinergic receptors in the brain

D Varenicline is the most effective treatment for smoking cessation

E The majority of smokers do not wish to stop smoking

Answer: D

More than two-thirds of smokers wish to stop. NRT increases the quit rate compared to placebo and can be given in combination with Buproprion or Varenicline. Varenicline is a partial agonist of the nicotinic anticholinergic receptors. Buproprion is an anti-depressant which increases the levels of noradrenaline and dopamine in the brain.

FURTHER READING

Goodacre, S., Cohen, J., Bradburn, M. et al. (2014). The 3Mg trial: a randomised controlled trial of intravenous or nebulised magnesium sulphate versus placebo in adults with acute severe asthma. *Health Technology Assessment* 18 (22): 1–28.

Hardinge, M., Annandale, J., Bourne, S. et al. (2015). British Thoracic Society guidelines for home oxygen use in adults. *Thorax* 70 (Suppl 1): 1–43.

Kew, K., Kirtchuk, L., Michell, C., and Griffiths, B. (2014). Intravenous magnesium sulfate for treating adults with acute asthma in the emergency department (intervention protocol). Cochrane Database of Systematic Reviews (CD010909), (5), doi:10.1002/14651858. CD010909.pub2.

National Institute for Health and Care Excellence (2013) Stop smoking services. NICE Guideline (PH10). Available at: www.nice.org.uk/guidance/ph10/resources/stop-smoking-services-1996169822917.

National Institute for Health and Care Excellence (2015) Smoking : reducing and preventing tobacco use. NICE guideline (QS82). Available at: www.nice.org.uk

Parrot, S., Godfrey, C., and Raw, M. (1998). Guidance for commissioners on the cost effectiveness of smoking cessation interventions. *Thorax* 53 (Suppl 5): S2–S38.

Poole, P., Chong, J., and Cates, C.J. (2015). Mucolytic agents versus placebo for chronic bronchitis or chronic obstructive pulmonary disease. Cochrane Database of Systematic Reviews (7), [online]): doi: 10.1002/14651858. CD001287.pub5.

Varney, V., Adeyemo, S., Parnell, H. et al. (2014). The successful treatment of hypercapnic respiratory failure with oral modafinil. *International Journal of COPD* 9: 413–419.

Zheng, J.-P., Kang, J., Huang, S.-G. et al. (2008). Effect of carbocisteine on acute exacerbation of chronic obstructive pulmonary disease (PEACE study): a randomised placebo-controlled study. *Lancet* 371 (9629): 2013–2018.

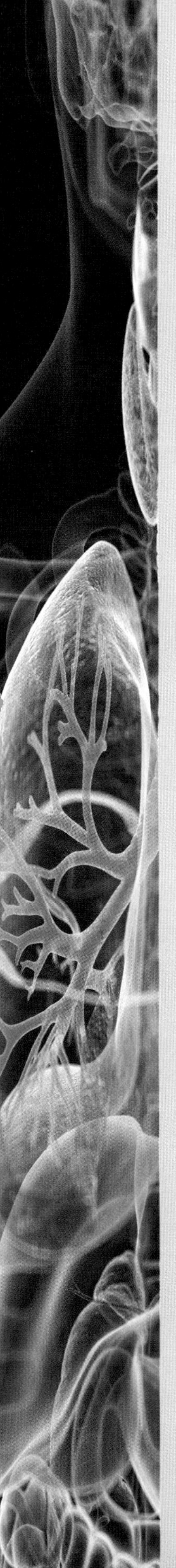

CHAPTER 4

Common respiratory investigations

Learning objectives

- To know what investigations are required to make a diagnosis in patients presenting with respiratory symptoms and signs
- To understand how samples of bloods, urine, pleural fluid, cerebrospinal fluid, and sputum can be useful in diagnosing respiratory conditions
- To be able to interpret peak expiratory flow, spirometry and lung function
- To understand the basic principles of imaging of the lung, including the chest X-ray, CT scan, CTPA, VQ scan, thoracic ultrasound, MRI scan, and PET scan
- To understand functional investigations, including the six-minute walk test, the shuttle test, and cardiorespiratory investigations
- To understand of investigations for sleep-related disorders, including overnight oximetry, sleep study, full polysomnography, and the multiple sleep latency test

Essential Respiratory Medicine, First Edition. Shanthi Paramothayan.

Companion website: www.wiley.com/go/paramothayan/essential_respiratory_medicine

Abbreviations

AAFB acid-alcohol-fast bacilli
ABG arterial blood gas
ABPA allergic bronchopulmonary aspergillosis
ACE angiotensin converting enzyme
ANCA anti-neutrophil cytoplasmic antibodies
AP artero-posterior
ARTP Association for Respiratory Technology and Physiology
ATS American Thoracic Society
BAL bronchoalveolar lavage
β-hCG β-human chorionic gonadotrophin
BTS British Thoracic Society
CAP community acquired pneumonia
CO carbon monoxide
COPD chronic obstructive pulmonary disease
CRP C-reactive protein
CSF cerebrospinal fluid
CT computed tomography
CTPA computed tomography pulmonary angiogram
CUS compressive ultrasound
CXR chest X-ray
EBUS endobronchial ultrasound-guided biopsy
ECG electrocardiogram
ECHO echocardiogram
EEG electroencephalograph
EGPA eosinophilic granulomatosis with polyangiitis
ELISA enzyme-linked immunosorbent assay
EOG electro-oculogram
ERS European Respiratory Society
ESR erythrocyte sedimentation rate
EUS endoscopic ultrasound
FDG ^{18F} Fluorodeoxy glucose
FeNO exhaled nitric oxide
FEV forced expiratory volume
FEV_1 forced expiratory volume in 1 second
FNA fine needle aspiration
FRC functional residual capacity
FVC forced vital capacity
GPA granulomatosis with polyangiitis
HAP hospital acquired pneumonia
HIV human immunodeficiency virus
HLA human leukocyte antigen
HRCT high-resolution computed tomography
IgE immunoglobin E
IGRA interferon gamma release assay
IH idiopathic hypersomnia
INR international normalised ratio
KCO transfer coefficient
LDH lactate dehydrogenase
MPO myeloperoxidase
MRI magnetic resonance imaging
MRPA magnetic resonance pulmonary angiogram
MSLT multiple sleep latency test
MTB *mycobacterium tuberculosis*
MVV maximal voluntary ventilation
NICE National Institute for Health and Care Excellence
NREM non-rapid eye movement
NSIP non-specific interstitial pneumonia
O_2 oxygen
OSA obstructive sleep apnoea
PCR polymerase chain reaction
PE pulmonary embolus
PEF peak expiratory flow
PET positron emission tomography
PPD purified protein derivative
PTH parathyroid hormone
pCO_2 partial pressure of carbon dioxide in blood
pO_2 partial pressure of oxygen in blood
RAST radioallergosorbent test
REM rapid eye movement
RV residual volume
RVC relaxed vital capacity
SIADH syndrome of inappropriate anti-diuretic hormone
SMWT six-minute walk test
SUV standardised uptake value
SWT shuttle walk test
TBNA transbronchial lymph node aspiration
TLC total lung capacity
TLCO carbon monoxide transfer factor
TST tuberculin sensitivity test
VA alveolar gas volume
VATS video-assisted thoracoscopy
VC vital capacity
VE exercise ventilation
VQ ventilation perfusion scan
ZN Ziehl-Neelsen stain

Laboratory tests

Blood tests can be helpful in the diagnosis of several respiratory conditions and in excluding other conditions. A full blood count is a basic blood test that is conducted in most patients who present to hospital with acute respiratory symptoms and in many patients who present to the outpatient department. Although rarely diagnostic alone, the results can be helpful when interpreted with the results of other investigations.

Patients with chronic anaemia (low haemoglobin) can present with breathlessness as the oxygen-carrying capacity of the blood is reduced. Anaemia can also exacerbate underlying lung disease. Primary polycythaemia rubra vera, a myeloproliferative disease associated with the JAK2 gene mutation, results in a haemoglobin greater than $18\,g\,dl^{-1}$ and a haematocrit of over 55%. Relative polycythaemia can occur secondary to dehydration. **Secondary polycythaemia** occurs as a physiological response to chronic hypoxaemia; there is an increase in the production of erythropoietin which stimulates the bone marrow to produce more red blood cells. This can occur in those living at high altitudes as part of adaptation and in those with any chronic lung disease, including chronic obstructive pulmonary disease (COPD), pulmonary hypertension, obstructive sleep apnoea (OSA), and carbon monoxide poisoning. It can also be associated with certain haemoglobinopathies, renal cell cancer, liver tumours, and von Hippel-Lindau disease.

Haemoglobin electrophoresis can confirm the diagnosis of a haemoglobinopathy, for example, sickle cell disease. Sickle cell crisis can result in an acute, life-threatening chest syndrome, which is discussed in Chapter 17. Haemoglobinopathies are a common cause of pulmonary hypertension, which is discussed in Chapter 11.

The white cell count may be elevated in patients with an acute infection, such as upper or lower respiratory tract infection, and acute sinusitis. The differential cell count can give important clues as to the underlying condition. The neutrophil count may be increased with bacterial infections, steroid therapy, and inflammatory diseases. The white cell count may be reduced with bone marrow suppression secondary to chemotherapy and with severe infection. Patients with neutropenia are at increased risk of respiratory tract infections. Neutropenia with a neutrophil count of less than 1 mmol/L predisposes to life-threatening sepsis.

A raised lymphocyte count in peripheral blood may be due to viral infection or *Mycobacterium tuberculosis* (MTB) infection. A low CD4 lymphocyte count is associated with human immunodeficiency virus (HIV) which predisposes to several respiratory tract infections, including pneumocystis jerovicii and is discussed in Chapter 8. Peripheral blood eosinophilia could be due to asthma, allergic conditions, eosinophilic granulomatosis with polyangiitis (EGPA) and parasitic infections. Causes of eosinophilia are discussed in Chapter 7.

A raised C-reactive protein (CRP) and erythrocyte sedimentation rate (ESR) can occur with any systemic infection, but may be raised with other inflammatory conditions, including rheumatological conditions and malignancy. Blood cultures should be taken in any patient who presents with symptoms and signs of sepsis, including those with severe community or hospital acquired pneumonia.

Measurements of urea, creatinine, and electrolytes are routinely done. Hyponatraemia may be associated with a syndrome of inappropriate anti-diuretic hormone (SIADH) which may be associated with small cell lung cancer (Chapter 9). Renal failure can occur in several respiratory/renal syndromes; eosinophilic granulomatosis with polyangiitis (EGPA), granulomatosis with polyangiitis (GPA) and Goodpasture's syndrome. If these conditions are suspected, anti-neutrophil cytoplasmic antibodies (ANCA) should be checked. These vasculitic conditions are discussed in Chapter 11. Patients with parenchymal lung disease of unknown cause or with CT showing non-specific interstitial pneumonia (NSIP) should have investigations for collagen vascular diseases, which will include an autoantibody screen. Liver function tests must be monitored in patients on antifungal drugs, such as itraconazole and voriconazole, and those on Azithromycin when used as a prophylactic antibiotic. Transient increase in alanine transaminase and alkaline phosphatase are often found in patients taking antibiotics.

A d-dimer test is often done as one of the investigations for suspected pulmonary embolus (PE), but this has low specificity as it is raised in many conditions, including malignancy, infection, and pregnancy. Therefore, it is only useful when it is negative. The role of d-dimer in diagnosing a PE is discussed in Chapter 11. Troponin levels may be elevated in severe PE because of right heart strain.

Raised corrected calcium is commonly seen in patients with lung cancer who have metastases to bone, and in squamous cell lung cancer due to exogenous parathormone secretion (see Chapter 9). Raised corrected calcium is seen in 10–20% of patients with active sarcoidosis because activated macrophages in the lung and lymph nodes synthesise vitamin D which increases calcium absorption in the gut. Patients with active sarcoidosis may have raised serum angiotensin converting enzyme (ACE) levels. This is not diagnostic of sarcoidosis but can be useful when monitoring response to treatment. Sarcoidosis is discussed in Chapter 7.

Various immunological tests are used to determine if there is immune deficiency in adults and children presenting with recurrent respiratory infections. Patients with bronchiectasis should have measurements of their immunoglobulins, including IgG subclasses (see Chapter 12). Mannose-binding lectin deficiency and defective anti-pneumococcal polysaccharide antibody response can predispose to recurrent respiratory infections.

Human immunodeficiency virus (HIV) infection can be the cause of recurrent respiratory tract infections and increases the risk of *Mycobacterium tuberculosis* infection. It is recommended that patients presenting with frequent or recurring respiratory infections, and those presenting with *Mycobacterium tuberculosis* infection, have an HIV test (see Chapter 8).

Patients with allergic asthma will have raised IgE levels, and those with high levels above 700 units ml^{-1} may benefit from treatment with Omalizumab (Xolair), a recombinant IgG1monoclonal antibody. IgE levels will also be greatly elevated in allergic bronchopulmonary aspergillosis (ABPA). In patients with asthma, a radioallergosorbent test (RAST) can be used to confirm an immune response to a specific allergen, for example, cat or house dust mite. Avian precipitants will be positive in patients who have hypersensitivity pneumonitis secondary to exposure to antigens from birds, including pigeons, parrots, and budgerigars.

Theophylline is used in the management of acute and chronic asthma and COPD, and is usually given at a dose of 400 mg daily. Theophylline has a narrow therapeutic range between 10 and 20 mg l^{-1}, with significant side effects if blood levels are high; therefore, levels should be monitored. Theophylline is metabolised in the liver by the cytochrome P450 system and therefore drug interactions are important (see Chapter 3).

A lymphoproliferative disorder is always in the differential diagnosis in patients presenting with lymphadenopathy, including bilateral hilar lymphadenopathy and an anterior mediastinal mass (see Chapter 16). In lymphoma, lactate dehydrogenase (LDH) will be increased. Tumour markers too may be helpful in the investigation of an anterior mediastinal mass. The β-human chorionic gonadotrophin (β-hcg) level may be elevated in those with a teratoma, which could be one of the causes of an anterior mediastinal mass (see Chapter 16).

A gamma-interferon test (QuantiFERON) is an important investigation in the diagnosis of *Mycobacterium tuberculosis*. This is discussed in Chapter 8.

There is evidence that Vitamin D is important in protecting against respiratory tract infections, including MTB infection. Measurement of 1, 25-dihydroxycholecalciferol levels, the active form of the vitamin, should be done in patients with recurrent infections and in those diagnosed with MTB. Supplementation should be offered to those found to have levels less than 50 nmol l^{-1}.

Arterial blood gas (ABG) measurements are essential in managing many respiratory conditions which present with respiratory failure. The interpretation of ABG is discussed in Chapter 13.

Sputum tests can be useful in the diagnosis of respiratory tract infections. Routine sampling of sputum is not recommended in the diagnosis of community acquired pneumonia (CAP) as there is a huge variation in the rate of positivity, from 10–80%. Staphylococcal aureus is easily cultured but haemophilus influenzae is harder to culture. If MTB is suspected, then three samples of sputum should be sent for *acid-alcohol-fast* bacilli (AAFB) and Ziehl-Neelsen (ZN) stain. If the patient is unable to cough up sputum or is unfit for bronchoscopy, induced sputum can be obtained by getting the patient to inhale hypertonic saline solution which will liquefy the secretions and cause violent coughing. Healthcare workers carrying out this procedure should take adequate precautions by doing it in a negative pressure room and by wearing masks, gowns, and gloves.

Analysis of **pleural fluid** is an important investigation in the diagnosis of pleural disease and is discussed in detail in Chapter 10. Pleural fluid obtained by aspiration or from pleural drainage must be sent for biochemistry (protein, lactate dehydrogenase and cholesterol), cytology, microbiology, and pH. An exudate suggests that the fluid is secondary to infection or malignancy and further investigations, such as a pleural biopsy, may be required. Tuberculous pleural effusion can be difficult to diagnose because there are very few organisms in the fluid, but a lymphocytic pleural fluid suggests MTB infection. Measurement of polymerase chain reaction (PCR), adenosine deaminase, and interferon-y levels in pleural fluid can be diagnostic of a

Mycobacterium tuberculosis pleural infection. Adenosine deaminase levels above 40 U l^{-1} is strongly suggestive of MTB. The pH of the fluid can be helpful in the diagnosis of an empyema.

Analysis of **cerebrospinal fluid (CSF)** for protein, glucose, ZN stain, and culture should be done in patients presenting with miliary tuberculosis as it is essential to diagnose tuberculous meningitis (see Chapter 8). The CSF may appear turbid, with elevated protein and lymphocytes and a very low glucose. Organisms are not often seen in the CSF, but PCR of CSF may be helpful if MTB is suspected.

Measurement of legionella and pneumococcal antigens in the urine of those presenting with CAP is recommended in the NICE guidelines and can guide management (see Chapter 8). This is a specific and sensitive test which remains positive even after treatment with antibiotics has been commenced. Three early morning urine samples are often sent for the diagnosis of MTB, but the yield is low except in genitourinary tuberculosis. Compound 490 may be present in the urine samples of patients with MTB, but further evaluation is required before this test becomes widely available.

Some 30–50% of patients with active sarcoidosis have hypercalciuria which can be measured by collecting a urine sample for 24 hours. If untreated, this may result in renal calculi and nephrocalcinosis. Patients with sarcoidosis who have hypercalcaemia and hypercalciuria may require immunosuppression.

A skin prick test is useful in patients suspected of having an atopic condition, such as asthma, eczema, or urticaria. It is a quick, safe, and inexpensive test compared to measuring allergen-specific immunoglobin E (IgE). A few drops of purified allergen extract are placed on the flexor surface of the forearm and the tip of a small stylet is pressed into the superficial epidermis through the drop of allergen. A positive reaction is when there is a weal with a surrounding erythematous flare after 15 minutes, and the size of this can be measured in millimetres. The reaction to the allergen is compared to the reaction from a drop of histamine (the positive control) and to a drop of normal saline control solution. An itchy weal will develop at the site of histamine within 10 minutes. This is demonstrated in the supplementary material (www.wiley.com/go/Paramothayan/Essential_Respiratory_Medicine).

The Mantoux test, also known as the tuberculin sensitivity test (TST), is a well-established investigation for suspected MTB and latent tuberculosis. Thus, 0.1 ml of purified protein derivative (PPD) is injected intradermally in the forearm of the patient and the size of the induration is measured after 48–72 hours. Individuals who have had the BCG vaccination will show a mild skin reaction at the site of injection. The Mantoux test is demonstrated in the supplementary material. The result of the Mantoux test must be interpreted carefully together with the results of the Interferon gamma release assay (IGRA), the clinical presentation of the patient, and the CXR, as discussed in Chapter 8.

Imaging of the lung

Chest X-ray (CXR) (Figure 4.1) is one of the commonest investigations undertaken. Although it lacks the sensitivity and specificity of more sophisticated imaging techniques, it is quick and easy to do, available in all hospitals, and relatively cheap, with only a low dose of radiation exposure. If an abnormality is found, it is important to review old CXRs if possible as some abnormalities may be due to previous infection, scarring, or surgery.

An erect, postero-anterior (PA) CXR (Figure 4.2) taken with the arms fully abducted, in full inspiration, with the X-ray beam travelling from back to front, will give optimal images. If the patient is unwell and unable to be upright, then an antero-posterior (AP) CXR can be done. The size of the heart cannot be accurately estimated with an AP CXR. A lateral CXR gives a good view of the structures lying behind the heart and the diaphragm, especially the hilar and perihilar structures which are usually not clear on a PA CXR (Figure 4.3, Figure 4.4).

When reviewing a CXR, it is important to look at it in a systematic way. If the CXR is not rotated, then the medial ends of the clavicles will be symmetrical, and the thoracic spines will appear straight. If the patient has taken a full inspiration and the exposure is adequate, then the lungs will appear black and the vertebral bodies will be visible. In full inspiration, the right hemidiaphragm will be 2 cm higher than the left hemidiaphragm as the liver pushes it up, and it will be intersected by the anterior part of the sixth rib. (Box 4.1) lists the features on the CXR that should be checked. Abnormalities in some areas are often missed; this

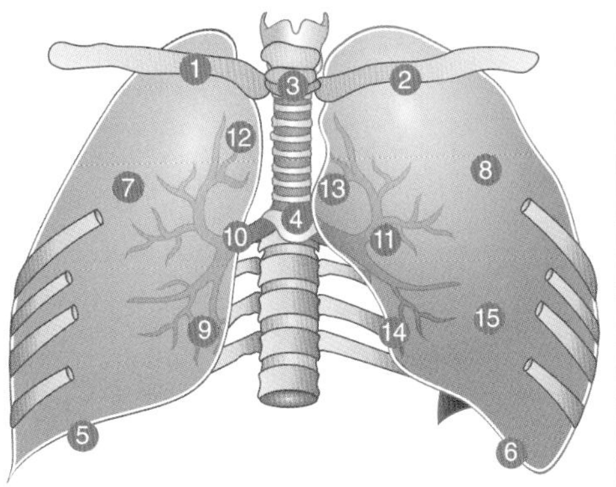

1. Right clavicle
2. Left clavicle
3. Trachea
4. Carina
5. Right diaphragm
6. Left diaphragm
7. Right lung
8. Left lung
9. Right heart border (right atrium)
10. Right hilum (bronchi, arteries and veins)
11. Left hilum (bronchi, arteries and veins)
12. Superior vena cava
13. Aortic arch
14. Left heart border (left ventricle)
15. Pulmonary vessels

Figure 4.1 Diagram of normal PA CXR with labels of structures.

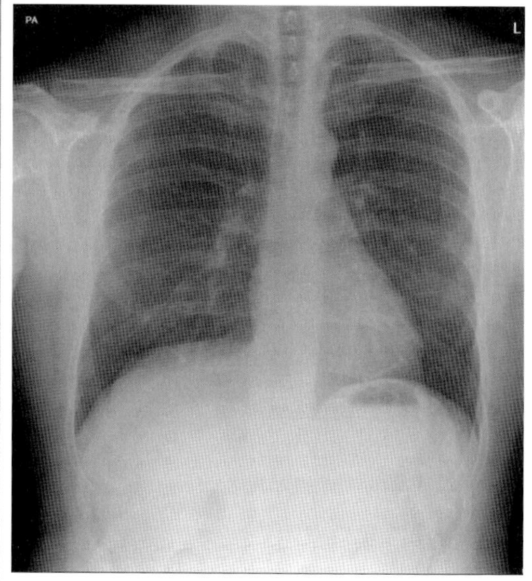

Figure 4.2 Normal PA CXR.

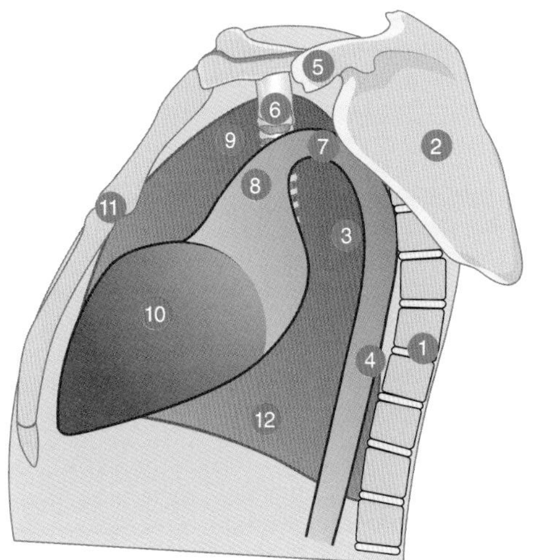

1. Thoracic vertebral bodies
2. Scapula
3. Pulmonary trunk and hilum
4. Descending aorta
5. Head of clavicle
6. Trachea
7. Aortic arch
8. Ascending aorta
9. Anterior mediastinum
10. Heart
11. Sternum
12. Diaphragm

Figure 4.3 Diagram of normal lateral CXR with labels of structures.

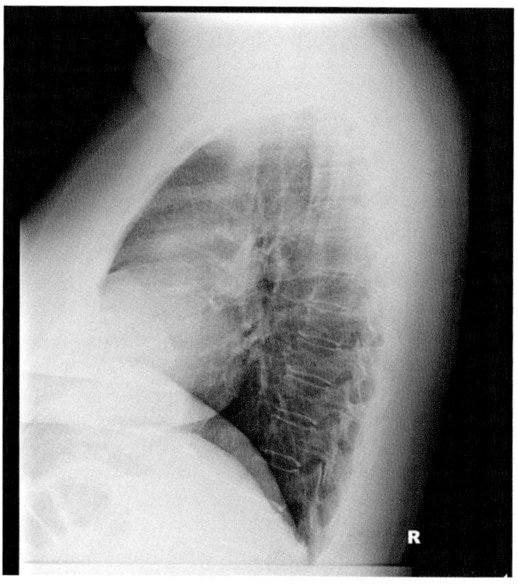

Figure 4.4 Normal lateral CXR.

Box 4.1 Interpretation of the CXR.

- Correct patient (name and date of birth)
- Date of CXR
- Correct labelling of right and left side
- Symmetry: medial ends of both clavicles and thoracic spines
- Adequate exposure: vertebral bodies visible
- Shape and bony structures of the chest wall
- Position of trachea
- Mediastinal contours
- Hila
- Size of lungs
- Lung markings
- Position and clarity of diaphragm
- Ribs and clavicle
- Soft tissue
- Heart size and cardiac silhouette
- Area behind the heart
- Lung apices
- First costochondral junctions
- Costophrenic angles

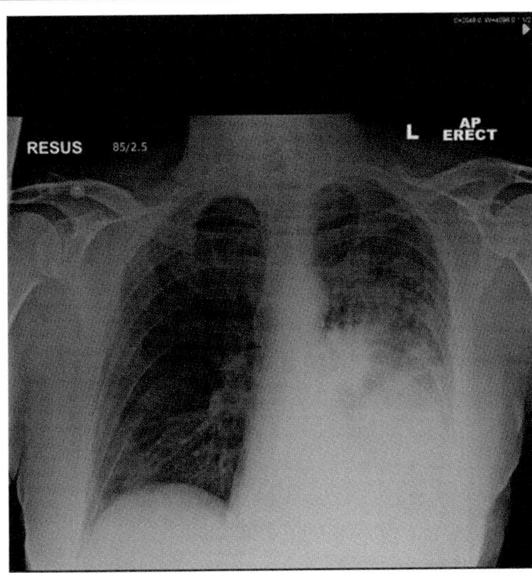

Figure 4.5 CXR showing consolidation left lower lobe with air bronchogram.

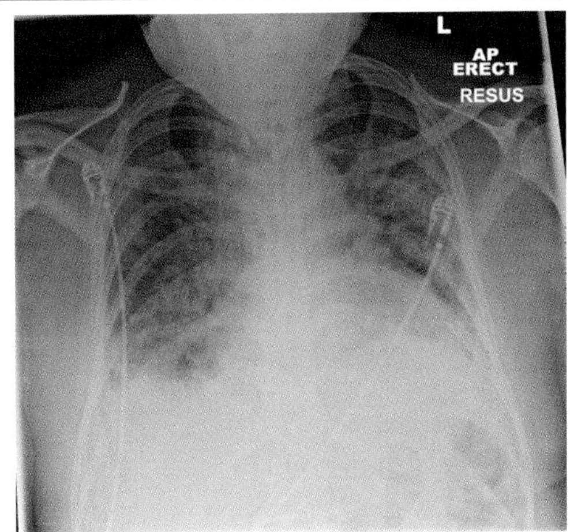

Figure 4.6 CXR showing pulmonary oedema.

includes the area behind the heart, the lung apices, the first costochondral junction, and the costophrenic angles.

A normal CXR appears black because the lungs are filled with air. In a normal CXR, the carina will be sharp. Splaying of the carina suggests subcarinal lymphadenopathy or an enlarged left atrium. The hila are composed of the pulmonary arteries, pulmonary veins, bronchi, and lymph nodes. The left hilum is 0.5–1.5 cm higher than the right hilum. The oblique fissure, which is visible in 60% of individuals, separates the upper and lower lobes of the left lung and the middle and lower lobes of the right lung. The horizontal fissure separates the upper and middle lobes of the right lung. The costophrenic angles are normally sharp and well delineated.

A lack of clarity, for example, along the heart borders or the diaphragm, suggests adjacent consolidation or collapse of the surrounding lung and is called the 'silhouette sign'. In the consolidated lung, air passing through a bronchus will show up against the opaque lung and is called an 'air bronchogram'. Figure 4.5 shows a CXR of a consolidated lung with an air bronchogram. Pulmonary oedema has the appearance of fluid in the alveoli, fissures and costophrenic angles and the presence of Kerley B lines. There will be areas of sub-segmental collapse, with atelectasis, linear lines, and horizontal lines. The cardiothoracic ratio may be greater than 50%, suggesting cardiomegaly. With pulmonary oedema, the shadowing starts at both hila and increases towards the periphery of the lungs in a 'bat's wing' distribution. Figure 4.6 shows a CXR with pulmonary oedema.

The CXR is often the first investigation to lead to a diagnosis of lung cancer. Abnormalities that suggest lung cancer include a lung mass, lobar collapse, pleural effusion, or a pulmonary nodule. The terms 'nodule' and 'mass" are often used interchangeably but a lesion less than 3 cm should be called a nodule and a lesion larger than 3 cm called a mass.

Features that are suspicious for malignancy include a large size, cavitation, spiculation, and increase in size over time (if previous imaging is available to compare with). The differential diagnoses, investigation, and management of pulmonary masses and pulmonary nodules are discussed in Chapter 9.

Cavitation is an area of radiolucency within a mass and the differential diagnosis includes squamous cell carcinoma, MTB, lung abscess, klebsiella pneumonia, *Staphylococcus aureus* pneumonia, GPA, and pulmonary infarct. Figure 4.7 shows a cavitating lesion.

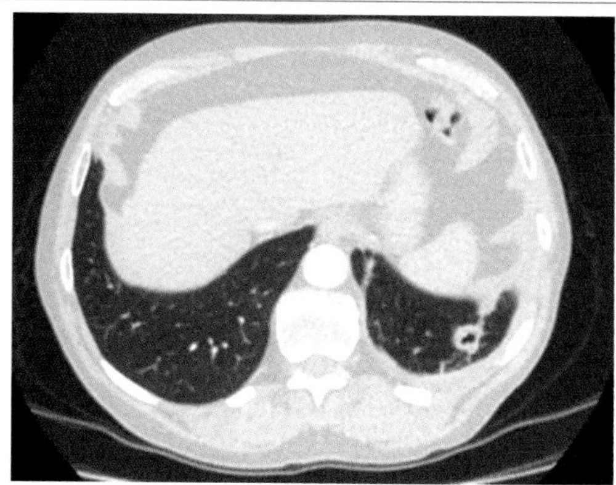

Figure 4.7 CXR showing a cavitating lesion left lower lobe.

Pulmonary nodules measuring 3–5 mm are called **miliary**, and the differential diagnosis of miliary nodules includes miliary tuberculosis (Figure 4.8), fungal infections, and chickenpox pneumonia (see Chapter 8).

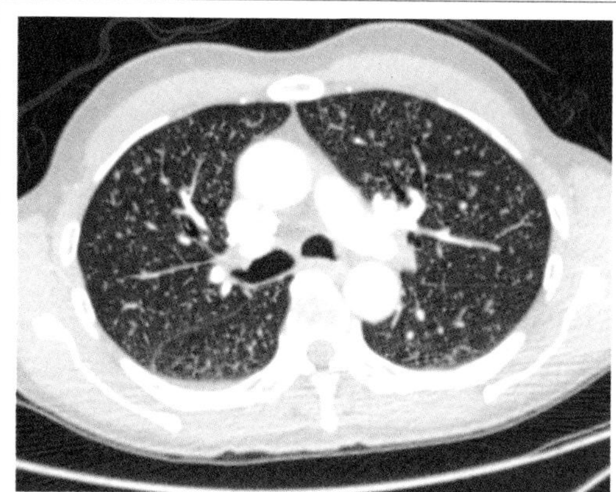

Figure 4.8 CT thorax showing miliary tuberculosis.

Collapse of a lobe of the lung occurs when there is no air entering that lobe, for example, when there is an endobronchial lesion in the bronchus, such as lung cancer, an inhaled foreign body, or even impacted mucus plug. Collapse of a lobe will also result in volume loss and compensatory expansion of the other lobes which results in increased transradiency of the adjacent areas of the lung.

A complete '**white out**' can occur either due to complete collapse of a lung, a large pleural effusion, extensive consolidation, or a combination of these. When there is complete collapse, the mediastinum (trachea and heart) will shift towards the side of the collapse and with a pleural effusion, the trachea will shift away from the effusion.

The radiological appearance which is characteristic for each lobar collapse is described in Box 4.2.

Consolidation of the lung results in opacification on the CXR. This can occur due to an infective process, such as pneumonia, or pulmonary haemorrhage, when air in the lung is replaced by semi-solid material, such as an exudate or blood. The appearance of consolidation can also be due to bronchoalveolar cell cancer (adenocarcinoma in situ) (Figure 4.16).

Idiopathic pulmonary fibrosis (usual interstitial pneumonia, UIP), results in the appearance of small lungs due to volume loss, with reticulonodular shadowing, but the changes are non-specific (Figure 4.17). An HRCT is required to identify the hallmark features of sub-pleural reticulation, honeycombing, and traction bronchiectasis.

Upper zone fibrosis, which can occur due to previous *Mycobacterium tuberculosis* infection, sarcoidosis and rarely in ankylosing spondylitis (less than 2%), can result in volume loss, resulting in tracheal deviation and elevation of the hila. The radiological changes associated with the different parenchymal lung diseases are discussed in Chapter 7.

In asthma, there may be hyperinflation of the lungs (Figure 4.18). In severe COPD, the CXR will show emphysematous lungs (Figure 4.19) and signs of hyperinflation. The CXR may appear normal in early bronchiectasis but with advanced disease the bronchi may appear dilated. A high-resolution computed tomography (HRCT) will be necessary to appreciate these changes. This is discussed in Chapter 12.

A pleural effusion (Figure 4.20) appears as an area of opacification in the lung, often with a meniscus. A small pleural effusion will result in the blunting of the costophrenic angle. A large pleural effusion will cause tracheal deviation and mediastinal shift away from the effusion. Pleural diseases are discussed in Chapter 11.

Box 4.2 CXR appearances with collapse of lobes.

- **Right upper lobe collapse**: elevation of the right hilum and the horizontal fissure (Figure 4.9). If collapse is due to a mass, then there will be the 'Golden S' sign
- **Right middle lobe collapse**: blurring of the right heart border (Figure 4.10). A lateral CXR will show the oblique and horizontal fissures coming together anteriorly to form a wedge (Figure 4.11)
- **Right lower lobe collapse**: blurring of the right hemidiaphragm and increased area of density behind the right heart shadow, with a shift of the heart to the right, and downward movement of the right hilum (Figure 4.12), A lateral CXR shows increased opacification in the posterior portion of the lower spine
- **Left upper lobe collapse**: the collapsed upper lobe moves forward and upwards, pulling the left lower lobe upwards and behind it (Figure 4.13). This appears as a veil within the left hemithorax without any sharp margins (Figure 4.14)
- **Left lower lobe collapse**: a triangular area of increased density behind the heart shadow, shift of the heart shadow to the left, blurring of the left hemidiaphragm, and increased transradiency of the left hemithorax because of compensatory expansion of the left upper lobe (Figure 4.15). This is called the sail sign

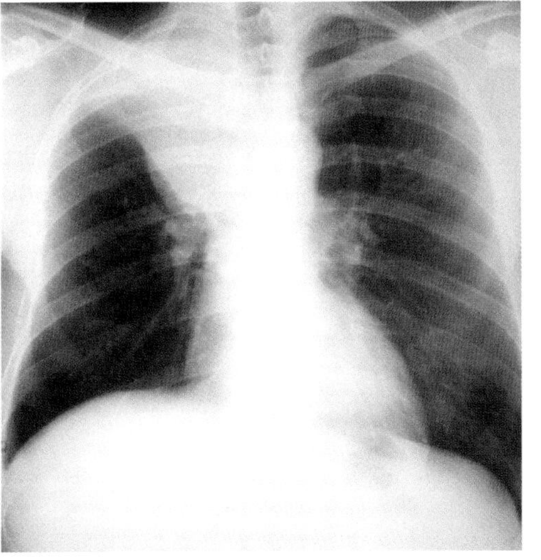

Figure 4.9 CXR showing right upper lobe collapse.

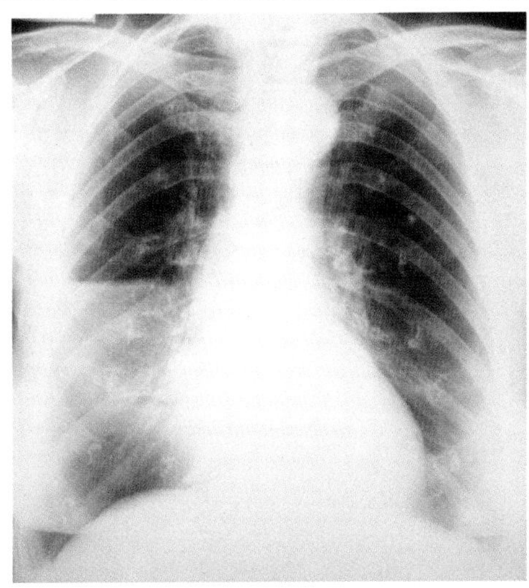

Figure 4.10 CXR (PA) showing right middle lobe collapse.

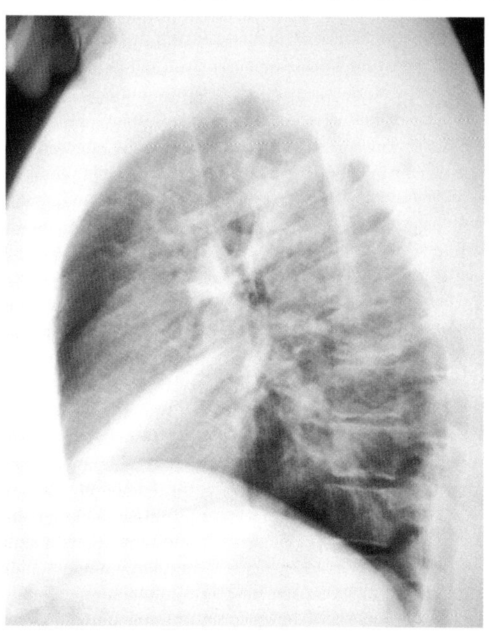

Figure 4.11 CXR (lateral) showing right middle lobe collapse.

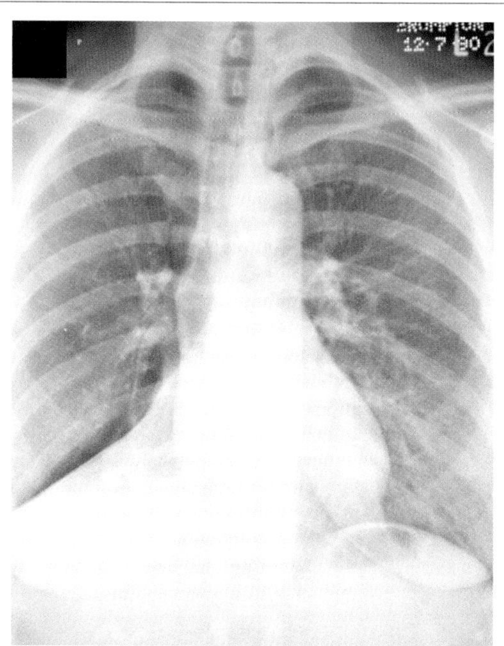

Figure 4.12 CXR (PA) showing right lower lobe collapse.

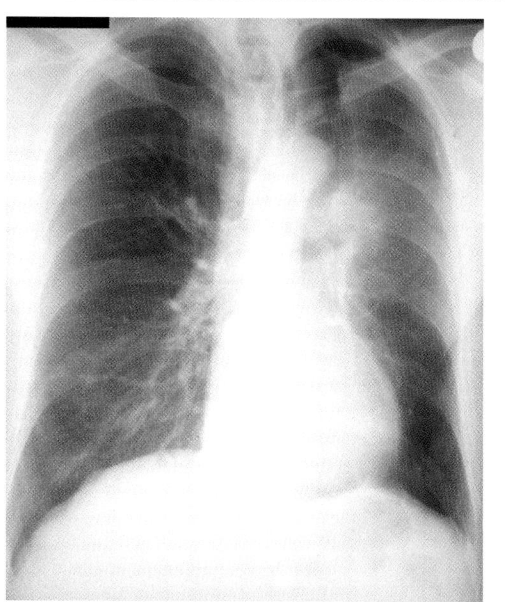

Figure 4.13 CXR (PA) showing left upper lobe collapse.

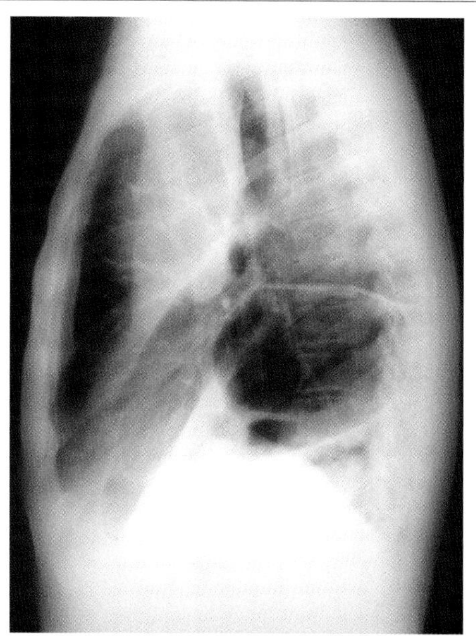

Figure 4.14 CXR (lateral) showing left upper lobe collapse.

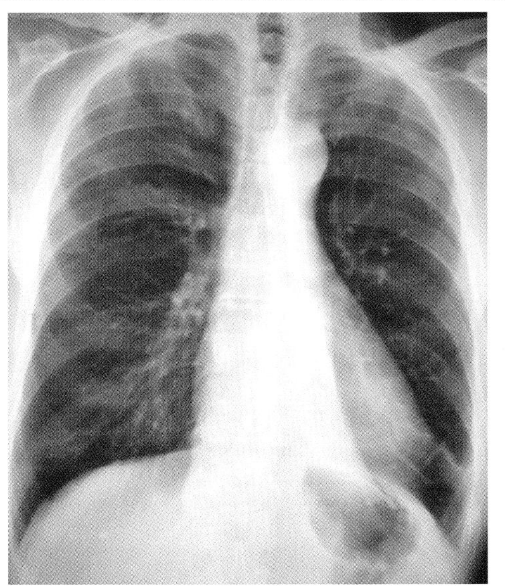

Figure 4.15 CXR showing left lower lobe collapse.

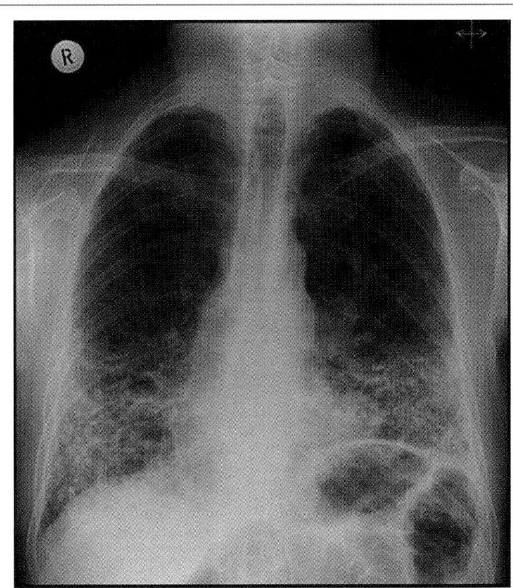

Figure 4.17 CXR showing idiopathic pulmonary fibrosis.

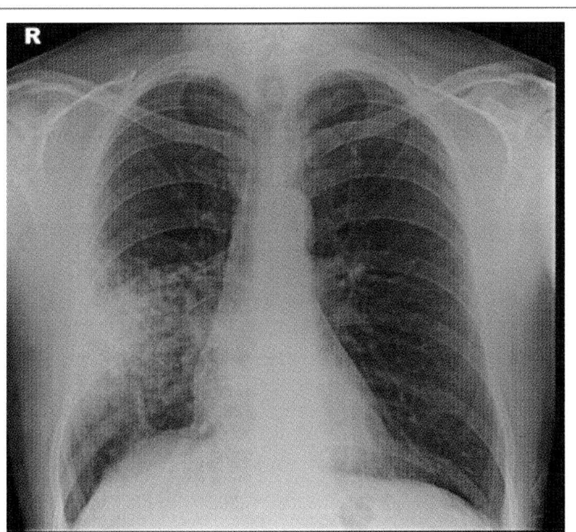

Figure 4.16 CXR showing right mid-zone consolidation.

CXR will also detect elevation of the diaphragm (Figure 4.21), although further imaging with CT and ultrasound will be required to determine the reason for this. CXR can show anterior and posterior mediastinal masses, although a CT will be required to show the structures in detail. The differential diagnosis, investigation, and management of mediastinal masses are discussed in Chapter 16.

A computed tomography scan (CT scan) is more sensitive and specific than a CXR and is required to see the structures of the thoracic cavity in detail (Figure 4.22). Iodine-containing contrast is given which will show as bright white when it fills the blood vessels. A CT of the thorax and abdomen is essential for the initial staging of lung cancer and when investigating pleural diseases (Figure 4.23, Figure 4.24). Spiral images are taken contiguously, and modern CT scanners can take images of the entire lung within 3–5 seconds. Modern scanners can detect nodules 3–4 mm in size. Low-dose chest CT will expose the patient to a lower dose of radiation, which is important in those who require regular CT scans to monitor pulmonary nodules or monitor the response to treatments. The contraindications for using iodine include renal failure, allergy to iodine or to previous contrast. The CT images associated with the different conditions are depicted in each chapter discussing various lung diseases.

A CT pulmonary angiogram (CTPA) is the main investigation for suspected pulmonary embolus. Images of the pulmonary arteries are seen and can detect central and segmental pulmonary emboli with good sensitivity and specificity (Figure 4.25). The iodine-containing contrast appears as bright white within the blood vessels and pulmonary

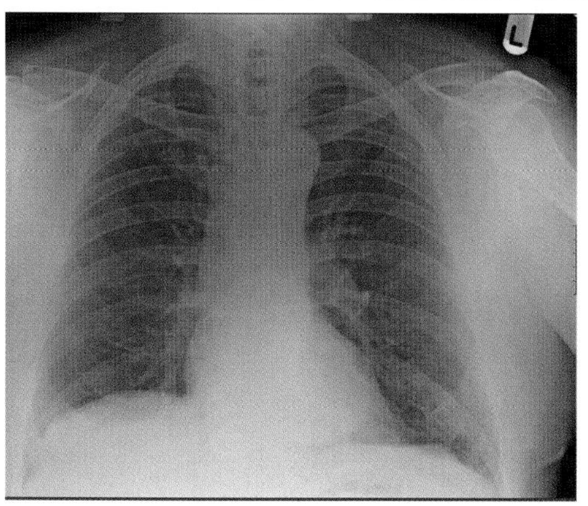

Figure 4.18 CXR showing hyperinflated lungs in asthma.

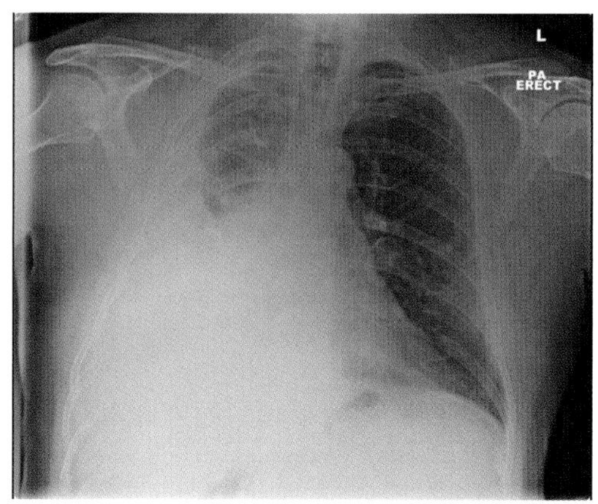

Figure 4.20 CXR showing a right-sided pleural effusion.

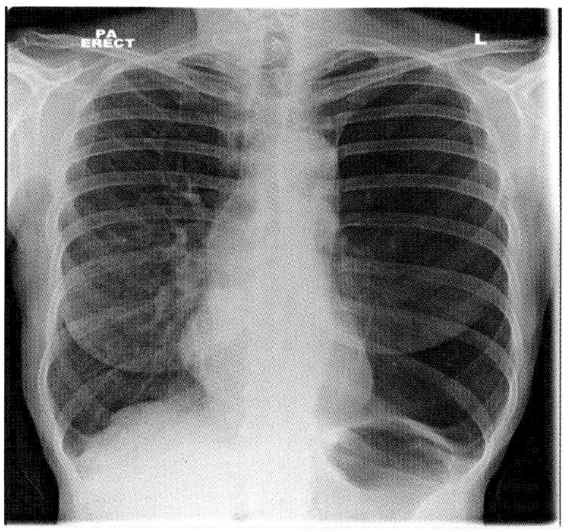

Figure 4.19 CXR showing emphysematous lungs in COPD.

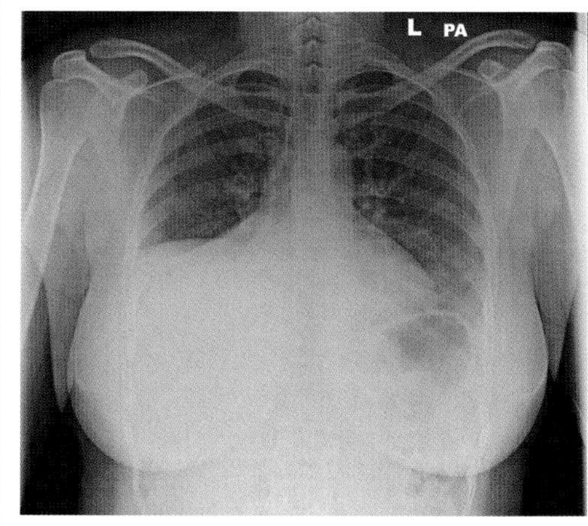

Figure 4.21 CXR showing elevation of the right hemidiaphragm.

emboli will appear as dark 'filling' defects. CTPA has replaced conventional pulmonary angiography as the investigation of choice in most patients with suspected pulmonary embolus (PE). The guidelines recommend avoiding CTPA in pregnant and young women, if possible. The investigation of PE is discussed in Chapter 13.

High-resolution CT (HRCT) takes images of the parenchyma every 10 mm, and is essential in the diagnosis of parenchymal lung diseases which are discussed in Chapter 7 (Figure 4.26). When the patient is prone, better images of the lung bases posteriorly are obtained. HRCT is also useful in diagnosing bronchiectasis and emphysema (Chapter 6), lymphangitis carcinomatosis (Chapter 9) and bronchiolitis obliterans.

A **positron emission tomography (PET) scan** is essential in the accurate staging of lung cancer. 18 fluoro-2-deoxy-glucose, which is an analogue of glucose, is injected and is taken up by rapidly metabolising cells, including cancer cells, which release positrons which are detected by a gamma camera. Dual PET/CT scans can correlate the FDG-avid areas with the anatomy. PET is good at detecting distant metastases, especially to adrenal glands and bone.

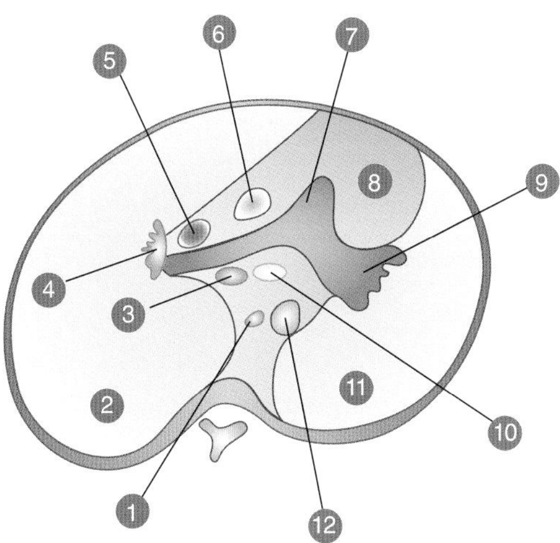

Figure 4.22 Diagram of normal CT thorax with labels of the structures.

A PET report states the FDG-avidity of the mass, nodules and lymph nodes which is expressed as SUVmax (Figure 4.27). The sensitivity of PET for lung cancer is 80% and the specificity is 97%. A PET scan cannot be done on patients with poorly controlled diabetes mellitus and elevated blood glucose levels.

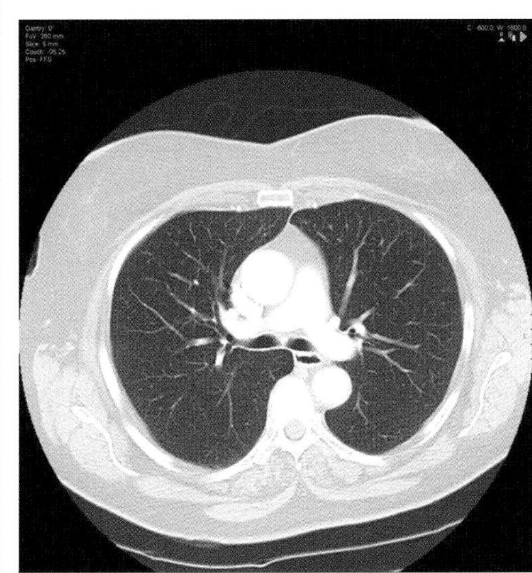

Figure 4.23 Normal CT thorax (lung windows).

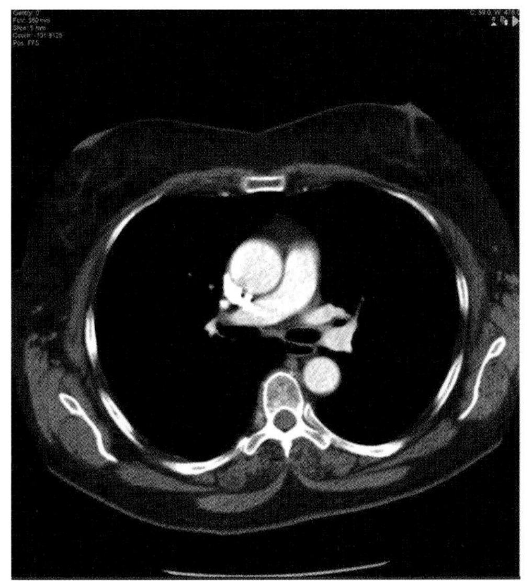

Figure 4.24 Normal CT thorax (mediastinal windows).

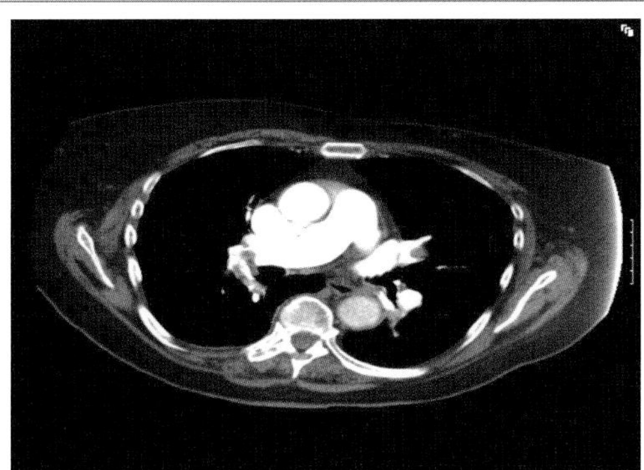

Figure 4.25 CTPA showing bilateral filling defects in multiple pulmonary emboli.

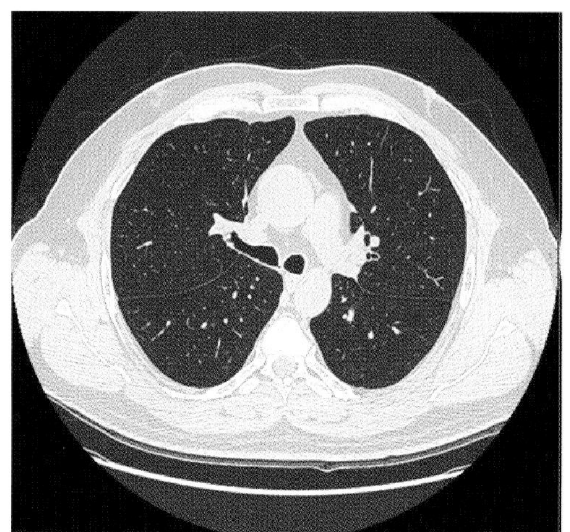

Figure 4.26 HRCT of normal lung.

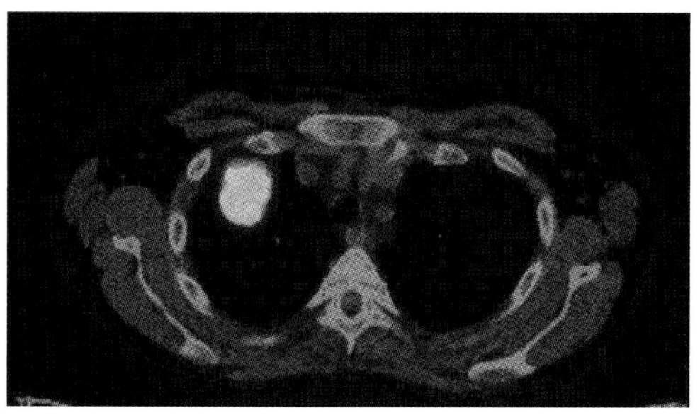

Figure 4.27 PET scan showing FDG-avid lesion in lung cancer.

A PET scan is an essential diagnostic test in the diagnosis and management of solitary pulmonary nodules and lymphadenopathy. It is not sensitive for nodules less than 8 mm. The heart and brain are metabolically active organs, so PET cannot reliably detect brain metastases. Carcinoid tumours, bronchoalveolar cell carcinoma (now called adenocarcinoma in situ), and some slowly-growing tumours may not be FDG-avid, so the results must be interpreted together with the clinical presentation and the results of all other investigations.

A **bone scan** is another nuclear medicine test which can detect bone metastases, osteomyelitis, and other bone disease, and is less expensive than a PET scan. Technetium-99m-methylene diphosphonate (MDP) is injected and the gamma rays emitted are detected.

A **ventilation perfusion (VQ) scan** is used to investigate acute and chronic pulmonary emboli (Figure 4.28). It has less sensitivity and specificity than CTPA, and many VQ scans are reported as 'indeterminate' but is the imaging of choice for women less than 40 years of age with suspected PE and for pregnant women. Perfusion-only scans can be done which will reduce the amount of radiation exposure. VQ scanning is also used for the investigation of chronic PE. The patient inhales a radioactively labelled inert gas (usually Xenon or technetium) to assess ventilation and then a radiolabelled contrast is injected to measure perfusion. If the patient has lung disease, such as COPD, then there will be 'matched defects' as areas of the lungs will be under-ventilated, and blood will be diverted away from these areas because of hypoxic vasoconstriction. If there are pulmonary emboli present, then there will be 'unmatched defects', with normal ventilation but no perfusion. Chapter 11 has images of VQ scans in PE. Quantitative VQ scans can also be used prior to lung resection to assess regional lung function and to estimate the amount of residual lung function.

A **thoracic ultrasound** is a simple, safe, non-invasive, and quick procedure which can be done at the bedside (Figure 4.29). It is particularly used for the investigation and management of pleural disease. It can show a pleural effusion, detect features of loculation and stranding, and is used to guide pleural aspiration and the insertion of a chest drain. Thoracic ultrasound can also be used to biopsy the pleura or a large lung mass. Diaphragmatic paralysis can be diagnosed by seeing the paradoxical upward movement of the diaphragm during inspiration. This, together with muscle studies, is used in the investigation of diaphragmatic palsy. Ultrasound of the liver may be indicated when liver metastases are suspected and can also be used to take a liver biopsy, which may be the way to make a histological diagnosis in some patients with poor lung function who cannot have a lung biopsy.

Magnetic resonance imaging (MRI) is a safe investigation as it does not expose the patient to radiation, but many find it difficult as it can be noisy and claustrophobic. MRI is contraindicated in those with a pacemaker or metal implants. MRI is good at giving anatomical clarity to some soft

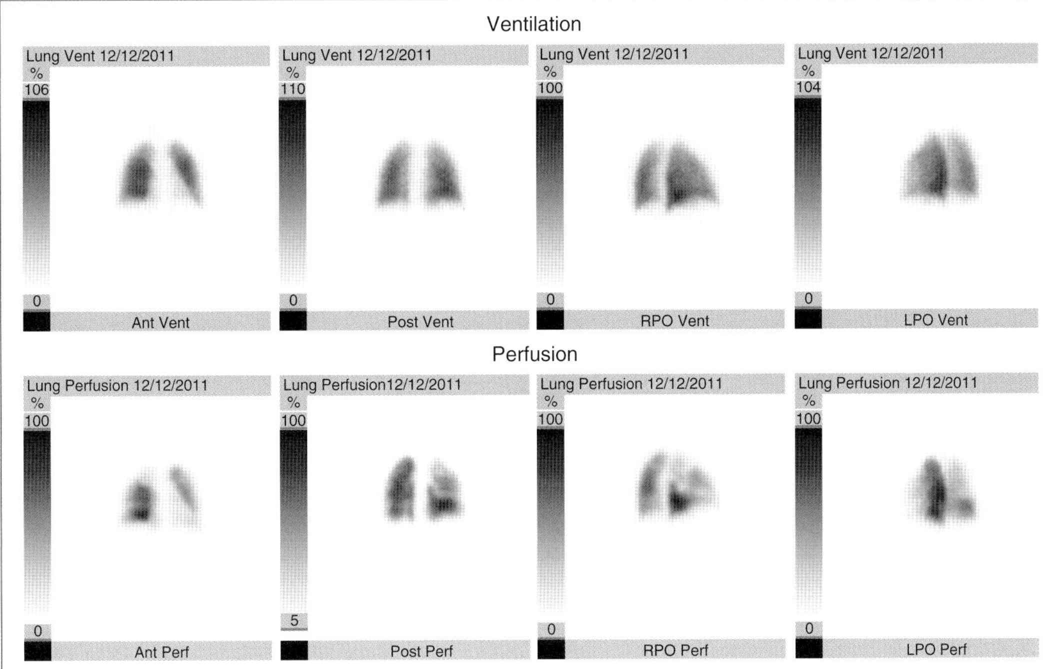

Figure 4.28 VQ scan showing perfusion defects consistent with pulmonary emboli.

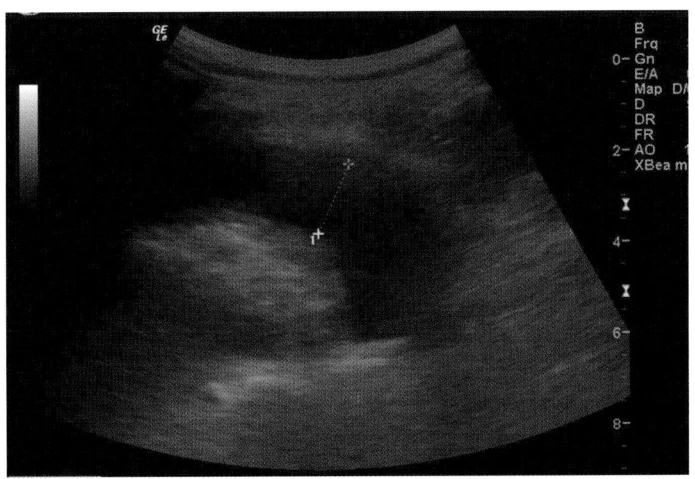

Figure 4.29 Thoracic ultrasound scan of a pleural effusion.

tissue structures, and to see if there is involvement of the chest wall with tumours. MRI can give useful information if thoracic surgery is being contemplated. MRI is the investigation of choice for suspected spinal cord compression.

Lung function tests

Lung function tests, which measure airflow, lung volumes, and gas exchange, are essential in the diagnosis and management of respiratory diseases. An individual's lung function will depend on their sex, ethnicity, age, height, and weight. The values obtained are compared to the predictive normal values which have been obtained from a large cohort of individuals and expressed as a percentage. The patient must be shown how to carry out the manoeuvre and the test should be repeated a few times to ensure reproducibility. The results of the lung function must be interpreted carefully together with information gleaned from the history, clinical examination, and radiology.

Dynamic lung volumes are easily measured in the outpatient setting and include peak expiratory flow (PEF), forced expiratory volume (FEV), forced vital capacity (FVC), and relaxed vital capacity (RVC). Patients should be advised to stop taking any inhalers for the duration of the action of the medication, for example, salbutamol for 4 hours and salmeterol for 12 hours. Patients should be asked to avoid smoking for at least 24 hours, not drink alcohol for at least 4 hours, not undertake vigorous exercise for at least 30 minutes and not consume any caffeine for at least 12 hours prior to the procedure. Other medication taken, for example, oral corticosteroids or theophylline, which will cause bronchodilation, should be noted.

The measurements should be made with the patient sitting on a high chair in non-restrictive clothing and with their dentures in, so long as these fit well. It is important to observe the patient during the manoeuvre to ensure that the technique is appropriate, that the mouthpiece is firmly held between the teeth and the lips, and that there is no air leak around the mouthpiece. The age, height, weight, and ethnicity of the patient are required to interpret the results from the available reference values. Values will be lower in the elderly.

Dynamic measurements are effort-dependent and can be manipulated by the patient. A low value will be obtained if the patient is weak, tired, or not motivated. A patient who conducts the manoeuvre by blowing against a closed glottis, or by coughing or spitting into the device, may get an artificially high reading.

Dynamic testing is contraindicated in those with haemoptysis, pneumothorax, severe hypertension, recent myocardial infarction, tachyarrhythmias, pulmonary embolus, aneurysms of thoracic or abdominal aorta, cerebral aneurysm, increased intraocular pressure, recent eye surgery or recent surgery to the abdomen or thorax.

A peak flow meter is a cheap, portable, and easy-to-use device (Figure 4.30) used to measure **peak expiratory flow (PEF)** in $L\,min^{-1}$, which is a measure of resistance to air flow through the larger airways. The patient is asked to take a full inspiration and then breathe out as hard and as fast as possible into the mouthpiece, with an open glottis, to measure the maximum flow rate. The PEF is reached within the first 100 milliseconds and is sustained for approximately 100 ms. This is demonstrated in the supplementary material.

The PEF will be reduced in those with obstructive airways disease, especially conditions

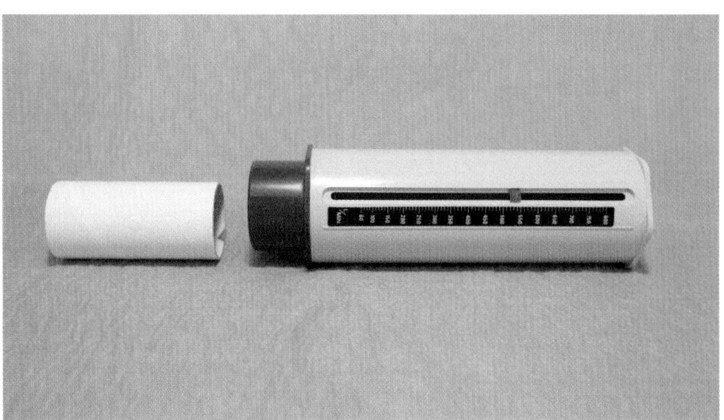

Figure 4.30 Peak flow meter.

that result in narrowing of the medium-sized and large airways such as asthma and COPD. As COPD is largely an irreversible condition, routine PEF monitoring is not usually recommended. Diurnal PEF monitoring is an important test in the diagnosis and monitoring of asthma, which is a reversible condition. In a patient suspected of having asthma, measurement of PEF in the morning and evening should be done over several weeks to see if there is a greater than 15% variability in readings, which is approximately 50 ml/L. The patient should also be given a peak flow diary card to document the readings and to write down the symptoms experienced. The normal diurnal variation is 8%. Figure 4.31 shows diurnal PEF measurements in an individual with poorly controlled asthma. PEF monitoring is essential in the self-management of asthma, guiding the patient as to when they may require oral corticosteroids or admission to hospital (see Chapter 6). PEF monitoring may be used to diagnose occupational asthma, which is discussed in Chapter 15.

PEF may also be reduced in diseases affecting the chest wall, such as neuromuscular diseases, kyphoscoliosis, and in conditions that affect the upper airways, such as tracheal tumour or a thyroid goitre. Therefore, PEF results cannot be interpreted on their own and spirometry testing is required.

Spirometry is cheap and easy to use in General Practice, in the outpatient department, and by the bedside. It is a measurement of the volume of air that can be exhaled during a forced expiration in one manoeuvre. The patient is asked to breathe in maximally to full inspiration and then exhale completely. The **forced expiratory volume in 1 second (FEV_1)** and the **forced vital capacity (FVC)** are measured and the FEV_1/FVC ratio is calculated (Table 4.1).

The FEV_1 is the volume of air that can be expired with forced expiration from maximal inspiration in the first second. The **vital capacity (VC)** is the total volume of air exhaled from maximal inspiration. It can be a forced exhalation with maximal effort (FVC) or a relaxed exhalation (RVC), and the best value can be used. Inspiratory vital capacity is the maximal volume of air inspired from full expiration. The recommendations for dynamic testing as described above should be adhered to. Sometimes a nose clip can be used if the patient has difficulty with the manoeuvre. As with PEF measurements, the best of three readings is taken.

FEV_1 and FVC are reproducible and the normal ranges for age, sex, height, and weight are well defined. As well as giving the numbers, most modern spirometers will give a print-out of the graph which should be examined as the shape of the

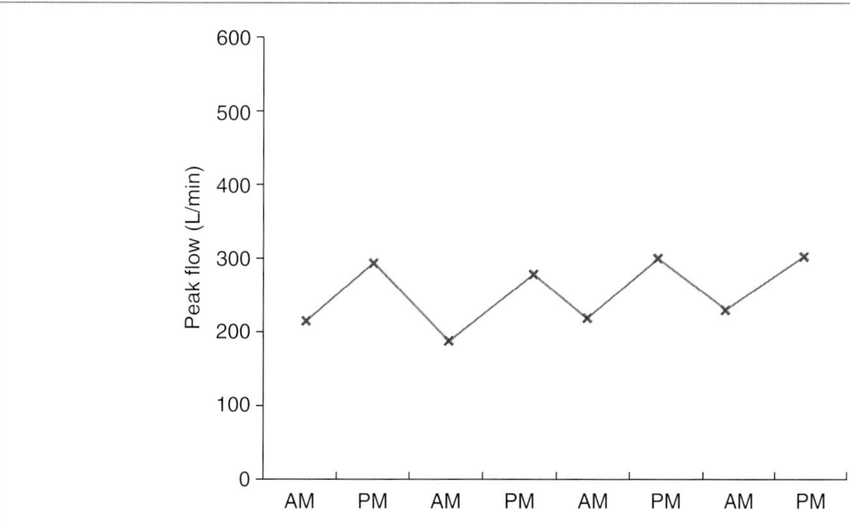

Figure 4.31 Peak flow readings showing diurnal variation.

Table 4.1 Interpretation of full lung function test.

Condition	FEV_1	FVC	FEV_1/FVC	TLC	TLCO	KCO
Asthma	↓↓	↔/↓	↓<0.7	↑	↔/↑	↑
Emphysema	↓↓	↓	↓<0.7	↑	↓↓	↓↓
Intra-pulmonary restrictive diseases	↓	↓↓	↔/↑	↓	↓↓	↔/↓
Extra-pulmonary restrictive diseases	↓	↓↓	↔/↑	↓	↓	↑

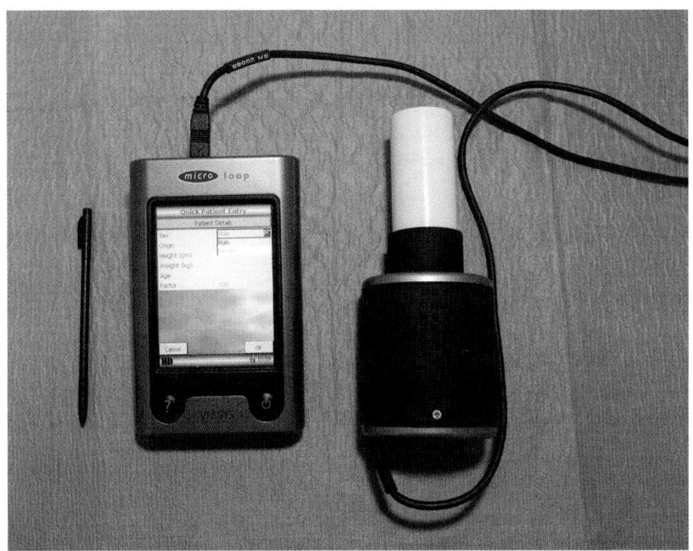

Figure 4.32 Handheld spirometer.

curve will vary according to the underlying condition (Figure 4.32).

In a healthy individual, the FVC and RVC are equal and should be exhaled within 4–6 seconds, with at least 70% of the air being expelled in the first second (FEV_1), so that the normal FEV_1/FVC ratio is 0.75–0.85 (75–85%). FEV_1 and FVC peak in adults in the third decade then decline by 30 ml/year. The FEV_1/FVC ratio may be less than 75% in the elderly with normal lungs.

The FEV_1/FVC ratio will distinguish between obstructive and restrictive lung disease, although further tests will be required to confirm the exact diagnosis. The values determine the severity and prognosis of the condition and can be used to monitor response to treatment. In obstructive conditions, such as asthma or COPD, when there is narrowing of the large and medium-sized airways, the FEV_1 (as with PEF) will be reduced. As air trapping occurs during forced expiration, FVC will be less than RVC and these patients may take up to 15 seconds to expel all the air. As FEV_1 is reduced more than FVC, the ratio of FEV_1/FVC is less than 0.7. Narrowing of the smaller, peripheral airways in bronchiectasis and bronchiolitis obliterans will result in a reduction

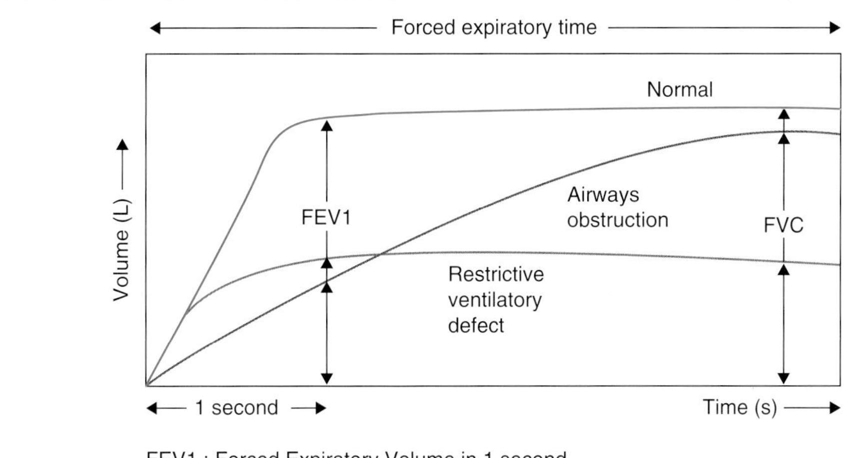

Figure 4.33 Spirometry in a normal individual and in obstructive and restrictive lung disease.

in airflow over the middle-half of expiration rather than the beginning of expiration. This is reported as PEF 25–75%.

In restrictive conditions, such as interstitial lung diseases, the FVC will be reduced because of decreased lung compliance. FEV_1 will also be reduced because there is less volume of air to expel, however, this is not reduced to the same extent as in an obstructive airways disease. Therefore, the FEV_1/FVC ratio will be normal or increased. Figure 4.33 shows spirometry findings in the normal individual and in those with airway obstruction and restriction.

VC will also be decreased in conditions affecting the chest wall, such as kyphoscoliosis and ankylosing spondylitis, and in conditions causing diaphragmatic or inspiratory muscle weakness, such as myopathies and myasthenia gravis. Measurement of static lung volumes is required to differentiate between parenchymal diseases and chest wall diseases causing restriction.

Bronchodilator reversibility testing of peak flow and spirometry should be done to differentiate between reversible and irreversible obstruction. Most laboratories will do this only if the initial spirometry or peak flow suggest obstruction. Some 200 mcg of salbutamol is inhaled, and the measurement taken 20 minutes later. The guidelines vary slightly in their diagnostic criteria for asthma. The Association for Respiratory Technology and Physiology/British Thoracic Society (ARTP/BTS) guidelines recommend a 160 ml increase in FEV_1 or 330 ml increase in VC, the European Respiratory Society (ERS) recommends a greater than 10% or 200 ml increase in predicted FEV_1 and the American Thoracic Society (ATS) recommends a 12% or 200 ml increase in baseline FEV_1 and FVC. A 15%, or 200 ml, increase in FEV_1 or FVC suggests some reversibility and a 20% or 400 ml increase after bronchodilator is convincing evidence of reversibility. Lack of reversibility does not rule out asthma but may suggest the need for a provocation test. Exercise can induce bronchoconstriction in a hyper-responsive patient, with a 15% reduction in PEF and FEV_1 post exercise. In individuals with diaphragmatic weakness, the supine VC will be 30% less than the erect VC as the contents of the abdomen push up against the diaphragm in the supine position.

The shape of the **flow-volume loop** can differentiate between extra-thoracic and intra-thoracic obstruction when there is narrowing of the upper airways. Flow is more effort-dependent at high lung volumes, so narrowing here will have the greatest effect on maximum expiratory flows. The volume of air inspired and expired is plotted against time. The starting point of full inspiration is to the left of the diagram, the expiratory flow appears above the horizontal line, and inspiratory flow below the line. At total lung capacity (TLC), the airways are most dilated and airway resistance is minimised, so the maximum peak expiratory flow is reached quickly after the start of the forced expiration.

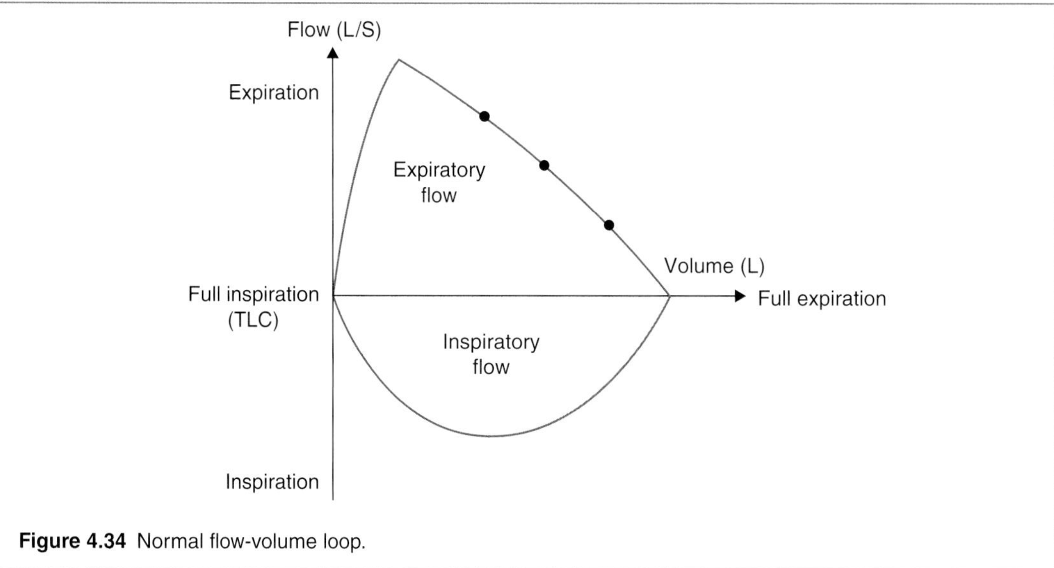

Figure 4.34 Normal flow-volume loop.

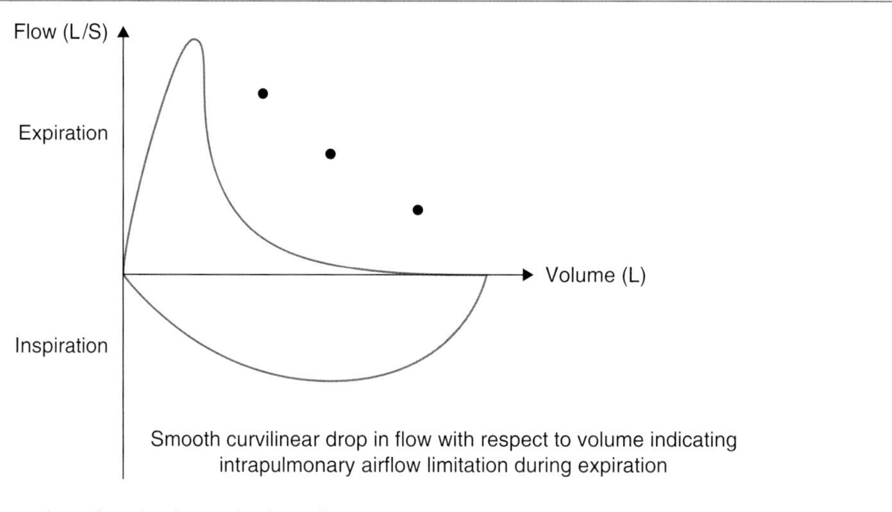

Figure 4.35 Flow-volume loop in obstructive lung disease.

As expiration continues, lung volumes progressively diminish, and airway resistance increases. The maximum flow achievable declines when no further air can be exhaled, and the flow reaches zero. At this point the loop reaches the horizontal axis. The inspiratory manoeuvre is more effort-dependent and less reproducible than the expiratory part, so the maximum inspiratory flow is less than the maximum expiratory flow. Figure 4.34 shows a normal flow-volume loop.

Figure 4.35 shows the flow-volume loop in obstruction; there is airflow limitation during expiration, but the inspiratory part is normal. Figure 4.36 shows the flow-volume loop in a restrictive condition where the inspiratory limb is abnormal. Figure 4.37 shows the flow-volume loop with mixed lung disease, for example, a patient with severe COPD and pulmonary fibrosis.

If there is extra-thoracic obstruction, for example, compression of the trachea by a goitre in the neck, then there is decapitation of the expiratory part of the loop with limitation of the inspiratory limb caused by tracheal narrowing during inspiration (Figure 4.38).

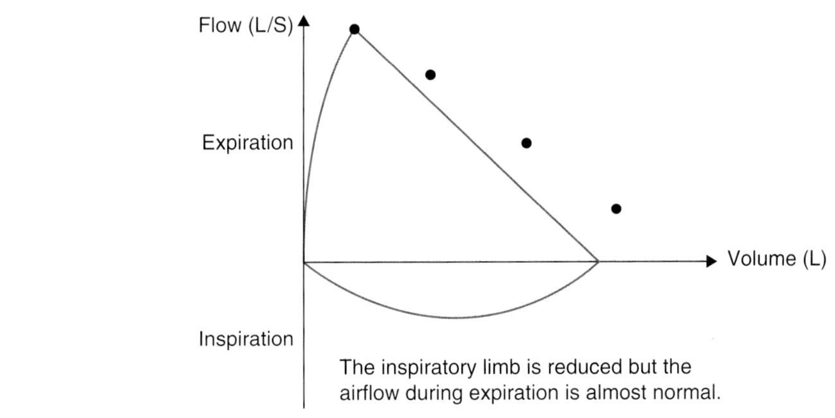

Figure 4.36 Flow-volume loop in restrictive lung disease.

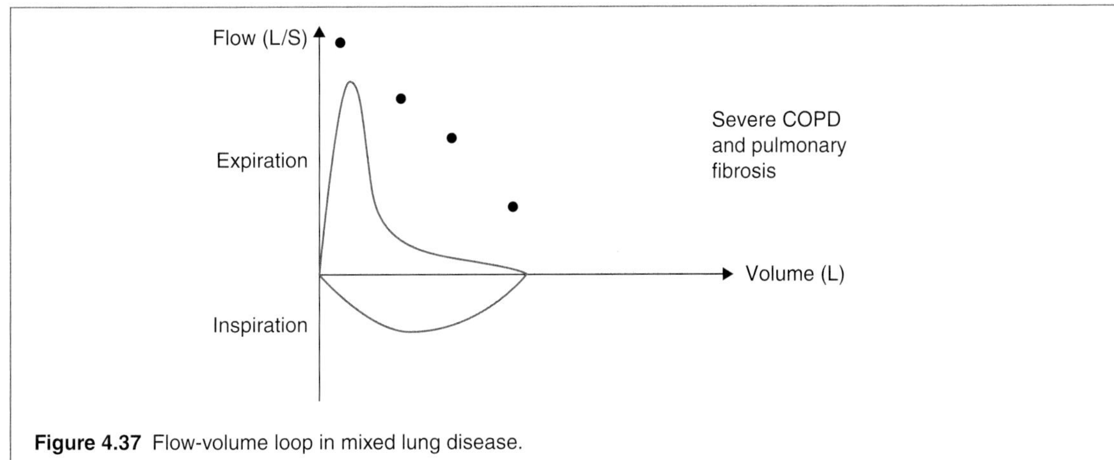

Figure 4.37 Flow-volume loop in mixed lung disease.

If the large airway obstruction is intra-thoracic, for example, a tracheal stricture, then there will be decapitation of the expiratory limb of the loop but minimal reduction in the intra-thoracic limb (Figure 4.39).

A fixed large airway obstruction can occur when there is tracheal stenosis caused by a tracheal tumour or previous intubation. The flow-volume shows flattening of both the inspiratory and expiratory limbs (Figure 4.40).

Static (absolute) lung volumes are required to make an accurate diagnosis, especially in those who have restriction on spirometry (Figure 4.41). The **total lung capacity (TLC)** is the total volume of air in the lungs after full inspiration, the **functional residual capacity (FRC)** is the volume of air left in the lungs at the end of normal tidal expiration and the **residual volume (RV)** is the amount of air left in the lungs after maximum expiration. The **vital capacity (VC)** is the volume of air expelled by full expiration after full inspiration. The **tidal volume (TV)** is the volume of air that enters and leaves the lungs during normal breathing.

Static lung volumes are measured in a Lung Function Laboratory using the helium dilution method or the whole-body plethysmography method. In the helium dilution technique, air with a known concentration of helium is breathed through a closed circuit and the volume of gas in the lungs is calculated from a measure of the dilution of the helium. Helium is an inert gas which is not absorbed or metabolised. The gas dilution method only measures gas in communication with the airways and underestimates TLC in patients

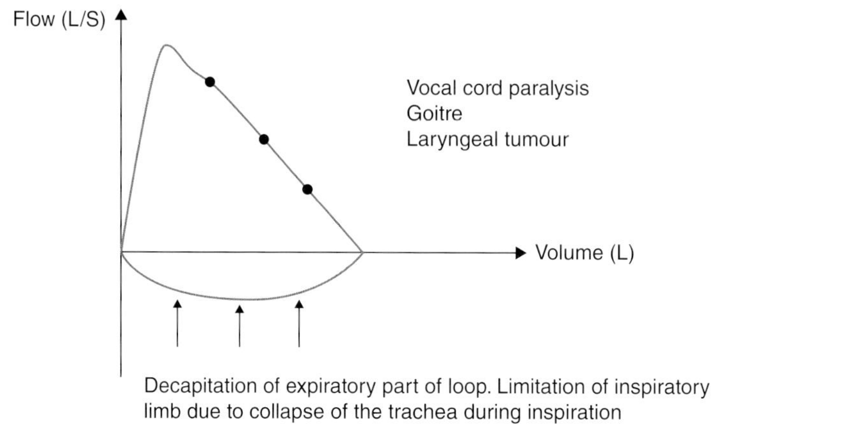

Figure 4.38 Flow-volume loop in variable extra-thoracic upper airway obstruction.

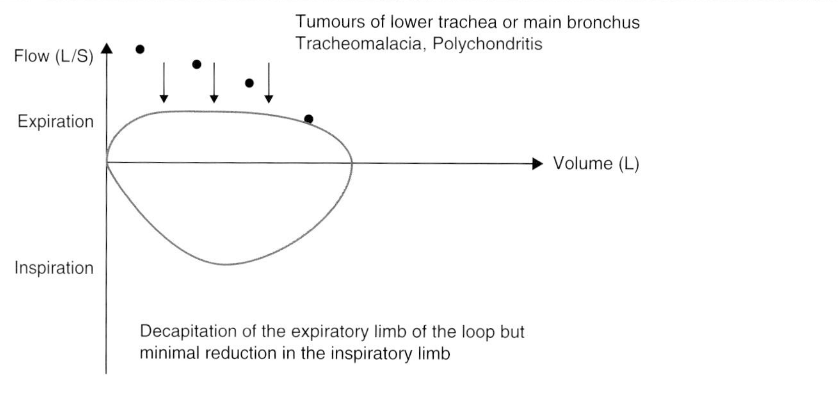

Figure 4.39 Flow-volume loop in variable intra-thoracic obstruction.

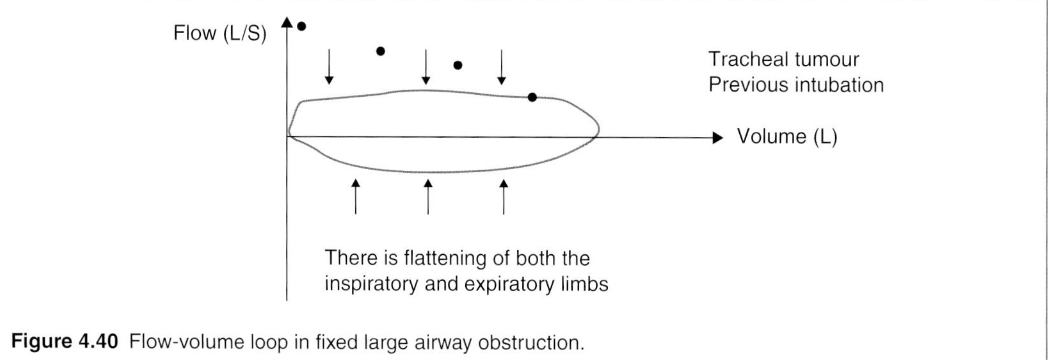

Figure 4.40 Flow-volume loop in fixed large airway obstruction.

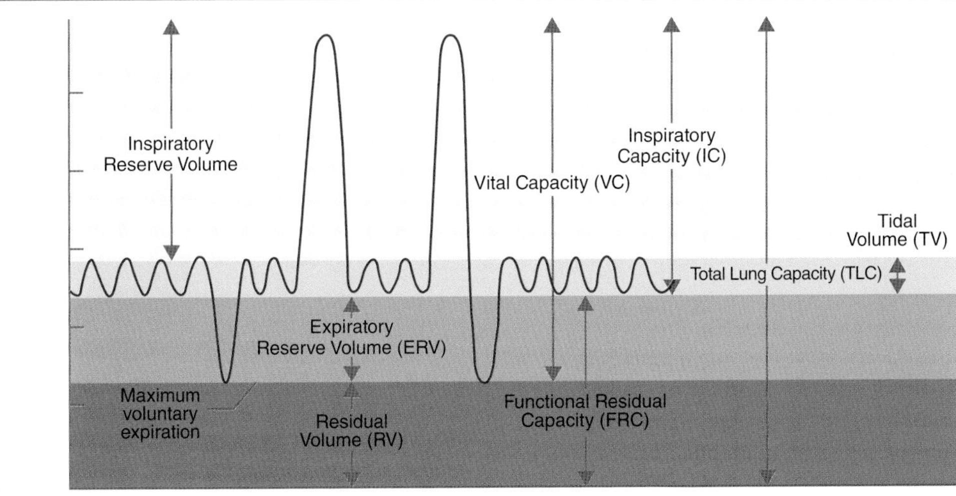

Figure 4.41 Static lung volumes: Total Lung Capacity (TLC), Expiratory Reserve Volume (ERV), Residual Volume (RV), Vital Capacity (VC), Functional Residual Capacity (FRC), Inspiratory Capacity (IC), Tidal Volume (TV).

with severe airway obstruction because of poorly ventilating bullae or those with cystic lung disease.

The whole-body plethysmography test uses a large airtight body box that allows the simultaneous determination of pressure-volume relationship in the thorax of a patient placed inside this box. When the plethysmograph is sealed, changes in lung volume are reflected by a change in pressure within the plethysmograph. Plethysmography tends to overestimate TLC because it measures all intra-thoracic gas, including gas in bullae, cysts, stomach, and oesophagus. The values obtained by either method are compared with the predicted values of individuals of the same age, sex, ethnicity, height, and weight and given as a percentage predicted.

TLC will be reduced in any intrapulmonary or extra-pulmonary restrictive disorder and increased in conditions that result in air-trapping. FRC will also be increased in conditions that cause airway obstruction, such as COPD. RV and FRC can distinguish between different types of restrictive conditions. Both RV and FRC will be decreased in parenchymal lung diseases whereas RV will be reduced but FRC will be normal in conditions causing respiratory muscle weakness and obesity.

A single-breath method is used to measure the **transfer coefficient factor for carbon monoxide (TLCO)**, also called the **diffusing capacity**, which is an estimate of the amount of CO which diffuses across the alveolar-capillary membrane. A very low concentration of CO is used as a surrogate for O_2. To measure TLCO we need to know the amount of CO transferred across/minute and the pressure gradient across the alveolar membrane. TLCO is a sensitive but not specific measurement.

The patient is asked to breathe in a mixture of helium and CO, then hold their breath for 10 seconds and then exhale completely. The volume of gas equivalent to the dead space (approximately 1500 ml) is discarded. The remaining sample is analysed for concentrations of helium and CO. Helium is not absorbed or metabolised as it is an inert gas. Therefore, the change in concentration of helium between the inspired and expired samples is the amount of gas dilution and is used to estimate the **alveolar gas volume (VA)**. The expired concentration of CO is lower than the inspired level as some of the CO is absorbed into the bloodstream. The rate of uptake of CO is calculated as the uptake/minute/unit of partial pressure of CO (mmol min^{-1} kPa^{-1}).

The **transfer coefficient (KCO)** is the transfer factor per unit alveolar volume (VA) and is also measured using the single breath-hold technique. TLCO = KCO/VA and is corrected for haemoglobin. KCO measures the transfer of CO in the alveoli that are ventilated. The non-ventilated alveoli are not measured as they do not contribute to the alveolar gas volume (VA).

TLCO is reduced by conditions which result in ventilation/perfusion mismatch. This includes conditions which impede blood flow, such as a pulmonary embolus, conditions that reduce the alveolar surface area, for example, bullous emphysema, and diseases that impede transport of oxygen across the capillary membrane as occurs in parenchymal lung diseases. KCO too will be decreased with these intrinsic lung diseases.

TLCO is also reduced by conditions which result in a reduction in the volume of healthy lung available to participate in gas transfer, for example, respiratory muscle weakness causing restriction, chest wall deformity, such as kyphoscoliosis, obesity and after a pneumonectomy. Unlike TLCO, KCO is not diminished by extrathoracic restrictive conditions and may be elevated as KCO only measures the transfer of CO in ventilated alveoli which have more than their normal share of blood as blood is diverted away from the non-ventilated alveoli. The greater blood volume increases CO absorption and gas transfer.

TLCO increases when the pulmonary capillary blood volume increases, for example, with a high cardiac output state, with polycythaemia, and pulmonary haemorrhage.

Respiratory muscle function tests are used to measure weakness of the respiratory muscles which can cause a restrictive ventilatory defect with decreased TLC and VC. In diaphragmatic palsy, the pressure of the abdominal contents pushing up against the weak diaphragm results in a 30% fall in VC when supine compared to the erect position. Two small balloon-tipped catheters, one measuring the oesophageal pressure and the other the gastric pressure, are inserted to measure the differences in pressure. Generalised respiratory muscle function may be assessed by measuring mouth pressures. Maximum inspiratory mouth pressure, Pi max, is measured during maximum inspiratory effort from a residual volume against an obstructed airway using a mouthpiece and transducer device. Maximum expiratory mouth pressure, Pe max, is measured during maximum expiratory effort from TLC.

Methacholine provocation testing can be used to measure the degree of airway responsiveness and is recommended in those who are suspected of having asthma but who have normal spirometry with no significant bronchodilator response. It is particularly useful in those with cough-variant asthma. The patient should be instructed to stop oral corticosteroids, theophylline, and inhaled medications for a few days before the procedure is undertaken. A baseline spirometry is done, then a small dose of methacholine is inhaled, and spirometry repeated. The dose of methacholine should be gradually increased and serial spirometry carried out. The concentration of methacholine required to provoke a 20% fall in FEV_1 is calculated. If this is less than 32 mg, then asthma is confirmed. This investigation is usually done in Respiratory Units and closely supervised, with bronchodilators available, as there is a risk of severe bronchoconstriction. Histamine can be used instead of methacholine.

Measurement of fractional **exhaled nitric oxide (FeNO)**, a marker of airway inflammation, is recommended by NICE in the diagnosis of asthma. It is a quick, simple, and non-invasive test, but the results must be used in conjunction with the results of other investigations. A negative test does not exclude asthma.

Exercise testing

Exercise (walking) tests are used to determine the severity, response to treatment, and prognosis in patients with chronic respiratory diseases, including COPD, pulmonary hypertension, diffuse parenchymal lung diseases, and in chronic heart failure. The procedure must be standardised, with clear instructions to each patient.

Exercise tests are an important part of the assessment of functional status and required in those who are being considered for lung transplantation, heart and lung transplantation, or lung volume reduction surgery. These measurements are often the primary end-point in trials looking at the efficacy of treatments in these conditions. Exercise testing is contraindicated in those who have had a recent myocardial infarction, those with severe angina, and those with uncontrolled hypertension.

The **six-minute walk test (SMWT)** is easy to do, safe and well tolerated, even in patients who have limited exercise tolerance. The patient is asked to walk along a straight line on a hard surface, on his/her own and the distance walked in six minutes is measured. The oxygen saturation and extent of breathlessness should be determined. The SMWT correlates well with pulmonary function tests, quality of life measures, and mortality. This is demonstrated in the supplementary material.

The **shuttle walk test (SWT)** requires the patient to walk back and forth between two markers set 10 metres apart in response to a pre-set timer. The timer beeps to indicate when the patient should have reached the marker. The interval between beeps will gradually decrease until the patient is unable to keep up. Both the SWT and the SMWT will improve with inhaled therapy for COPD and with pulmonary rehabilitation. Oxygen saturation should be measured at rest and during the SMWT and the SWT. The oxygen saturation correlates with disease severity and can be used to monitor the progression of the disease and any improvement with treatment.

Cardiopulmonary exercise testing is an important investigation in the assessment of patients with breathlessness, and is used to determine disease severity. The ventilatory reserve can be measured by examining the relationship between peak exercise ventilation (VE) and the maximal voluntary ventilation (MVV). It is not within the scope of this textbook to discuss this in any further detail.

Sleep studies

Several investigations are available for patients presenting with sleep disordered breathing. The simplest is an **overnight oximetry** when an oximeter probe is placed on the patient's finger overnight. A drop of 4% or more in the oxygen saturation is abnormal and the number of these desaturations every hour can be measured. More than 15 desaturations per hour is diagnostic of obstructive sleep apnoea, although the exact criteria vary from laboratory to laboratory.

Polysomnography is more sensitive and specific and involves overnight measurement of oxygen saturation, thoracic and abdominal movement, snoring, pulse, and blood pressure. This can be done in the patient's home using a portable device. Full polysomnography is indicated if a more complex sleep disorder, such as restless leg or central sleep apnoea, is suspected. This is conducted in a sleep laboratory and involves measuring the stages of sleep using an electroencephalograph (EEG). During normal sleep, 25% of the activity will be rapid eye movement (REM) sleep and the rest is non-rapid eye movement sleep (NREM). Muscle activity and eye movements are measured using an electromyogram (EMG) and electro-oculogram (EOG) and are important in the diagnosis of restless leg syndrome and other sleep-related disorders which are discussed in Chapter 14.

The **multiple sleep latency test (MSLT)** is used to determine the degree of daytime somnolence and is important in the diagnosis and management of narcolepsy and idiopathic hypersomnia (IH). The patient is placed in a dark room during daytime and asked to lie down to sleep. A normal individual will take 10–20 minutes to fall asleep, whereas an individual with narcolepsy or IH will fall asleep in less than 8 minutes. Once the individual falls asleep, he/she should we woken up after 15 minutes. The patient will have five scheduled naps during the day, each separated by two hours.

Cardiology investigations

An **electrocardiogram (ECG)** is an important basic investigation in patients presenting with chest pain, breathlessness, and syncope. Patients with these symptoms are often referred to the respiratory clinic. Cardiac causes, including ischaemic heart disease, hypertensive disease, valvular heart disease, and arrhythmias must be excluded. The ECG will be abnormal in those presenting with pulmonary embolus, with the commonest finding being sinus tachycardia. ECG features of right heart strain, right bundle branch block, right axis deviation and S1Q3T3 are also indicative of pulmonary embolus, which is discussed in Chapter 11. The ECG will be abnormal in patients with pulmonary hypertension and cor pulmonale.

An **echocardiogram** measures the structure and function of the left and right side of the heart, the structure of the pulmonary arteries, the structure and function of the valves, and the pericardium. Patients with pulmonary hypertension will have a raised pulmonary artery pressure (PAP), estimated by measuring the tricuspid regurgitant wave, and right ventricular hypertrophy. Pulmonary hypertension is discussed in Chapter 11.

Invasive investigations

A **nose and throat examination (nasendoscopy)** is carried out for the investigation of a chronic cough. It is safe and easy to do, has little morbidity and can be done without sedation using local anaesthetic. This can be used to directly visualise the nasal passages to look for evidence of infection, crusting, abnormal nasal pathology, and nasal polyps. The oropharynx can be examined for evidence of candida, acid reflux and cobblestoning. Nasendoscopy can also be used to look at the movement of the vocal cords and diagnose vocal cord palsy and vocal cord dysfunction,

A **bronchoscopy** is an invasive test that is essential in the diagnosis, treatment and management of lung malignancies, infections, and interstitial lung diseases. Flexible fibre-optic bronchoscopy is done as a day case. It is safe in most patients, with a low complication rate. It is conducted under sedation (intravenous midazolam) and local anaesthetic (lignocaine), with careful monitoring of the pulse rate and oxygen saturation. It is used to examine the appearances of the nasal passages, oropharynx, epiglottis, and vocal cords. After instillation of adequate lignocaine to the vocal cords, the trachea, carina and right and left bronchial trees can be directly visualised to the fourth and fifth divisions of the endobronchial tree. Vocal cord palsy, tumours of the vocal cord, tracheal tumours, tracheomalacia, and endobronchial tumours can be seen at bronchoscopy.

Biopsies and brushings can be taken from the area of abnormality. Significant bleeding can occur when biopsies are taken, especially from abnormal tissue, so the clotting and platelet count should be checked prior to taking biopsies. The position of the tumour can give information about the operability of the tumour. Bronchoscopy is also indicated for the removal of a foreign body, more common in small children who may inhale it. Samples of bronchoalveolar lavage (BAL) taken at bronchoscopy are commonly used in the investigation of lung cancer and lower respiratory tract infections. Cytology from lavage and brushings, and histology from endobronchial biopsies are used to diagnose lung cancer, including bronchoalveolar cell carcinoma (adenocarcinoma *in situ*) and carcinoid tumour of the lung. Microbiological analysis is used to diagnose respiratory tract infections, including MTB, and pneumocystis jerovici, particularly when sputum is not available. The differential cell count in the lavage fluid can be helpful in the diagnosis of several respiratory diseases, including asthma, COPD, sarcoidosis, and interstitial lung diseases. Transbronchial biopsy is used in the diagnosis of diffuse parenchymal lung disease, including sarcoidosis, and is discussed in Chapter 7.

Therapeutic suctioning at bronchoscopy clears increased volumes of mucopurulent or purulent secretions and allows better aeration of the lungs. Transbronchial lymph node aspiration (TBNA) and endobronchial ultrasound-guided biopsy (EBUS) of lymph nodes are minimally invasive tests which are now widely available to obtain biopsies from enlarged hilar, mediastinal, and subcarinal lymph nodes which may be enlarged due to malignancy (including lymphoma), MTB, or sarcoidosis.

When there is significant narrowing of the bronchus with tumour or granulation tissue, laser or cryotherapy can be used to reduce the narrowing, at least temporarily. This is a palliative procedure in patients with lung cancer and can improve breathlessness. In some cases, an endobronchial stent can be inserted to improve ventilation of the airways. Endobronchial radiotherapy can also be used. A rigid bronchoscopy conducted under general anaesthetic may be required for more complicated procedures, especially if there is a significant risk of bleeding or airway compromise. Thoracic surgical back-up should be available.

Peripheral lung nodules and masses can be sampled by fine needle aspiration (FNA) under CT or ultrasound guidance (Figure 4.42). Lymph nodes outside the thoracic cavity, for example, in the supraclavicular fossa, can also be sampled, either by FNA or Trucut biopsy, which give larger samples for histological analysis. In the diagnosis of lung cancer, it may be easier to biopsy other areas of abnormality, such as liver, bone, or subcutaneous nodules.

If pleural disease is suspected, then aspiration of pleural fluid under thoracic ultrasound is undertaken and fluid sent for cytology, microbiology, and biochemistry. This is discussed in greater detail in Chapter 10. Chest drain will be required for drainage of large pleural effusions and a chemical pleurodesis can be carried out in those with recurrent malignant pleural effusions who are not fit for

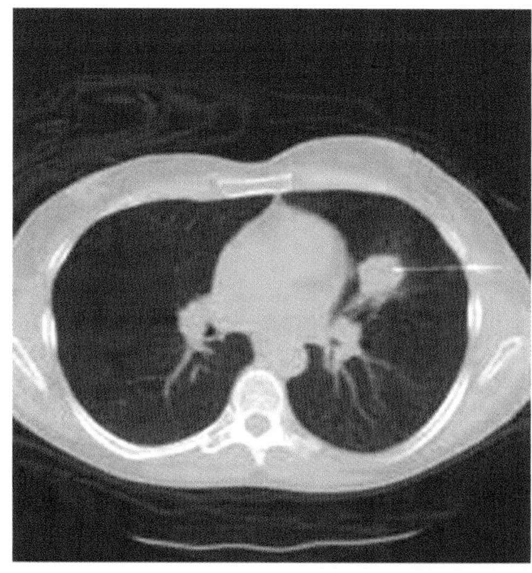

Figure 4.42 CT-guided FNA of lung mass with needle in pulmonary lesion.

a surgical pleurodesis. A pleural biopsy can also be conducted under CT guidance when a pleural malignancy is suspected.

Medical thoracoscopy can be done under intravenous sedation and the pleural space can be examined for evidence of malignancy, biopsies taken, and pleurodesis carried out. For those with pleural disease, a video-assisted thoracoscopic surgery (VATS) is often the investigation of choice but will require a general anaesthetic and will be carried out by the thoracic surgeon. The pleural cavity can be directly visualised, biopsies taken, and surgical pleurodesis carried out. The VATS procedure can be used to take lung biopsies, perform wedge resection, and lobectomy. A full thoracotomy will be needed for a pneumonectomy. The thoracic surgeon can also sample mediastinal lymph nodes at mediastinoscopy.

A right heart catheter is used to measure the right heart pressure in patients with pulmonary hypertension and to monitor the effect of the treatments for pulmonary hypertension. Other invasive procedures include the insertion of a stent for superior vena cava obstruction, emergency cricothyroidectomy for upper airway obstruction, tracheostomy for those requiring long term invasive ventilation, and surgical embolectomy for patients with massive pulmonary embolus who do not respond to thrombolysis or in whom thrombolysis is contraindicated.

Miscellaneous investigations

A variety of genetic tests, including prenatal testing, are available for the diagnosis of cystic fibrosis, primary ciliary dyskinesia, and α-1 antitrypsin deficiency. HLA B27 testing may be positive in patients with ankylosing spondylitis.

SUMMARY OF LEARNING POINTS

- A variety of investigations are available to aid the diagnosis of patients presenting with respiratory symptoms and signs.
- Many of the blood tests are non-specific but can rule out other causes of the symptoms; for example, anaemia can contribute to breathlessness.
- Radiological investigations are essential in the diagnosis of respiratory diseases.
- The CXR is the commonest radiological investigation worldwide and can be helpful in many conditions, including pneumonia and lung cancer.
- CT thorax gives information about the main structures in the thorax and mediastinum, including masses and lymph nodes, and is an essential investigation in the diagnosis of lung cancer, pleural disease, and mediastinal tumours. A CT-guided biopsy can be done to take samples from tumours and the pleura.
- The CTPA will detect acute pulmonary emboli by visualising the pulmonary arteries up to the segmental arteries.
- The HRCT is necessary in diagnosing parenchymal lung diseases, including pulmonary fibrosis and sarcoidosis.
- The VQ scan is less specific and sensitive than a CTPA for diagnosing pulmonary emboli but is indicated in young women and pregnant women as it exposes them to less radiation. It is also the investigation of choice if chronic pulmonary emboli are suspected.
- The PET scan uses ^{18}fluoro-deoxyglucose, a glucose analogue, which is taken up by rapidly metabolising cells. It is essential in the staging of lung cancers and other malignancies. It can detect local and distant metastases but is not good at detecting brain metastases.
- Thoracic ultrasound is a non-invasive investigation used in the investigation of pleural disease and to guide the insertion of a needle for pleural aspiration, pleural biopsy and for chest drain insertion.
- An MRI scan of the thorax is important in the diagnosis of mediastinal masses and chest wall disease, including invasion by tumour, spinal cord compression and brain metastases.
- Lung function tests are essential in the diagnosis of many respiratory diseases, in determining the prognosis and in monitoring progression and response to treatment. This includes peak expiratory flow measurement, spirometry and measurement of static lung volumes; total lung capacity, residual volume, and functional residual capacity.

- Measurements of transfer coefficient and the transfer factor are essential in approximating the diffusion of oxygen through the capillary membrane from the alveolus and can differentiate between parenchymal and extra-thoracic causes of a restrictive lung disease.
- Sleep studies are used to diagnose sleep-related disorders, which include obstructive sleep apnoea, central sleep apnoea, periodic limb disorders, narcolepsy, and idiopathic hypersomnia. This includes overnight oximetry, overnight sleep study, polysomnography and multiple sleep latency test.
- Exercise testing is important in assessing the functional status of a patient with respiratory disease. This includes the six-minute walk test and the shuttle test. It gives prognostic information, is used to monitor response to treatment and is the primary end-point in many trials in respiratory disease.
- An ECG is important in diagnosing cardiac conditions, including ischaemic heart disease, arrhythmias, and right heart strain which can occur after a pulmonary embolus and with pulmonary hypertension.
- An echocardiogram is important in the diagnosis and management of pulmonary hypertension and in the assessment of the severity of a pulmonary embolus.
- Bronchoscopy is an important investigation in the diagnosis of lung cancer, respiratory infections and interstitial lung diseases. Histology can be taken at biopsy, cytology by bronchial brushings and bronchoalveolar lavage. Samples from lavage can also be sent for microbiological analysis and for differential cell count.
- Pleural procedures include simple ultrasound-guided pleural aspiration, pleural drainage, medical thoracoscopy, and video-assisted thoracoscopic procedures used to visualise the pleura, take biopsies, and to carry out pleurodesis.

MULTIPLE CHOICE QUESTIONS

4.1 Which of the following is NOT associated with lung cancer?

A Hypercalcaemia
B Hyponatraemia
C Raised CRP
D Raised d-dimer
E Raised IgE

Answer: E

All the above can be found with lung cancer apart from IgE which will be raised in allergic conditions, including asthma and ABPA.

4.2 Which of the following investigations is most likely to yield a diagnosis in a patient presenting with a malignant pleural effusion?

A Bronchoalveolar lavage
B Pleural fluid cytology
C Transbronchial biopsy
D Tumour markers
E VATS pleural biopsy

Answer: E

A VATS pleural biopsy allows for direct visualisation of the pleura and biopsies can be taken for histology. Pleural fluid cytology may be diagnostic, but not in most cases. Histology is always preferable to cytology. The other investigations are not indicated for a pleural effusion, although bronchoalveolar lavage and transbronchial biopsy may be helpful if there is an endobronchial lesion. Tumour markers are not helpful in making the diagnosis.

4.3 What are the CXR features of right upper lobe collapse?

A Blurring of the right heart border
B Blurring of the right hemidiaphragm
C Depression of the right hilum
D Elevation of the horizontal fissure
E Elevation of the right hemidiaphragm

Answer: D

When the right upper lobe collapses, the rest of the right lung is shifted upwards. This means that the horizontal fissure, which divides the right upper and middle lobes, and the right hilum are elevated. Blurring of the right heart border is found with right middle lobe collapse and blurring of the right hemidiaphragm is seen with right lower lobe collapse.

4.4 **Which of the following conditions is NOT associated with a cavitating mass on CXR?**

A Bronchoalveolar cell carcinoma (adenocarcinoma *in situ*)
B Lung abscess
C *Mycobacterium tuberculosis* infection
D Squamous cell carcinoma
E *Staphylococcus aureus* pneumonia

Answer: A

Bronchoalveolar cell carcinoma looks consolidative, with patchy, white shadowing. All the other conditions listed are in the differential diagnosis for a cavitating lesion. Other conditions that result in a cavitating mass include vasculitic conditions and pulmonary infarct.

4.5 **Which of the following statements about a PET scan is true?**

A Contraindicated in a patient with chronic renal failure
B Contraindicated in a patient who is allergic to seafood
C Excellent at detecting brain metastases
D Sensitivity for lung cancer is 99%
E Specificity for lung cancer is 97%

Answer: E

Positron emission tomography (PET) uses ^{18}fluoro-deoxy glucose and not iodine-containing contrast. This radioactive glucose analogue is taken up by rapidly metabolising cells, including cancer cells. Slow-growing tumours, such as carcinoid or bronchoalveolar cell tumour (adenocarcinoma *in situ*) may not be PET-avid. PET cannot reliably detect metastases in metabolically active organs like the brain and heart. The sensitivity of PET in detecting lung cancer is 80% and the specificity is 97%.

4.6 **Which of the following statements about ventilation/perfusion (VQ) scanning is true?**

A Many VQ scans are reported as indeterminate
B Matched defects suggest chronic pulmonary emboli
C It is more sensitive at detecting acute pulmonary emboli than CTPA
D It should be avoided in pregnant women
E It is the investigation of choice in COPD

Answer: A

Many VQ scans are reported as indeterminate so that further imaging with CTPA is often required, as it is less sensitive than CTPA. Matched defects are found when there is reduced ventilation and therefore perfusion, for example, in COPD. VQ scanning is therefore not indicated in chronic lung diseases. A VQ scan is the investigation of choice for a pregnant woman suspected of having a pulmonary embolus as this exposes her and the foetus to less radiation than a CTPA. A perfusion scan alone can be considered in this group.

4.7 **Which of the following combination of findings is consistent with emphysema?**

A ↓FEV_1, ↓TLC and ↑TLCO
B ↓FEV_1, ↑TLC and ↓TLCO
C ↓FEV_1, ↑TLC and ↑TLCO
D ↑FEV_1, ↓TLC and ↓TLCO
E ↑FEV_1, ↓TLC and ↑TLCO

Answer: B.

Emphysema is an obstructive airways disease and therefore FEV_1 will be reduced. As there is air-trapping and there will be bullae, the total lung capacity will be increased. The transfer coefficient (TLCO) will be reduced as the alveolar-capillary interface is destroyed.

4.8 **The following combination of findings in lung function testing suggest which of these conditions? ↓FVC, normal FEV_1/FVC ratio, ↓TLCO and ↑KCO.**

A Asthma
B Bronchiectasis
C COPD
D Obesity
E Pulmonary fibrosis

Answer: D

The decreased FVC rules out asthma, bronchiectasis, and COPD which are obstructive conditions. In any parenchymal lung disease, the FEV_1/FVC ratio may be normal or increased, but the TLCO and KCO will be reduced. In extrathoracic conditions, such as obesity, neuromuscular diseases and musculoskeletal diseases the TLCO will be reduced but the KCO will be increased.

4.9 Which of the following investigations is most likely to confirm a diagnosis of diaphragmatic palsy?

A Arterial blood gas measurement
B CT thorax and abdomen
C Lateral CXR
D Lying and standing vital capacity
E Shuttle walk

Answer: D

Individuals with unilateral diaphragmatic palsy may be relatively asymptomatic except when supine or underwater, for example, swimming or in a bath, because of the pressure of the abdominal contents pushing up against the weak diaphragm. ABG will be normal. The CXR and CT thorax will show elevation of the hemidiaphragm but this, by itself, is not diagnostic of diaphragmatic palsy. A reduction by 20% in the VC when supine suggests diaphragmatic palsy. Diaphragmatic muscle studies will then confirm this.

4.10 A multiple sleep latency test (MLST) is used to diagnose which condition?

A Central sleep apnoea
B Insomnia
C Narcolepsy
D Obstructive sleep apnoea
E Periodic limb movement

Answer: C

MSLT, which measures how quickly someone falls asleep during the daytime, is used to diagnose narcolepsy and idiopathic hypersomnia. A sleep study is required to diagnose OSA and a full polysomnography with EEG and EMG monitoring is required to diagnose central sleep apnoea and periodic limb movement.

FURTHER READING

Albert, R.K., Spiro, S.G., and Jett, J.R. (1999). *Comprehensive Respiratory Medicine*. London: Mosby.

American Thoracic Society (ATS), Crapo, R.O., Casaburi, R. et al. (2002). ATS statement: guidelines for the six-minute walk test. *American Journal of Respiratory and Critical Care Medicine* 166 (1): 111–117.

American Thoracic Society and American College of Chest Physicians (2003). ATS/ACCP statement on cardiopulmonary exercise testing. *American Journal of Respiratory and Critical Care Medicine* 167 (2): 211–277.

British Thoracic Society and the Association of Respiratory Technicians and Physiologists (1994). Guidelines for the measurement of respiratory function: recommendations of the British Thoracic Society and the Association of Respiratory Technicians and Physiologists. *Respiratory Medicine* 88 (3): 165–194.

Brown, C.D. and Wise, R.A. (2007). Field tests of exercise in COPD: the six-minute walk test and the shuttle walk test. *COPD: Journal of Chronic Obstructive Pulmonary Disease* 4 (3): 217–223.

Gibson, G.J. (2009). *Clinical Tests of Respiratory Function*, 3e. London: Hodder Arnold.

Hansell, D. (2003). Thoracic imaging. In: *Respiratory Medicine* (ed. G. Gibson, D. Geddes, U. Costabel, et al.), 316–351. London: W. B. Saunders.

Hansell, D.M. and Armstrong, P. (2005). *Imaging of the Diseases of the Chest*, 4e. Edinburgh: Elsevier Mosby.

Kinnear, W.J.M. (1997). *Lung Function Tests: A Guide to their Interpretation*. Nottingham: Nottingham University Press.

Lima, D.M., Colares, J.K.B., and Da Fonseca, B.A.L. (2003). Combined use of the polymerase chain reaction and detection of adenosine deaminase activity on pleural fluid improves the rate of diagnosis of pleural tuberculosis. *Chest* 124 (3): 909–914.

Newall, C., Evans, A., Lloyd, J. et al. (2000). *ARTP Spirometry Handbook*. Birmingham: Association for Respiratory Technology and Physiology.

Quanjer, P. (1983). Standardized lung function testing: report of Working Party. *Bulletin européen de physiopathologie respiratoire* 19 (Suppl 5): 45–51.

Smith, A.D., Cowan, J.O., Filsell, S. et al. (2004). Diagnosing asthma. *American Journal of Respiratory and Critical Care Medicine* 169 (4): 473–478.

Stradling, P. and Stradling, J.R. (1991). *Diagnostic Bronchoscopy: A Teaching Manual*, 6the. Edinburgh: Churchill Livingstone.

Villegas, M.V., Labrada, L.A., and Saravia, N.G. (2000). Evaluation of polymerase chain reaction, adenosine deaminase, and interferon? In pleural fluid for the differential diagnosis of pleural tuberculosis. *Chest* 118 (5): 1355–1364.

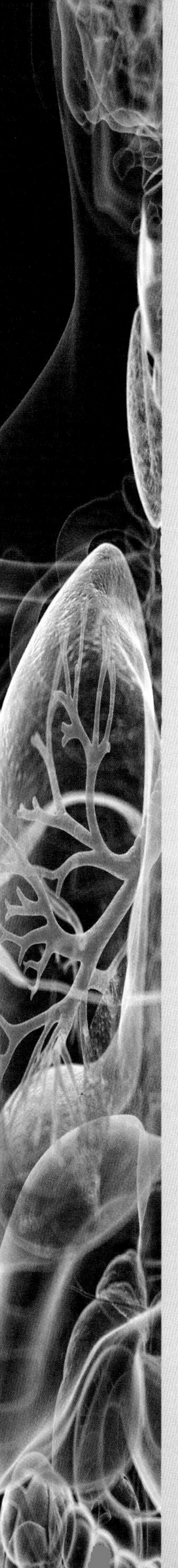

CHAPTER 5

Common presentations of respiratory disease

Learning objectives

- To understand how to take a comprehensive respiratory history
- To know how to carry out a respiratory examination
- To understand the differential diagnosis of breathlessness
- To recognise the differential diagnosis of pleuritic chest pain
- To learn about the differential diagnosis of cough
- To understand the differential diagnosis and management of haemoptysis
- To learn about the differential diagnosis and management of upper airways obstruction
- To understand how to conduct a pre-operative respiratory assessment
- To recognise the respiratory problems in a post-operative patient
- To know how to conduct a respiratory assessment of an acutely ill patient

Essential Respiratory Medicine, First Edition. Shanthi Paramothayan.

Companion website: www.wiley.com/go/paramothayan/essential_respiratory_medicine

Abbreviations

ABG	arterial blood gas
ACE	angiotensin converting enzyme
BiPAP	bilevel positive airways pressure
CO_2	carbon dioxide
COPD	chronic obstructive pulmonary disease
CPAP	continuous positive airways pressure
CT	computed tomography
CTPA	computed tomography pulmonary angiogram
CXR	chest X-ray
DVT	deep vein thrombosis
ECG	electrocardiogram
GORD	gastro-oesophageal reflux disease
HDU	high dependency unit
HIV	human immunodeficiency virus
HRCT	high-resolution computed tomography
ITU	intensive care unit
MRC	Medical Research Council
NIV	non-invasive ventilation
OSA	obstructive sleep apnoea
PE	pulmonary embolus
PND	paroxysmal nocturnal dyspnoea
SLE	systemic lupus erythematosus
TED	thromboembolic disease
TVF	tactile vocal fremitus
TVR	tactile vocal resonance
VQ	ventilation perfusion scan
VR	vocal resonance

Respiratory history

The aim of taking the respiratory history is to construct a sensible differential diagnosis. The clinical examination will then help to narrow the differential diagnosis and determine which investigations are required to confirm the suspected diagnosis in most cases.

Taking a detailed history in a fluent way is an important skill to learn and will improve with experience. While medical students are taught to take the history in a certain order, this is not critical so long as the history is comprehensive, and the relevant points are covered. A structured approach is, however, essential. Box 5.1 lists the important points to take in a patient presenting with respiratory symptoms or signs. This is demonstrated in the supplementary material (www.wiley.com/go/Paramothayan/Essential_Respiratory_Medicine).

Box 5.1 Important points in a respiratory history.

- Demographic information
- Presenting complaint or main symptom
- Associated symptoms
- History of presenting complaint
- Past medical history
- Smoking history
- Occupational history
- Recreational history
- History of atopy and allergy
- Family history
- Drug history
- Allergy to medication
- Systemic symptoms

Demographic information includes the age, sex, ethnicity, and country of origin of the patient. This is important as certain conditions are more prevalent in males or females, and several respiratory conditions are more common in people from certain countries and ethnic backgrounds.

It is important to elicit what the presenting complaint is, including the onset, nature, severity, and duration of the symptom. It is important to understand what factors exacerbate or relieve the symptom, whether the patient has suffered from this symptom before and if the cause was ever found. It is important to ask about associated respiratory symptoms and systemic symptoms, such as fever, malaise, night sweats, joint pains, rashes, and weight loss, as this information can lead to the correct diagnosis.

Past medical history is always relevant and should include a history of prematurity, immunisations, childhood illnesses, tuberculosis, and contact with anyone with *Mycobacterium tuberculosis*. A history of previous malignancies and cardiac problems is particularly important.

Smoking is a significant risk factor for several lung diseases, so a detailed history of smoking should be obtained. The number of pack years should be calculated as this can quantify the risk. Patients should be asked about exposure to passive smoking at home, at work, and in social situations. A comprehensive occupational history is important as exposure to industrial dusts, chemicals, asbestos, and silica can result in the development of pulmonary fibrosis, occupational asthma, and hypersensitivity pneumonitis. It may be necessary to ascertain the occupational history of the spouse if there is concern about mesothelioma. History of recent travel abroad may be relevant when the patient presents with symptoms of infection or eosinophilia.

Patients with atopy and allergy may present with symptoms of cough, breathlessness, and wheeze, and may also suffer with nasal symptoms. These patients may have a history of hay fever or eczema. Many people are allergic to a variety of inhaled allergens, for example, house dust mite, which can be demonstrated by doing a skin prick test. It is important to ask about their home environment, whether they have any pets and if their house is damp. Some patients who are exposed to bird 'bloom' can develop hypersensitivity pneumonitis, often called 'bird fancier's lung'.

A detailed drug history is essential as many drugs can have an adverse effect on the lungs in a variety of ways. This is discussed in Chapter 3. Radiotherapy to the thorax can result in fibrosis, either acutely or many years later. Patients should be specifically asked whether they take or have taken any recreational drugs or any over-the-counter medications.

Ascertaining information about the family history is important as certain respiratory conditions can be inherited, for example, cystic fibrosis, primary ciliary dyskinesia, and alpha 1-antitrypsin. The predisposition to develop lung cancer and asthma is also inherited.

In Box 5.2 the differential diagnosis of common respiratory symptoms is discussed.

Box 5.2 Common respiratory symptoms.

- Breathlessness
- Cough
- Haemoptysis
- Chest pain
- Wheezing
- Snoring

Breathlessness

Breathlessness is a common presentation with a wide differential diagnosis. **Dyspnoea** is the term for difficulty in breathing and **tachypnoea** means breathing at an increased respiratory rate. A normal respiratory rate at rest is between 12 and 16 breaths per minute but will, of course, increase with exertion. **Orthopnoea** describes difficulty with breathing when lying flat and may be secondary to cardiac failure, chronic obstructive pulmonary disease (COPD), obstructive sleep apnoea (OSA) or diaphragmatic palsy. **Paroxysmal nocturnal dyspnoea (PND)** describes the sudden onset of breathlessness, with the patient gasping, requiring them to sit upright in bed. This occurs most commonly with pulmonary oedema, but patients with severe OSA often report waking up gasping for breath. **Apnoea** means cessation of breathing for more than 10 seconds and may occur repeatedly in OSA. **Kussmaul breathing**, often described as 'air hunger', is deep and laboured breathing that occurs with severe metabolic acidosis, for example, diabetic ketoacidosis or chronic renal failure, when the respiratory centre is stimulated to blow off carbon dioxide as a compensatory mechanism. **Cheyne-Stokes respiration** occurs in patients with severe heart failure and in those with central sleep apnoea due to the oscillation in the level of carbon dioxide in the blood; there is a cyclical pattern of breathing, from hypoventilation, even apnoea, to hyperventilation.

The onset of breathlessness can be acute or chronic in nature. Table 5.1 lists some common causes of acute and chronic breathlessness.

When asking patients about their symptom of breathlessness, it is essential to establish whether this was acute or gradual in onset, whether it occurs at rest or on exertion. If it occurs on exertion, then it is important to find out how far they can walk and whether their breathlessness affects their activities of daily living. The severity of breathlessness can be graded using the Medical Research Council's Dyspnoea Grade (MRC Grade) which is described in Box 5.3. The BORG scale can also be used to grade perceived breathlessness, especially in the context of exercise testing. Other important points in the history include the overall duration of breathlessness, whether it is progressively getting worse, whether there is any diurnal variation, or if it is worse when lying down. Patients with

Table 5.1 Causes of breathlessness.

System	Acute onset (minutes to hours)	Sub-acute onset (hours to days)	Chronic onset (weeks to months)
Respiratory	Pulmonary embolus Pneumothorax Acute asthma Upper airway obstruction Foreign body inhalation Epiglottitis Anaphylaxis Hypersensitivity pneumonitis	Exacerbation of asthma Exacerbation of COPD Community acquired pneumonia Bronchiectasis Hypersensitivity pneumonitis Idiopathic pulmonary fibrosis Sarcoidosis Chronic pulmonary emboli	COPD Lung cancer Pleural effusion Idiopathic pulmonary fibrosis Sarcoidosis COPD Any interstitial lung disease Pulmonary hypertension Obstructive sleep apnoea
Cardiac	Pulmonary oedema Ruptured heart valves Myocardial infarction Arrhythmia Aortic dissection Cardiac tamponade	Left ventricular failure Congestive cardiac failure Pericardial effusion Arrhythmia	Congestive cardiac failure Cardiomyopathy
Neuromuscular	Guillain-Barré Botulism	Poliomyelitis Diaphragmatic palsy Myasthenia gravis	Diaphragmatic palsy Poliomyelitis Motor neurone disease Muscular dystrophies Multiple sclerosis Myasthenia gravis Amyotrophic lateral sclerosis

Musculoskeletal	Traumatic fracture Costochondritis	Chest wall disease Post-thoracic surgery	Chest wall disease Kyphosis Scoliosis Chest wall surgery (thoracoplasty)
Central nervous system	Acute stroke	Acute stroke	Parkinson's disease
Metabolic	Diabetic ketoacidosis Ethylene glycol poisoning Salicylate poisoning	Diabetic ketoacidosis Chronic renal failure Salicylate poisoning	Chronic renal failure
Endocrine	Thyrotoxicosis Phaeochromocytoma	Hypothyroidism	Large goitre
Haematology			Chronic anaemia
Psychological	Panic attack Hyperventilation	Anxiety	Chronic anxiety Phobias
Physiological	Strenuous exercise Acute mountain sickness Deep sea diving	Mountain sickness Pregnancy	Mountain sickness Obesity

Box 5.3 The MRC Dyspnoea grade.

1. No breathlessness except on strenuous exertion
2. Breathless when walking fast or uphill
3. Not able to keep up with contemporaries on level ground and needs to stop for breath
4. Stops for breath after 100 m or after a few minutes on level ground
5. Breathless at rest or on minimal exertion, such as dressing

diaphragmatic weakness will complain of breathlessness when lying flat and when under water, for example, swimming, as the abdominal contents push up on the diaphragm, reducing ventilation. Collateral history from a member of the family who has observed the patient can be very useful.

Management of severe breathlessness

Breathlessness can be life-threatening and anyone presenting with this will need immediate attention. The patient should be assessed quickly with regards to the airways and breathing, have their oxygen saturation and arterial blood gas measured, and commenced on the appropriate amount of oxygen through the correct device. If a respiratory arrest is imminent, then the anaesthetist should be called urgently with view to intubation. If intubation and ventilation are not necessary, the patient should have continuous monitoring of oxygen saturation, serial measurement of arterial blood gases, a chest X-ray, and an electrocardiogram (ECG). The management of type 1 and type 2 respiratory failure is discussed in Chapter 13.

Cough

Cough is a violent, forceful, protective reflex provoked by the stimulation of receptors in the larynx, trachea and bronchial tree to remove inhaled irritants, including secretions. Violent coughing can result in cough syncope due to reduction in venous return and cerebral perfusion.

Acute cough is a common presentation to General Practice, is often secondary to a respiratory infection and therefore self-limiting. When taking a history of cough from a patient, it is important to ask whether the cough is acute or chronic, dry or productive, the duration of the cough, whether the patient is a smoker, and whether the patient has any associated symptoms.

Box 5.4 Causes of dry cough in non-smoker with normal CXR.

- Cough-variant asthma
- Gastro-oesophageal reflux disease (GORD)
- Postnasal drip
- Allergy (includes hay fever)
- Post infection
- Medication (angiotensin converting enzyme (ACE) inhibitors)
- Dry mouth
- Foreign body
- Chronic throat clearing
- Psychogenic

Patients with a chronic cough, which affects 8% of the population, are often referred for a specialist opinion. Chronic cough (more than six weeks in duration) may be due to several different pathologies, for example, asthma, COPD, or lung cancer. In many cases, there are multiple causes for the cough. It is important to ask about the volume, content, and colour of any sputum produced as this can give clues as to the aetiology of the cough. Yellow or green sputum usually indicates a bacterial infection, persistently green and foul-smelling sputum may suggest bronchiectasis, and large volumes of watery sputum (bronchorrhoea) can occur in those with bronchoalveolar cell carcinoma (Adenocarcinoma in situ).

Patients who present acutely with a productive cough and other symptoms, such as breathlessness and fever, may have a more serious respiratory tract infection, such as community acquired pneumonia, and may require antibiotics. As well as a careful physical examination, they will need blood tests to check the inflammatory markers, and a chest X-ray (CXR) to see if there are any signs of consolidation. A sputum sample should be sent for microscopy, culture, and sensitivity and to look for *acid-alcohol-fast* bacilli. Patients with recurrent chest infections should have further investigations (see Chapters 6 and 8).

Box 5.4 lists the possible causes of a dry cough in a non-smoker with a normal CXR.

A careful history and examination should point to the most likely diagnosis. If cough-variant asthma is suspected, then a chest X-ray, spirometry, skin prick testing, peak flow homework, methacholine challenge, and high-resolution computed tomography (HRCT) may be required to exclude other pathology and to confirm the diagnosis. Treatment with inhaled steroids should result in the resolution of the cough. If GORD is suspected, then pH studies may be required, although many doctors will prescribe a trial of a proton pump inhibitor to see if there is improvement. If a post-nasal drip is felt to be the most likely cause, then a CT sinus may be helpful. Antihistamines and steroid nasal sprays given in the head-down position should improve the cough. If the likely cause of the cough is not clear, then a nose and throat examination may be helpful in determining whether there are any signs of acid reflux, infection, cobblestoning (which might indicate chronic throat clearing), nasal pathology, and to rule out a foreign body in the airways.

Post-infectious coughs are common and can persist for months. Treatment with oral or inhaled steroids for a minimum of two weeks can result in an improvement in symptoms. In cases of cough secondary to allergy, it is important to identify the triggers and remove them if possible. Antihistamines may also be helpful. Up to 20% of patients on an ACE inhibitor can develop a dry, irritating cough; this may not necessarily occur immediately after commencing the medication.

Most smokers have a persistent 'smoker's' cough and those with COPD and chronic bronchitis have a daily productive cough, mainly in the mornings. However, a persistent cough is the commonest symptom of lung cancer, so a careful history, a clinical examination, and a chest X-ray should be conducted in all patients with a smoking history. Patients with damage to the vagus nerve or with recurrent laryngeal nerve palsy may present with a 'bovine' cough which is a non-explosive cough due to an inability to close the glottis. These patients will also have a hoarse voice or dysphonia. These patients should have a computed tomography (CT) thorax and a bronchoscopy.

Haemoptysis

Coughing up blood indicates lung pathology and is alarming for the patient. Occasionally epistaxis, haematemesis, or bleeding from the gums can be misinterpreted as haemoptysis, so a careful history with specific questions about the nature of the blood must be obtained. In most cases, fresh, red blood mixed with sputum indicates lung pathology. Dark, altered blood may be of gastrointestinal origin.

Infection and inflammation of the respiratory tract are the commonest cause of small volume haemoptysis and patients will have other symptoms and signs of infection, including cough and fever. Bronchiectasis, pulmonary tuberculosis, and aspergilloma are also in the differential diagnosis for haemoptysis. Sputum microscopy and culture are essential to identify the causative organism and to test for antibiotic sensitivities. Haemoptysis is a common presentation of lung cancer, so patients at risk of lung cancer should be investigated quickly with a chest X-ray followed by a CT thorax and a bronchoscopy. Sputum cytology may have a role in patients who are suspected of having lung cancer but who are too frail for invasive tests. Table 5.2 lists the causes of haemoptysis.

Bleeding secondary to a biopsy at bronchoscopy is common and usually settles after a few minutes. Topical adrenaline, 10 ml of 1 : 10,000, should be administered slowly and directly to the site of bleeding while monitoring the patient's pulse and blood pressure. If the bleeding does not settle, then the patient will have to be managed as described below for life-threatening haemoptysis. Patients having a bronchial biopsy, or a CT-guided biopsy should be informed that they could cough up blood for several days post procedure. If there is evidence of continuous, but non-life-threatening bleeding, then they should be discharged home on oral Tranexamic acid, an antifibrinolytic agent, 1–1.5 g twice or three times a day.

Management of life-threatening haemoptysis

The term massive haemoptysis should be avoided as the definition of what this is varies widely in the literature and it is impossible to quantify the amount of blood loss, as much of the blood may be in the lungs. Most experts agree that the term life-threatening haemoptysis is preferable and the definition is bleeding of >200 ml in 24 hours which results in airway obstruction and abnormal gas exchange, which does not stop, and which causes haemodynamic compromise. The cause of death from uncontrolled haemoptysis would be from asphyxiation.

Table 5.2 Causes of haemoptysis.

Malignancy (see Chapter 9)
Carcinoma of lung
Carcinoma of trachea
Infection (see Chapter 8)
Mycobacterium tuberculosis
Aspergilloma
Community acquired pneumonia
Aspiration pneumonia
Lower respiratory tract infection
Bronchiectasis
Cystic fibrosis
Lung abscess
Histoplasmosis
Vascular (see Chapter 11)
Pulmonary emboli
Arterio-venous malformation
Hereditary haemorrhagic telangiectasia
Goodpasture's syndrome
Polyangiitis (Wegener's granulomatosis)
Autoimmune
SLE pneumonitis
Sarcoidosis
Behçet's disease
Cardiac
Pulmonary oedema
Mitral stenosis
Miscellaneous
Coagulopathies
Anticoagulant therapy
Trauma, including violent coughing
Inhalation of foreign body
Pulmonary haemosiderosis
Pulmonary endometriosis
Broncholithiasis

Life-threatening haemoptysis is rare, estimated as <1.5% of all cases of haemoptysis. In the past, pulmonary tuberculosis and bronchiectasis were the common causes, now lung cancer, aspergilloma, and cystic fibrosis are the commonest causes. In these cases, the bleeding occurs due to erosion in the bronchial artery. The mortality depends on the age of the patient, any underlying lung and cardiac disease, the rate of bleeding and the ability of the patient to clear the blood from the airways. Mortality may be up to 25% in those managed conservatively and up to 20% with surgery, although the estimates vary greatly in the literature.

Patients presenting with life-threatening haemoptysis must be managed in the intensive care unit or high dependency unit by intensivists and respiratory physicians. The patient will require immediate resuscitation with intravenous fluids, airway protection, oxygen supplementation, cross-matched blood, fresh frozen plasma, and the correction of any coagulopathy. Bloods should also be sent for urgent vasculitic screen.

Tranexamic acid has been shown to reduce overall bleeding time, the duration of bleeding, and the overall volume of blood loss, with no short-term thromboembolic complications. Intravenous tranexamic acid should be given as a slow infusion at a dose of 100 mg min^{-1} followed by 25–50 mg kg^{-1} over 24 hours.

If the patient is haemodynamically stable, then an urgent computed tomography pulmonary angiography (CTPA) should be carried out to exclude pulmonary embolus and to identify any obvious masses or cavities. The source of the bleeding should be identified, ideally with rigid bronchoscopy, although this may not be easy if there is a lot of blood, and the patient may require selective lung intubation before this can be carried out. Topical adrenaline, a potent vasoconstrictor, may reduce the bleeding and endobronchial tamponade may be effective in stemming the flow of blood. The patient should be nursed lying on the side of the bleeding lung.

The source of the bleeding can be identified by bronchial angiography with embolization of the bronchial artery. Early discussion with a thoracic surgeon is important as surgical resection of the affected part of the lung may be required if the bleeding cannot be stopped. Chronic haemoptysis secondary to lung cancer can be treated by palliative radiotherapy. Patients in whom the source of bleeding cannot be identified are managed conservatively.

Chest pain

Chest pain is a common and worrying symptom. It can be due to significant pathology, so should always be taken seriously. When taking the history of chest pain, it is important to be specific about the nature of the pain, the onset, duration, site, radiation, periodicity, exacerbating factors, and relieving factors.

Chest pain of cardiac origin is generally described as a dull ache with radiation down the left arm, towards the jaw or to the back. Patients with cardiac-sounding pain may also describe breathlessness. Pain arising from the gastrointestinal system (epigastrium, liver, gall bladder, spleen) can radiate to the chest and the shoulders and this can be confused with cardiac or respiratory pain.

Musculoskeletal pain, which is pleuritic in nature, is worse with inspiration and with movement and there will be musculoskeletal tenderness on palpation. The patient may complain of breathlessness if he or she is unable to fully expand his or her lungs due to the pain. Musculoskeletal pain can occur secondary to chest wall trauma and the pain can be severe if ribs have been fractured.

Costochondritis occurs due to inflammation of the costochondral, costosternal, or sternoclavicular joints and is a common cause of musculoskeletal chest pain in young adults. Costochondritis is commoner in females and in patients with fibromyalgia. It is self-limiting, with symptoms resolving within eight weeks. The term Tietze's syndrome is used when there is swelling of these joints. Bornholm disease is caused by Coxsackie virus B, which results in muscle aches and pains in the chest wall.

Chest pain secondary to respiratory pathology is usually pleuritic in nature. It is described as sharp and stabbing and aggravated by inspiration and coughing. It occurs due to inflammation of the pleura from any cause. Rubbing of the visceral and parietal pleura against each other stimulates the nerve endings. Crackles may be heard when there is 'pleurisy' of any aetiology. Pleuritic chest pain responds well to non-steroidal anti-inflammatory drugs which should be prescribed regularly, so long as there are no contra-indications.

Table 5.3 lists common causes of pleuritic chest pain and the basic investigations that would be required.

Table 5.3 Common causes of pleuritic chest pain.

Onset	System	Diagnosis	Investigations
Acute (minutes to hours)	Respiratory	Pneumothorax Pulmonary embolus	Chest X-ray CTPA or VQ scan
Acute (minutes to hours)	Musculoskeletal	Trauma Rib fractures Costochondritis Tietze's syndrome	Chest X-ray CT thorax Clinical examination
Sub-acute (hours to days)	Respiratory	Pneumothorax Pulmonary embolus Pleural effusion	Chest X-ray CTPA or VQ scan
Sub-acute (hours to days)	Musculoskeletal	Costochondritis Tietze's syndrome Bornholm disease	Clinical examination
Chronic (days to weeks)	Respiratory	Pneumothorax Community acquired pneumonia SLE pneumonitis Pleural effusion	Chest X-ray Chest X-ray CT thorax Clinical examination Chest X-ray CT thorax Pleural ultrasound
Chronic (days to weeks)	Musculoskeletal	Costochondritis Tietze's syndrome Bornholm disease Chest wall infiltration with tumour	Clinical examination CT thorax MRI thorax

Patients with lung cancer may have chest wall infiltration with tumour which can cause severe pain. Metastases to ribs and bones can also cause severe pain. In these cases, there are likely to be several other symptoms and signs and abnormal radiology. Patients with malignant mesothelioma (see Chapter 9) often present with a persistent dull ache in their chest which progressively gets worse over time. Pain secondary to lung cancer or malignant mesothelioma often requires high doses of opioid drugs to control it. Palliative radiotherapy is also indicated as a treatment for bony pain.

Wheeze

Wheeze is a high-pitched whistling sound made when the airways are narrowed and can occur during inspiration or expiration. Patients may not complain of wheeze but may report breathlessness or chest tightness. Family members may report that they have heard wheezing.

Widespread, polyphonic, expiratory wheezing is commonly associated with obstructive airways disease, such as asthma or COPD. Diurnal symptoms or symptoms made worse with exercise or cold air suggest a reversible cause, such as asthma. Patients with an occupational cause of asthma will report breathlessness and wheezing while at work which improves when they are away from the work environment. Similarly, those who are allergic to pets usually feel better when they are away from the animal. Patients who develop wheezing secondary to obstructive airways disease will improve with bronchodilators and corticosteroids. Cardiac failure can present with widespread wheeze, sometimes termed 'cardiac asthma'. A monophonic wheeze can be a sign of a fixed obstruction which may be secondary to endobronchial narrowing, for example, with tumour. Wheezing can be audible from the end of the bed, but usually requires a stethoscope to be heard.

Patients with vocal cord dysfunction present with what appears to be a wheeze. However, all the noise is generated in the throat from closure of the vocal cords which move paradoxically and there will be no wheeze heard on auscultation of the chest. The diagnosis and management of this are discussed in Chapter 6.

Hoarse voice

Many viral and bacterial infections can result in a brief period of laryngitis which improves over a few days and weeks. A persistent hoarse voice indicates inflammation or damage to the larynx or to its nerve supply. The left recurrent laryngeal nerve has a long course through the left hemithorax (see Chapter 2) and can be damaged by trauma, thoracic and neck surgery (particularly thyroid surgery), and lung cancer. Persistent hoarse voice in a smoker requires immediate investigation with CXR, CT thorax, and a bronchoscopy.

Snoring

Snoring is a common symptom during sleep which is often not pathological. It describes a sound made by the turbulent flow of air through narrowed upper airways. Snoring is often positional, usually worse when lying on the back, exacerbated by alcohol and sedatives, and worse in older people with lax muscles, and in those who are overweight. It can become a problem when it disturbs the patient's sleep or their partner's sleep. Such patients are often referred for polysomnography to rule out obstructive sleep apnoea. This is discussed in Chapter 14, and is demonstrated in the supplementary material.

Examination of the respiratory system

Examination of the respiratory system should be thorough and systematic. It is important to observe the patient from the end of the bed, if possible, positioned at a 45° angle. The respiratory rate at rest should be counted. A normal respiratory rate is between 12 and 16 breaths per minute at rest. The tidal volume is 500 ml with a minute ventilation rate of 6 L min^{-1}. Expiration, which is a passive process, takes slightly longer than inspiration, which is an active process. Hyperinflation will result in a prolonged expiratory phase of breathing.

From the end of the bed, with the patient taking a deep breath in, it is possible to note any abnormality or asymmetry of the chest wall and whether one side of the chest moves less than the other (Figure 5.1). The side that moves less is always the side with the pathology. Observation should also be made of pursed-lip breathing, use of

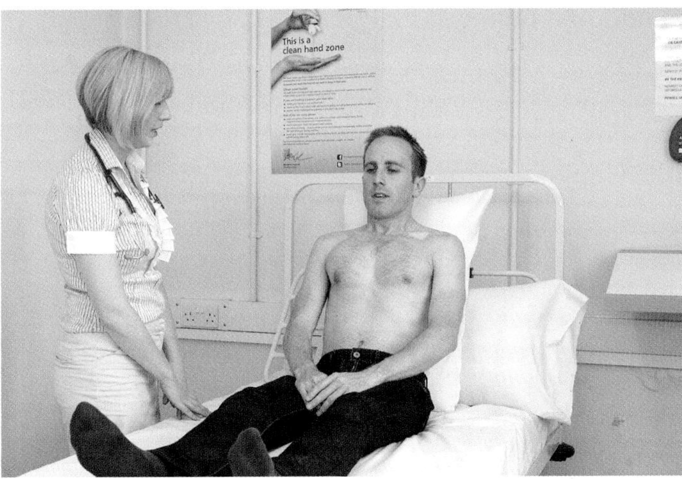

Figure 5.1 Observing chest expansion on inspiration.

Box 5.5 Chest wall deformities.

- ***Pectus excavatum* (funnel chest)** is a congenital abnormality of the anterior chest wall due to abnormal development of the sternum and ribs. It occurs in every 300–400 births, is commoner in males and may be associated with Marfan's syndrome and Ehlers-Danlos syndrome. This can compromise breathing if severe, and can cause chest pain
- ***Pectus carinatum* (pigeon chest)** is an inherited deformity of the chest wall due to overgrowth of cartilage, resulting in protrusion of the sternum and ribs. It is commoner in men and becomes obvious during puberty. If severe, it can affect breathing
- **Kyphosis** is a common chest wall deformity. The adolescent type, called Scheuermann's disease, occurs when several vertebrae become wedged together. It is common in the elderly due to degenerative changes, osteoporotic fractures, or spondylolisthesis. It can result in chest discomfort and difficulty breathing. If severe, it can impair rib movement. It is a cause of restrictive lung disease and type 2 respiratory failure
- **Scoliosis** is the abnormal lateral curvature of the spine. It can be congenital, is commoner in females, and becomes worse during puberty. Due to abnormal movement of the chest wall it can result in reduced lung volumes and type 2 respiratory failure

accessory muscles, intercostal recession, and tracheal tug, all of which are signs of hyperinflation.

Box 5.5 lists some common chest wall deformities which can cause abnormal breathing and lead to the development of respiratory failure.

Box 5.6 lists what to look for in the hands and nails and the causes of clubbing.

Cardiovascular examination should include taking the pulse and the blood pressure and to determine whether there are any signs of right heart failure: elevated jugular venous pressure, signs of pulmonary hypertension (loud P2, right ventricular heave), and peripheral oedema. A displaced apex beat may suggest mediastinal shift, for example, with a large pneumothorax or pleural effusion.

The patient should be examined for evidence of lymphadenopathy which could be due to infective causes (viral, bacterial, *Mycobacterium tuberculosis*), malignancy (lung cancer, lymphoma), HIV or sarcoidosis. Nodes in the submental, submandibular, cervical, supraclavicular, pre-auricular, post-auricular, and occipital areas should be examined. If any lymph nodes are palpated, then the axilla

Box 5.6 Hand and nail changes.

- Nicotine staining indicates cigarette smoking
- Clubbing: differential diagnosis includes bronchial carcinoma, idiopathic pulmonary fibrosis, bronchiectasis, emphysema, and lung abscess. Non-respiratory causes include cyanotic heart disease, endocarditis, atrial myxoma, liver cirrhosis, inflammatory bowel disease, and coeliac disease. Clubbing can be familial and idiopathic. Patients with finger clubbing usually also have clubbing of their toe nails (Figure 5.2)
- Peripheral cyanosis can indicate cardiac or respiratory pathology
- Fine tremor could indicate over-use of β_2-agonist medication or thyrotoxicosis
- CO_2 retention tremor (asterixis) is a coarse, flapping tremor suggestive of excessive amounts of carbon dioxide in the bloodstream in patients with type 2 respiratory failure (Figure 5.3). The patient should be asked to extend their arms and wrists out and keep their fingers apart for at least 30 seconds. Other clinical signs of CO_2 retention include a bounding pulse, drowsiness, and irritability

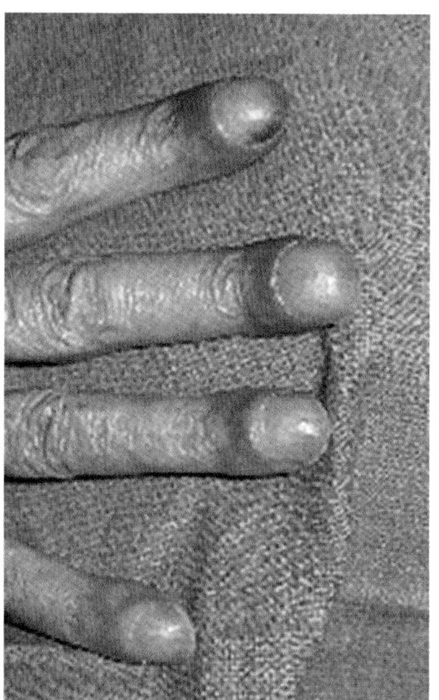

Figure 5.2 Clubbing of the finger nails and tar staining. *Source: ABC of COPD*. 3rd edition, Figure 3.3.

and inguinal areas should also be examined for lymphadenopathy (Figure 5.4).

The trachea should be examined by inserting the index and middle fingers in the suprasternal notch to look for signs of deviation which could be due to extra-thoracic or intra-thoracic causes. Extra-thoracic causes of tracheal deviation include a large, retrosternal thyroid goitre, which can also cause significant tracheal compression or lymphadenopathy. Intra-thoracic causes of tracheal deviation (Figure 5.5, Figure 5.6) include pneumothorax and pleural effusion, which will push the trachea away from the side in which they occur. Upper lobe collapse, which may be due to endobronchial obstruction or chronic apical fibrosis, can cause tracheal deviation towards the side of the lesion.

The conjunctiva should be examined to look for pallor suggestive of anaemia, and the mucous membranes of the mouth, lips, and tongue examined for telangiectasia and central cyanosis. Cyanosis is seen when there is >5 g dl^{-1} of deoxygenated haemoglobin present. Horner's syndrome (ptosis, miosis, enophthalmos, and anhidrosis) (Figure 5.7) suggests damage to the sympathetic chain in the neck, for example, by a Pancoast's tumour (see Chapter 9). Bilateral ptosis is suggestive of Myasthenia Gravis and eye signs secondary to thyroid disease may be obvious. General inspection of the skin may show bruising and thinning secondary to steroid therapy, markers of autoimmune disease (for example psoriatic plaques), or erythema nodosum on the shins.

Examination of the chest

Close examination of the chest includes noting any scars which might indicate previous surgery, chest drain insertion, or radiotherapy. A reduction in the crico-sternal distance may suggest hyperinflation. Note should be made of signs of superior vena cava obstruction, which includes distended, engorged, pulseless veins in the neck, a jugular venous pressure that is fixed and raised, collateral veins on the chest and arms, and facial oedema.

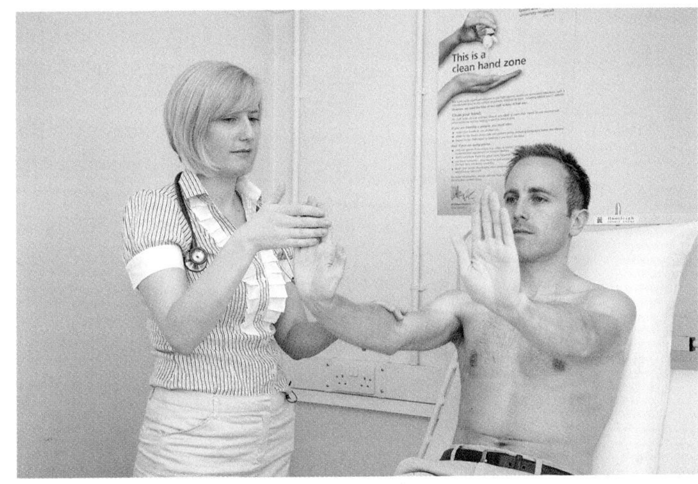

Figure 5.3 Checking for CO_2 retention flap.

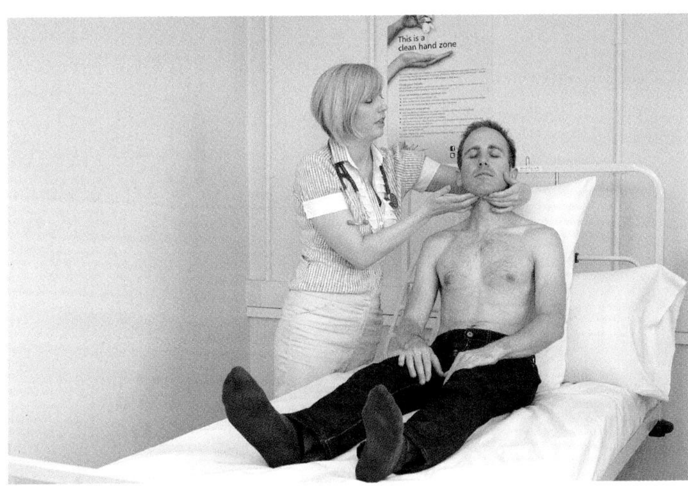

Figure 5.4 Checking for lymphadenopathy.

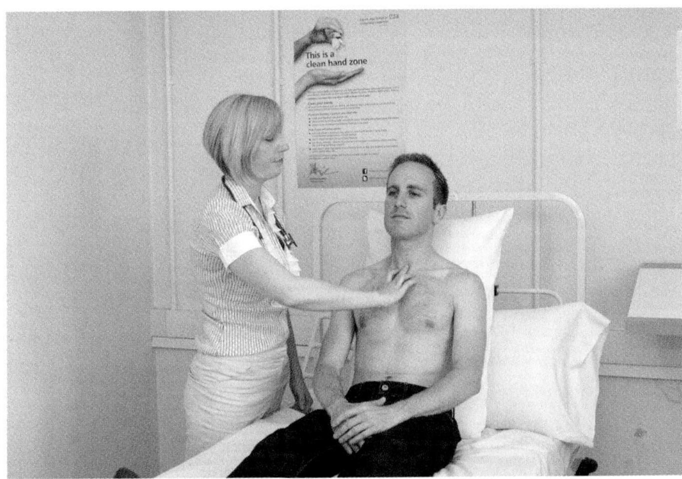

Figure 5.5 Checking for tracheal deviation.

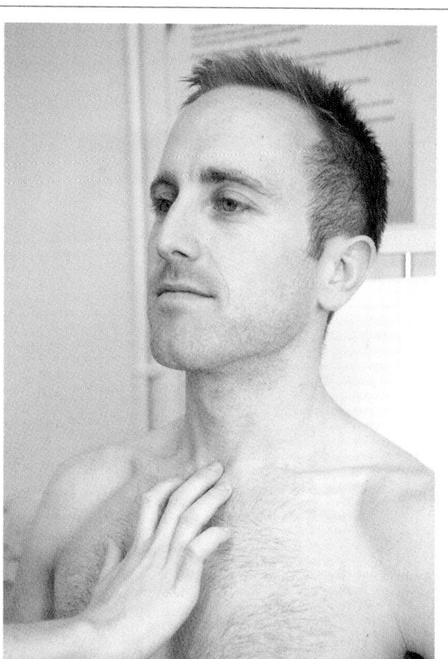

Figure 5.6 Close-up view showing how to check for tracheal deviation.

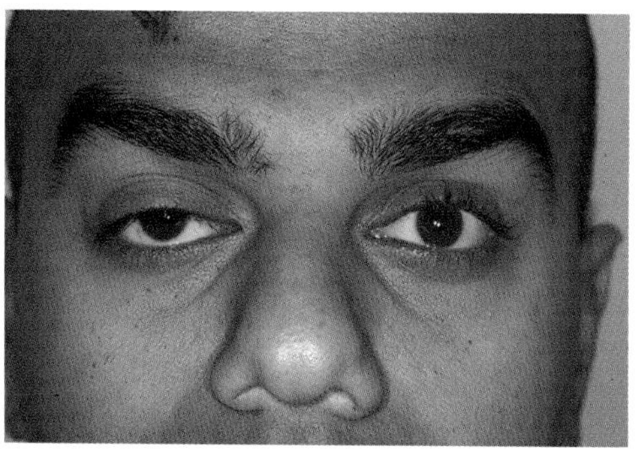

Figure 5.7 Unilateral (right-sided) Horner's syndrome showing ptosis, miosis, and aniscoria (difference in size of the pupils between the two eyes).

Chest expansion should be conducted anteriorly and posteriorly using both hands in the upper and lower chest wall and comparing the left to the right side. The hands should be placed firmly on the chest wall with the fingers spread apart and with the thumbs in the midline. The patient should be asked to take a deep breath in and the movement apart of the thumbs noted to see if the chest expands normally. Again, note should be made of any asymmetry in chest expansion as this suggests pathology on that side (Figure 5.8, Figure 5.9).

Chest expansion will be reduced bilaterally in conditions affecting both lungs, such as COPD or pulmonary fibrosis, the former due to hyperinflation and the latter due to reduced lung compliance. Asymmetry of chest expansion suggests pathology affecting one side of the lung, for example, pneumonia or pleural effusion (Figure 5.10). Weakness of the diaphragmatic muscles may result in the abdominal wall moving paradoxically inwards during inspiration.

Percussion should be conducted anteriorly and posteriorly in a systematic and symmetrical way, covering the upper, middle, and lower zones of the thorax. The middle finger should be placed flat against the chest wall and should be tapped firmly using a finger from the other hand (Figure 5.11, Figure 5.12). Normal lungs are full of air and the percussion sound is resonant. When there is consolidation (fluid or debris in the alveolar sacs) or if there is a pleural effusion, then there will be dullness on percussion. The percussion note will be hyper-resonant with a large pneumothorax.

Auscultation is usually done using the diaphragm of the stethoscope (Figure 5.13). Normal lungs, full of air, transmit low frequency sounds. Normal breath sounds are described as vesicular.

The listener should describe whether the wheeze occurs during inspiration, expiration, or throughout the respiratory cycle, whether it is monophonic or polyphonic, and in which zones of the chest it can be heard. Polyphonic wheezes, usually heard throughout the lung fields, indicate obstructive airways disease (asthma, COPD, bronchiectasis) but can also be heard with cardiac failure. A monophonic wheeze heard in a fixed position indicates a fixed obstruction, for example, a tumour.

Crackles are caused when the respiratory bronchioles open, and occur when the lungs have reduced compliance. Coarse crackles can be due to pulmonary oedema or bronchiectasis and fine crackles suggest an interstitial abnormality, such as occurs in idiopathic pulmonary fibrosis. Crackles due to secretions will clear on coughing.

Lungs which have consolidation will transmit high frequency sounds. Bronchial breathing, a harsh sound, indicates an air-fluid interface as

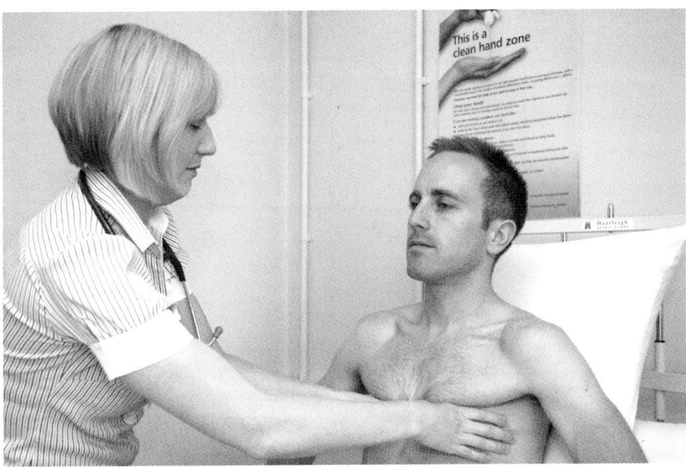

Figure 5.8 Checking for chest expansion upper anterior chest.

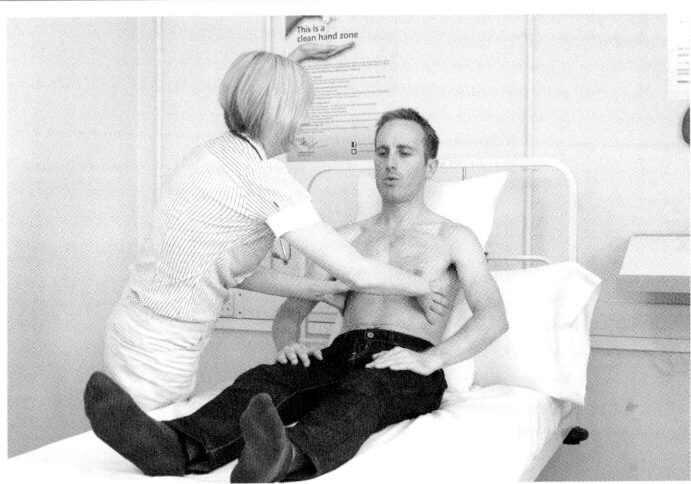

Figure 5.9 Checking for chest expansion lower anterior chest.

might be found in pneumonia or on top of a pleural effusion.

Tactile vocal fremitus (TVF) and vocal resonance (VR) detect the transmission of sound from the lungs to the periphery. The patient is asked to say '99' or '111' and the transmission of the sound is felt either as vibration using the lateral surface of the hands or heard through the stethoscope. TVF and VR will be reduced with a pleural effusion and increased in consolidation. A high-pitched 'bleating' sound, called aegophony, can be heard in areas of consolidation. When patients with consolidation are asked to whisper '99', then the high-pitched consonants of speech may be heard (whispering pectoriloquy).

A pleural rub is described as a 'squeaky' sound, like the sound of new leather. This is suggestive of pulmonary infarction, for example, after a pulmonary embolus.

Abnormal respiratory sounds can be heard on: www.easyauscultation.com, YouTube, or https://www.med.ucla.edu. The supplementary video demonstrates how to take a respiratory history and conduct a respiratory examination.

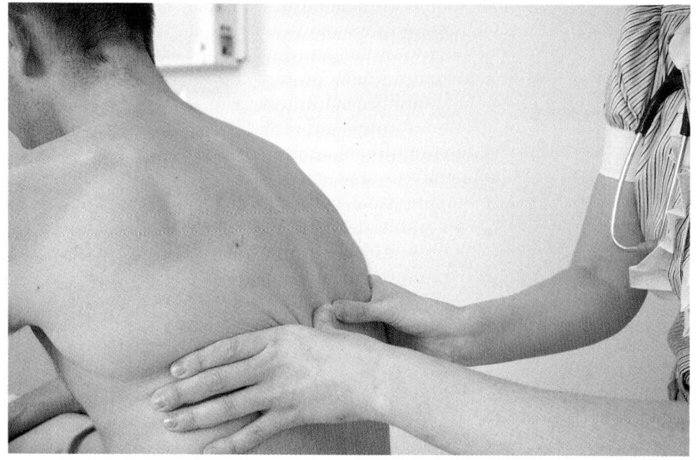

Figure 5.10 Checking for chest expansion posteriorly.

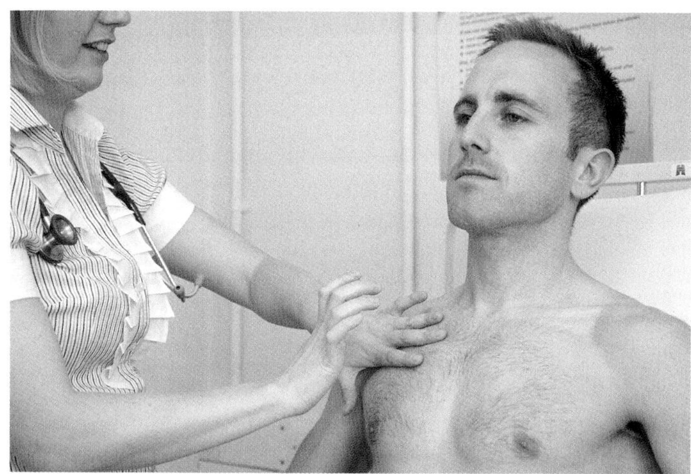

Figure 5.11 Percussion of the chest anteriorly.

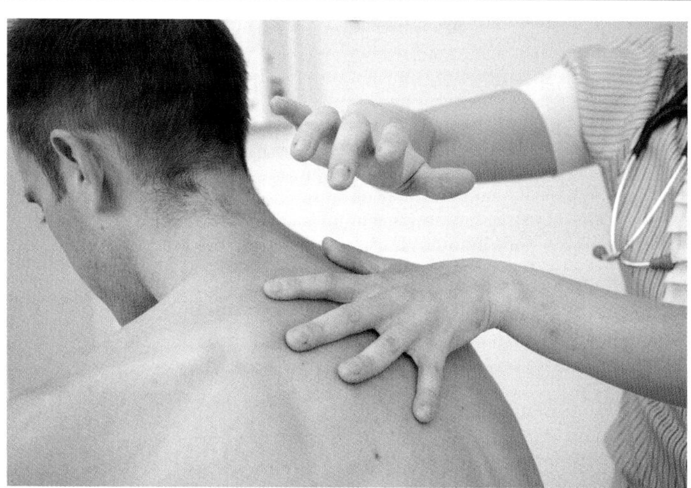

Figure 5.12 Percussion of the chest posteriorly.

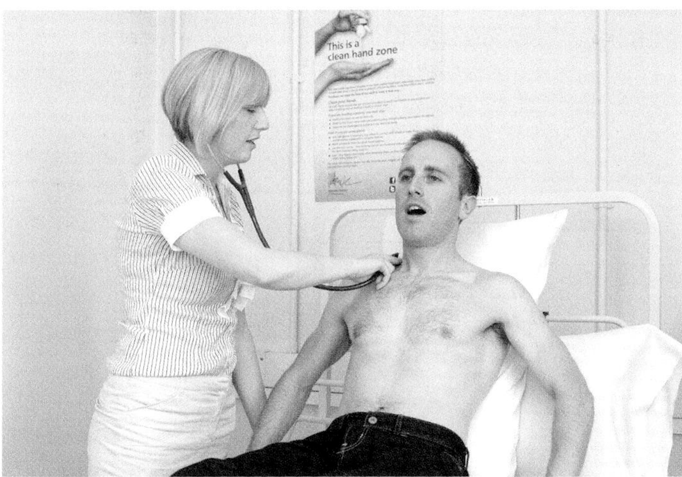

Figure 5.13 Auscultation of the lungs.

Table 5.4 lists abnormal findings on examination of the chest and what pathology this might indicate.

Pre-operative respiratory assessment

The surgeon and anaesthetist will require some information about the patient's cardiac and respiratory systems prior to carrying out surgery, particularly if this involves a general anaesthetic. While the anaesthetist will usually assess the patient and make the final decision, they will expect basic respiratory information to be available.

In a patient who has no respiratory problems, this usually includes documentation of a normal respiratory examination, oxygen saturation, and chest X-ray result. In patients who have underlying respiratory disease, a more comprehensive evaluation will be required, and senior respiratory opinion is often sought. The results of full lung function tests, including diffusing capacity, and the results of an arterial blood gas test will be required. Many elderly patients with chronic lung disease are found to be unfit for surgery involving general anaesthetic. For patients with poor lung function in whom surgery with a general anaesthetic cannot be avoided, optimisation of lung function with inhaled therapy, nebulised bronchodilators, and chest physiotherapy is advised. Patients who use a continuous positive airways pressure (CPAP) or bilevel positive airways pressure (BiPAP) machine, for example, for OSA or chronic type 2 respiratory failure, should be advised to bring that with them to the hospital. Such patients should be managed in the high dependency unit or intensive care unit.

Post-operative respiratory problems

Major surgery causes significant physiological changes in the body. In the immediate post-operative period, pain, opioid analgesia, and immobility will result in reduced coughing and the pooling of secretions in the lungs. This can cause atelectasis and increase the risk of pulmonary infection. This can be significant, especially after major abdominal surgery. Patients who have had surgery often develop breathlessness. This should be assessed in a systematic way with clinical examination, CXR, and arterial blood gas (ABG) examination.

Patients with known chronic lung disease may require respiratory support post-operatively. Some may require CPAP, non-invasive ventilation (NIV) or intubation. The majority will benefit from nebulised bronchodilators, mucolytic agents, and chest physiotherapy to clear secretions and reduce the risk of atelectasis.

Post-surgery immobility is an increased risk factor for deep vein thrombosis and pulmonary embolus. Patients should be prescribed prophylactic low molecular weight heparin or thromboembolic disease (TED) stockings to prevent this. Doctors looking after patients who have had surgery should be aware of the risk of thromboembolic disease.

Patients are often unable to take adequate oral fluids and are prescribed intravenous fluids. If too much fluid is prescribed without an assessment of fluid status, then the patient may go into acute pulmonary

Table 5.4 Abnormalities on examination of the lungs.

Condition	General observation	Chest expansion	Percussion	TVF and VR	Auscultation
Asthma	Tachypnoea Audible wheeze	Hyperinflated	Normal	Normal	Polyphonic wheeze
COPD	Tachypnoea Pursed-lip breathing	Hyperinflated	Normal	Normal	Polyphonic wheeze
Pneumonia	Fever Tachypnoea	Reduced on side of consolidation	Dull on side of consolidation	Increased	Coarse crackles Bronchial breathing Whispering pectoriloquy Aegophony
Pleural effusion	Tachypnoea Tracheal deviation away from side of effusion	Reduced on side of effusion	Dull on side of effusion (stony dull)	Reduced	Reduced breath sounds
Pulmonary fibrosis	Tachypnoea Clubbed	Reduced	Normal	Normal	Fine late-inspiratory crackles
Lobar collapse	Tachypnoea Tracheal deviation towards the side of collapse	Reduced on side of collapse	Normal	Normal	Reduced breath sounds on side of collapse
Pneumothorax	Tachypnoea Tracheal deviation away from side of pneumothorax	Reduced on side of pneumothorax	Hyper-resonant	Reduced	Reduced breath sounds on side of pneumothorax

oedema, resulting in breathlessness, especially if the patient is elderly and has cardiac problems.

Respiratory assessment of an acutely ill patient

Sudden and severe respiratory compromise resulting in respiratory failure is a common problem in hospitals. Such a patient will need clinical examination to elicit the cause of the respiratory failure. Oxygen should be given through the correct device and at the correct rate after measurement of the arterial blood gas (PO_2, PCO_2, pH and bicarbonate) to determine whether it is type 1 or type 2 respiratory failure. Further investigations should include a CXR, a CT scan, an ECG, and echocardiogram to make a definite diagnosis. A senior medical opinion will be required. The management of respiratory failure is discussed in Chapter 13.

Stridor is an alarming sign to observe in a patient as it suggests impending upper airway obstruction. The sound is worse on inspiration and can be heard without a stethoscope. There are several causes of stridor. Inhalation of a foreign body can cause airway obstruction. A bang on the back of the chest or the Heimlich manoeuvre will be required to remove the object. In children, gentler manoeuvres are advised. Epiglottitis can cause swelling of the upper airways and is a medical emergency which might require intubation by an experienced anaesthetist. Smoke inhalation can also cause severe burns and oedema of the upper airways resulting in obstruction. Anaphylaxis is another cause of upper airway obstruction that will need to be managed with intramuscular adrenaline (0.5 ml of a 1 : 1000 solution), chlorpheniramine, 10–20 mg IV, hydrocortisone 100–500 mg IV and inhaled β2-agonist for bronchospasm.

SUMMARY OF LEARNING POINTS

- A comprehensive history and thorough clinical examination will lead to the correct diagnosis in most cases.
- Breathlessness can be due to many different causes and does not always indicate lung pathology.
- Cough is a common symptom. A sensible algorithm should be used to make the diagnosis.
- Common causes of a dry cough in a non-smoker with a normal CXR include asthma, GORD, postnasal drip, ACE inhibitor, and post-infectious cough.
- Cough is the commonest presentation of patients with lung cancer, so smokers with persistent cough should have a CXR.
- Pleuritic chest pain indicates inflammation of the pleural surface from any of several causes, including infection, malignancy, and infarction.
- The differential diagnosis of pleuritic chest pain includes pneumothorax, pulmonary embolus, and community acquired pneumonia, so a CXR is required.
- The differential diagnosis for haemoptysis includes infection, malignancy, vasculitides, and coagulopathies.
- Causes of upper airway obstruction include epiglottitis, inhaled foreign body, smoke inhalation, and anaphylaxis. Patients will present with stridor and will require intubation.
- Post-operative respiratory problems include atelectasis, pneumonia, pulmonary embolus, and pulmonary oedema if too much intravenous fluid is given in patients with cardiac dysfunction.

MULTIPLE CHOICE QUESTIONS

5.1 Which one of the following statements is true?

A Breathlessness always indicates a problem with the lungs
B Breathlessness when lying flat always indicates heart failure
C Breathlessness should be graded using the MRC scale
D Breathlessness in pregnancy is always worrying
E All breathless patients need oxygen

Answer: C

Breathlessness may indicate lung pathology, but can also be due to problems with other systems of the body such as the heart, muscles, or thoracic cage. A detailed history and careful examination is required to make a diagnosis. Although orthopnoea, which is breathlessness when lying flat, is often associated with heart failure, it can also occur with COPD, OSA, and diaphragmatic palsy. Breathlessness in pregnancy can be physiological due to the increased demands as well as due to the enlarged uterus pushing up on the diaphragm. Only patients who are hypoxic need oxygen.

5.2 Which of the following statements is true?

A All patients with a cough should have a CXR
B Normal spirometry excludes asthma as a cause of dry cough
C Bronchiectasis usually presents with a dry cough
D Persistent cough in a smoker is a worrying symptom
E GORD is a common cause of productive cough

Answer: D

Smokers who have a persistent cough (longer than three weeks) should have a clinical examination and a CXR to exclude lung cancer. Cough-variant asthma is common and spirometry may be normal. GORD and postnasal drip are common causes of a dry cough. Not all patients with a cough need a CXR, only if there are clinical concerns, such as weight loss, haemoptysis, and if the patient has been a smoker.

5.3 A 55-year-old man presents with haemoptysis. A CXR shows a cavitating lesion. Which of the following diagnoses will you exclude?

A Aspergilloma
B Community acquired pneumonia
C Granulomatosis with polyangiitis (Wegener's)
D Non-small cell lung cancer
E Sarcoidosis

Answer: E

All the above, except sarcoidosis, can present with haemoptysis and a cavitating lesion. Infections with *Staphylococcus aureus* and *Streptococcus millieri* develop cavities.

5.4 A 26-year-old woman presents with pleuritic chest pain and breathlessness and is found to have pain on palpation of her sternum and chest wall. The most likely diagnosis is which of the following?

A Asthma
B Costochondritis
C Gastro-oesophageal reflux
D Pneumothorax
E Pulmonary embolus

Answer: B

The most likely diagnosis with this presentation is costochondritis or Tietze's syndrome. Clearly the patient will require a thorough examination and investigations, including a chest X-ray, ECG, and measurement of oxygen saturation to exclude the other conditions.

5.5 Dullness on percussion and an increased vocal resonance indicate which pathology?

A Lung cancer
B Pleural effusion
C Pneumonia
D Pneumothorax
E Pulmonary oedema

Answer: C

Dullness on percussion with increased VR indicates consolidation which occurs with pneumonia.

5.6 Finger clubbing and fine crackles on auscultation are indicative of which condition?

A Bronchiectasis
B Idiopathic pulmonary fibrosis
C Lung abscess
D Pneumonia
E Pulmonary oedema

Answer: B

Clubbing and fine crackles occur in idiopathic pulmonary fibrosis. Clubbing can occur in bronchiectasis, but the crackles are coarse. Clubbing can also occur with lung abscess but no crackles will be heard. Coarse crackles may be heard in both pneumonia and pulmonary oedema.

5.7 A tension pneumothorax on the right hemithorax will result in which condition?

A Tracheal deviation to the left and decreased breath sounds on the left
B Tracheal deviation to the right and decreased breath sounds on the right
C Tracheal deviation to the right and hyper-resonance on percussion on the right
D Tracheal deviation to the left and hyper-resonance on percussion on the right
E Tracheal deviation to the left and increased breath sounds on the right

Answer: D

A pneumothorax on the right side will push the trachea away towards the left side and there will be mediastinal shift to the left. Percussion on the right side will be hyper-resonant and there will be reduced breath sounds on the right.

5.8 Which clinical features indicate a large left pleural effusion?

A Tracheal deviation to the left, decreased breath sounds, and dullness on percussion on the left
B Tracheal deviation to the right, decreased breath sound, and dullness on percussion on the left
C Tracheal deviation to the right, decreased breath sounds, and dullness on percussion on the right
D Tracheal deviation to the left, increased breath sounds, and dullness on percussion on the left
E Tracheal deviation to the right, increased breath sounds on the right, and dullness on percussion on the left

Answer: B

A large pleural effusion will push the trachea away to the right. There will be reduced chest expansion, reduced breath sounds, and dullness on percussion on the left side.

5.9 Which clinical features indicate right upper lobe collapse?

A Tracheal deviation to the right with reduced chest expansion on the right
B Tracheal deviation to the right with reduced chest expansion on the left
C Dullness to percussion on the right with increased tactile vocal fremitus
D Hyper-resonance on the right with decreased breath sounds on the right
E Dullness to percussion on the left with decreased breath sounds on the right

Answer: A

Right upper lobe collapse will cause tracheal deviation towards the right, with decreased chest expansion and reduced breath sounds on the right.

5.10 A patient with vocal cord dysfunction usually presents with which condition?

A Crackles
B Haemoptysis
C Pleuritic chest pain
D Upper airway noise
E Wheeze on auscultation

Answer: D

Patients with vocal cord dysfunction complain of breathlessness and wheeze, even at rest, but auscultation of the lungs is usually normal. They close off their throat and vocal cords, so they generate a noise that may resemble stridor.

FURTHER READING

Conlan, A.A. and Hurwitz, S.S. (1980). Management of massive haemoptysis with the rigid bronchoscope and cold saline lavage. *Thorax* 35 (12): 901–904.

Jean-Baptiste, E. (2000). Clinical assessment and management of massive hemoptysis. *Critical Care Medicine* 28 (5): 1642–1647.

Kreit, J.W. (2004). Hemoptysis. In: *Clinical Respiratory Medicine*, 2e (ed. R. Albert, S. Spiro and J.R. Jett), 253–254. Philadelphia, PA: Mosby.

Lordan, J.L., Gascoigne, A., and Corris, P.A. (2003). The pulmonary physician in critical care: illustrative case 7, assessment and management of massive haemoptysis. *Thorax* 58 (9): 814–819.

Morice, A.H., McGarvey, L., and Pavord, I. (2006). Recommendations for the management of cough in adults. *Thorax* 61 (Suppl 1): i1–i24.

Uflacker, R., Kaemmerer, A., Neves, C., and Picon, P.D. (1983). Management of massive hemoptysis by bronchial artery embolization. *Radiology* 146 (3): 627–634.

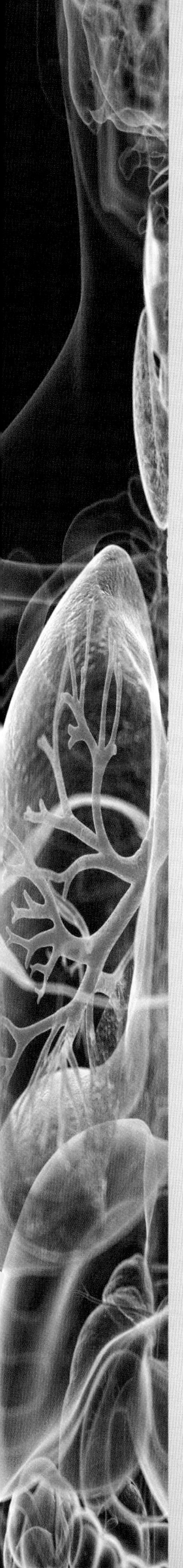

CHAPTER 6

Obstructive airways disease

Learning objectives

- To understand the aetiology and epidemiology of asthma
- To learn about the diagnosis and differential diagnosis of asthma
- To understand the management of acute and chronic asthma
- To recognise the risk factors for fatal asthma
- To understand the aetiology and epidemiology of chronic obstructive pulmonary disease (COPD)
- To understand the diagnosis and differential diagnosis of COPD
- To understand the management and prognosis of COPD
- To understand the management of acute exacerbation of COPD
- To have some understanding of the diagnosis and management of α-1 antitrypsin deficiency (α-1ATD)
- To understand the diagnosis and management of allergic bronchopulmonary aspergillosis (ABPA)
- To understand the diagnosis and management of vocal cord dysfunction
- To understand the diagnosis and management of hyperventilation syndrome

Essential Respiratory Medicine, First Edition. Shanthi Paramothayan.

Companion website: www.wiley.com/go/paramothayan/essential_respiratory_medicine

Abbreviations

α-1AT	α-1 antitrypsin
α-1ATD	α-1 antitrypsin deficiency
ABG	arterial blood gas
ABPA	allergic bronchopulmonary aspergillosis
ACQ	Asthma Control Questionnaire
ADAPT	Antitrypsin Deficiency Assessment and Programme for Treatment
AHR	airway hyper-responsiveness
BHR	bronchial hyper-responsiveness
BiPAP	bilevel positive airway pressure
CAP	community acquired pneumonia
CAT	COPD Assessment Test
CBT	cognitive behavioural therapy
CO	carbon monoxide
CO_2	carbon dioxide
COPD	chronic obstructive pulmonary disease
CXR	chest X-ray
DNA	deoxyribonucleic acid
ECRHS	European Community Respiratory Health Survey
EGPA	eosinophilic granulomatosis with polyangiitis
FEV_1	forced expiratory volume in one second
FVC	forced vital capacity
GINA	Global Initiative for Asthma
GOLD	Global Initiative for Chronic Obstructive Lung Disease
GP	General Practitioner
HAD	Hospital Anxiety and Depression questionnaire
HDM	house dust mite
HDU	high dependency unit
HRCT	high-resolution computed tomography
HV	hyperventilation
ICS	inhaled corticosteroid
ICU	intensive care unit
Ig	immunoglobulin
IgE	immunoglobin E
ISAAC	International Study of Asthma and Allergy in Children
JVP	jugular venous pressure
KCO	transfer coefficient
LABA	long-acting β_2-agonist
LTOT	long term oxygen therapy
LVRS	lung volume reduction surgery
MRC	Medical Research Council
NICE	National Institute for Health and Care Excellence
NIV	non-invasive ventilation
NO	nitric oxide
NO_2	nitric dioxide
NRAD	National Review of Asthma Deaths
NRT	nicotine replacement therapy
NSAIDS	non-steroidal anti-inflammatory drugs
O_3	ozone
OCS	oral corticosteroids
PEF	peak expiratory flow
PVFM	paradoxical vocal fold motion
QOL	quality of life
RAST	radioallergosorbent test
RV	residual volume
SABA	short-acting β_2-agonist
SIGN	Scottish Intercollegiate Guidelines Network
SO_2	sulphur dioxide
Th1	T-helper lymphocytes 1
Th2	T-helper lymphocytes 2
TLC	total lung capacity
TLCO	transfer factor for carbon monoxide (diffusing capacity)
UK	United Kingdom
VATS	video-assisted thoracoscopic surgery
VCD	vocal cord dysfunction

Introduction

Diseases that cause airway obstruction include asthma, chronic obstructive pulmonary disease (COPD), and bronchiectasis. Bronchiectasis is a suppurative lung disease associated with frequent infective exacerbations. This is discussed in Chapter 12.

Asthma and COPD are common conditions that account for a significant amount of morbidity in the general population, requiring frequent visits to the General Practitioner (GP). Patients with these conditions present with breathlessness, which is worse on exertion, a cough, and chest tightness. These symptoms may be present all the time, as in COPD, or may be intermittent and variable, as in asthma. Patients with asthma and COPD are prone to exacerbations, usually triggered by infection, often requiring hospitalisation.

The differential diagnosis for obstructive airways disease includes α-1 antitrypsin deficiency (α-1 ATD), allergic bronchopulmonary aspergillosis (ABPA), hyperventilation (HV), and vocal cord dysfunction (VCD). The diagnosis of these conditions can be made by taking a detailed history, clinical examination, appropriate radiology (CXR, HRCT), spirometry, and lung function testing with reversibility. Other investigations, such as a methacholine challenge, measurement of immunoglobulin E and aspergillus IgG levels can clarify the diagnosis.

Asthma

Definition

Asthma is a reversible, obstructive airways disease caused by inflammation, hyper-responsiveness, and narrowing of the bronchial tree in a susceptible individual, secondary to a variety of stimuli.

Epidemiology

The exact prevalence of asthma worldwide is unknown because of historic differences in definition, diagnostic criteria, and methods of data collection. The International Study of Asthma and Allergies in Children (ISAAC) and the European Community Respiratory Health Survey (ECRHS) have been monitoring the prevalence of asthma worldwide and have reported an increase since the 1960s, with significant variation between countries. The increased prevalence is mainly in urbanised Western countries, and there are several hypotheses as to the possible reasons for this trend.

The estimated incidence of asthma is 2.6–4/1000 individuals per year in the United Kingdom (UK) and the prevalence is 3–34% worldwide. This equates to approximately 8% of adults and 20% of children with asthma. Mortality from asthma is 4/100 000 in the UK, with 1500 deaths every year.

Children with asthma are usually atopic, have had bronchial hyper-responsiveness (BHR) and wheezing for at least 12 months, and demonstrate variability in peak expiratory flow readings. Many children with evidence of BHR and wheeze, particularly those under 5 years of age, are incorrectly diagnosed as having asthma. Viral respiratory tract infections and passive smoking, particularly maternal cigarette smoking, are risk factors for BHR and wheezing. There is some evidence that neonates who go on to develop asthma later in life have worse lung function in infancy.

Airway hyper-responsiveness (AHR), which includes BHR, is an abnormally exaggerated response to stimuli such as infection, cold air, or exercise, resulting in the contraction of the bronchial smooth muscle. The degree of bronchoconstriction can be measured by the dose of methacholine or histamine required to cause a 20% fall in forced expiratory volume in one second (FEV_1) as discussed in Chapter 4.

Not all individuals with AHR will develop asthma, but because many will have symptoms of dry cough and wheeze when exposed to these triggers, it can be difficult to differentiate between AHR and mild asthma. In adults, the main differential diagnosis for asthma is chronic bronchitis; therefore, adult patients with a history of cigarette smoking should have investigations, including a chest X-ray (CXR) and spirometry with reversibility testing, to establish the correct diagnosis.

A family history of asthma is an important risk factor for developing asthma, even in non-atopic children, with 60% of the susceptibility to asthma being inherited. Twin studies have shown a 19% concordance in monozygotic twins and 4.8% concordance in dizygotic twins. The prevalence of asthma is greater in boys compared to girls, reaching a peak at puberty. The prevalence of asthma in females gradually increases with age, so that it is equal to that in men between the ages of 20 and 40, thereafter becoming more common in females. The reason for this difference is not clear. It has been postulated that it may reflect smaller relative airway size, increased atopy, and differences in the reporting of symptoms in boys.

The **aetiology of asthma** is multifactorial; airway inflammation occurs when a genetically susceptible individual with atopy is exposed to certain environmental factors. **Atopy** is the tendency to produce high amounts of immunoglobulin E (IgE) when exposed to small amounts of an antigen. These patients will demonstrate positive reactions to antigens on skin prick testing. Atopic individuals have a high prevalence of asthma, allergic rhinitis, urticaria, and eczema.

Atopy and asthma show polygenic inheritance and genetic heterogeneity, with gene linkages on chromosome 11q13. The genes responsible for the different components of asthma, such as IgE production, BHR and cytokine production, are found on chromosomes 5q, 7, 11q, 12q, 16, 17, and 21q. The ADAM33 gene on chromosome 70p13, which is a disintegrin and a metalloprotease gene, is involved in the structural airway components of asthma, such as airway remodelling. Expression of this gene may lead to the development of chronic persistent asthma, with irreversible airway obstruction and excess decline in FEV_1 over time.

Environmental factors appear to be important in the development of asthma. The ISAAC study found an increased association between wheeze and atopy in developed, urbanised countries. As people spend more time inside, concentrations of indoor allergens become more important than outdoor allergens. This is particularly important in young children as allergen exposure early in life may be important in determining sensitisation. Exposure to the house dust mite (HDM) *Dermatophagoides pteronyssinus* (found in high concentrations in carpets, soft furnishings, and bedding) in early life may be associated with an increased likelihood of sensitisation to HDM by preschool age. Sensitisation to pet-derived allergens (cat, dog, rabbit) is also common.

There is some evidence that exposure to bacterial and viral antigens in very early life may result in allergen sensitisation and the development of asthma. There appears to be a link between exposure to respiratory syncytial virus, human rhinovirus, mycoplasma pneumonia infections, and the development of asthma.

The hygiene hypothesis, in contrast, postulates that lack of childhood infections results in altered T-cell function and a tendency to develop asthma. Some epidemiological studies have shown that close contact with animals in early life may decrease the prevalence of asthma and allergy, perhaps by the provocation of immune tolerance. The results of studies on domestic allergen avoidance, which are very difficult to conduct, are inconsistent. Atmospheric pollution can worsen asthma, but there is no evidence that it is a cause of asthma. Occupational asthma accounts for 15% of cases of asthma and is discussed in Chapter 15.

Atopic individuals produce IgE antibodies to specific allergens which can be measured in the serum. Skin prick testing can also be used to demonstrate allergy to a specific allergen. A video demonstrating how skin prick testing is performed is found in the supplementary material (www.wiley.com/go/Paramothayan/Essential_Respiratory_Medicine). Serum levels of IgE correlate better with AHR and asthma severity than skin prick testing which correlates better with allergic rhinitis. It is common for atopic individuals to be sensitive to more than one allergen. Individuals with asthma are highly likely to have other atopic conditions, such as allergic rhinitis and atopic dermatitis (eczema). Approximately a third of children with atopic dermatitis will go on to develop asthma in adolescence.

Pathophysiology of asthma

Airway inflammation, caused by various cytokines, results in reversible obstruction throughout the tracheobronchial tree. The reversibility distinguishes asthma from COPD. In a sensitised, atopic individual, inhalation of an allergen results in a two-phase response consisting of an early reaction, reaching its climax in about 20 minutes, and a late reaction, developing 6–12 hours later. In the early response, T-helper lymphocytes have an important role in the regulation of the inflammatory response. Th2 cells secrete pro-inflammatory interleukins, which leads to the release of high levels of allergen-specific IgE antibodies by plasma cells. The IgE antibodies bind to receptors on mast cells and eosinophils and stimulate them to release preformed mediators, including histamine, prostaglandins, platelet-activating factor, tryptase, major basic protein, eosinophil cationic protein, eosinophil protein X, heparin, and cysteinyl leukotrienes. These mediators cause bronchoconstriction within minutes.

The late phase reaction is the result of infiltration of the smooth muscle layer by eosinophils, basophils, neutrophils, monocytes, and dendritic cells, which cause patchy desquamation of the epithelial cells. There is also an increase in the number of mucus glands, goblet cell hyperplasia and hypertrophy, and hyperplasia of the airway smooth muscle. Cytokines released by Th2 Helper cells results in further contraction of the airway smooth muscle, increased permeability of the blood vessels, and increased mucus secretion. Acute inflammation results in oedema and mucus-plugging of the bronchial tree. In contrast, the Th1 cells produce cytokines that down-regulate the atopic response.

Narrowing of bronchi of different calibres results in polyphonic wheezing. Narrowing of the smaller airways with a diameter of less than 2 cm leads to closure of these airways at low lung volumes, resulting in air trapping, an increase in residual volume (RV), an increase in total lung capacity (TLC), and dynamic hyperinflation. High-resolution computed tomography (HRCT) images of the thorax can demonstrate the heterogeneous narrowing of the airways. Bronchoconstriction can also occur through reflex neural mechanisms.

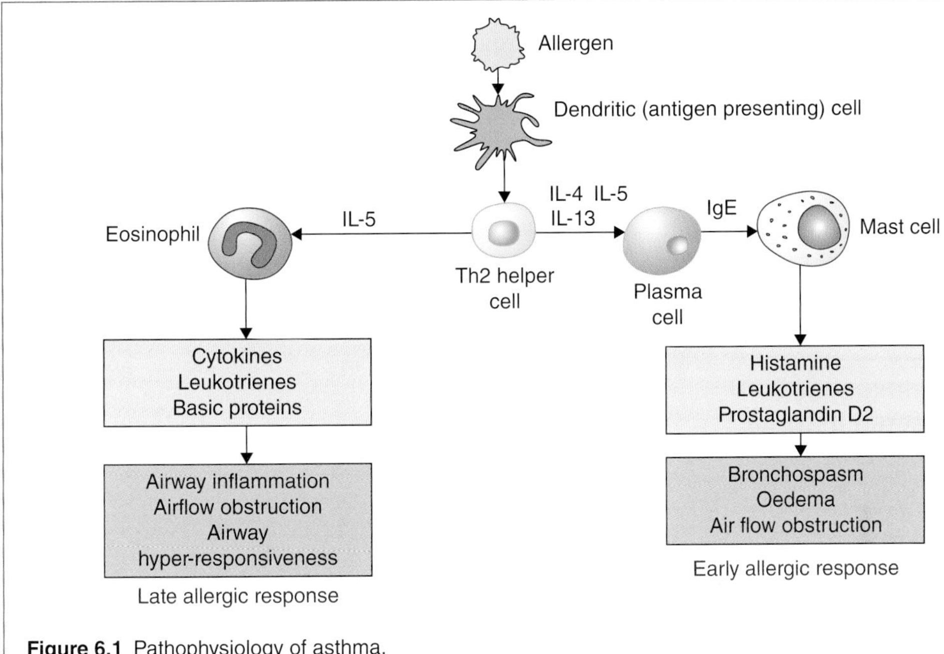

Figure 6.1 Pathophysiology of asthma.

While eosinophils are associated with acute asthma, neutrophils are more prevalent in steroid-dependent asthma, and are associated with chronic, persistent airway inflammation and structural changes. With increased severity and chronicity of asthma, there is remodelling of the airways, with collagen deposition and fibrosis of the airway wall, resulting in fixed narrowing and a decreased response to bronchodilator medication (Figure 6.1).

Clinical presentation

Asthma is a variable, reversible condition and therefore it can be difficult to make a reliable diagnosis between exacerbations when the individual is well. Chronic asthma can result in progressive disease and irreversible airway obstruction.

Clinical history: Patients with asthma present with symptoms of cough, chest tightness, breathlessness, and wheeze. These symptoms are variable and intermittent and may be precipitated by triggers at home or at work. There may be diurnal variation in symptoms, with peak flow measurements usually worse in the mornings compared to the evenings. The differential diagnosis of a patient with breathlessness and wheeze includes bronchiectasis, COPD, allergic bronchopulmonary aspergillosis (ABPA), α-1 antitrypsin deficiency (α-1 ATD), and left ventricular failure.

Cough-variant asthma is common. Patients will present with a persistent dry cough, particularly at night, but with no breathlessness or wheeze. Clinical examination, a CXR, and spirometry may be normal in these individuals. The differential diagnosis of a dry cough in a non-smoker with a normal CXR includes acid reflux, post nasal drip, use of non-steroidal anti-inflammatory drugs, use of angiotensin converting enzyme (ACE) inhibitors for the treatment of hypertension, inhaled foreign body, and post-infectious cough. Vocal cord dysfunction (VCD) and hyperventilation (HV) can be difficult to differentiate from asthma and are discussed later in this chapter.

The clinician should ask the patient about a history of atopy, which includes hay fever, allergic rhinitis, and eczema, and about a family history of atopy. They should document in detail any environmental factors that may be triggering the asthma, both at home and at work. A history of smoking and passive smoking is important.

Clinical examination may be normal in between exacerbations. In patients with severe chronic asthma, there may be signs of hyperinflation as described in Chapter 5. Individuals with childhood asthma, especially if undertreated, may develop a chest deformity. During an acute asthma attack, the patient will be breathless at rest, with increased pulse and respiratory rates, and polyphonic expiratory and inspiratory wheeze due to the narrowing of bronchi of different sizes. In life-threatening asthma, the patient may become cyanosed, have a silent chest, and become bradycardic.

Box 6.1 lists the investigations that may be required in a patient presenting with symptoms of unexplained cough and or breathlessness. Some of these investigations are to rule out other causes of these symptoms and are described in Chapter 4.

Box 6.1 Investigations in suspected asthma.

- Blood tests: Full blood count, IgE, radioallergosorbent test (RAST) if a specific allergy is suspected
- Skin prick test to allergens: tree pollen, grass pollen, dog, cat, horse, feather, HDM, aspergillus fumigatus
- CXR
- HRCT
- Peak expiratory flow (PEF) and PEF homework
- Spirometry
- Full lung function test with reversibility
- Methacholine provocation test
- Exhaled nitric oxide (FeNO)
- Sputum analysis
- Nose and throat examination
- Bronchoscopy

Patients with atopy and asthma often have a mildly raised peripheral blood eosinophilia and raised IgE. Results of skin prick testing must be interpreted carefully as a positive result merely indicates that the patient is sensitised to that allergen and has the potential to develop symptoms when exposed to that allergen. RAST measures the level of circulating IgE to an antigen, for example, cat. Skin prick test positivity to aspergillus fumigatus and positive aspergillus fumigatus IgE and IgG suggests allergic bronchopulmonary aspergillosis (ABPA). Further investigations, including an HRCT and sputum samples for aspergillus, would be indicated. Eosinophilic granulomatosis with polyangiitis (EGPA), formerly known as Churg-Strauss syndrome, can masquerade as asthma, and should be suspected if there is a very high eosinophilic count in peripheral blood and the patient appears to be steroid- dependent. This condition is discussed in Chapter 11.

PEF measurements may show diurnal variation in asthma (Figure 6.2), with a lower value in the morning compared to the evening. PEF homework, which means that the patient keeps a record of their PEF measurements taken in the mornings and the evenings for several weeks, can be helpful. A 20% or greater variability between mornings and evenings suggests asthma.

Spirometry will be obstructive, with a reduced FEV_1 and an FEV_1/FVC ratio of less than 70%.

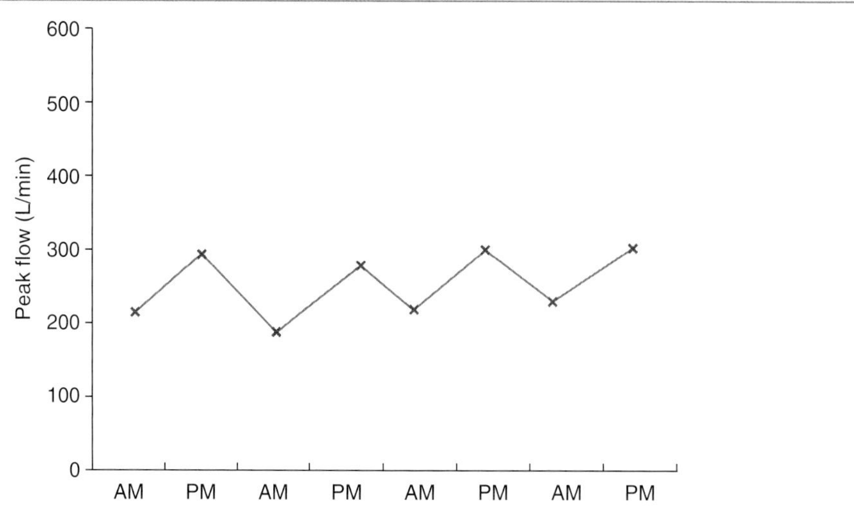

Figure 6.2 Diagram of PEF chart in poorly controlled asthma showing diurnal variation.

See Chapter 4 for the interpretation of spirometry. Improvement in symptoms and in spirometry 20 minutes after a bronchodilator is administered (200 μg inhaled salbutamol or 2.5 mg of nebulised salbutamol) is diagnostic of asthma if the FEV_1 increases by at least 15% of the baseline value or by more than 200 ml. Spirometry values are also used to establish the severity of asthma, which determines the management. Patients with chronic asthma and COPD will have little or no reversibility when given bronchodilators, as they have a fixed obstruction.

Full lung function tests with reversibility can give additional information. In those with chronic asthma, the residual volume (RV) and total lung capacity (TLC) will be increased due to air trapping, but there will be no impairment of gas exchange, so the transfer factor for carbon monoxide (TLCO) will be normal. There may be evidence of small airway disease with a reduction in FEV 25%, FEV 50% and FEV 75%.

Spirometry and lung function tests may be normal in patients with mild asthma in between exacerbations and in those with cough-variant asthma. Additional hyper-reactivity testing with methacholine or histamine can be diagnostic. This is described in Chapter 4. The concentration of the drug that results in a 20% decrease in FEV_1 can be calculated. Exercise can also be used to provoke airway hyperresponsiveness. Exhaled NO levels are increased in patients with asthma and bronchiectasis but will be normal in VCD and hyperventilation, so can be useful in differentiating between these conditions.

The CXR may be normal in mild asthma (Figure 6.3), but may be hyperinflated in chronic asthma, with increased lung volumes and flat diaphragms. The CXR may appear normal in patients with mild bronchiectasis and ABPA, so an HRCT should be considered if these conditions are suspected (Figure 6.4 shows a HRCT in asthma). Differential cell count from induced sputum may show an eosinophilia in asthma. The presence of aspergillus may suggest ABPA.

Nose and throat examinations can be helpful when a patient presents with a persistent dry cough as this will detect evidence of acid reflux, oral candida, and post nasal drip. Nasal polyps may suggest asthma, which is often associated with sensitivity to aspirin. Abnormal adduction of vocal cords during inspiration, made worse by exercise, suggests VCD. Ultrasound of the vocal cords can also show abnormal adduction during inspiration suggestive of VCD.

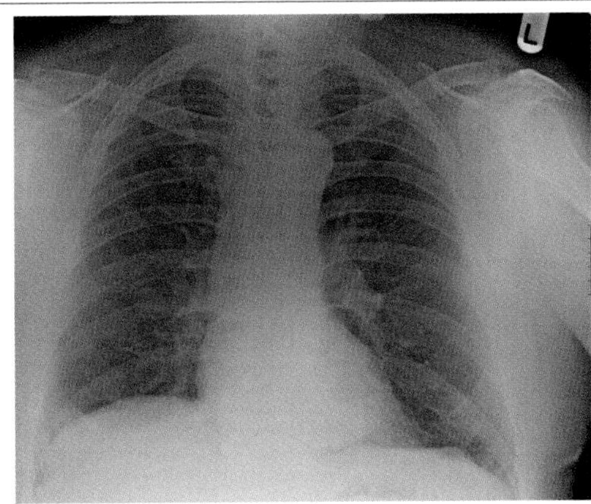

Figure 6.3 CXR in asthma.

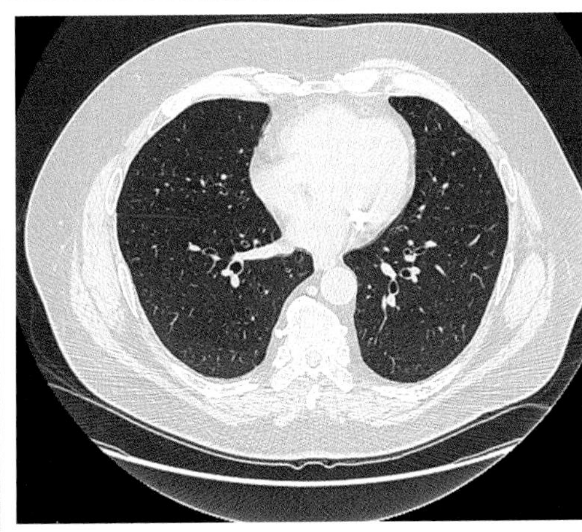

Figure 6.4 HRCT in asthma.

Bronchoscopy with lavage for microbiology may be helpful if an infection is suspected. It is also important to exclude an inhaled foreign body which can be a cause of persistent cough and monophonic wheeze, especially in children. Therapeutic suctioning can clear mucus plugging which can occasionally result in lobar collapse in asthma, resulting in persistent cough, wheeze, and breathlessness.

The algorithm for the diagnosis of asthma is given in Appendix 6.A.

Management of asthma: The aim is to obliterate the symptoms of asthma so that the individual has a good quality of life, with normal exercise tolerance, and no exacerbations. This can be achieved by avoiding allergens that trigger exacerbations and using the appropriate inhaled therapy.

The aim of **inhaled therapy** is to reduce the need for reliever inhaler with no limitation in physical activity. Well-controlled asthma means that the patient requires short-acting β_2-agonist (SABA) less than two days in a week, and less than two nights a month. Appropriate inhaled therapy should achieve the best lung function possible with the minimum of side effects. There should be no more than one exacerbation per year requiring OCS and no hospital admissions.

Inhaled therapy should be prescribed as recommended by NICE/Scottish Intercollegiate Guidelines Network (SIGN), with a stepwise increase in therapy. If the asthma is poorly controlled, then treatment should be 'stepped up'. When there is better control, then 'stepping-down' therapy can be considered. The mechanism of action of the drugs used to treat asthma, their side effects and interactions, inhaler devices, and nebulisers are discussed in Chapter 3. The management of asthma is given in Appendix 6.B.

Step 1: mild, intermittent symptoms. Reliever short-acting β_2-agonist (SABA) such as salbutamol or terbutaline used as and when required. If the patient requires them more than twice a day, then move to step 2.

Step 2: Regular prevention therapy. Add ICS 200–800 $\mu g\,day^{-1}$.

Step 3: Add-on therapy. Commence long-acting β_2-agonist (LABA), or increase dose of inhaled corticosteroid (ICS) to 800 $\mu g\,day^{-1}$, or consider leukotriene inhibitor.

Step 4: Persistent poor control. Consider increasing dose of ICS further, or add theophylline.

Step 5: Severe symptoms, frequent or continuous use of OCS. Use lowest dose of OCS, maintain ICS at 2000 $\mu g\,day^{-1}$

ICS are the most effective preventative drugs in adults and children for maintaining control in asthma. They should be prescribed to all who have had exacerbations or nocturnal asthma, and those using β-2 agonist more than twice a day. A reasonable starting dose is 400 $\mu g\,day^{-1}$ for adults and should be titrated for effective control.

Patients at Step 4 or Step 5 should be referred to the respiratory physician. Other conditions, such as ABPA or bronchiectasis, will need to be excluded. Individuals with poor asthma control despite treatment with adequate doses of inhaled corticosteroid (ICS), long-acting β_2-agonist (LABA), and leukotriene inhibitor may require a higher dose of ICS, up to 2000 $\mu g\,day^{-1}$. Oral theophylline, a weak bronchodilator, can be introduced at Step 4, usually at a dose of 400 mg daily. The mechanism of action of theophylline, contraindications for its use, side effects, and drug interactions are discussed in Chapter 3.

Some patients with severe asthma appear to be steroid-dependent and experience worsening of their symptoms when the dose of OCS is reduced below a dose of 10 mg daily. Conditions such as EGPA, COPD, and ABPA should be excluded. Compliance and inhaler technique should always be checked.

Patients with allergic asthma have high concentrations of IgE which leads to the secretion of cytokines and mediators which cause bronchoconstriction. Omalizumab (Xolair) is a recombinant humanised immunoglobulin G1 monoclonal antibody that binds to the circulating IgE, forming immune complexes that are cleared by the reticuloendothelial system. Omalizumab prevents IgE from binding to receptors on mast cells, eosinophils, and basophils, thus reducing the effect of the late phase response, with decreased production of cytokines. Omalizumab is indicated for the treatment of patients with asthma who are not controlled at Step 5, who require frequent courses of OCS, and who have high levels of IgE. It is given subcutaneously in a hospital setting as there is a risk of anaphylaxis in 1–2/1000.

There is evidence to support the hypothesis that vitamin D deficiency can worsen the control of asthma. Therefore, patients with vitamin D deficiency should be prescribed supplements. Bronchial thermoplasty, a procedure available in a few centres, is a technique whereby radio-frequency waves are used to apply heat through a bronchoscope to reduce the amount of smooth muscle in the bronchial wall mucosa, resulting in reduced bronchoconstriction. This has been shown to improve asthma control in some patients with severe asthma who are not well controlled with other treatments. The long term benefits and risks of this treatment are not fully understood.

Role of doctor or asthma nurse: Patients with asthma should have regular reviews (at least once every six months) by a trained healthcare professional. He/She should assesses their symptoms, their compliance with therapy, any over-use of short-acting β_2-agonist (SABA), possible under-use of ICS, conduct spirometry, and assess their inhaler technique. The patient should have a self-management plan which describes what medication to take, how to increase the medication when symptoms deteriorate, and what to do if they experience an exacerbation. The management plan should include the role of PEF monitoring, with advice to take oral corticosteroids (OCS) and seek medical help if their PEF drops below 75% of their best or predicted PEF. Patients should be aware of environmental triggers and should avoid these as much as possible. Patients who smoke should be advised to quit, and nicotine replacement therapy (NRT) prescribed, as discussed in Chapter 3. Patients with asthma should have an annual influenza vaccination and a pneumococcal vaccination. Regular review by a doctor or specialist nurse has been shown to improve daily control of asthma symptoms with a reduction in the risk of near-fatal or fatal asthma exacerbation. Patients with moderately severe or severe asthma should have a supply of OCS to take in an emergency.

The Global Initiative for Asthma (GINA) suggests asking the following questions to assess symptom control over the past four weeks as listed in Box 6.2. There are other validated questionnaires to assess symptom control, including the Asthma Control Questionnaire (ACQ-5) score and the ACT score.

Box 6.2 GINA assessment of symptoms control.

1. Daytime asthma symptoms more than 2 × week
2. Any night-time waking 2 × week due to asthma
3. Reliever needed for asthma >2 × week
4. Any limitation of normal activity due to asthma

None of the above: asthma is well controlled.
1–2 of the above: asthma partly controlled.
1–4 of the above: asthma poorly controlled.

Box 6.3 lists some of the recognised triggers for acute asthma.

Box 6.3 Triggers for acute asthma.

Environmental

• Animal-derived allergen	• Cigarette smoking
• Bird-derived allergen	• Passive cigarette smoking
• House dust mite (HDM)	• Fireplace smoke
• Pollen	• Chlorine (household cleaners, swimming pools)
• Grass	• Paints
• Mould	• New furnishings releasing volatile compounds
• Atmospheric pollution	• Exercise
• Ozone (SO_2, NO_2, O_3)	• Cold air
• Perfumes, hair sprays	

Drugs

• Aspirin	• β-blockers
• NSAIDS	• Sulphite (wine, vinegar, dried fruit)

Infection

• Viral respiratory tract infection	• Bacterial respiratory tract infection

Hormonal

• Premenstrual	• Pregnancy
• Stress	

Avoidance of triggers: Patients should be advised to either avoid or reduce exposure to any triggers that have been identified. If a skin prick test or RAST test confirms allergy to an animal, then exposure should be removed or limited. If the patient is allergic to HDM, then they should be advised to remove carpets and reduce the amount soft furnishings which harbour HDM. Mattress and pillow protectors can be purchased which may help. Individuals with any drug reaction should avoid those medications. Patients should be advised to avoid scented perfumes, air sprays, hair sprays, and aerosols.

Thunderstorms can trigger an asthma exacerbation by lifting allergens into the air and by disrupting pollen grains into smaller allergenic particles, which are more easily inhaled. High pressure, with warm, dry, still air, results in an accumulation of airborne pollutants, including particulates, such as ozone (O_3), nitric dioxide (NO_2), and sulphur dioxide (SO_2), as well as pollen and fungal spores, which can trigger an asthma attack. Desert dust contains crystalline silica and can be transported across large parts of the globe in a storm. Temperature and humidity may play a role in exercise-induced asthma. Inhalation of cold, dry air can result in bronchoconstriction caused by water loss and cooling of the airways after a rapid flow of blood into the airway blood vessels, resulting in oedema. Hot, humid air can also lead to bronchoconstriction mediated by the vagal system.

If the trigger to an asthma attack cannot be avoided, then the patient should be advised to take a dose of bronchodilator, for example, prior to exercise. Patients should be advised to warm up gradually before exercise. Leukotriene antagonists are recommended for patients with exercise-induced asthma. For those with severe atopy, antihistamines might help with symptom control.

Worsening of asthma symptoms prior to or during menstruation has been reported in 20–40% of women with asthma. It is postulated that this is due to the increase in the levels of oestrogen and progesterone. Aspirin sensitivity may be more prevalent in women with perimenstrual asthma. Hormonal treatment with the oral contraceptive pill has not been found to be helpful. Although no clear trial data exists, leukotriene antagonists may be helpful in this group of patients. During pregnancy, asthma can get worse in a third of patients, remain the same in a third, and get worse in a third. Management of asthma is the same as in the non-pregnant individual.

Non-selective β-blockers (for example, those prescribed in eye drops), aspirin, and NSAIDs are responsible for acute exacerbation in 3–5% of adults. Those with nasal polyposis are at a higher risk of aspirin sensitivity. Depression and chronic stress can worsen the control of asthma. Parental depression and stress are associated with severe asthma in children.

Viral infections, especially influenza and respiratory syncytial virus, are common causes of asthma exacerbations. Therefore, patients with asthma should be advised to have the influenza vaccination. Food allergies can cause asthma if the aerolised allergen, in the form of steam, vapour, or sprays is inhaled. Sulphite sensitivity can cause asthma symptoms, but not in an IgE-mediated way.

Prognosis of asthma: Most patients with asthma remain reasonably stable with only one or two exacerbations every year which can be managed with oral corticosteroids (OCS) and antibiotics if there is evidence of a bacterial respiratory tract infection. In the UK, 20% of patients with asthma account for 80% of the overall costs of managing asthma, amounting to one billion pounds every year.

Acute asthma exacerbation can be severe and life-threatening. Approximately 1500 people die each year from acute asthma in the UK. Many of these deaths are preventable, as published in the National Review of Asthma Deaths (NRAD) in 2012. Near-fatal exacerbations can occur in those even with mild asthma and can be of slow or rapid onset. Deaths occur for the following reasons: failure to recognise the severity of the asthma attack, delay in starting appropriate treatment, under-prescription of inhaled corticosteroids, discharging the patient too early, and delay in referring the patient to the intensive care unit (ICU). Deaths also occur because of poor compliance by the patient and because patients and doctors often under-estimate the risk of a fatal asthma attack. The term 'brittle asthma' is used to describe those with significant diurnal PEF variability despite adequate treatment and those who suffer sudden, unexpected exacerbations. Box 6.4 lists those patients who have risk factors for fatal asthma. Box 6.5 lists the presentation of patients with a severe asthma exacerbation who require careful assessment and possible admission. Box 6.6

Box 6.4 Risk factors for fatal asthma.

• Recent exacerbation	• Sensitivity to NSAID and aspirin
• Recent hospital admission	• Poor perception of dyspnoea
• Previous ICU admission with intubation	• Over-use of SABA
• Requiring >3 types of asthma medication	• Under-use of ICS
• Dependence on OCS	• Delay in seeking medical help
• Poor compliance	• Brittle asthma

Box 6.5 Patients requiring admission to hospital from asthma.

- Worsening symptoms of breathlessness, wheeze, and cough
- Nocturnal symptoms of breathlessness, wheeze, and cough
- Increasing use of β_2-agonist reliever
- Poor response to OCS
- Peak expiratory flow <75% predicted or best
- Pregnant
- Living alone
- Previous near-fatal asthma
- Brittle asthma
- Psychological problems, including evidence of poor compliance

describes the clinical features of acute, severe asthma and life-threatening asthma.

These features suggest impending respiratory arrest.

Management of acute asthma: The doctor should take a thorough history if possible, noting the important points described above. Treatment should be commenced without delay. Auscultation of the chest and blood pressure measurement should be done periodically to ensure that there is improvement. Oxygen saturation should be monitored continuously and serial ABG measurements made. Box 6.7 lists the urgent investigations usually done in the emergency department. Box 6.8 describes the medication given to a patient with acute severe asthma exacerbation.

Box 6.6 Features of acute severe asthma and life-threatening asthma.

Acute severe asthma

• Peak expiratory flow (PEF) ≤50% predicted	• Pulse rate >110 beats min^{-1}
• Unable to complete sentences in one breath	• Polyphonic wheeze
• Respiratory rate >25 breaths min^{-1}	• $paCO_2$ normal and rising on serial ABG

Life-threatening asthma

• PEF<35% predicted or unrecordable	• SpO_2<92% on air
• Feeble respiratory effort	• Exhaustion
• Cyanosis	• Confusion
• Silent chest	• Rising $PaCO_2$
• Bradycardia	• Hypotension

Monitoring of patients with severe acute asthma: Patients who present with symptoms of a severe asthma exacerbation should be monitored closely in the high dependency unit (HDU) or ICU and will require regular clinical assessment and urgent review by a senior doctor. The oxygen saturation should be maintained above 92% and high flow oxygen can be given if required. Serial ABG measurements should be done as indicated by the patient's clinical status. Patients with acute asthma will have a high respiratory rate and therefore become hypocapnic as they blow off CO_2. A normal or rising $PaCO_2$ (>4.6 kPa) and a pH of less than 7.35 would be cause for concern. If the patient does not improve within 1 hour of initial management, then intubation and ventilation may be required to prevent respiratory arrest.

Box 6.7 Urgent investigations for acute asthma.

- Chest X-ray to exclude consolidation, pneumothorax, and pleural effusion
- Oxygen saturation with continuous monitoring
- Baseline ABG on air if $SpO_2 < 92\%$ with repeat ABG test to monitor $PaCO_2$ level and pH
- ECG every 30 minutes
- Blood tests to measure full blood count, urea and electrolytes, C-reactive protein, and aminophylline level if on aminophylline

Referral to the intensive care team and the on-call anaesthetist should be made urgently. Non-invasive ventilation (BiPAP) is not usually indicated for patients with respiratory failure secondary to asthma.

It is essential that patients who present with severe asthma and are admitted to hospital are assessed carefully prior to discharge. Box 6.9 lists key points to consider before discharge.

National Review of Asthma Deaths (NRAD): A confidential enquiry into over 200 asthma deaths in 2012 concluded that many of these deaths were preventable. Most of the deaths of young people occurred in the summer and in the winter of elderly patients. Most patients who died had chronic,

Box 6.8 Immediate treatment for acute asthma.

- Oxygen 40–60% given via a Hudson mask to maintain SpO_2 between 94% and 98%. Patients with asthma do not usually retain CO_2 secondary to oxygen therapy. Continuous monitoring of oxygen saturation
- Salbutamol 2.5–5 mg via oxygen-driven nebuliser at a flow rate of 6 L min^{-1}. Repeat dose at 15-minute intervals if no improvement. Continuous nebulisation if required. When a nebuliser is not available, salbutamol can be given via a large volume spacer
- Ipratropium bromide (atrovent), 500 µg at 6-hourly intervals, driven via oxygen-driven nebuliser at a flow rate of 6 L min^{-1}. The combination of salbutamol and ipratropium bromide results in a much greater bronchodilatation than salbutamol alone
- Corticosteroids can be given orally (prednisolone 40–50 mg daily) or intravenously (hydrocortisone 200 mg initially and then 100 mg 6 hourly). Prednisolone should be given as quickly as possible and continued for at least two weeks; a tapering reduction in dose is not required. Steroids have been shown to reduce mortality in asthma exacerbation
- Intravenous magnesium sulfate 2 g (8 mmol) in 250 ml sodium chloride 0.9% over 1 hour. It causes relaxation of airway smooth muscle
- Intravenous fluids with potassium supplements if necessary, as hypokalaemia can develop secondary to β_2-agonist usage
- Intravenous aminophylline, 250 mg in 100 ml sodium chloride 0.9% over 30 minutes as a loading dose, followed by an infusion (750 mg/24 hours); blood concentration of aminophylline should be monitored if the infusion is continued for over 24 hours. Bolus of aminophylline should not be given to patients who are already on oral preparations of this drug. Lower doses should be used in patients with heart failure, hepatic failure, and in those taking drugs which are cytochrome P450 enzyme inhibitors, such as cimetidine, ciprofloxacin, and erythromycin
- Antibiotics if symptoms and signs of a bacterial respiratory tract infection
- Intravenous β_2-agonist, salbutamol 3–20 µg min^{-1} or terbutaline 1.5–5 µg min^{-1} infusion, can be considered for patients with life-threatening asthma who are not improving despite management so far listed. There is no strong evidence that the intravenous route is better than the inhaled route. Cardiac monitoring will be required as intravenous β_2-agonists can cause cardiac arrhythmias
- Intravenous methylprednisolone, 80 mg in 100 ml sodium chloride 0.9% over 1 hour, can be given if patient not responding to the above treatments and can be repeated daily for up to three days
- Intubation and ventilation if patient shows signs of life-threatening asthma

Box 6.9 Checklist prior to discharge.

- The PEF should be more than 75% of their predicted or best and PEF diurnal variability should be less than 25%
- The nebulised therapy should have been stopped for at least 24 hours and the patient stable on their discharge medication for at least 24 hours
- The patient should be on appropriate inhalers (ICS and LABA) and the inhaler technique must be checked
- The patient should be discharged home on a short course of oral prednisolone
- The patient should be given a peak flow meter and a self-management plan
- The side effects of the drugs prescribed should be discussed
- The patient should be strongly advised to stop smoking and referred to a smoking cessation clinic
- The patient should be advised to have an annual influenza vaccination
- The patient should be advised to avoid triggers which cause exacerbation
- Follow-up appointment with the GP, community or hospital respiratory teams should be organised within two weeks of discharge

severe asthma which was not being appropriately managed, with insufficient inhaled or oral steroids, and excessive use of SABA and LABA on their own. Nearly half the deaths occurred in patients who had had a previous hospital admission. These high-risk patients were not being reviewed regularly and had not been referred to a specialist. There was a lack of compliance from some patients, lack of education about their condition, with only 23% having a written self-management plan. Many of these patients had an underlying psychological problem. During an exacerbation, there was a failure by the patient and health care professional to recognise the severity of the condition and manage it appropriately. The majority developed their symptoms of asthma exacerbation over a 48-hour period, which means that there should have been sufficient time to intervene.

Chronic asthma: A proportion of patients with asthma go on to develop irreversible airway obstruction, which is less responsive to OCS. These patients will have chronic symptoms of breathlessness, cough, and wheeze, and it can be difficult to distinguish them from those with COPD. These individuals develop structural changes in the airways, with permanent damage to the epithelium, increase in the number of goblet cells, thickening of the lamina reticularis (the sub-basement membrane), increased smooth muscle mass and formation of extracellular matrix. This process is called remodelling and causes distortion of the airways. Management is as for asthma and COPD.

Chronic obstructive pulmonary disease (COPD)

COPD is characterised by progressive airflow obstruction which is not fully reversible and does not change markedly over several months. In 90% of cases, COPD develops because of damage caused by cigarette smoking. The total number of cigarettes smoked daily over the number of years, which can be calculated as the number of pack years, indicates the risk of developing COPD. Cigar and pipe smoking also increase the risk of COPD, but to a lesser extent than cigarette smoking. Other risk factors for developing COPD include passive smoking, occupational exposure to dusts, coal mining, air pollution, and smoke from indoor cooking fires. α-1 antitrypsin deficiency (α-1ATD) accounts for 1% of cases of COPD. This is discussed later in this chapter.

COPD increases with age, being particularly prevalent in those over the age of 65 years. The ageing process itself results in a decline in FEV_1 of about 30 ml/year after the age of 30, but smoking accelerates this decline (Figure 6.5).

Only 15–25% of individuals who smoke develop COPD, therefore genetic factors which confer susceptibility are implicated. Exactly what these are is unclear. COPD is commoner in urban areas compared to rural areas and is more prevalent in lower socio-economic groups, particularly in those with poor nutrition.

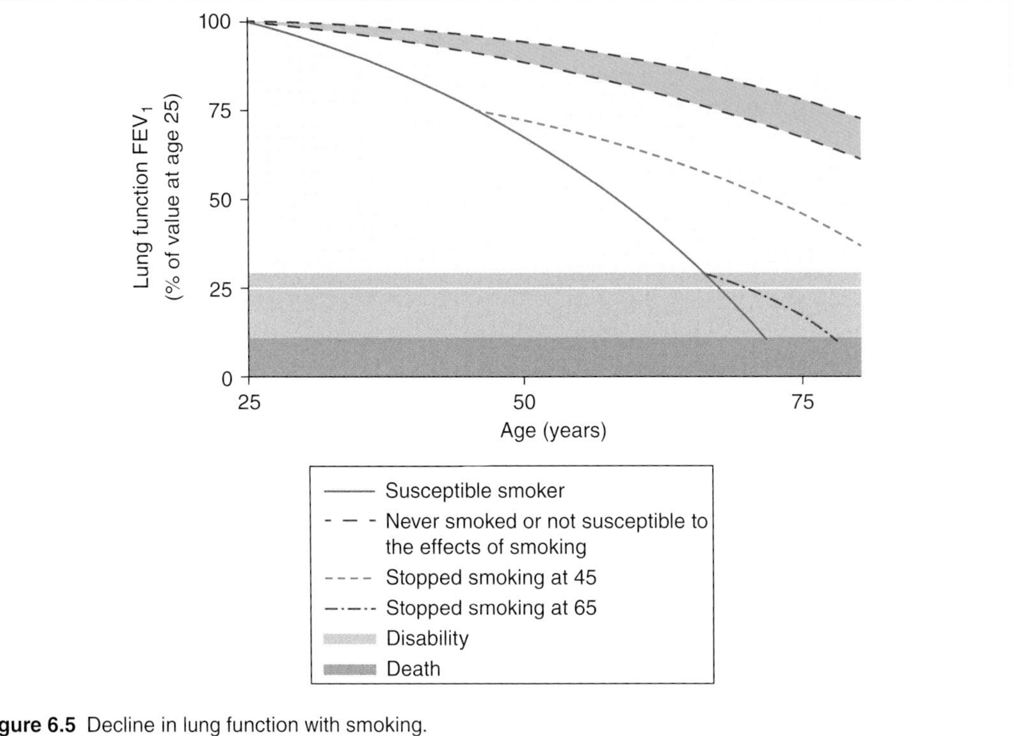

Figure 6.5 Decline in lung function with smoking.

Worldwide, COPD is responsible for considerable morbidity and mortality. The number of young people who have started smoking has increased in Eastern Europe, China, and India in the past few decades. It is predicted that by 2020 COPD will be the third commonest cause of death worldwide. In the UK, approximately three million people have COPD, 15% of men and 5% of women. Many individuals with COPD are undiagnosed and therefore not treated. COPD exacerbations are responsible for a third of hospital admissions, and COPD causes around 30 000 deaths every year in the UK. It is a huge economic burden on the NHS, estimated as almost one billion pounds every year. COPD has a significant effect on patients' quality of life and their ability to continue with their normal activities.

Pathophysiology of COPD: Patients with COPD present primarily with symptoms of chronic bronchitis (chronic productive cough) and emphysema (severe breathlessness on exertion) (Figure 6.6). Cigarette smoke activates neutrophils in the lungs which invade the bronchial mucosa and secrete proteases, including elastase and collagenase, which damage the alveoli, resulting in the formation of bullae. In healthy lungs, enzymes that counteract these proteases, such as the enzyme α-1AT, maintain a balance, so that healthy lung tissue is not damaged. However, in the lungs of smokers, the increased production of proteases compared to anti-proteases results in the destruction of the alveolar sacs, with the formation of large bullae, particularly in the upper zones of the lungs. This progresses to the development of widespread emphysema. Much of the alveolar surface of the lung is destroyed and not available for gas exchange; this can be measured as a reduction in TLCO and KCO. The ventilation/perfusion mismatch results in an increase in the alveolar-arterial gradient (A-a gradient) and hypoxaemia. Hypoxic pulmonary vasoconstriction results in raised pulmonary artery pressure and, over time, leads to pulmonary hypertension and right heart failure (cor pulmonale).

Patients with chronic bronchitis develop inflammation of the airways with fixed structural changes. There is an increase in the number of goblet cells and hypertrophy of the goblet cells, resulting in the production of viscous mucus which is hard to clear. This mucus acts as a culture medium

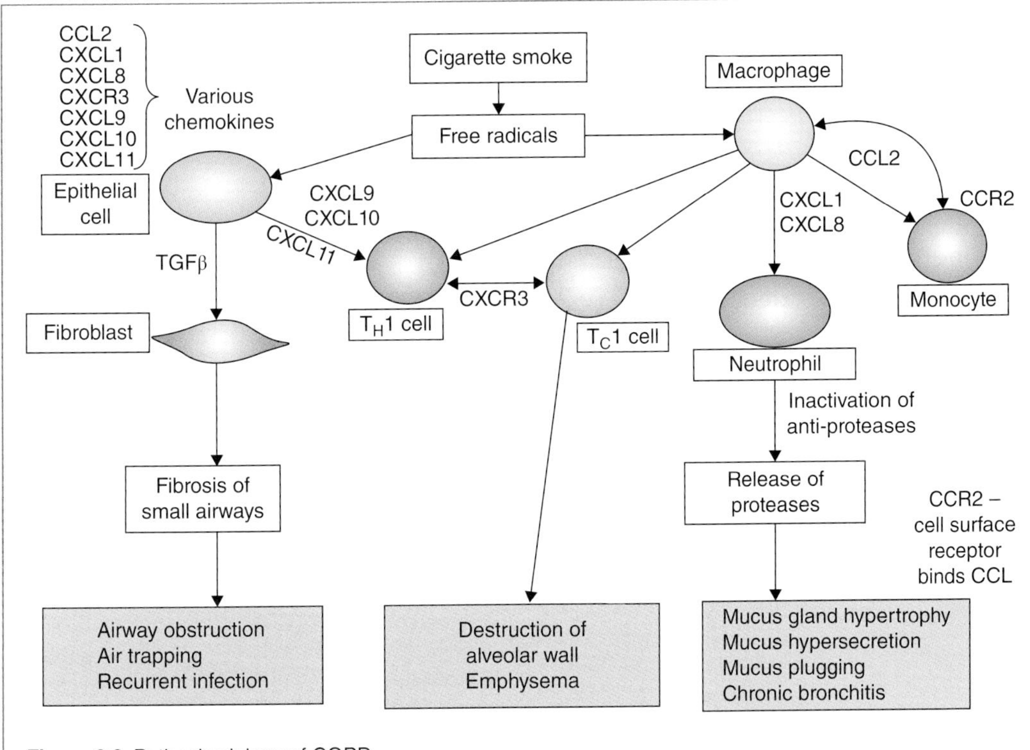

Figure 6.6 Pathophysiology of COPD.

for infective organisms. Damage to cilia affects the host defence mechanisms, which also predisposes to recurrent respiratory tract infections. Recurrent infections lead to further inflammation of the lungs, and a decline in lung function.

Mechanical changes result in increased airway resistance and a loss of the elastic recoil of the lungs, so that they collapse on expiration, causing air trapping and hyperinflation. This increases the work of breathing; therefore, the patient needs to use accessory muscles of breathing to overcome the resistance and adopts pursed-lip breathing to force the air out.

Clinical presentation of COPD: Box 6.10 lists the symptoms and signs of COPD. In mild COPD, clinical examination may be normal but as the condition gets worse, signs will become apparent, especially during an exacerbation. Patients who develop type 2 respiratory failure may show signs of CO_2 retention. Patients with severe COPD may have the signs of cor pulmonale, which is right heart failure secondary to chronic lung disease. This will result in pulmonary hypertension.

It is important to determine the extent of breathlessness as this correlates with the severity of COPD. Baseline measurement can be helpful in determining the prognosis and in assessing the impact of any treatment. The Medical Research Council (MRC) Dyspnoea Scale is commonly used and is described in Box 6.11. Other measures which can be used to determine the extent of breathlessness include the shuttle test and the 6-minute walk test, which are described in Chapter 4. There are several validated questionnaires which can be used to assess overall function, quality of life (QOL), and impact of the disease. The St. George's Respiratory Questionnaire is a validated, comprehensive, disease-specific, health-related score used in many trials, but too lengthy to use in routine clinical practice. The COPD Assessment Test (CAT), which is an 8-item measure of the patient's symptoms, can be used to assess and monitor patients' symptoms at each clinic visit.

A diagnosis of COPD should be suspected in any individual over the age of 40 years who presents with symptoms of breathlessness and has a

Box 6.10 Symptoms and signs of COPD.

Symptoms
- Breathlessness on exertion (dyspnoea)
- Wheeze
- Frequent lower respiratory tract infections
- Chronic productive cough

Signs
- Tachypnoea (respiratory rate > 25 breaths min^{-1})
- Tachycardia (> 100 beats min^{-1})
- Barrel chest
- Use of accessory muscles
- Increased anteroposterior diameter of thoracic cage
- Pursed-lip breathing
- Cyanosis
- Prolonged expiratory phase of respiration
- Polyphonic expiratory wheeze
- CO_2 retention: confusion, irritability, flapping tremor, bounding pulse, papilloedema
- Cor pulmonale: raised JVP, peripheral oedema
- Pulmonary hypertension: loud P2 and right ventricular heave
- Reduced muscle mass
- Cachexia

Box 6.11 MRC dyspnoea scale.

Grade 1	breathless only on strenuous exertion
Grade 2	breathless when walking up a slight hill
Grade 3	breathless when walking on flat ground
Grade 4	breathless on walking 100 metres
Grade 5	breathless on dressing or undressing

history of cigarette smoking. Spirometry showing an FEV_1/FVC ratio of less than 70% predicted post administration of a short-acting bronchodilator confirms the diagnosis of COPD. The Global Initiative for Chronic Obstructive Lung Disease (GOLD) and NICE define severity of COPD as Mild, Moderate, Severe, and Very Severe, based on the spirometry values when the FEV_1/FVC is less than 70% predicted.

Mild	$FEV_1 \geq 80\%$
Moderate	FEV_1 50–79%
Severe	FEV_1 30–49%
Very severe	$FEV_1 \leq 30\%$

Other investigations in the diagnosis of COPD: To establish that the airway obstruction is irreversible, spirometry should be done after giving a SABA. Reversibility testing after a trial of corticosteroids is not recommended in the diagnosis of COPD. Full lung function tests will show that the total lung capacity (TLC) and the residual volume (RV) are increased due to air trapping and static hyperinflation. The destruction of alveoli, with a reduction in surface area for gas exchange, will result in a reduction in transfer factor for CO (TLCO) and transfer coefficient (KCO). Interpretation of the lung function test in COPD is discussed in Chapter 4.

Pulse oximetry may be normal in mild COPD, but may gradually drop to below 90%, initially on exertion, and then at rest. Patients experiencing an exacerbation will frequently have a low oxygen saturation. Patients who have oxygen saturation less than 92% when breathing room air will require the measurement of arterial blood gas (ABG) to ascertain the PaO_2 and $PaCO_2$ levels. Patients with oxygen saturation level below 90%, and who are found to be in type 1 or type 2 respiratory failure, will require careful oxygen therapy to prevent respiratory acidosis (see Chapter 13).

A CXR is recommended in all patients presenting with symptoms suggestive of COPD to exclude other conditions which can present with similar symptoms, including community acquired pneumonia, pneumothorax, lung cancer, pulmonary embolus, and heart failure. In COPD, particularly if the patient has emphysema, the CXR will show hyperinflation, with flat diaphragms, increased retrosternal airspace, and an elongated cardiac shadow (Figure 6.7). When there is significant bullous

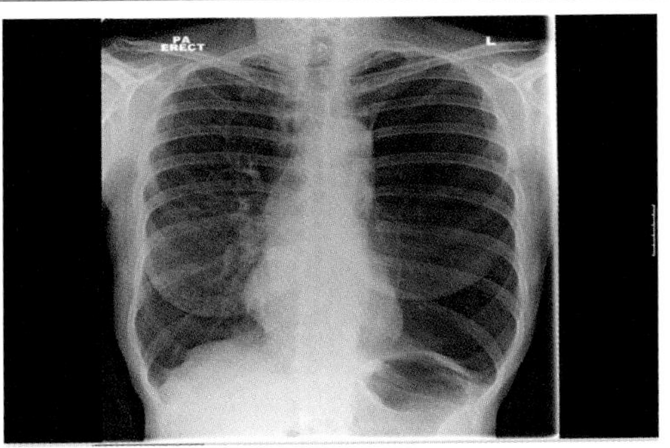

Figure 6.7 CXR in COPD showing hyperinflation.

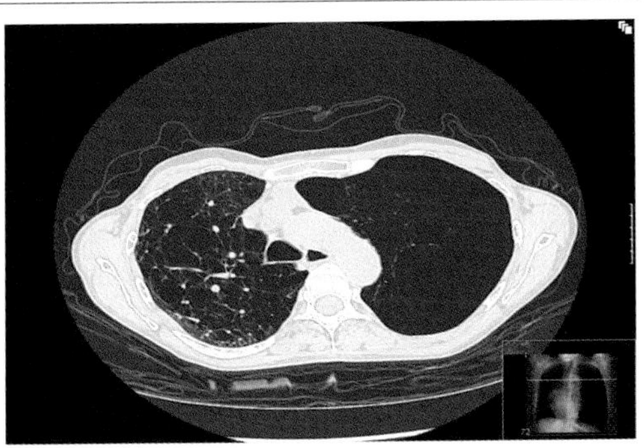

Figure 6.8 HRCT showing a large bulla in left lung in severe emphysema.

Box 6.12 Smoking cessation actions.

ASK:	identify smokers at every visit
ADVISE:	every patient who smokes to quit
ASSESS:	assess their willingness to quit
ASSIST:	provide access to counselling and prescribe pharmacotherapy
ARRANGE:	follow-up

disease, the lung fields may appear black. An HRCT will show centrilobular emphysema, predominantly in the upper zones when due to cigarette smoking (Figure 6.8). α-1ATD is associated with pan acinar emphysema in the lower lobes and is discussed later in this chapter.

A patient presenting for the first time with symptoms of breathlessness should have full blood count, and urea and electrolytes measured. Patients with severe, long-standing COPD can develop secondary polycythaemia due to chronic hypoxia. This can exacerbate the development of pulmonary hypertension.

Objective measurement of exercise capacity with the shuttle walk test or 6-minute walk test can be of prognostic value and an important component of the body mass index, airflow obstruction, dyspnea and exercise (BODE) index, which is used when selecting patients for lung volume reduction surgery or lung transplantation. Exercise capacity falls significantly in the year before death. Measurement of inspiratory, expiratory, and quadricep muscle strength is not normally indicated in routine clinical practice but may be part of the investigations required prior to transplantation.

The aim of **management of COPD** is to prevent progression of the disease, relieve symptoms, improve the quality of life, reduce morbidity, and prevent hospital admissions. It includes lifestyle changes, most importantly smoking cessation, pharmacological treatment, pulmonary rehabilitation, nutrition, and psychological support. Patients with severe COPD may require long term oxygen therapy (LTOT). Some patients, especially those who are under the age of 60 years with no significant co-morbidities, should be referred for consideration of lung transplantation. Patients with chronic type 2 respiratory failure can be managed with domiciliary non-invasive ventilation (NIV) and LTOT. There should be recognition of severe, end-stage COPD. The doctor should have a discussion with the patient and their family members about palliation, referral to the hospice, and 'Do Not Attempt Resuscitation (DNAR)' decisions.

Smoking cessation is the only intervention that reduces the progression of the disease and the risk of death. The earlier the diagnosis of COPD is made, and the earlier the patient stops smoking, the better the outcome. The GOLD guidelines recommend that all healthcare professionals should ensure that they ask the 5 A questions as listed in Box 6.12.

The pharmacological agents used to help people to stop smoking are discussed in Chapter 3.

Large, multi-centre, international studies have concluded that **inhaled therapy** improves symptoms, improves QOL, and reduces the number of exacerbations and hospital admissions. These trials have not shown that inhaled therapy reduces the decline in lung function or reduces mortality. Benefit from inhaled therapy is seen mainly in those with moderate and severe COPD.

Inhaled therapy includes SABA, such as salbutamol and terbutaline, LABA, such as salmeterol and formoterol, short-acting anticholinergic drugs, such as ipratropium bromide, long-acting anticholinergic drugs, such as tiotropium and aclidinium and inhaled corticosteroids (ICS).

SABA and LABA improve symptoms and reduce the risk of exacerbations, especially when they are combined. Combining bronchodilators with different modes of pharmacological action gives sustained bronchodilation with fewer side effects. LABA are more effective at symptom control and in reducing exacerbations than the short-acting drugs. ICS are also recommended for patients with moderate or severe COPD ($FEV_1 < 60\%$ predicted) who have experienced at least two exacerbations in the previous year, although the dose-response relationships is unknown in COPD. ICS, when combined with a LABA, has been shown to improve symptoms, quality of life (QOL), and reduce frequency of exacerbations and hospital admissions. They do, however, increase the risk of non-fatal pneumonia. A combination of ICS, LABA, and LAMA (often called triple therapy) is recommended for those with severe COPD.

The flowchart of inhaled therapy in COPD (see Appendix 6.C) describes the management of mild and severe COPD as per the NICE Guidelines. The pharmacology of the inhaled drugs, their side effects, drug interactions, and the devices used to deliver these drugs is discussed in Chapter 3.

Roflumilast, a phosphodiesterase-4 inhibitor, has been shown to reduce exacerbations in those with moderate and severe COPD. Theophylline, a phosphodiesterase-5 inhibitor, can also be considered in those with moderate and severe COPD who are still symptomatic despite optimal inhaled therapy. Slow-release preparations are used in COPD, but theophylline has a narrow therapeutic range with a high risk of toxicity which is dose-related. A mucolytic drug, such as carbocisteine, can improve the symptom of chronic, productive cough in some, but not all, patients.

Pulmonary rehabilitation has been shown to be an effective intervention when a patient is discharged from hospital after an acute exacerbation. Pulmonary rehabilitation improves breathlessness, exercise tolerance, muscle strength, and QOL, especially in those with dyspnoea and a Medical Research Council (MRC) score of 3–5. Pulmonary rehabilitation includes exercises to strengthen the deconditioned muscles of the arms, legs, and muscles of respiration. An eight-week programme, comprising of aerobic exercises three times a week, is carried out by trained nurse specialists and physiotherapists. The exercise programme should be continued for maximum and ongoing benefit.

Relaxation techniques, including yoga and cognitive behavioural therapy (CBT), can help the patient gain more control of their breathing and reduce the symptom of dyspnoea. Chest physiotherapy and postural drainage, including the use of a flutter valve, can help expectorate the thick secretions that are part of the symptomatology of COPD.

Patients with severe COPD are often in a catabolic state and appear cachectic due to the increased work of breathing. The BODE index, which is a measure of body mass index (BMI), airflow obstruction, dyspnoea, and exercise capacity, can be of prognostic value and used in determining patients suitable for lung transplantation. Nutritional support improves muscle strength and health status as measured by the St. George's Respiratory Questionnaire.

Chronic illnesses predispose to anxiety and depression. The Hospital Anxiety and Depression (HAD) questionnaire can be used to assess this. Patients should be referred for psychological support. Patients with respiratory conditions often run support groups, such as the 'Breathe Easy Club', which many find beneficial. It is recommended that all patients over the age of 65 with COPD and those with $FEV_1 < 40\%$ are offered the influenza and pneumonia vaccinations which will reduce the risk of serious respiratory illnesses and death.

LTOT should be commenced in patients who develop pulmonary hypertension and hypoxia. The ECG will show right axis deviation and a dominant R wave in V1 indicating right ventricular hypertrophy. An echocardiogram can estimate the pulmonary artery pressure and the function of the right heart. Type 1 respiratory failure, with a $PaO_2 < 7.3$ kPa at rest or a PaO_2 of <8 kPa with evidence of peripheral oedema, polycythaemia, or pulmonary hypertension, are indications for starting LTOT. Two measurements of the ABG should be done three weeks apart when the patient has recovered from an exacerbation and is stable. Patients on LTOT should be encouraged to use it for at least 15 hours in a 24-hour period (including while they are asleep) as this improves survival. LTOT is not a treatment for breathlessness and should be used with caution in those who continue to smoke. NIV together with LTOT can be considered in patients with chronic type 2 respiratory failure secondary to COPD. LTOT is discussed in more detail in Chapter 3.

There are several surgical treatments for severe emphysema. Bullectomy is the removal of redundant lung tissue which allows adjacent lung parenchyma to expand more effectively by reducing static hyperinflation. Lung volume reduction surgery (LVRS) is recommended for those with emphysema affecting the upper lobes and low exercise capacity but with no significant co-morbidities. LVRS can be done as a video-assisted thoracoscopic surgery (VATS) procedure. LVRS decreases hyperinflation, improves elastic recoil and airflow limitation and the efficiency of respiratory muscle, thus reducing air trapping. These procedures improve symptoms, QOL, and survival compared to medical treatment alone if suitable patients are selected. Bronchoscopic lung volume reduction, which involves the placement of a valve into the bronchus, is a non-surgical alternative for patients with heterogeneous emphysema on CT, FEV_1 between 15% and 45%, and hyperinflation (TLC > 100% predicted and RV > 150% predicted). Patients who are appropriately selected show improvement in symptoms and exercise tolerance but appear to have an increased frequency of exacerbations and haemoptysis.

Patients who have heterogeneous emphysema, with FEV_1 of less than 20%, TLCO <20%, and a BODE index of 5–10, should be referred for consideration of a single lung transplant if they are less than 65 years or for a double lung transplant if they are less than 60 years. They must have stopped smoking for at least six months, be able to participate in a pulmonary rehabilitation programme, have no significant co-morbidities, and be motivated.

Patients with COPD should be regularly reviewed by either a doctor or a nurse who assesses their clinical state, documents any exacerbations, checks spirometry to determine the rate of decline, reviews medication and the side effects of medication, and checks the inhaler technique. Attention should be paid to the patient's nutrition and mental state and referral to dietician and psychiatrist made as appropriate. Patients with COPD often have co-morbidities which should be diagnosed and treated. Lung cancer is the commonest cause of death in patients with mild COPD.

Diagnosis of exacerbation of COPD: an exacerbation results in worsening symptoms of breathlessness, cough, and systemic symptoms, such as fever, reduced appetite, and reduced mobility. Exacerbations are commonly due to viral or bacterial infections, changes in the weather, and atmospheric pollution. Exacerbations are commoner in the winter months.

The frequency of exacerbations has prognostic implications. Risk factors for exacerbations and hospital admissions include severe COPD (the lower the FEV_1, the more likely to have an exacerbation), and previous exacerbations. Patients with a certain phenotype appear to have an increased risk of experiencing exacerbations. A cohort of patients present to hospital with apparent exacerbation for psychosocial reasons. Each true exacerbation results in a decline in lung function, with more than 55 ml/year of lung capacity lost compared to 30 ml/year which occurs as part of the ageing process. The all-cause mortality three years after hospitalisation approaches 50%. Preventing exacerbations and treating exacerbations aggressively will improve the prognosis of patients with COPD.

Management of exacerbation of COPD: these patients are often brought to hospital by ambulance and managed initially in the emergency department as they can be critically unwell. They will be tachypnoeic, tachycardic and hypoxic and may develop type 1 or type 2 respiratory failure, with a risk of respiratory arrest. The differential diagnosis of this presentation includes pneumothorax (see Chapter 10), lung cancer (see Chapter 9), pulmonary embolism (see Chapter 11) and cardiac causes, including arrhythmias and heart failure.

A national COPD audit has shown that patients referred to the respiratory team and managed in a respiratory unit fare better than those under non-specialist teams. Some patients with severe COPD

Box 6.13 Management of exacerbation of COPD.

- Controlled oxygen (through venturi mask)
- Nebulised short-acting β_2-agonist
- Nebulised short-acting anticholinergic bronchodilator
- Systemic corticosteroids (oral or intravenous)
- Aminophylline (oral or intravenous)
- Mucolytic agent
- Chest physiotherapy
- Antibiotics if evidence of bacterial infection
- Diuretics
- Anti-coagulation
- Anxiolytics
- Nutrition
- Non-invasive ventilation
- Intubation and ventilation if reversible cause
- Palliation

exacerbation may need to be in the HDU or the ICU. Box 6.13 lists the management of exacerbation of COPD.

Patients with an exacerbation of COPD are often hypoxic and in respiratory failure. As many of these patients are at risk of developing type 2 respiratory failure, controlled oxygen therapy via a venturi mask is indicated based on the arterial blood gas result. Ideally, the baseline ABG should be taken on air, but if the patient is very hypoxic, then the baseline ABG should be taken on oxygen, but note should be made of the exact amount of inspired oxygen so that the ABG result can be interpreted accurately. This is also important when monitoring the patient's ABG results. Oxygen should be prescribed on the drug chart so that the oxygen saturation is kept between 88% and 92%. The ABG should be checked after 30 minutes to ensure that there is no acute CO_2 retention. Patients with an exacerbation of COPD and type 2 respiratory failure will require non-invasive ventilation (NIV) using BiPAP.

Nebulised salbutamol should be given at least four times in 24 hours but can be given every few hours. A dose of 2.5 mg or 5 mg can be used, depending on the size of the patient. The nebuliser solution should be driven by 6 L air, with supplemental oxygen given through a nasal cannula for those who are hypoxic. The main side effects of β_2-agonists are tremor, tachycardia, and hypokalaemia. Some patients cannot tolerate salbutamol, and terbutaline is an alternative SABA.

Nebulised ipratropium bromide, a short-acting, antimuscarinic, anticholinergic drug, should be given at a dose of 500 μg every six hours, driven by 6 L air and supplemental oxygen as required. While on nebulised SAMA, any LAMA that they usually take should be stopped. Systemic corticosteroids should be prescribed as they shorten the recovery time and decrease the risk of relapse. 40 mg of oral prednisolone given for five days is as effective as intravenous hydrocortisone, which can be given to those who are unable to take oral medication. The patient should continue to take their usual ICS during this period.

Aminophylline can be given orally at a dose of 225 mg twice a day, or intravenously with a loading dose of 5 mg kg^{-1} to a maximum of 500 mg over 30 minutes via a rate-controlled device if the patient is not already on aminophylline. Aminophylline can cause tachycardia and cardiac arrhythmias, therefore cardiac monitoring and checking the blood level of aminophylline are important. The side effects and drug interactions are discussed in Chapter 3.

Mucolytic agents can help expectorate viscous mucus, but long term studies in COPD have not been conclusive, with little evidence of a significant benefit. Carbocisteine, 750 mg three times daily, could be prescribed to patients with viscous sputum who have difficulty expectorating. In stable COPD, only those who appear to be benefitting should continue with it. Saline nebulisers, an Acapella device, and chest physiotherapy may be more effective in clearing sputum than carbocisteine alone. N-acetyl cysteine, which has antioxidant properties, has not been shown to be beneficial in this group of patients.

Patients who have symptoms of a bacterial chest infection, with an increase in the volume of sputum and change in the colour of the sputum, should be given antibiotics dictated by local guidelines. Many of these patients will have a raised white cell count, with a neutrophilia, and raised CRP. The differential diagnosis for this presentation includes community acquired pneumonia: patients with community acquired pneumonia (CAP) will have clinical signs of consolidation and radiological evidence of consolidation. If the patient has symptoms and signs of a bacterial chest infection, sputum should be sent for culture if possible. *Haemophilus influenzae, Streptococcus pneumonia*, and *Moraxella catarrhalis* are common pathogens in COPD as they often colonise the respiratory tract. Some 50% of patients with COPD have bacteria colonisation in the lower respiratory tract when they are stable. Exacerbation may be due to the acquisition of new strains of bacteria. Treatment of bacterial infections with antibiotics leads to faster recovery time and reduces the risk of relapse after discharge.

If the patient develops acute type 2 respiratory failure with acidosis (pH < 7.35), they must be started on BiPAP and monitored closely on a respiratory ward or HDU by a team experienced in the management of type 2 respiratory failure. A decision regarding the ceiling of care and resuscitation should be made after careful consideration of the facts, discussion with the respiratory physician, intensivist, the patient, and their family members. The management of type 2 respiratory failure is discussed in Chapter 13.

Patients with severe, end-stage COPD, who are not responding to treatment, should be referred to the palliative care team and should be placed on the end-of-life register. They may benefit from opioids to ease breathlessness.

Discharging a patient admitted with an exacerbation of COPD: patients should be off their nebulised treatment and have oxygen saturation above 88% on exertion. They should be on appropriate inhaled therapy and their inhaler technique should be checked. They should be discharged home on a reducing course of oral prednisolone at a rate of 5 mg every three to seven days. Some patients with COPD will require a longer course of prednisolone than those with asthma. Patients who are hypoxic will require assessment for long term oxygen therapy (LTOT) three weeks after discharge when they are stable. It is dangerous for patients who continue to smoke to have oxygen at home. Patients should be strongly encouraged to stop smoking, should be offered nicotine replacement therapy (NRT), and referred to the smoking cessation clinic.

NICE guidelines recommend pulmonary rehabilitation, so all patients referred with an exacerbation should be mobilised early and referred for pulmonary rehabilitation. These patients should have an annual influenza vaccination and pneumococcal vaccination every 10 years. For those patients who have recurrent exacerbations despite optimal treatment, bronchiectasis should be excluded (see Chapter 12). A three-month trial of prophylactic Azithromycin, given three times a week, may decrease the frequency of exacerbations in this group. This should be prescribed cautiously in those with liver function abnormalities, tinnitus, or hearing loss.

α-1 Antitrypsin Deficiency

Clinical presentation: patients with α-1 antitrypsin deficiency (α-1ATD) present with symptoms of progressively worsening breathlessness, wheeze, and infective exacerbations. Results of investigations will be consistent with a diagnosis of COPD, with obstruction on spirometry and little reversibility. The CXR and HRCT will show predominantly basal emphysema.

α-1ATD is the cause of emphysema in 1–2% of cases. It should be suspected in anyone younger than 40 with a family history of emphysema, and emphysema predominantly affecting the lung bases. It is often under-diagnosed. Typically, these individuals are not heavy smokers, but even minimal smoking increases the risk of developing emphysema. The WHO recommends that all patients under the age of 40, and all adolescents with asthma, are investigated for α-1ATD.

Pathophysiology: α-1AT is a 52 kDa serine protease inhibitor which is synthesised in the liver and secreted into the bloodstream. It binds irreversibly to trypsin (and other enzymes) and inactivates them. Neutrophil elastase digests damaged, ageing cells and bacteria, and is important in the healing process of normal lungs. α-1AT inactivates elastase and protects the lungs from too much damage. Low levels of α-1AT result in alveolar damage and the formation of bullae. Smoking activates neutrophil elastase and inactivates α-1AT, so worsens alveolar damage and the development of emphysema.

Genetics of α-1ATD: α-1ATD is a relatively common inherited condition with a frequency of 1 : 2500 worldwide and 1 : 2000 in Caucasians. The gene for α-1AT is on chromosome 14 and mutations at the protease inhibitor (Pi) locus lead to a single amino acid substitution which results in reduced levels of the enzyme in the serum. Glutamine to lysine mutation on position 342 results

Box 6.14 Enzyme activity in α-1ATD.

PiMM:	100% activity of α-1AT (normal)	PiMZ:	60%
PiMS:	80%	PiSZ:	40%
PiSS:	60%	PiZZ:	10–15%

in PiZ genotype and glutamine to valine mutation on 264 results in PiS.

α-1ATD is an autosomal recessive condition with co-dominant inheritance, so that each allele is responsible for 50% of the circulating α-1AT level. Phenotypic expression is variable. Those who are heterozygous are carriers and do not manifest the disease, but those who are homozygous will develop the condition. Approximately 80 allelic variants have been described. Normal α-1AT gene is called M. Abnormal variants are A–L or N–Z, and produce different amounts of the protein. Box 6.14 lists the levels of enzyme activity with the different alleles. A serum concentration <15–20% of normal values suggests homozygous α-1ATD.

Some 95% of Caucasians have PiMM and 1 in 20 are PiMZ. 95% of deficiency states resulting in clinical manifestations are PiZZ; 60–70% with PiZZ develop emphysema at a young age, and this is made more likely by smoking.

α-1ATD is the commonest cause of liver disease in infants and children, affecting 10%. It also affects 15% of adults, being more common in men than in women. The abnormal protein accumulates in hepatocytes, causing chronic hepatitis, cirrhosis, and hepatocellular carcinoma. Liver function tests will show a cholestatic picture and a liver biopsy will show characteristic PAS-positive (periodic acid Schiff) inclusions in hepatocytes.

Diagnosis of α-1ATD: clinicians should have a low threshold for investigating patients who present with early onset emphysema and who have a family history of emphysema. α-1AT concentrations in blood, measured by quantitative immunoprecipitation, will show low levels, the normal range is 1.10–2.10. α-1AT phenotype can be measured by isoelectric focusing and DNA studies can confirm the diagnosis. The WHO recommends screening in areas with a high prevalence of the disease and for those with a family history.

Management of α-1ATD: smoking cessation should be strongly advised. Management is as for COPD, as outlined earlier in this chapter. Some patients will progress rapidly to requiring LTOT. Single or double lung transplantation are options in those with progressive disease. Augmentation therapy with α-1AT protein, which can be inhaled as an aerosol spray or given intravenously, is recommended for those with emphysema and will reduce the decline in FEV_1. It is not helpful in liver disease. Recombinant α-1AT given weekly has not yet been shown to confer significant clinical benefit. Patients with α-1AT liver disease should avoid alcohol and should be vaccinated for hepatitis A and B. Liver transplantation should be considered.

Patients with α-1AT deficiency should be referred to a recognised national centre, such as the Antitrypsin Deficiency Assessment and Programme for Treatment (ADAPT), and be enrolled onto a Registry so that they can participate in trials, have assessment of their carrier status, and be referred for genetic counselling.

Allergic bronchopulmonary aspergillosis (ABPA)

ABPA should be suspected in patients with a long history of asthma that does not respond to standard therapy. Patients will present with breathlessness, a cough productive of thick, mucopurulent sputum plugs, and recurrent infections. The differential diagnosis includes COPD and bronchiectasis. CT thorax will show the characteristic central bronchiectasis (Figure 6.9).

ABPA is not an infection, but an exaggerated T-helper cell reaction to aspergillus fumigatus. Blood tests will show peripheral eosinophilia (see Chapter 7 for causes of eosinophilia), very high plasma IgE levels, and precipitating and specific antibodies to Aspergillus fumigatus. Skin prick tests will be positive for aspergillus and sputum may also grow aspergillus.

Management of ABPA is as for bronchiectasis (see Chapter 12). In addition, patients should receive antifungal treatment for 16 weeks, either voriconazole or itraconazole, and a high dose of prednisolone, with careful monitoring of liver function test.

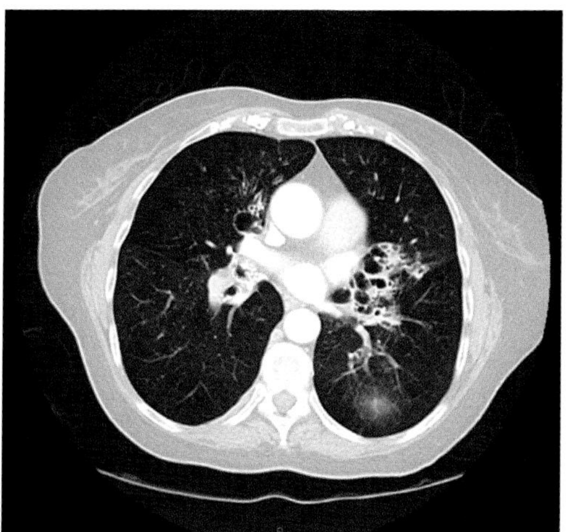

Figure 6.9 HRCT in ABPA showing proximal bronchiectasis.

Box 6.15 Aetiology of vocal cord dysfunction.

• Asthma	• Neurological injury
• Exercise	• Irritants
• Laryngopharyngeal reflux	• Psychological disorders

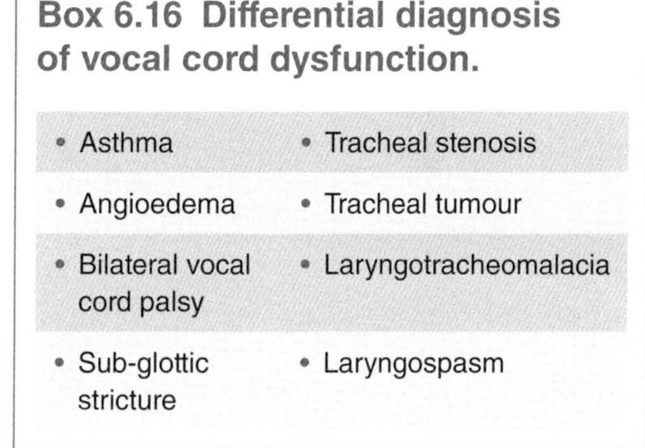

Box 6.16 Differential diagnosis of vocal cord dysfunction.

• Asthma	• Tracheal stenosis
• Angioedema	• Tracheal tumour
• Bilateral vocal cord palsy	• Laryngotracheomalacia
• Sub-glottic stricture	• Laryngospasm

Vocal cord dysfunction

Definition: Vocal cord dysfunction (VCD), or paradoxical vocal fold motion (PVFM), occurs due to abnormal movement of the vocal cords. During normal breathing, the true vocal cords abduct during inspiration, allowing air to enter the trachea and partially adduct during expiration. In VCD, there is an abnormal adduction of the vocal cords on inspiration.

Clinical presentation: VCD is commoner in women compared to men and can affect patients of all ages. Patients with VCD complain of breathlessness and persistent wheeze at rest and on exertion. They may also complain of throat tightness, dysphonia, a choking sensation, dysphagia, and rhinosinusitis. They often have a diagnosis of asthma or COPD but continue to complain of symptoms despite optimal treatment with inhalers. Patients present to the emergency department with what appears to be loud wheeze and stridor. Auscultation of the chest will not reveal any wheeze as in acute asthma. As this condition is often not recognised, patients with VCD often have unnecessary treatments, including high doses of corticosteroids, intubation, and ventilation. Clinical observation will reveal inspiratory stridor. VCD can occur secondary to a variety of conditions. Box 6.15 lists some of these.

Diagnosis: the differential diagnosis of VCD is listed in Box 6.16. Clinical history and examination will suggest VCD. Laryngoscopy or bronchoscopy are the diagnostic tests of choice. These investigations will show abnormal adduction of the vocal cords during inspiration which may be exacerbated after exertion. Examination will also exclude a subglottic stricture and tracheal stenosis. Ultrasound of the vocal cords may be diagnostic if there is no concern about a stricture or tumour.

Methacholine challenge will be normal and will exclude asthma. Flow volume loops will show evidence of extra-thoracic airway obstruction, with flattening of the inspiratory loop.

Management of VCD: VCD should be managed with a combination of reassurance, education, behavioural therapy, and speech therapy. Amitriptyline, used 'off licence', at a starting dose of 10 mg, taken two hours before going to sleep, appears to relax the vocal cords, with improvement over 7–28 days. The dose can be increased weekly by 10 mg, to a maximum dose of 70 mg. Most patients respond to a dose of between 10 mg and 40 mg over three to six months, and the dose can be reduced once the vocal cords relax. Amitriptyline will also correct the insomnia which is associated with this condition. The main side effects occur at higher doses and include dry mouth and fatigue. Caution is also advised in using amitriptyline in patients with severe prostatic hypertrophy. Patients should be advised to drive with care because of possible drowsiness.

Hyperventilation syndrome (HV)

Hyperventilation (HV) syndrome is a condition associated with an increase in minute ventilation, so that the patient presents with intermittent episodes of breathlessness. As there are no clear diagnostic criteria, it is difficult to estimate the incidence and prevalence. The diagnosis is often made after excluding other causes of breathlessness. The differential diagnosis of hyperventilation syndrome includes panic attacks and anxiety disorders, although it is not clear whether the psychological condition is primary or secondary. The prevalence of hyperventilation is higher in those with underlying psychological problems than it is in the normal population, and a detailed clinical history may reveal a psychological cause. It is commoner in women compared to men. Box 6.17 lists the common symptoms of hyperventilation syndrome.

Patients presenting with hyperventilation report difficulty taking a breath in, and may be found to take slow, deep breaths. Patients with panic or anxiety disorder will breathe rapidly and take shallow breaths. They will also report these symptoms after exercise and the extent of their symptoms will not correlate to the level of the exercise. These patients also report symptoms of anxiety and fear. The control of breathing is discussed in Chapter 2.

Box 6.17 Symptoms of hyperventilation syndrome.

- Breathlessness at rest
- Light-headedness
- Chest pain
- Paraesthesia
- Palpitations
- Carpo-pedal spasm

It is postulated that patients who present with hyperventilation have increased sensitivity to CO_2 and an increased respiratory drive when feeling anxious or distressed. This results in reduced $PaCO_2$, respiratory alkalosis, and a reduction in cerebral blood flow which leads to paraesthesia, headache, and light-headedness. Respiratory alkalosis results in changes to the level of ionised calcium, and reduced binding to albumin, which can result in tetany.

Diagnosis of hyperventilation syndrome: acute respiratory and cardiac conditions will need to be excluded with a detailed history, examination, and investigations as discussed in Chapter 5. The history will be one of intermittent breathlessness, with no clear pattern, and normal physical examination and investigations. A clinical presentation suggestive of hyperventilation and no features to suggest an alternative diagnosis is sufficient to make the diagnosis. However, most patients will have a CXR, ECG, spirometry, and measurement of oxygen saturation at rest and on exertion, to rule out other conditions. Convincing the patient that there is no other serious medical condition can be difficult.

Management of hyperventilation syndrome: the main management is with psychological therapies, including behavioural therapy and breathing retraining as part of pulmonary rehabilitation. Patients who present with an episode of acute hyperventilation should be reassured after excluding other causes. They should be taken to a quiet area and an attempt should be made to keep them calm and breathe at a normal rate. A small dose of a sedative drug may be beneficial. As patients who are hyperventilating will be hypocapnic, breathing into a paper bag has long been advocated as part of the management, as this results in an increase in the CO_2 level in the blood. However, this cannot be recommended as there is a significant risk of hypoxia. Referral to a psychiatrist for management of anxiety and depression should be considered. β-blockers and benzodiazepines may be beneficial in some patients. Yoga and Buteyko techniques may be helpful in reducing hyperventilation by reducing the respiratory rate.

SUMMARY OF LEARNING POINTS

- Obstructive airways diseases are common causes of morbidity and mortality worldwide.
- Atopy is an inherited tendency to produce large amounts of IgE when exposed to an allergen.
- Asthma is an atopic condition in which exposure to an allergen results in an exacerbation in a genetically susceptible individual.
- Asthma is a reversible condition caused by airway inflammation; the reversibility distinguishes it from COPD.
- Acute asthma exacerbations are managed with nebulisers, systemic steroids, magnesium sulfate, high flow oxygen, and intravenous aminophylline.
- Patients with acute asthma should be monitored closely with regular clinical assessments, including serial ABG measurements.
- Patients who are not improving or deteriorating, with normalising of the $PaCO_2$, should be referred urgently for intubation and ventilation.
- Chronic asthma can develop in patients who have been under-treated; these patients will respond less to bronchodilators as there are fixed, structural changes in the airways.
- There are approximately 1500 asthma deaths in the UK every year.
- Most deaths from asthma are preventable: inadequate use of preventative inhalers, over-use of SABA, lack of recognition of deterioration by patient and doctor, poor compliance.
- COPD is a significant cause of morbidity and mortality worldwide.
- The risk factors for COPD include cigarette smoking, passive smoking, occupational exposure to dusts, and atmospheric pollution.
- The diagnosis of COPD is made when the FEV_1/FVC ratio is less than 70% on spirometry.
- COPD severity can be categorised by spirometry as mild, moderate, severe, and very severe.
- The severity of COPD guides management, predicts the frequency of exacerbations and the risk of death.
- Smoking cessation is the most important intervention for patients with COPD.
- Inhaled therapy with SABA, LABA, SAA, LAM, and ICS should be offered in all cases, depending on symptoms and FEV_1. A combination of inhalers is more effective than individual drugs.
- Pulmonary rehabilitation should be offered to patients with COPD with an MRC score of 3 or more and improves symptoms, exercise tolerance, and QOL.
- Mucolytic agents can be useful in some patients with COPD, but the evidence for their use is minimal.
- Roflumilast, a phosphodiesterase-4 inhibitor, improves symptoms and prognosis in patients with severe COPD.
- Theophylline, a non-selective phosphodiesterase inhibitor, has a moderate bronchodilator effect, so could be considered in addition to inhaled therapy but the drug has a narrow therapeutic range and has significant side effects and drug interactions.
- α-1ATD is an inherited condition with autosomal codominance. Patients with homozygous disease develop basal emphysema and liver disease.
- Management of α-1ATD is as for emphysema. Intravenous augmentation therapy and lung transplantation can also be considered.
- Vocal cord dysfunction is a common condition which is often misdiagnosed as acute asthma.
- The diagnosis of VCD is made by observing the movement of the vocal cords during inspiration.
- Management of VCD is with speech and language therapy and amitriptyline.
- Hyperventilation is associated with anxiety and is commoner in women than in men.
- Hyperventilation should be managed with reassurance, CBT, β-blockers, and benzodiazepines.

MULTIPLE CHOICE QUESTIONS

6.1 Which of the following investigations is most likely to be abnormal in a patient with mild asthma?

A CXR
B Eosinophil count in peripheral blood
C Exhaled NO
D Methacholine challenge
E Spirometry

Answer: D

CXR and spirometry are likely to be normal in mild asthma in between exacerbations. The eosinophil count and exhaled NO, which is a measure of airway inflammation, are likely to be normal. Methacholine provocation test is the most sensitive of these investigations at detecting airway hyper-responsiveness.

6.2 Which of the following is recommended in the management of asthma?

A Desensitisation to allergen
B Leukotriene receptor inhibitor at Step 2 of the guidelines
C Non-invasive ventilation for respiratory failure
D Pulmonary rehabilitation
E Vaccination against influenza virus

Answer: E

Patients with asthma are usually atopic and should avoid any allergens that cause an exacerbation, but desensitisation is not recommended. Leukotriene receptor inhibitor should be considered in those who have not responded to adequate doses of ICS and LABA, especially those with high IgE and exercise-induced and aspirin-sensitive asthma, so at Step 3. Patients who develop type 1 respiratory failure will require intubation if they do not improve with management. Pulmonary rehabilitation is indicated for patients with COPD and not asthma.

6.3 Which of the following is a feature of life-threatening asthma?

A $PaCO_2$ <4 kPa
B PEF >75% predicted
C Polyphonic wheeze
D Silent chest
E Tachycardia

Answer: D

Patients with asthma initially present with polyphonic wheeze and type 1 respiratory failure. As they are tachypnoeic, they will blow off CO_2, which may be low. If there is inadequate treatment or no response to treatment, the patient will tire. In life-threatening asthma, the $PaCO_2$ will rise, and may be at the higher end of the normal range, >4.5 kPa. At this stage, there is little air entering or leaving the lungs, so-called 'silent chest'. The patient is likely to be bradycardic.

6.4 Which of the following is a risk factor on its own for fatal asthma?

A Moderately severe asthma
B Lower respiratory tract infection
C No hospital admissions with asthma
D Poor perception of dyspnoea
E Under-use of SABA

Answer: D

Patients with mild, moderate, and severe asthma are at risk of fatal asthma if their condition is inadequately treated, if they have poor perception of their symptoms and if they do not understand how to manage it. Lower respiratory tract infections may exacerbate asthma, but is not a risk factor for a fatal asthma attack by itself. Under-use of SABA indicates good control of symptoms as does no previous hospital admissions. NRAD found that patients who had a poor perception of dyspnoea were at risk of death.

6.5 Which of the following investigations is essential in the diagnosis of COPD?

A Arterial blood gas.
B CXR
C HRCT
D Spirometry
E Reversibility testing

Answer: D

The diagnosis of COPD is made when a symptomatic patient has FEV_1 <80% predicted or FEV_1/FVC <70%. ABG, CXR, and HRCT may be normal in mild COPD. Reversibility testing is not indicated in COPD, although it may be useful in patients in whom there is uncertainty about whether they have asthma or COPD.

6.6 Which of the following has been shown to have NO benefit in a patient with COPD?

A Aminophylline
B Inhaled corticosteroids
C Leukotriene antagonist
D Pulmonary rehabilitation
E Smoking cessation

Answer: C

There is strong evidence for the benefit of smoking cessation and pulmonary rehabilitation in patients with COPD. Inhaled corticosteroids, together with LABA, have been shown in large, multi-centre trials to improve the symptoms and reduce the frequency of exacerbations in those with moderate and severe COPD. Aminophylline appears to have a bronchodilator effect and can be used in those who are symptomatic despite the use of inhaled therapy. Leukotriene antagonists have no role in COPD but are used in Step 3 of asthma management.

6.7 Which of the following is indicated for the management of acute exacerbation of COPD?

A CPAP
B High flow oxygen
C Intravenous salbutamol
D Intravenous magnesium sulfate
E Non-invasive ventilation

Answer: E

CPAP is a way to deliver oxygen in severe type 1 respiratory failure. CPAP and high flow oxygen are not indicated in hypoxic patients with COPD because of the risk of CO_2 retention and the development of type 2 respiratory failure. Intravenous salbutamol and magnesium sulfate are not used in an acute exacerbation of COPD, but can be occasionally used, with caution, in an exacerbation of asthma. NIV is the treatment of choice in a patient who develops type 2 respiratory failure because of COPD exacerbation.

6.8 Which of the following statements about α-1ATD is true?

A α-1ATD is an autosomal dominant condition
B α-1ATD never occurs in children
C Augmentation therapy with intravenous protein does not improve lung function
D Emphysema mainly affects the upper lobes of the lungs
E Lung transplantation is the best treatment for severe disease

Answer: E

α-1ATD affects 10% of neonates, presenting with liver disease. It is the commonest cause of liver disease in this age group and presents with abnormal liver function tests. It is an autosomal recessive condition with co-dominance. Intravenous α-1AT improves lung function, but transplantation is the best option for severe disease. The emphysema affects the lower lobes, unlike the emphysema in COPD, which affects the upper lobes.

6.9 Which of the following statements about ABPA is true?

A Chest physiotherapy is not required
B Corticosteroids are not indicated
C CXR will show cavitation with a fungal ball
D IgE level in blood will be very high
E Treatment is with standard antibiotics as used for community acquired pneumonia

Answer: D

Patients with ABPA present with breathlessness, cough, and wheeze. Management is as for bronchiectasis, so includes chest physiotherapy. CXR may appear normal but HRCT will show proximal bronchiectasis. A cavitating lesion with a fungal ball is seen with aspergilloma, not ABPA. The IgE levels will be very high (>1000iU). Antifungal treatment is recommended (voriconazole, itraconazole).

6.10 Which of the following statements about VCD is true?

A Methacholine challenge will be abnormal
B Patients with VCD cough up a lot of purulent sputum
C Patients with VCD should be treated with high doses of corticosteroids
D Sub-glottic stricture should be excluded
E The vocal cords are paralysed in VCD

Answer: D

Patients with VCD are often mis-diagnosed as having asthma or COPD and receive high doses of steroids which do not improve the symptoms. Methacholine challenge will be normal as there is no airway hyper-responsiveness or bronchoconstriction. These patients do not cough up sputum. Subglottic strictures and tracheal stenosis should be excluded at bronchoscopy. There is no paralysis of the vocal cords, but abnormal adduction during inspiration.

Appendix 6.A Diagnosis of asthma

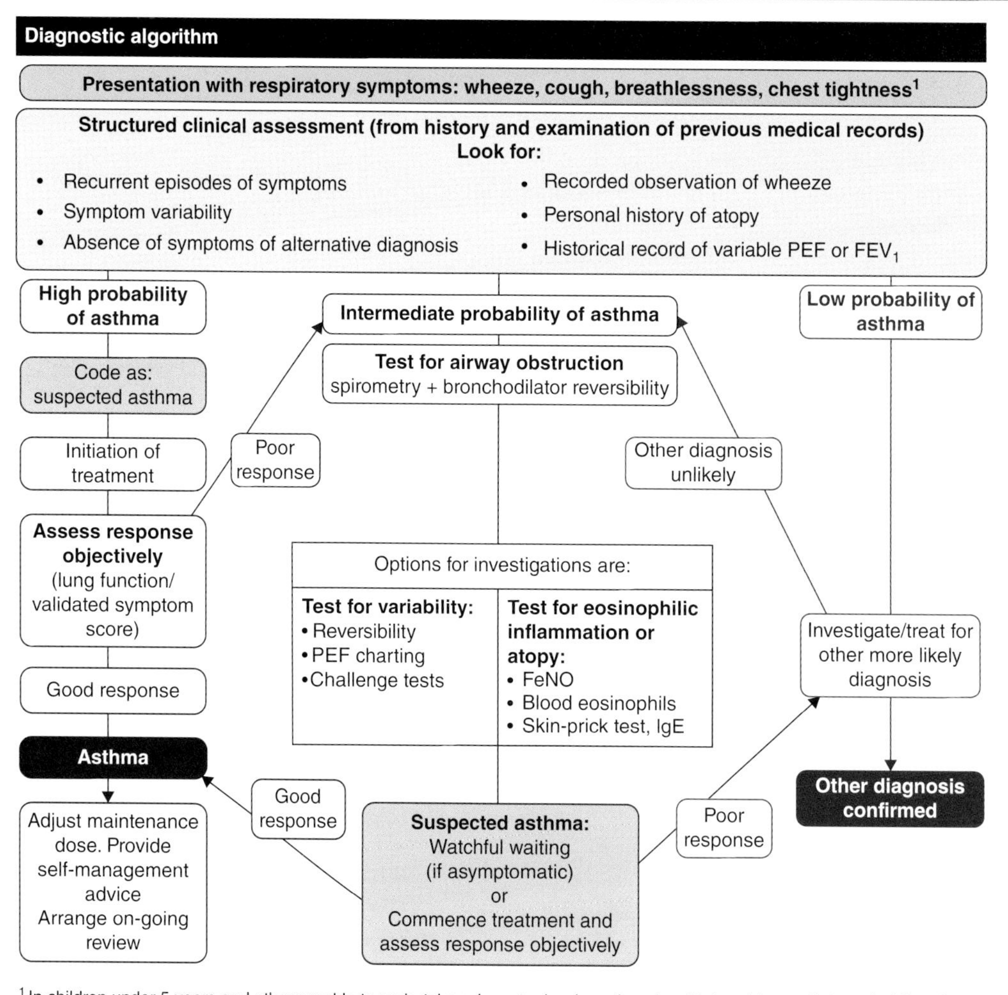

[1] In children under 5 years and others unable to undertake spirometry in whom there is a high or intermediate probability of asthma, the options are monitored initiation of treatment or watchful waiting according to the assessed probability of asthma.

Figure 6.A.1 Diagnostic algorithm for presentation with respiratory symptoms.

Appendix 6.B Management of asthma

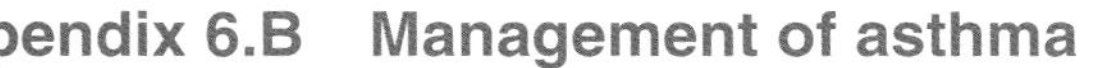

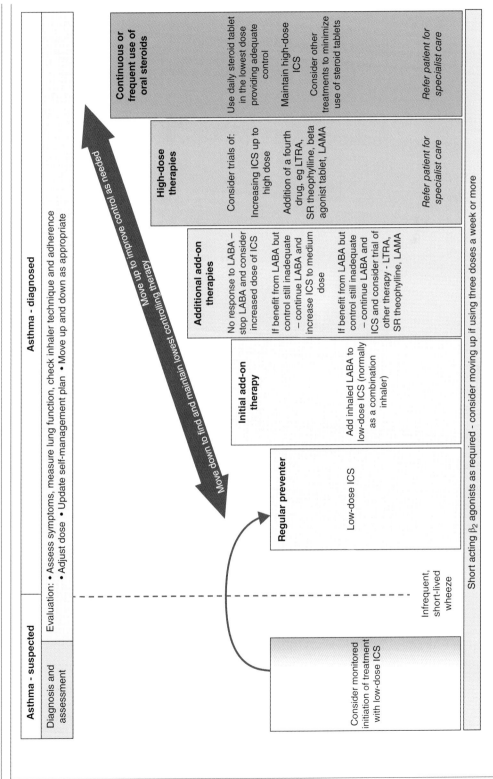

Figure 6.B.1 Summary of asthma management in adults.

Appendix 6.C Management of COPD

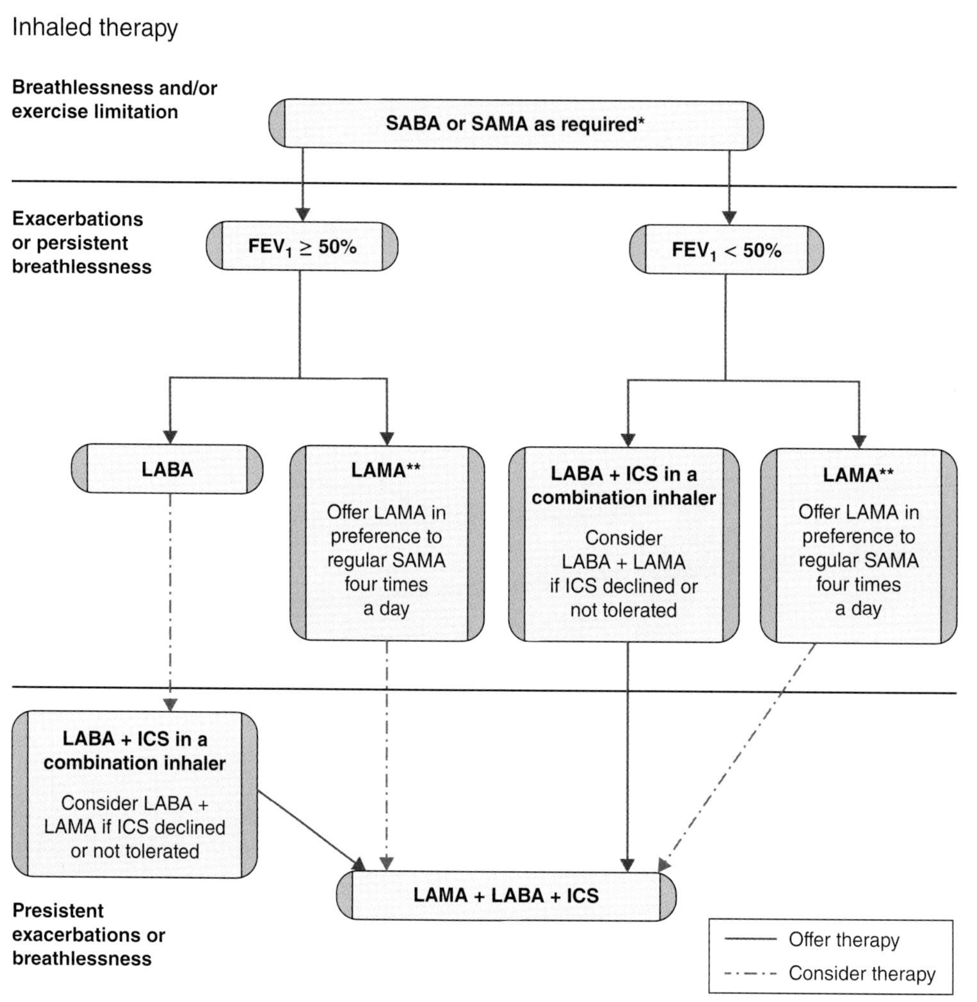

- Choose a drug based on the person's symptomatic response and preference, the drug's side effects, potential to reduce exacerbations and cost.
- Do not use oral corticosteroid reversibility tests to identify patients who will benefit from inhaled corticosteroids.
- Be aware of the potential risk of developing side effects (including non-fatal pneumonia) in people with COPD treated with inhaled corticosteroids and be prepared to discuss this with patients.

*SABA as required may continue at all stages, **Discontinue SAMA
SABA, Short-Acting Beta$_2$ Agonist; SAMA, Short-Acting Muscarinic Antagonist
LABA, Long-Acting Beta$_2$ Agonist; LAMA, Long-Acting Muscarinic Antagonist
ICS, Inhaled Corticosteroid

Figure 6.C.1 Diagnostic algorithm for inhaled therapy.

FURTHER READING

American Thoracic Society (ATS) and European Respiratory Society (2003). American Thoracic Society/European Respiratory Society statement: standards for the diagnosis and management of individuals with alpha-1 antitrypsin deficiency. *American Journal of Respiratory and Critical Care Medicine* 168 (7): 818–900.

Asthma UK (2017). Asthma UK website. Available at: www.asthma.org.uk (accessed 13 March 2017).

Bolton, C.E., Bevan-Smith, E.F., Blakey, J.D. et al. (2013). British Thoracic Society guideline on pulmonary rehabilitation in adults. *Thorax* 68 (Suppl 2): iii–30.

ten Brinke, A., Zwinderman, A., Sterk, P. et al. (2001). Factors associated with persistent airflow limitation in severe asthma. *American Journal of Respiratory and Critical Care Medicine* 164 (5): 744–778.

British Thoracic Society (2014). Quality standards for pulmonary rehabilitation in adults. *British Thoracic Society Reports* 6 (2): 1–32.

British Thoracic Society, Pulmonary Rehabilitation Guideline and Group (2013). BTS guideline on pulmonary rehabilitation in adults. *International Journal of Respiratory Medicine* 68 (2): 1–31.

Brochard, L., Mancebo, J., Wysocki, M. et al. (1995). Noninvasive ventilation for acute exacerbations of chronic obstructive pulmonary disease. *New England Journal of Medicine* 333 (13): 817–822.

Buist, A.S., Burrows, B., Cohen, A. et al. (1989). Guidelines for the approach to the patient with severe hereditary alpha-1-antitrypsin deficiency. *American Review of Respiratory Disease* 140 (5): 1494–1497.

COPD Assessment Test and GlaxoSmithKline (2016). COPD assessment test website. Available at: http://www.catestonline.org (accessed 13 March 2017).

Flenley, D.C. (1978). Interpretation of blood-gas and acid-base data. *British Journal of Hospital Medicine* 20 (4): 384–386. 388, passim.

Gelb, A.F., Schein, A., Nussbaum, E. et al. (2004). Risk factors for near-fatal asthma. *Chest* 126 (4): 1138–1146.

Gibson, P.G., Powell, H., Coughlan, J. et al. (2003). Self-management education and regular practitioner review for adults with asthma. *The Cochrane Database of Systematic Reviews* 1: CD001117.

Global Initiative for Asthma (GINA) (2015). Global strategy for asthma management and prevention [online]. Available at: www.ginasthma.com.

Global Initiative for Asthma (GINA). (2017). Global initiative for asthma – GINA [online]. Available at: http://ginasthma.org (accessed 13 March 2017).

Global Initative for Chronic Obstructive Lung Disease (2006). Global Strategy for the diagnosis, management and prevention of chronic obstructive pulmonary disease 2006: Global initiative for chronic obstructive lung disease. Available at: http://www.who.int/respiratory/copd/GOLD_WR_06.pdf (accessed 13 March 2017).

Global Initative for Chronic Obstructive Lung Disease (2016). GOLD website. Available at: http://goldcopd.org (accessed 13 March 2017).

Halbert, R.J., Natoli, J.L., Gano, A. et al. (2006). Global burden of COPD: systematic review and meta-analysis. *European Respiratory Journal* 28 (3): 523–532.

Hardinge, M., Annandale, J., Bourne, S. et al. (2015). British Thoracic Society guidelines for home oxygen use in adults. *Thorax* 70 (Suppl 1): 1–43.

Hornsveld, H.K., Garssen, B., Dop, M.J. et al. (1996). Double-blind placebo-controlled study of the hyperventilation provocation test and the validity of the hyperventilation syndrome. *Lancet* 348 (9021): 154–158.

Howell, J.B. (1990). Behavioural breathlessness. *Thorax* 45 (4): 287–292.

Jones, M., Harvey, A., Marston, L., and O'Connell, N.E. (2013). Breathing exercises for dysfunctional breathing/hyperventilation syndrome in adults. *The Cochrane Database of Systematic Reviews* 5: CD009041.

Kew, K., Kirtchuk, L., Michell, C., and Griffiths, B. (2014). Intravenous magnesium sulfate for treating adults with acute asthma in the emergency department (intervention protocol). *Cochrane Database of Systematic Reviews* 1.

Kramer, N., Meyer, T.J., Meharg, J. et al. (1995). Randomized, prospective trial of noninvasive positive pressure ventilation in acute respiratory failure. *American Journal of Respiratory and Critical Care Medicine* 151 (6): 1799–1806.

Martin, T., Hovis, J., Costantino, J. et al. (2000). A randomized, prospective evaluation of noninvasive ventilation for acute respiratory failure. *American Journal of Respiratory and Critical Care Medicine* 161 (3 Pt 1): 807–813.

Meyers, B.F. and Patterson, G.A. (2003). Chronic obstructive pulmonary disease. 10: Bullectomy, lung volume reduction surgery, and transplantation for patients with chronic obstructive pulmonary disease. *Thorax* 58 (7): 634–638.

Morris, M.J. and Christopher, K.L. (2010). Diagnostic criteria for the classification of vocal cord dysfunction. *Chest* 138 (5): 1213–1223.

National Institute for Health and Care Excellence (2008). Stop smoking services. NICE Public Health Guideline (PH10) [online]. Available at: www.nice.org.uk/guidance/ph10/resources/stop-smoking-services-1996169822917 (accessed 13 March 2017).

National Institute for Health and Care Excellence (2010). Chronic obstructive pulmonary disease. NICE Clinical Guidelines (CG101) [online]. Available at: doi:10.1038/nrdp.2015.76.

National Institute for Health and Care Excellence (2013). Quality standard for asthma, NICE Guideline (QS25) NICE Quality Standard 25, (February), p. 48 [online]. Available at: www.nice.org.uk/guidance/qs25.

National Institute for Health and Care Excellence (2015). Smoking: reducing and preventing tobacco use. NICE Guideline (QS82), (March). Available at: www.nice.org.uk/guidance/qs82

National Review of Asthma Deaths (NRAD), Healthcare Quality Improvement Partnership (HQIP), Clinical Outcome Review Programmes (CORP) and Royal College of Physicians (2014). Why asthma still kills: the National Review of Asthma Deaths (NRAD) [online]. Available at: http://www.cdc.gov/vitalsigns/Asthma/?s_cid=vitalsigns_065%5C, http://www.ncbi.nlm.nih.gov/pubmed/26076339, http://www.thieme-connect.de/DOI/DOI?10.1055/s-0032-1326964.

Nava, S., Ambrosino, N., Clini, E. et al. (1998). Noninvasive mechanical ventilation in the weaning of patients with respiratory failure due to chronic obstructive pulmonary disease: A randomized, controlled trial. *Annals of Internal Medicine* 128 (9): 721–728.

Newman, K.B., Mason, U.G. IIIrd, and Schmaling, K.B. (1995). Clinical features of vocal cord dysfunction. *American Journal of Respiratory and Critical Care Medicine* 152 (4 Pt 1): 1382–1386.

O'Driscoll, B.R., Howard, L.S., Davison, A.G., and British Thoracic Society (2008). BTS guideline for emergency oxygen use in adult patients. *Thorax* 63 (Suppl 6(October)): vii–i68.

Parrot, S., Godfrey, C., and Raw, M. (1998). Guidance for commissioners on the cost effectiveness of smoking cessation interventions. *Thorax* 53 (Suppl 5): S2–S38.

Pingleton, S.K. (1988). Complications of acute respiratory failure. *American Review of Respiratory Disease* 137 (6): 1463–1493.

Plaza, V., Serrano, J., Picado, C. et al. (2002). Frequency and clinical characteristics of rapid-onset fatal and near-fatal asthma. *European Respiratory Journal* 19 (5): 846–852.

Poole, P.J. and Black, P.N. (2006). Mucolytic agents for chronic bronchitis or chronic obstructive pulmonary disease. *The Cochrane Database of Systematic Reviews* 3: CD001287.

Rabe, K.F., Hurd, S., Anzueto, A. et al. (2007). Global strategy for the diagnosis, management, and prevention of chronic obstructive pulmonary disease: GOLD executive summary. *American Journal of Respiratory and Critical Care Medicine* 176 (6): 532–555.

Rodrigo, G.J., Neffen, H., and Castro-Rodriguez, J.A. (2011). Efficacy and safety of subcutaneous omalizumab vs placebo as add-on therapy to corticosteroids for children and adults with asthma: A systematic review. *Chest* 139 (1): 28–35.

Royal College of Physicians (2008). *Non-invasive Ventilation in Chronic Obstructive Pulmonary Disease: Management of Acute Type 2 Respiratory Failure: National Guidelines, Number 11*. London: Royal College of Physicians of London.

Scottish Intercollegiate Guidelines Network Society, British Thoracic Society, Royal College of Physicians, Healthcare Improvement Scotland, Education for Health and Asthma UK (2016). British Guideline on the Management of Asthma: A National Clinical Guideline (SIGN 153), Scottish Intercollegiate Guidelines Network (September).

Varney, V., Adeyemo, S., Parnell, H. et al. (2014). The successful treatment of hypercapnic respiratory failure with oral modafinil. *International Journal of COPD* 9: 413–419.

Voelker, R. (2012). Asthma forecast: why heat, humidity trigger symptoms. *JAMA* 308 (1): 20.

Zheng, J.-P., Kang, J., Huang, S.-G. et al. (2008). Effect of carbocisteine on acute exacerbation of chronic obstructive pulmonary disease (PEACE study): a randomised placebo-controlled study. *Lancet* 371 (9629): 2013–2018.

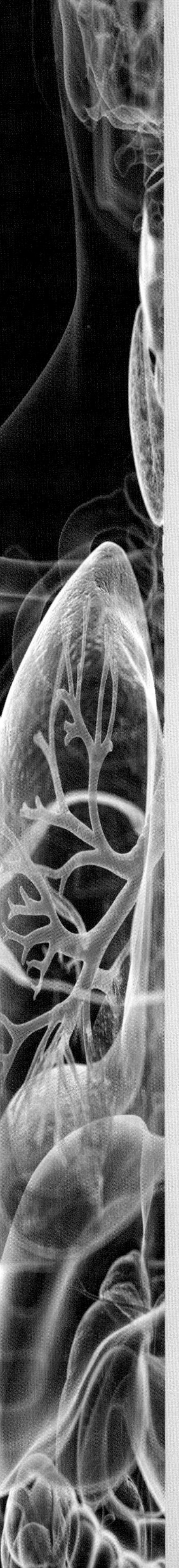

CHAPTER 7

Diffuse parenchymal lung disease

Learning objectives

- To understand the classification of diffuse parenchymal lung diseases (DPLD)
- To appreciate the aetiology and pathophysiology of DPLD
- To be aware of the clinical presentation of DPLD
- To understand the investigations required to make the diagnosis of a specific type of DPLD
- To appreciate the differential diagnosis of DPLD
- To understand the clinical presentation, diagnosis, and management of Idiopathic Pulmonary Fibrosis (IPF)
- To understand the clinical presentation, diagnosis, and management of Non-specific Interstitial Pneumonia (NSIP)
- To understand the clinical presentation, diagnosis, and management of sarcoidosis
- To have a basic understanding of the diagnosis and management of other, rarer DPLD
- To understand the differences in prognosis of the different types of DPLD

Essential Respiratory Medicine, First Edition. Shanthi Paramothayan.

Companion website: www.wiley.com/go/paramothayan/essential_respiratory_medicine

Abbreviations

ABPA	allergic bronchopulmonary aspergillosis
ACE	angiotensin converting enzyme
AIP	acute interstitial pneumonia
ARDS	acute respiratory distress syndrome
ATS	American Thoracic Society
BAL	bronchoalveolar lavage
BCG	Bacilli Calmette-Guérin
BHL	bilateral hilar lymphadenopathy
BOOP	bronchiolitis obliterans organising pneumonia
BTS	British Thoracic Society
COP	cryptogenic organising pneumonia
CRP	C-reactive protein
CTD	connective tissue disease
CXR	chest X-ray
DIP	desquamative interstitial pneumonia
DPLD	diffuse parenchymal lung disease
EAA	extrinsic allergic alveolitis
EBUS	endobronchial ultrasound
ECMO	extracorporeal membrane oxygenation
ERS	European Respiratory Society
ESR	erythrocyte sedimentation rate
FEV_1	forced expiratory volume in one secnd
FVC	forced vital capacity
GM-CSF	granulocyte-macrophage colony-stimulating factor
HIV	human immunodeficiency virus
HLA	human leukocyte antigen
HP	hypersensitivity pneumonitis
HRCT	high-resolution computed tomography scan
IFN	interferon
IIP	idiopathic interstitial pneumonia
IL	interleukin
ILD	interstitial lung disease
IPF	idiopathic pulmonary fibrosis
LAM	lymphangioleiomyomatosis
LDH	lactate dehydrogenase
LIP	lymphoid interstitial pneumonia
MCTD	mixed connective tissue disease
MHC	major histocompatibility complex
NAC	N-acetyl cysteine
NSIP	non-specific interstitial pneumonia
OCS	oral corticosteroids
PAP	pulmonary alveolar proteinosis
PAS	periodic acid Schiff
PLCH	pulmonary Langerhans cell histiocytosis
RB-ILD	respiratory bronchiolitis interstitial lung disease
SLE	systemic lupus erythematosus
TBLB	transbronchial lung biopsy
TLCO	transfer factor for carbon monoxide
TNF	tumour necrosis factor
TSC	tuberous sclerosis complex
UIP	usual interstitial pneumonia
VATS	video-assisted thoracoscopic surgery
VEGF-D	vascular endothelial growth factor
VC	vital capacity

Introduction

Diffuse parenchymal lung diseases (DPLDs) are a heterogeneous group of about 200 different non-neoplastic conditions characterised by inflammation and fibrosis of the alveoli, the distal airways, and interstitium from a variety of insults. In the early stages, the inflammatory alveolitis may be responsive to corticosteroids, but if untreated, most of these conditions will progress to irreversible lung fibrosis that is not responsive to corticosteroid therapy. These conditions are all restrictive lung diseases characterised by a reduction in forced vital capacity (FVC), an increase in the FEV_1/FVC ratio, and a reduction of the transfer factor for carbon monoxide (TLCO). These conditions present with parenchymal radiological abnormalities, and the distribution of these changes may point to the diagnosis. Histology of samples taken from transbronchial biopsy, video-assisted thoracoscopic surgery (VATS), or surgical lung biopsy is usually required to make a definitive diagnosis. The treatment and prognosis vary considerably for the different types of DPLD, so it is essential to make the correct diagnosis.

In the historical terminology used to classify interstitial lung diseases, ILD and DPLD are imprecise terms based on clinical, radiological, or histological features. These terms are still used interchangeably in old text books and can be confusing. The new classification aims to correlate the clinical presentation more accurately with the radiological and histological findings. Box 7.1 lists the common DPLD.

Diagnosis of DPLD

In the following section, an approach to a patient presenting with a possible DPLD will be outlined. Patients with a DPLD will present with a history of

Box 7.1 Classification of common diffuse parenchymal lung diseases.

Figure 7.1 shows the classification of DPLD:

- Eosinophilic pneumonias
- Hypersensitivity pneumonitis (extrinsic allergic alveolitis)
- Idiopathic interstitial pneumonias (IIP)
- Lymphangioleiomyomatosis (LAM)
- Langerhans cell histiocytosis (histiocytosis X)
- Pulmonary alveolar proteinosis
- Pulmonary amyloidosis
- Sarcoidosis

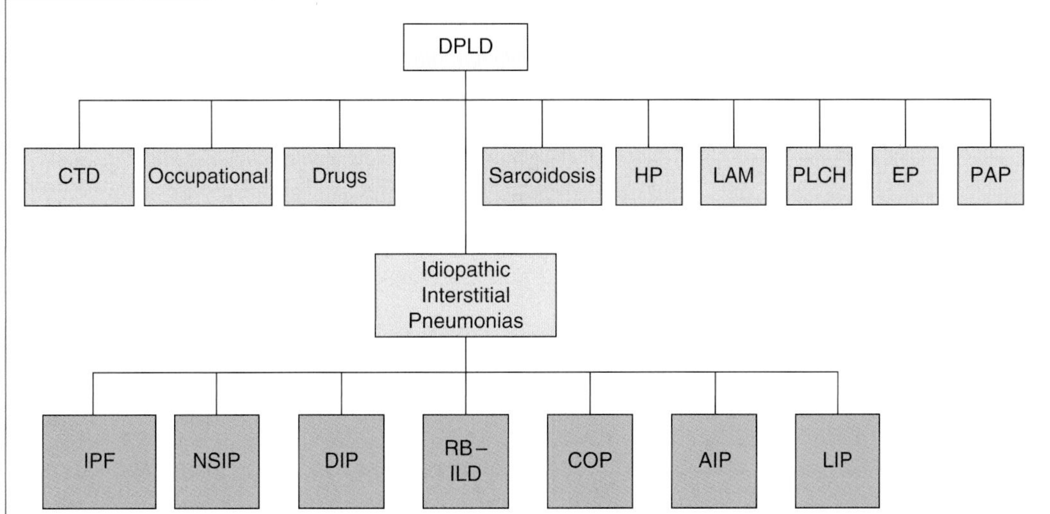

Figure 7.1 Classification of diffuse parenchymal lung disease (DPLD).

worsening breathlessness, cough, and other symptoms according to the underlying condition. It is important to obtain a detailed history and to conduct a thorough examination as this is likely to give clues as to the aetiology and the possible diagnosis. Box 7.2 summarises the important points to elicit in the history and Box 7.3 presents the important features to note on clinical examination.

A comprehensive occupational history is essential as exposure to inorganic dusts, organic dusts, and toxins is a common cause of alveolar damage. Lung damage secondary to occupational, recreational, and environmental exposure is discussed in more detail in Chapter 17. Drugs commonly associated with DPLD are listed in Box 7.4.

Investigations in a patient suspected of a DPLD

All patients with a suspected DPLD will require some basic investigations, including a chest X-ray, a high-resolution CT scan of the thorax (HRCT),

Box 7.2 History of patient presenting with DPLD.

- Duration of symptoms (acute, subacute, chronic)
- Full occupational history, particularly exposure to asbestos, silica, mouldy hay
- Pets, especially pigeon, parakeet, budgerigar
- Drugs
- Exposure to radiation
- Toxins, for example, paraquat
- Symptoms suggestive of collagen vascular disease
- HIV
- Family history of interstitial lung disease

Box 7.3 Clinical examination of a patient suspected of DPLD.

- Respiratory rate
- Finger clubbing
- Fine, late inspiratory, bibasal crackles
- Features of autoimmune disease
- Signs of cor pulmonale in advanced disease
- Oxygen saturation at rest and on exertion

Box 7.4 Drugs associated with DPLD.

- Amiodarone
- Chemotherapy agents
- Methotrexate
- Naproxen
- Nitrofurantoin
- Sulphonamides

The pulmonary side effects of some of these commonly used drugs are discussed in Chapter 3. A full list of drugs that affect the lungs can be found on www.pneumotox.com.

blood tests (which may include autoantibodies, serum angiotensin converting enzyme (ACE), and serum precipitins) and full lung function tests, including transfer factor for carbon monoxide (TLCO). In some cases, depending on the differential diagnosis and the results of the HRCT, patients may need a bronchoscopy with bronchoalveolar lavage (BAL) to exclude infection and to determine the differential cell count. HRCT changes can be diagnostic in chronic eosinophilic pneumonia, acute eosinophilic pneumonia, sarcoidosis, and allergic bronchopulmonary aspergillosis (ABPA).

A histological diagnosis will be required in many cases to make a definite diagnosis which will determine the management and prognosis. Small pieces of lung tissue obtained by a transbronchial biopsy may be sufficient to make a diagnosis of sarcoidosis, but a VATS lung biopsy taken from different lobes may be required when other conditions, for example, non-specific interstitial pneumonia (NSIP) or pulmonary amyloidosis, are suspected. In advanced disease, histology may be unhelpful as it will only show non-specific lung fibrosis without any clues as to the aetiology. In some cases, for example, in a patient presenting with typical clinical and radiological features of idiopathic pulmonary fibrosis (IPF), histology will not be necessary.

Patients with DPLD will have opacities on their CXR. The differential diagnosis, therefore, always includes infection, malignancy, and heart failure. The common DPLDs (see Box 7.1) have different aetiologies, management, and prognosis and will be discussed in more detail. In 10% of cases, the DPLDs remain unclassified, even with extensive investigations. This makes it difficult to treat and predict the prognosis. As with all DPLDs, careful monitoring over time is required to see how the condition progresses.

Idiopathic interstitial pneumonias (IIP)

Idiopathic interstitial pneumonias (IIP) constitute a group of inflammatory and fibrotic lung diseases, often of unknown aetiology. The classification used is that adopted by the American Thoracic Society/European Respiratory Society International Multidisciplinary Consensus and the British Thoracic Society and is listed in Box 7.5. The prognosis of the idiopathic interstitial pneumonias varies according to the specific type of IIP. While some respond well to immunosuppression, many have a severe and relentless course, progressing to type 1 respiratory failure and death (Figure 7.2).

Pathophysiology

The interstitium, which is the space between the epithelial and endothelial basement membranes, becomes infiltrated by inflammatory cells which

Box 7.5 Classification of idiopathic interstitial pneumonias.

- Idiopathic pulmonary fibrosis (IPF)
- Non-specific interstitial pneumonia (NSIP)
- Cryptogenic organising pneumonia (COP)
- Acute interstitial pneumonia (AIP)
- Respiratory bronchiolitis-associated interstitial lung disease (RB-ILD)
- Desquamative interstitial pneumonia (DIP)
- Lymphoid interstitial pneumonia (LIP)

can also affect the airspaces, the peripheral airways, the blood vessels, and their respective epithelial and endothelial linings. This can result in abnormal collagen deposition and proliferation of fibroblasts. It is postulated that the host's immune system plays an important role in the development of an IIP.

Idiopathic pulmonary fibrosis (IPF)

IPF, previously called cryptogenic fibrosing alveolitis, is a distinctive type of chronic fibrosing interstitial pneumonia of unknown aetiology which is limited to the lungs. The incidence of IPF is 7–16/100 000 per year, with a prevalence of 14–40/100 000 which increases with age, approaching 175/100 000 in those over 75 years. It is rare in patients younger than 50 years old and is twice as common in men as in women. It accounts for 25% of all ILD.

The aetiology of IPF is unknown, but an association with previous exposure to environmental dusts, such as metal and wood, has been found in some epidemiological studies. There is also an association with smoking. Immunological factors may be important, and it appears to run in some families. Several gene mutations, including mutations in the promoter region of a mucin gene (MUC 5B) and the telomerase and surfactant genes, are associated with sporadic and familial pulmonary fibrosis. Some 30% of patients with IPF have autoantibodies, such as rheumatoid factor, in their serum. This suggests that IPF is a form of connective tissue disease primarily affecting the lungs.

There is no cure for IPF, which progresses relentlessly to respiratory failure, with a median survival of 2.8 years from diagnosis. Approximately 2500

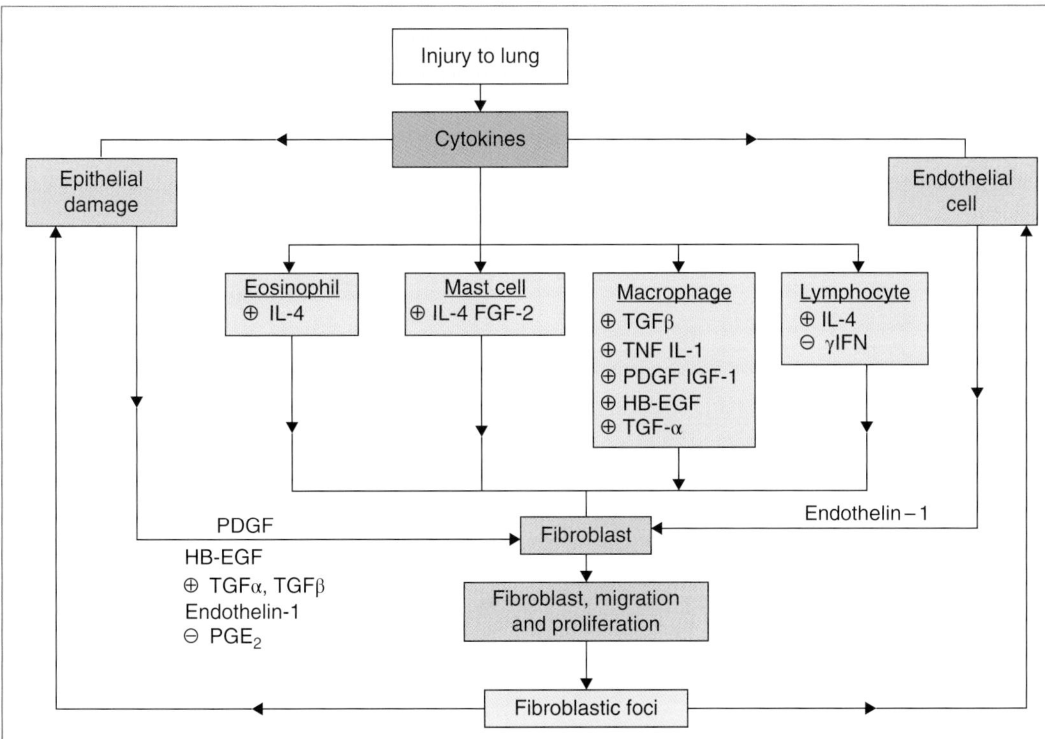

Figure 7.2 Pathophysiology of pulmonary fibrosis.

people die of IPF each year in the UK. There is some evidence that IPF increases the risk of lung cancer. It is essential to exclude other IIP, such as NSIP, which may respond better to treatment with corticosteroids and which may have a better prognosis.

Clinical presentation of IPF

Patients with IPF present with progressively worsening breathlessness, initially on exertion, then at rest. They may have a dry cough and complain of fatigue, malaise, and weight loss. These symptoms are non-specific and could apply to any of the IIPs or DPLDs. Symptoms suggestive of a connective tissue disease, such as Raynaud's, joint paints, rashes, and dysphagia, point to NSIP.

In IPF, clinical examination will reveal tachypnoea, clubbing in 50% of patients and fine, late-inspiratory, basal crackles on auscultation. Crackles are usually first audible at the lung bases in the posterior axillary line. In advanced disease, patients may develop clinical signs of cor pulmonale, which includes a raised jugular venous pressure, a parasternal heave, a loud P2, peripheral oedema, and low oxygen saturation.

Investigations in IPF

A chest X-ray will show reduced lung volumes with reticulonodular shadowing at the lung bases (Figure 7.3). An HRCT will typically show areas of reticulation, predominantly at the lung bases in a sub-pleural distribution with evidence of honeycombing, traction bronchiectasis, and architectural distortion (Figure 7.4, Figure 7.5). In IPF, there is minimal evidence of ground glass opacities although these can develop during acute exacerbations. The HRCT is atypical in 30% of cases and a lung biopsy will be required to confirm the diagnosis.

A lung function test will show a restrictive pattern with decreased vital capacity, increased FEV_1/FVC ratio and a reduced TLCO. Bronchoalveolar lavage will reveal a neutrophilia, the extent of which corresponds to the reticular changes on HRCT. This is indicative of, but not diagnostic of, IPF.

Blood tests should be sent for full blood count, urea and electrolytes and autoimmune profile.

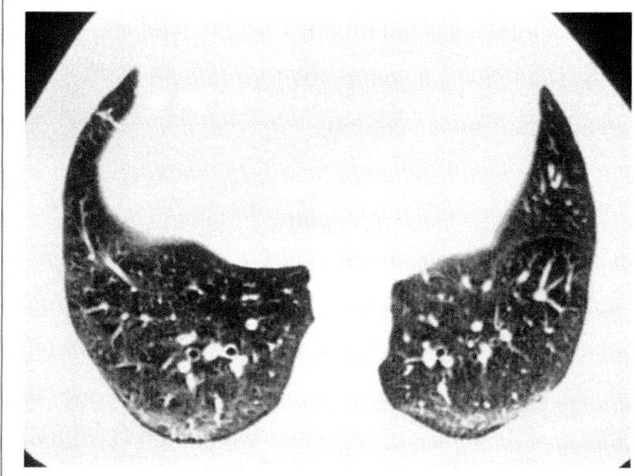

Figure 7.4 HRCT thorax showing bibasal fibrosis of idiopathic pulmonary fibrosis (IPF).

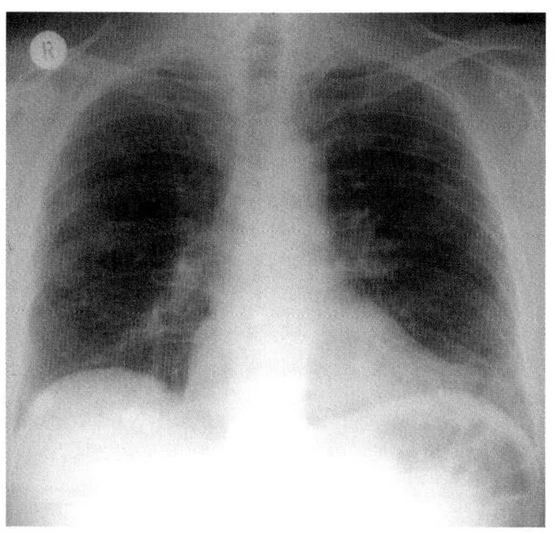

Figure 7.3 CXR of idiopathic pulmonary fibrosis (IPF).

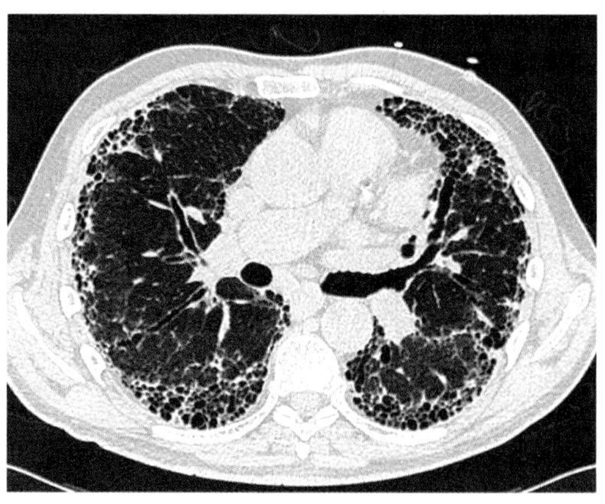

Figure 7.5 HRCT thorax showing fibrosis and honeycombing in advanced idiopathic pulmonary fibrosis (IPF).

If there is clinical evidence of pulmonary hypertension, then an ECG and an echocardiogram should be conducted. A six-minute shuttle test is an objective way to determine the degree of oxygen desaturation on exertion and is used as a primary end-point in trials looking at treatments for IPF.

With advanced disease, arterial blood gas sampling will confirm type 1 respiratory failure with hypoxia ($PaO_2 < 8$ kPa) and normo or hypocapnoea ($PaCO_2 < 6$ kPA). The alveolar-arterial gradient will be increased. (The calculation is described in Chapter 13.)

The diagnosis of IPF is usually made on the clinical history, clinical examination, and HRCT. The British Thoracic Society (BTS) guidelines recommend that if the history and HRCT are consistent with a diagnosis of IPF, then histology is not required. In patients with established IPF, histology is unlikely to be helpful as it will only show end-stage fibrotic changes with no clues as to the aetiology. If there are any unusual features in the presentation, for example, the patient is younger than 50 years old, or the radiological appearance is atypical, then a lung biopsy is recommended.

The histological appearance in IPF is described as '*usual interstitial pneumonia*' (UIP) (Figure 7.6). The lung parenchyma will have a heterogeneous appearance with patchy areas of normal lung, areas of mild interstitial inflammation, fibrosis, and honeycombing. Fibroblast activation results in the formation of fibroblastic foci at the margins of normal lung composed of dense collagen. Areas of honeycombing are composed of cystic, fibrotic air spaces lined by bronchiolar epithelium filled with mucin, and associated with smooth muscle hyperplasia. The areas of interstitial inflammation are patchy and consist of lymphocytes, plasma cells and histiocytes associated with hyperplasia of type 2 pneumocytes.

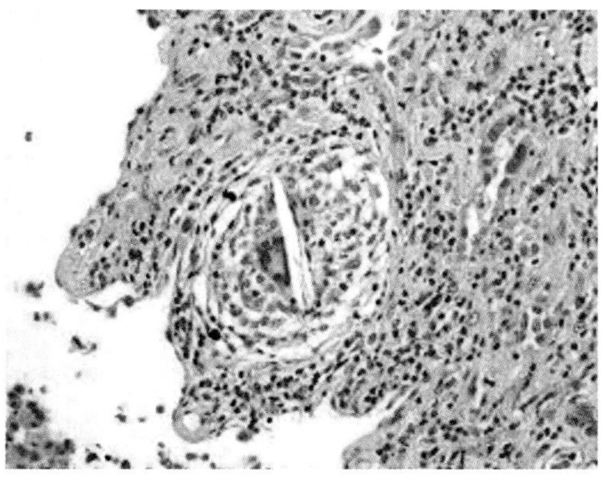

Figure 7.6 Histology of lung showing usual interstitial pneumonia (UIP) in IPF.

Management and prognosis in IPF

The prognosis in IPF is poor with no curative treatment. Most patients die of type 1 respiratory failure within five years. A multidisciplinary approach to diagnosis and management is important and suitable patients should be referred for participation in multicentre trials.

For decades, patients with IPF were treated with corticosteroids, azathioprine, and N-acetyl cysteine (triple therapy) but the PANTHER trial was stopped early because the results showed that patients in the triple therapy arm had increased mortality compared to the control group. Glutathione, a pulmonary antioxidant, is reduced in the bronchoalveolar fluid of patients with IPF. N-acetyl cysteine (NAC), a glutathione precursor with antioxidant properties, has been shown to replace glutathione levels in bronchoalveolar lavage fluid in patients with IPF. The IFEGENIA trial showed that the addition of NAC attenuated decline in FVC and TLCO compared to prednisolone and azathioprine, but more recent trial data (PANTHER) has shown no improvement with NAC compared to placebo. The current recommendation is that patients with IPF are not commenced on triple therapy, although those established on it can continue if they are stable.

Pirfenidone has anti-fibrotic, anti-inflammatory, and antioxidant properties *in vitro*. In recent trials (CAPACITY and ASCEND), pirfenidone has been shown to reduce the decline in vital capacity by 45% over a period of 24–72 weeks, amounting to about 120 ml of vital capacity over a year. Pirfenidone reduced the risk of disease progression and death by 43% and there was an increase in the number of patients with stable FVC. Pirfenidone has significant side effects, including nausea and photosensitivity, but these were tolerated by most patients. NICE has recommended the use of pirfenidone for patients with mild to moderate IPF and FVC of 50–80% predicted, but only in certain regional centres in the UK.

Nintedanib, an orally active tyrosine kinase inhibitor, has been shown in multi-centre trials

(INPULSIS 1 and 2) to halt the decline in FVC and may delay the time to first exacerbation. It is indicated in patients with IPF who have a vital capacity of between 50% and 80% predicted. Nintedanib has significant side effects, including diarrhoea, nausea, abdominal pain, and weight loss. As with pirfenidone, it can only be prescribed in regional centres.

Several other drugs are currently being trialled for the treatment of IPF. These include IFN-y, anti-TGF-β therapies, relaxin, lovastatin, ACE inhibitors, leukotriene receptor antagonists, endothelin receptor antagonists, and anti-TNF-α therapies. There is some evidence that micro-aspiration may play a role in the development of IPF and that treatment with a proton pump inhibitor increases survival. Although a preliminary study suggested benefit with warfarin, a recent study has suggested increased mortality in patients on warfarin, so this is no longer recommended. A lung transplant, either a double or single, may be considered in a patient younger than 60 years.

Patients with IPF can have acute exacerbations, with a sudden decline in vital capacity (VC) and development of severe hypoxaemia requiring high flow oxygen. In these patients, infection should be excluded and those with bacterial infection should receive intravenous antibiotics. Pneumothorax can be a cause of sudden deterioration. Acute exacerbations may be responsive to intravenous pulsed methylprednisolone given over three days, followed by a high dose of oral corticosteroids (OCS). Patients with advanced IPF should be offered palliative care, which includes long term oxygen therapy and opiates for severe breathlessness and cough.

Asbestosis, pulmonary fibrosis secondary to inhalation of asbestos fibres, can present with similar clinical and radiological features, but it is important to make the correct diagnosis as patients with asbestosis may be eligible for compensation. This is discussed in Chapter 15.

Non-specific interstitial pneumonia (NSIP)

NSIP is called '*non-specific*' because the histological features differ from those of the other idiopathic interstitial pneumonias. It occurs equally in men and women, typically in the fifth and sixth decade of life. NSIP is distinct radiologically and pathologically from IPF and has a better prognosis than IPF (Figure 7.7).

Some 88% of patients with NSIP have clinical features of an undifferentiated connective tissue disease, including sicca symptoms, arthralgia, dysphagia, Raynaud's symptoms, and gastro-oesophageal reflux. These patients may also have positive serological tests for rheumatoid factor, antinuclear antibodies, or antibodies to SSA, SSB, RNP, Jo-1 and SCL-70, although NSIP may

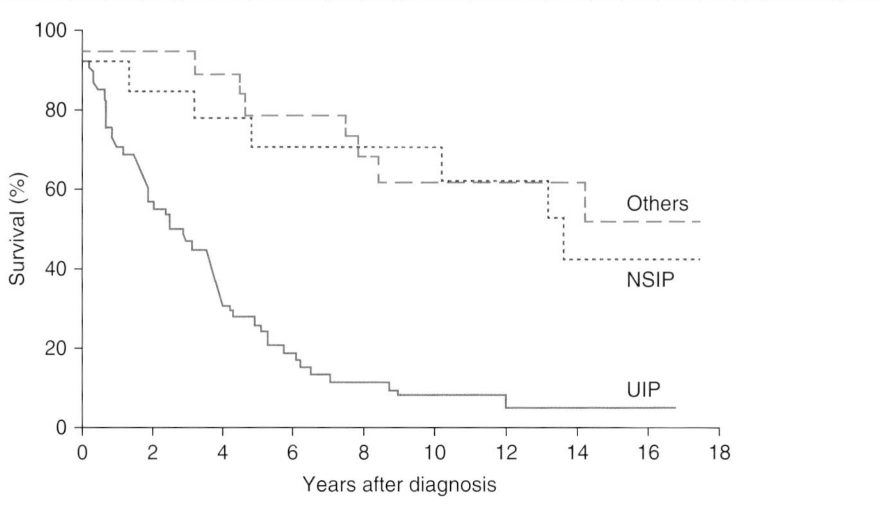

Figure 7.7 Prognosis in UIP, NSIP, and other fibrotic lung diseases.

Box 7.6 Aetiology of NSIP.

Connective tissue diseases

- Ankylosing spondylitis
- Behçet's disease
- Dermatomyositis
- Human immunodeficiency virus (HIV) infection
- Microscopic polyangiitis
- Mixed connective tissue disease (MCTD)
- Polymyositis
- Rheumatoid arthritis
- Sjögren's syndrome
- Systemic lupus erythematosus (SLE)
- Systemic sclerosis

Drugs associated with NSIP

- Amiodarone
- Carmustine
- Chlorambucil
- Flecanide
- Methotrexate
- Nitrofurantoin
- Statin

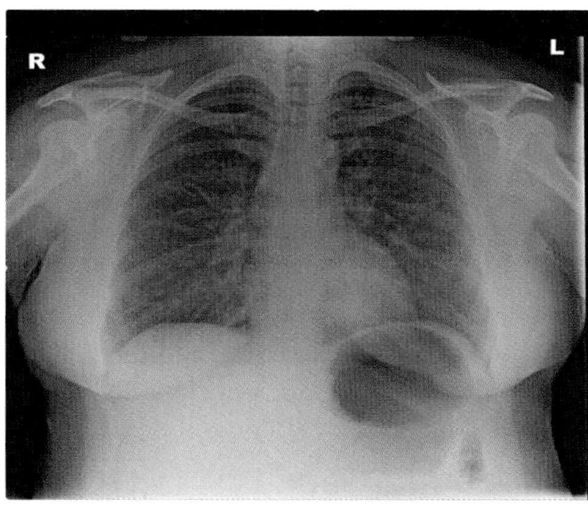

Figure 7.8 CXR of non-specific interstitial pneumonia (NSIP) showing interstitial shadowing.

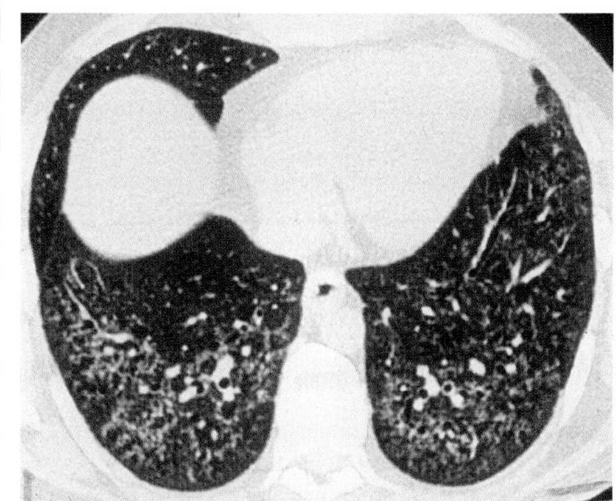

Figure 7.9 HRCT thorax showing ground glass changes of non-specific interstitial pneumonia (NSIP).

precede a diagnosis of a collagen vascular disease by several months or years. Radiologically, NSIP may resemble hypersensitivity pneumonitis (HP) or cryptogenic organising pneumonia (COP). Box 7.6 shows the aetiology of NSIP.

Clinical presentation of NSIP

Patients present with progressively worsening breathlessness, cough, and pleuritic chest pain, which develop over weeks to months. About a third of patients with NSIP may describe flu-like symptoms, including myalgias. They may report symptoms suggestive of a CTD, such as rashes, arthralgia, fatigue, sicca syndrome (dry eyes and mouth), and weight loss.

Clinical examination may reveal tachypnoea, bibasal crackles, and features of an underlying CTD. Clubbing is rare. Patients may be hypoxic or desaturate on exertion.

Investigations in NSIP

The CXR may appear normal in the early stages, but bilateral interstitial opacities will eventually develop (Figure 7.8). HRCT will show abnormalities, even when the CXR appears normal, typically diffuse, bilateral, basal, and subpleural ground glass changes (Figure 7.9). A minority of patients with NSIP will develop irregular, linear, reticular opacities, traction bronchiectasis, and volume loss. Honeycombing, which is a feature of UIP, is rare and may suggest advanced disease which is less responsive to treatment. The differential diagnosis for ground glass opacification is wide, therefore a surgical lung biopsy taken from several lobes is recommended.

NSIP is characterised by inflammatory changes in the lung parenchyma resulting in the ground glass changes seen on HRCT, and there is good correlation between the HRCT changes and the histological features. NSIP can be sub-classified into fibrotic or cellular types. In cellular NSIP there is interstitial infiltration of mononuclear cells with minimal fibrosis on lung biopsy and a better response to immunosuppression. BAL will show a non-specific lymphocytosis (50%) with an increase in the number of neutrophils and eosinophils. Dendritic cells, which play a role in the immune response through antigen presentation, are found in greater numbers in biopsies of patients with NSIP compared to UIP, and are found close to CD4 and CD8 lymphocytes. Fibrotic NSIP resembles UIP, is less responsive to immunosuppression than cellular NSIP, and has a worse prognosis.

Lung function shows a restrictive pattern with reduced vital capacity and a decrease in gas transfer. FVC and TLCO can predict the prognosis and can be useful in monitoring disease progression and response to treatment.

NSIP can resemble hypersensitivity pneumonitis (HP) clinically, radiologically, and histologically, although HP typically has granulomata and multinucleated giant cells. Focal areas resembling the changes seen in cryptogenic organising pneumonia (COP) can also occur.

Management of NSIP

If an underlying cause is found, for example, a drug, then this should be stopped. Infection should always be excluded by taking a BAL. Evidence for hypersensitivity pneumonitis should be sought by BAL and serum precipitins. Investigations to diagnose an underlying CTD should be conducted. In idiopathic NSIP, fewer than 20% of patients will improve or stabilise without therapy, but these patients will need careful monitoring with serial lung function and HRCT, initially every three months.

NSIP is more responsive to immunosuppressive treatment than IPF and has a better prognosis. Oral prednisolone at 1 $mg\,kg^{-1}\,day^{-1}$ should be started in patients who do not improve spontaneously. Patients with severe symptoms and worsening lung function can be treated with pulsed intravenous methylprednisolone, 1000 $mg\,day^{-1}$ for three days, followed by oral prednisolone, 40–60 mg daily. The steroids should be gradually tapered, aiming to reach 5–10 $mg\,day^{-1}$ on alternate days by the end of 12 months. Up to a third of patients will relapse when the steroids are stopped. High doses of corticosteroids have significant side effects, and these should be considered (see Chapter 3).

Azathioprine, starting at 50 $mg\,day^{-1}$, and increasing by 25 mg increments every 7–14 days up to 200 $mg\,day^{-1}$, can be given additionally to those who need a steroid-sparing agent or who have an incomplete response to steroids. Cyclophosphamide can be considered for those with severe lung disease secondary to CTD or those who have progressed despite steroids+/azathioprine. Oral cyclophosphamide can be given at a dose of 1.5–2 $mg\,kg^{-1}\,day^{-1}$ up to a maximum of 200 $mg\,day^{-1}$ as a single dose. Cyclophosphamide has significant side effects which limits its use in the long term. Mycophenolate mofetil can also be used for interstitial lung disease secondary to a connective tissue disorder and Rituximab is used as a rescue therapy in NSIP. A lung transplant can be considered with severe NSIP that is progressive despite immunosuppressive therapy. Patients on immunosuppressive therapy should have regular monitoring of their full blood count and a liver function test. Pneumocystis jiroveci infection is common in immunosuppressed individuals, so prophylactic co-trimoxazole is recommended.

Prognosis in NSIP

The overall response to therapy and prognosis in NSIP is good compared to UIP, with a median survival of 56 months compared to a median survival of 33 months in UIP. Some 66% will improve or remain stable after five years of treatment with a 15–25% mortality at five years.

Serial pulmonary function testing gives better prognostic information than imaging or histopathology, with the TLCO being the most sensitive prognostic indicator.

Cryptogenic organising pneumonia (COP)

Cryptogenic organising pneumonia (COP) is also called bronchiolitis obliterans organising pneumonia (BOOP). It occurs equally in men and women, with a peak incidence in the mid-fifties, and is commoner in smokers compared to non-smokers. The exact incidence and prevalence are unknown.

Patients often present after a lower respiratory tract infection with cough, malaise, fever, and dyspnoea, which can persist for several weeks and months. These patients are often diagnosed as having community acquired pneumonia and are treated with antibiotics despite the lack of evidence of a bacterial pneumonia. Symptoms can progress, with patients developing myalgias, weight loss, worsening breathlessness, and respiratory failure. Clinical examination may reveal crackles in the lungs, but clubbing is rare.

CXR and the HRCT thorax show unilateral or bilateral areas of patchy consolidation in 90% of cases (Figure 7.10, Figure 7.11). Less common findings include nodules with air bronchograms, reticulonodular shadowing or ground glass shadowing which can resemble NSIP. Blood tests may show a raised ESR and a neutrophilia, and a BAL will show 40% lymphocytes with an increase in the proportion of neutrophils and eosinophils. Transbronchial biopsy or open lung biopsy may be required if the diagnosis is in doubt and will show alveolar ducts and alveoli with intraluminal polyps and intra-alveolar buds of organising fibrosis.

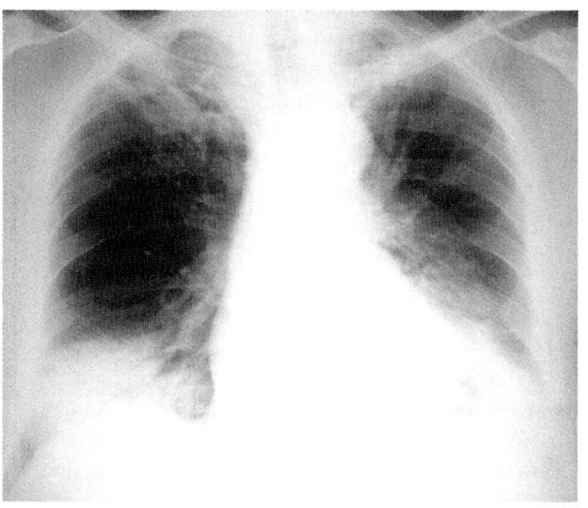

Figure 7.10 CXR in cryptogenic organising pneumonia (COP) showing areas of consolidation.

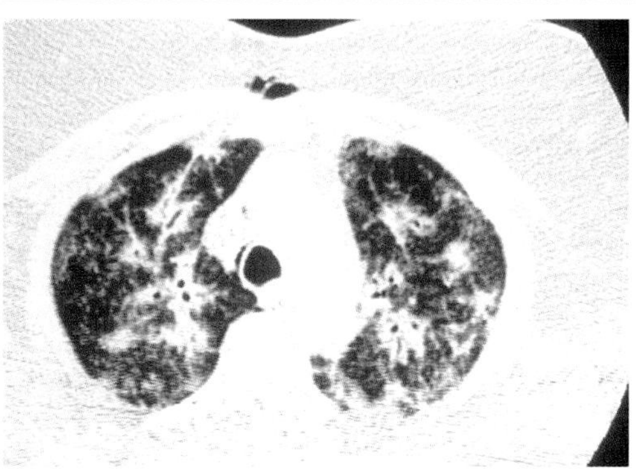

Figure 7.11 CT thorax showing extensive areas of consolidation in cryptogenic organising pneumonia (COP).

The differential diagnosis of COP includes pneumonia, sarcoidosis, bronchoalveolar cell carcinoma (adenocarcinoma *in situ*), eosinophilic pneumonia, NSIP, and atypical infection. In COP, no pathogen will be identified from a BAL and there will be no clinical or radiological improvement with antibiotics. Most patients with COP show a dramatic improvement with oral corticosteroids, although it is common for relapse to occur when the dose of steroids is reduced, so six months of treatment may be required. Stronger immunosuppression may be required in some cases.

Desquamative interstitial pneumonia (DIP)

DIP is relatively rare, accounting for about 8% of ILD, although the exact incidence and prevalence are unknown. It was called 'desquamative' as it was thought to be due to desquamation of alveolar macrophages on lung biopsy. However, it is now known to be due to the accumulation of intra-alveolar macrophages. It mainly affects smokers in the fourth and fifth decades and is twice as common in men as in women. It is unclear whether those exposed to passive smoking have an increased risk. There is also an association with connective tissue diseases. Patients present with breathlessness and a dry cough which develops over weeks and months and can progress to respiratory failure. Some 50% of patients develop clubbing.

A lung function test will reveal a mild reduction in lung volumes but a moderate reduction in transfer factor. The CXR may be normal in 20% of cases and the HRCT will show ground glass shadowing, predominantly in the lower zones with a peripheral distribution. In one-third of cases, the HRCT will progress to honeycombing (Figure 7.12). A BAL will show increased alveolar macrophages with granules of 'smoker's pigment' consisting of intracellular yellow, golden, brown, or black smoke particles. Histology will show macrophage accumulation in the distal airspaces and infiltration of alveolar septae with plasma cells and eosinophils.

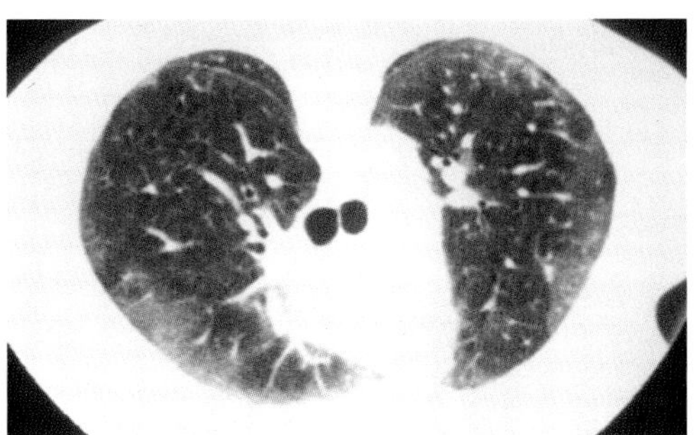

Figure 7.12 CT thorax of desquamative interstitial pneumonia (DIP) showing areas of fibrosis.

The differential diagnoses include RB-ILD, sarcoidosis, hypersensitivity pneumonitis (HP), and pneumocystis jiroveci infection. The prognosis is good with smoking cessation and oral corticosteroids, with a 70–80% 10-year survival.

Respiratory bronchiolitis interstitial lung disease (RB-ILD)

RB-ILD and DIP are similar clinically, radiologically, and pathologically and have a similar prognosis, although RB-ILD affects the lung in a more diffuse manner than DIP. Many consider RB-ILD to be an early form of DIP. Although the exact incidence and prevalence are unknown, it accounted for about 20% of biopsy-proven ILD cases in the Mayo Clinic. RB-ILD occurs most commonly in the fourth and fifth decades in smokers with a greater than 30-pack a year history, and is twice as common in men as in women.

Patients, usually smokers, present with dyspnoea and cough, and the CXR will show fine reticulonodular shadowing at the lung bases in 80% of cases (Figure 7.13). A lung biopsy will show pigmented, intraluminal macrophages within the respiratory bronchioles which contain iron-rich, granular, golden-brown particles. These macrophages are surrounded by peribronchiolar infiltrate of lymphocytes and histiocytes containing coarse, black pigment. As with DIP, RB-ILD is responsive to steroids and has a good prognosis in those who stop smoking.

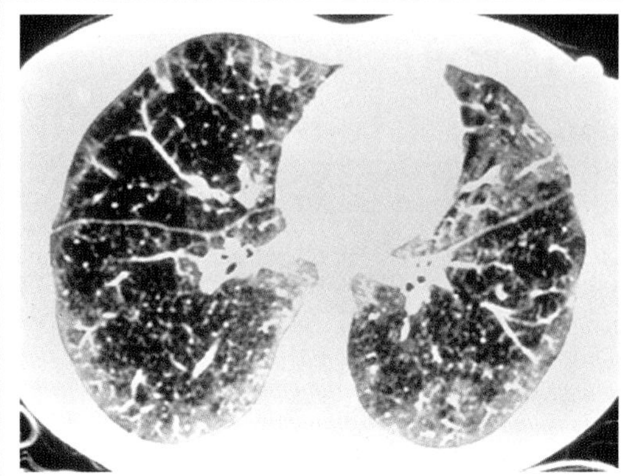

Figure 7.13 CT thorax of respiratory bronchiolitis-interstitial lung disease (RBILD).

Lymphoid interstitial pneumonia (LIP)

LIP is a rare form of ILD, considered to be a pulmonary lymphoproliferative disorder, often associated with HIV infection, hypogammaglobulinaemia, severe combined immunodeficiency, and collagen vascular diseases, particularly rheumatoid arthritis and Sjögren's. LIP is commoner in females in their fifth decade. Patients present with cough and dyspnoea which develops over months. Systemic symptoms include fever, weight loss, chest pain, and arthralgia. Clinical examination may reveal crackles in the lungs.

LIP is characterised by a diffuse lymphocytic interstitial infiltrate. It can be difficult to distinguish between lymphoma and LIP histologically, but immunocytochemistry and molecular analysis can separate neoplastic infiltrates from LIP. Blood tests often show mild anaemia and dysproteinaemia, with polyclonal increase in gammaglobulins or monoclonal increase in IgG or IgM in 75% of cases. The CXR shows alveolar shadowing at the lung bases or diffuse honeycombing. The HRCT shows ground glass opacities with perivascular cysts, perivascular honeycombing, reticular opacities, and lung nodules. The BAL will show lymphocytosis, and a lung biopsy will reveal dense lymphoid infiltrates. Corticosteroids may improve symptoms, but there is little evidence that it can reverse pulmonary fibrosis.

Acute interstitial pneumonia (AIP)

AIP, also called Hamman-Rich syndrome, is an aggressive form of ILD characterised by rapidly progressive diffuse alveolar damage. It is indistinguishable from ARDS secondary to sepsis and shock (see Chapter 17) and has a similar poor prognosis. Exacerbation of IPF can also present in a similar way, although in that case there will be underlying histological features of UIP. AIP has equal sex preponderance and can occur at any age, with a mean age of 50. The exact incidence and prevalence are unknown. Genetic and immunological factors may be important.

AIP is often preceded by a short history (three weeks) of upper respiratory tract viral infection, with patients presenting with cough, severe breathlessness, myalgia, malaise, and fever. Clinical examination will reveal widespread, diffuse crackles, signs of consolidation, and worsening hypoxaemia. The CXR and the CT thorax will show bilateral patchy airspace opacification with air bronchograms, ground-glass changes, bronchial dilatation, and architectural distortion, especially in the later organising stage of the disease. Lung function will show a restrictive pattern with reduced transfer factor. The BAL will show an increase in total cells, with haemorrhage secondary to alveolitis and hyaline membrane formation as seen in ARDS. A lung biopsy will reveal extensive fibroblast proliferation with thickening of the alveolar septa, the proliferation of atypical type 2 pneumocytes, and hyaline membrane formation within the alveolar walls.

AIP has a high mortality of more than 50%, with patients progressing rapidly to respiratory failure within one to three months of onset of illness. As in ARDS, treatment is with ventilatory support and prevention of secondary infection. Corticosteroids have not been shown to alter the natural history of the disease. ECMO may have a role in supporting oxygenation and preventing further damage to the lungs. Survivors usually progress to pulmonary fibrosis. Recurrence of AIP can occur.

Eosinophilic lung disease

Eosinophils predominantly dwell in tissues with a mucosal epithelial interface, such as the lungs, the gastrointestinal system, and the genitourinary system. The usual eosinophil count in peripheral blood is $<0.4 \times 10^9 l^{-1}$ which accounts for 1.3% of the circulating white cell count. The peripheral eosinophil count does not indicate the extent of eosinophilic infiltration of organs. Eosinophils are not found in the lungs of healthy individuals, so a finding of an eosinophilia of greater than 10% on a BAL is pathological.

Pulmonary eosinophilic diseases are a group of disorders which present with breathlessness, productive cough, and wheeze secondary to infiltration of the lung parenchyma by eosinophils which secrete inflammatory cytokines which damage the alveoli. In some cases, patients can develop systemic symptoms of fever, night sweats, weight loss, and myalgia. Some of these conditions may be associated with a peripheral blood eosinophilia, although in several serious eosinophilic conditions, the peripheral eosinophil count may be normal.

As with all the DPLD, it is essential to obtain a detailed history of any new drugs, including recreational drugs, occupational exposure to toxins and chemicals, travel to areas where parasitic diseases are endemic, and any history of allergy or atopy. Bacterial pneumonia is a serious consideration in these patients as it presents with the same symptoms and can be radiologically difficult to rule out, but pneumonia usually results in a neutrophilia and an eosinopenia secondary to the elevated endogenous corticosteroid levels.

In eosinophilic lung diseases, the chest X-ray is often normal, but may show parenchymal infiltrates, usually in a bilateral and peripheral distribution (Figure 7.14). The term 'infiltrate'

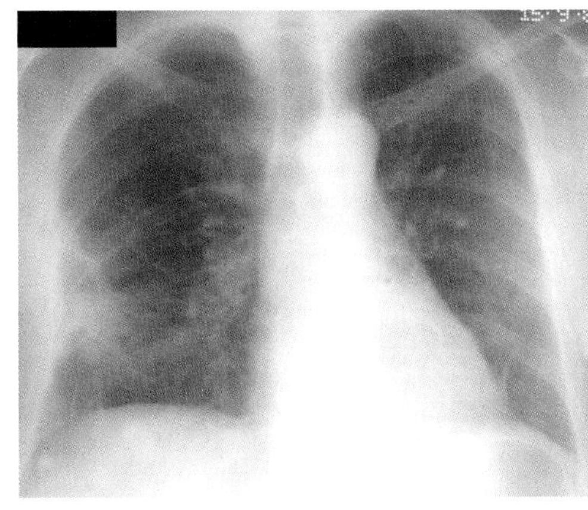

Figure 7.14 CXR of eosinophilic pneumonia showing interstitial shadowing.

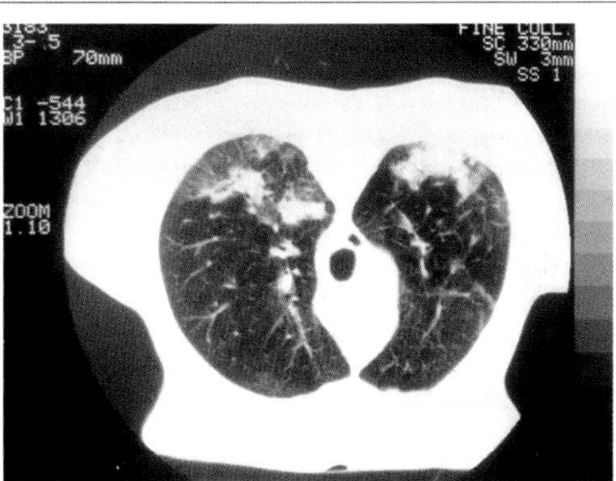

Figure 7.15 CT thorax of eosinophilic pneumonia showing areas of consolidation.

implies areas of consolidation within the parenchyma. The HRCT is much more sensitive at detecting subtle ground glass and other parenchymal changes, although in most cases of pulmonary eosinophilic diseases, the radiological appearances are non-specific. The differential diagnoses for the radiological appearances of eosinophilic pulmonary disease include IPF, sarcoidosis, HP, and COP (Figure 7.15).

Sputum samples can be helpful in determining the presence of eosinophils, which implies lung involvement, and in detecting larvae of parasites. BAL fluid should always be sent for microbiological analysis to exclude bacterial, fungal, and parasitic infections and for cytology to look for an underlying malignant cause, such as bronchoalveolar cell carcinoma (adenocarcinoma *in situ*). A diagnosis of eosinophilic pneumonia is likely if the differential cell count of BAL shows >10% eosinophils. A transbronchial biopsy may not yield samples that are adequate, so either a VATS or open lung biopsy may be necessary to demonstrate eosinophilic infiltration.

Measurement of total serum immunoglobin E (IgE) may be helpful when asthma or ABPA are likely, as IgE-mediated eosinophil production is induced by leukotrienes, histamine, and IL5, which are released by mast cells and basophils. Aspergillus-specific IgE and IgG measurement is recommended if the clinical and radiological features suggest ABPA. Auto-antibody testing should be done, as an underlying connective tissue disease is always a possibility with this presentation. Serum antifilarial IgG should be measured if the clinical features suggest helminth infection.

Table 7.1 lists the differential diagnosis of eosinophilic pulmonary diseases and describes the typical features of each of these.

Allergy to drugs, atopic diseases, and malignancy are the commonest causes of peripheral eosinophilia in the UK. Worldwide, parasitic infections account for most cases of peripheral eosinophilia. Appendix 7.A lists some of the commonly implicated drugs. Toxins and inhaled recreational drugs can also be associated with eosinophilia and are discussed in Chapter 15. ABPA is discussed in more detail in Chapter 6 and EGPA is discussed in more detail in Chapter 11.

Management of pulmonary eosinophilia depends on the severity of symptoms and the exact diagnosis. Infection must be excluded prior to commencing corticosteroids which are very effective in reducing the peripheral eosinophil count within hours. Therefore, if an eosinophilic condition is suspected, investigations should be carried out prior to starting corticosteroid treatment.

Sarcoidosis

Sarcoidosis is a multisystem disease characterised by the development of non-caseating granulomatous lesions in the affected organs. It is the commonest diffuse parenchymal lung disease worldwide and affects men and women in the third to fifth decades. The prevalence is 3/100 000 in Caucasians, 47/100 000 in African Americans and rises to 64/100 000 in Scandinavians. The markedly different prevalence between races, familial clustering, and a significantly increased incidence in monozygotic twins suggest a genetic predisposition. Studies have suggested linkage to a section within MHC on the short arm of chromosome 6. HLA Dr11, 12, 14, 15 and 17 confer susceptibility to the disease, whereas HLA DR1 and DR4 are protective.

It is postulated that sarcoidosis results from an abnormal immunological reaction to a poorly degradable antigen, with granulomas forming around the antigen to prevent dissemination. The frequent involvement of the lungs suggests that the antigen enters the body through inhalation. The ACCESS study, a case-control aetiological study of sarcoidosis, found some evidence that the antigen may be a remnant of microbial organisms, including Mycobacterium species, Propionibacterium acnes, and herpes. There is also some evidence implicating organic dusts, metals, minerals,

Table 7.1 Causes of eosinophilia.

Condition	Clinical presentation	Onset	Peripheral blood	Eosinophilic lung involvement	Skin involvement	Other organ involvement	Radiological changes
Allergic asthma, common Good prognosis	Dyspnoea Wheeze	Weeks to months	Mild eosinophilia Raised IgE	None	None	None	Hyperinflated
Allergy, common Good prognosis	Dyspnoea Wheeze	Hours to days	Eosinophilia Raised IgE Positive RAST to allergen	None	Positive skin prick tests to allergens, rash	Upper airways Skin Gastrointestinal tract	Normal
ABPA, relatively common Usually not fatal but difficult to eradicate	Dyspnoea Wheeze Cough Systemic symptoms	Weeks to months	Eosinophilia, Raised IgE, Raised aspergillus IgG, Positive aspergillus skin prick test	None	Positive skin prick to aspergillus	None	Proximal bronchiectasis with bronchial wall thickening, mucous plugging, and areas of atelectasis.
Eosinophilic granulomatosis with polyangiitis (EGPA) previously called Churg-Strauss Syndrome. Significant morbidity and mortality if untreated	Breathlessness Wheeze Rhinitis Fever Malaise Weight loss	Weeks to months	Eosinophilia	Eosinophilic lung infiltration	Eosinophilic infiltration resulting in rash, palpable purpura, and nodules	Eosinophilic infiltration of upper airways, kidneys, gastrointestinal tract, heart, and peripheral nervous system	Bilateral, peripheral pulmonary infiltrates, pleural effusion

(Continued)

Table 7.1 (*Continued*)

Condition	Clinical presentation	Onset	Peripheral blood	Eosinophilic lung involvement	Skin involvement	Other organ involvement	Radiological changes
Hypereosinophilic Syndrome (HES). Rare, some associated with an abnormality of the tyrosine kinase fusion protein. Fatal if untreated. OCS effective. Mepolizumab if associated with genetic abnormality Splenectomy	Fever Weight loss Cough Dyspnoea Night sweats Pruritis	Weeks to months	Very high peripheral eosinophil count ($>1.5 \times 10^9 l^{-1}$	High eosinophils, some of which are abnormal with a decrease in number and size of granules	Eosinophilic infiltration of skin	Eosinophilic tissue infiltration of many organs: heart, peripheral nervous system, and spleen. Increased risk of thromboembolic disease	Patchy ground glass opacities and areas of consolidation
Acute Eosinophilic Pneumonia. Idiopathic, can cause diffuse alveolar damage and progress to ARDS and respiratory failure. Responds to corticosteroids	Severe dyspnoea Non-productive cough Fever Hypoxia Myalgia	Rapid onset, over a few days	Normal peripheral eosinophil count initially, but may increase over time	Very high eosinophils in sputum and BAL (>25%)	None	None	Non–specific ground glass opacification with areas of consolidation, interlobular septal thickening, and pleural effusion
Chronic Eosinophilic Pneumonia. Idiopathic, commoner in women and non-smokers, may be commoner in those who have had radiotherapy for breast cancer. Responds to corticosteroids but can be recurrent	Dyspnoea Productive cough, Haemoptysis Wheeze Fever Weight loss Night sweats. In 50% asthma-like symptoms precede development of eosinophilia	Weeks to months	Peripheral eosinophilia in 80%	High eosinophils in sputum or BAL (> 40%). Nodular mucosal lesions with necrotising eosinophilic inflammation	None	None	Characteristic bilateral, consolidative, and ground glass areas which are peripheral and in the middle and upper zones. Pleural changes can occur

Tropical pulmonary eosinophilia occurs in those who have travelled abroad. Secondary to immune response to the parasites Wucheria bancrofti and Brugia Malayi, endemic in Asia and South America. Characterised by remissions and relapses. Successfully treated with diethylcarbamazine	Dyspnoea Productive cough Wheeze Chest pain Haemoptysis Fever Fatigue Weight loss	Weeks to months.	Significant peripheral eosinophilia > $3 \times 10^9 l^{-1}$. Serum IgE> 1000 $kU l^{-1}$ and increase titres of antifilarial IgG	Eosinophils in sputum and BAL	None	Gastrointestinal tract	Normal in 70% but showing diffuse reticulonodular opacities and mediastinal lymphadenopathy in 30%
Simple pulmonary eosinophilia (Löffler's syndrome), now used to describe acute onset pulmonary eosinophilia. Originally described in cases secondary to parasitic infection with Ascaris lumbricoides, strongyloidis stercoralis, ancyclostoma duodenale or necator americanus. Treatment with antihelminth drugs	Cough Malaise Anorexia Rhinitis Night sweats Fever Dyspnoea Wheeze	Over days to weeks	Low level peripheral eosinophilia	Sputum may be blood-tinged and show eosinophils, larvae, and Charcot-Leyden crystals	None	Gastrointestinal system	Flitting opacities ranging in size from a few mm to a few cm. Clear spontaneously after several weeks
Drug-induced	Cough Dyspnoea Hypoxia	Hours to days of taking new drug	Peripheral eosinophilia	None	Skin rash, infiltration of skin	None	Normal

solvents, pesticides, and wood stoves. There appears to be an association with tuberculosis and lymphoma.

In sarcoidosis, there is accumulation of CD4 lymphocytes within the organs involved, with a corresponding depletion in CD4 cElls peripherally. This anergy results in a delayed type 4 hypersensitivity response. Patients with sarcoidosis will have a negative reaction to tuberculin testing, even when they have had a previous Bacilli Calmette-Guérin (BCG) vaccination.

IL-2, IL-12 and IFN-γ activate T helper cells and have been shown to result in granuloma formation and exacerbation of sarcoidosis. High levels of IL-12, which is known to play an important role in the immunological response to intracellular organisms, have been found in the bronchial washings of patients with sarcoidosis. Genetic defects in IL-12 receptor decrease granuloma formation and increase the susceptibility to atypical mycobacterial infections. TNF-α is a non-specific, but potent, pro-inflammatory cytokine in sarcoidosis.

Clinical presentation of sarcoidosis

Sarcoidosis can present acutely or chronically. In many cases the diagnosis is made incidentally in an asymptomatic patient.

Acute sarcoidosis (Löfgren's syndrome)

Acute sarcoidosis typically occurs in young patients in their twenties and thirties. This type of presentation is more likely to occur in women, particularly in those of Irish and Nordic descent, and has a good prognosis. Box 7.7 lists the symptoms and signs of acute sarcoidosis (Figure 7.16, Figure 7.17). The differential diagnosis for this presentation is wide and includes viral or bacterial infection, mycobacterium tuberculosis infection, lymphoma, and autoimmune conditions.

Chronic sarcoidosis

Chronic sarcoidosis presents more insidiously and can affect one or several organs. The lungs are affected in 90% of cases, and in 50% of cases only the lungs are affected. In 10% of cases, there is only cutaneous involvement. Symptoms of pulmonary sarcoidosis include breathlessness, reduced exercise tolerance, cough, fatigue, anorexia, and weight loss. Examination of the chest will reveal reduced

Box 7.7 Symptoms and signs of acute sarcoidosis.

Symptoms	Signs
Fever	
Arthralgia	
Myalgia	
Rash	Erythema nodosum
Eye pain and redness	Anterior uveitis
Dyspnoea	
Night sweats	
Fatigue	
Weight loss	

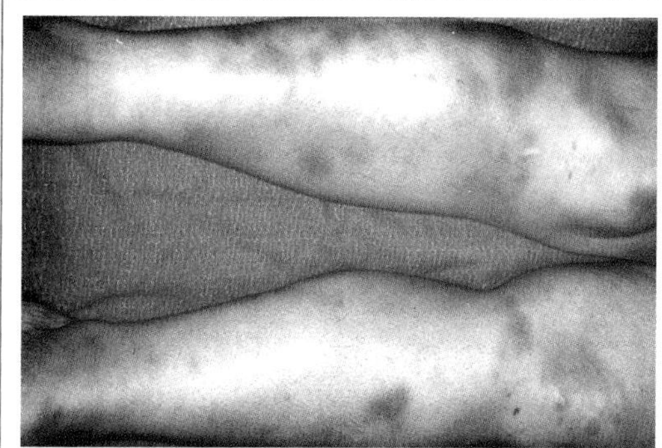

Figure 7.16 Erythema nodosum.

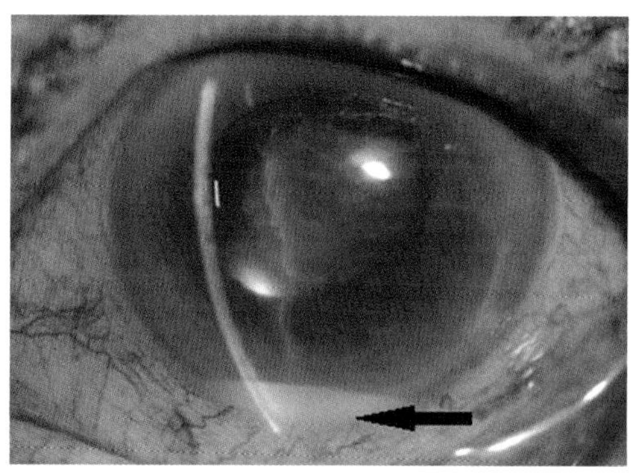

Figure 7.17 Anterior uveitis with arrow showing hypopyon.

lung expansion consistent with a restrictive process and crackles in 20% of patients. The differential diagnosis includes any of the diffuse parenchymal lung diseases.

The finding of an abnormal chest X-ray with bilateral hilar lymphadenopathy (BHL) in an asymptomatic individual is a common presentation of sarcoidosis. Other common presentations of sarcoidosis include hypercalcaemia and abnormal liver function tests.

Sarcoidosis can affect several organs in the upper respiratory tract, including the larynx, the pharynx, sinuses, and the post-nasal space, causing nasal obstruction, rhinosinusitis, nasal crusting, anosmia, epistaxis, and nasal polyposis. The differential diagnosis includes granulomatous polyangiitis (see Chapter 11) and asthma (see Chapter 6).

Multisystem sarcoidosis

Sarcoidosis can affect most of the organs in the body. Box 7.8 lists the organs involved.

Investigations

A comprehensive history, including a full occupational history and family history, should be ascertained. The diagnosis of sarcoidosis is made with a correlation between clinical presentation, radiological, and histopathological features.

Radiology

The lungs are involved in 90% of cases, so the CXR will be abnormal in the majority. Box 7.9 shows the different stages of pulmonary sarcoidosis (Figure 7.18, Figure 7.19, Figure 7.20, Figure 7.21, Figure 7.22, Figure 7.23, Figure 7.24, Figure 7.25).

Box 7.9 Radiological staging of pulmonary sarcoidosis.

Chest X-ray stage	
Stage 0	Normal chest X-ray (5–10%)
Stage 1	Bilateral hilar lymphadenopathy (45–65%)
Stage 2	BHL and pulmonary infiltrates (25–30%)
Stage 3	Pulmonary infiltrates without BHL (15%)
Stage 4	Pulmonary fibrosis

Box 7.8 Organs involved in multisystem sarcoidosis.

- **Skin:** lupus pernio in 25%, maculopapular eruption, plaques, nodules, and scar infiltration
- **Lymph nodes:** palpable in 30%
- **Eyes:** 26–50% develop anterior uveitis, posterior uveitis, retinal vasculitis, keratoconjunctivitis, conjunctival follicles
- **Muscle and joints:** 10–15% develop joint pain and swelling, muscle pain
- **Liver:** hepatomegaly in 12%, resulting in abnormal liver function test and granulomas
- **Spleen:** splenomegaly in 7%
- **Heart:** cardiomyopathy, third degree heart block, arrhythmias, sudden death
- **Bone:** bone cysts affecting hands and feet, dactylitis, osteolytic or osteosclerotic lesions
- **Salivary glands:** parotid and submandibular gland involvement in 4%
- **Lacrimal glands:** involvement in 1%
- **Kidneys:** nephrocalcinosis, renal calculi, acute nephritis
- **Gastrointestinal system, including pancreas:** involvement in 1%
- **Reproductive system:** although rare, involvement of testes can cause infertility. Sarcoidosis can become active after pregnancy
- **Central nervous system:** neurosarcoidosis can present with granulomatous meningitis (elevated lymphocyte count in cerebrospinal fluid), cranial and/or peripheral nerve palsies, seventh nerve palsy, space-occupying lesion resulting in obstructive hydrocephalus and seizures. Posterior pituitary involvement may cause diabetes insipidus

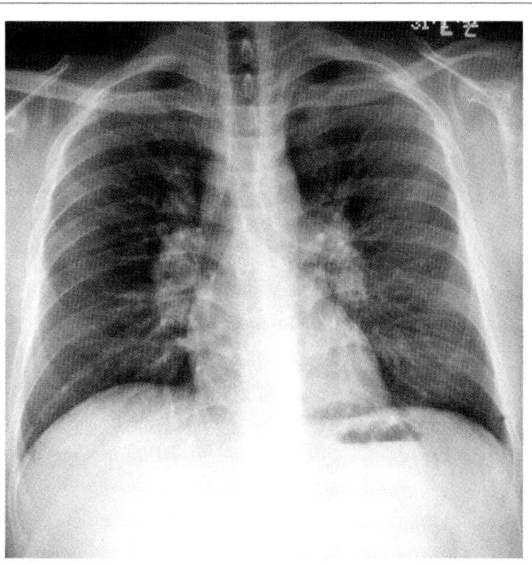

Figure 7.18 CXR of stage 1 pulmonary sarcoidosis showing BHL.

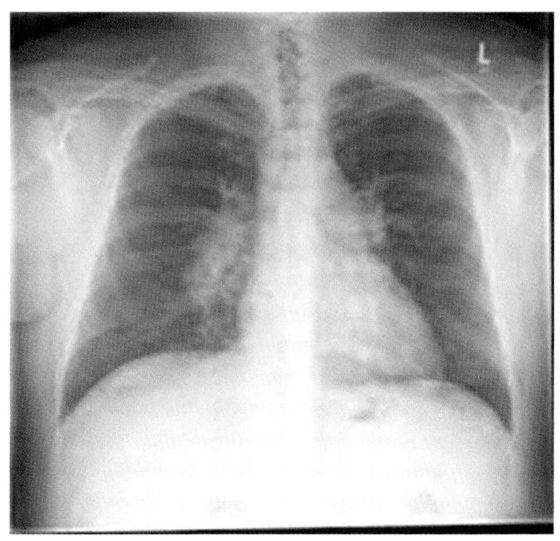

Figure 7.20 CXR of stage 2 pulmonary sarcoidosis with BHL and pulmonary infiltrates.

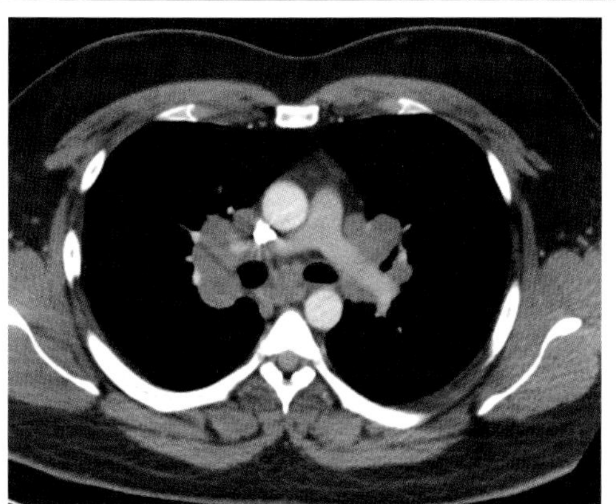

Figure 7.19 CT thorax of stage 1 pulmonary sarcoidosis showing bilateral hilar lymphadenopathy (BHL).

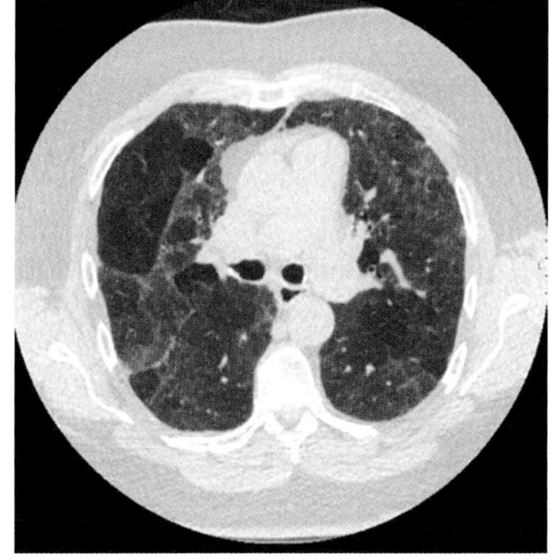

Figure 7.21 CT thorax of stage 2 pulmonary sarcoidosis with BHL and pulmonary infiltrates.

The differential diagnosis of bilateral hilar lymphadenopathy (BHL) includes mycobacterium tuberculosis infection and lymphoma. Rarer differentials in those with occupational exposure include silicosis and berylliosis (see Chapter 15). Coccidioidomycosis and histoplasmosis can occur in endemic areas in North America.

The HRCT scan of the thorax is more sensitive than a CXR and may show interstitial changes, even when the CXR appears normal. Typical HRCT features, which occur in 60–70% of cases, include nodules (called 'beading') in a perilymphatic or bronchovascular distribution, forming along the subpleural surface, along fissures and interlobular septae. The lung parenchyma in the upper and middle zones is affected, with sparing of the lung bases. Lymph nodes in the hilar and paratracheal region may be enlarged and calcified.

In stages 3 and 4 sarcoidosis, progressive pulmonary fibrosis results in reticulonodular shadowing, with volume loss of the upper lobes, displacement of the interlobar fissure, hilar

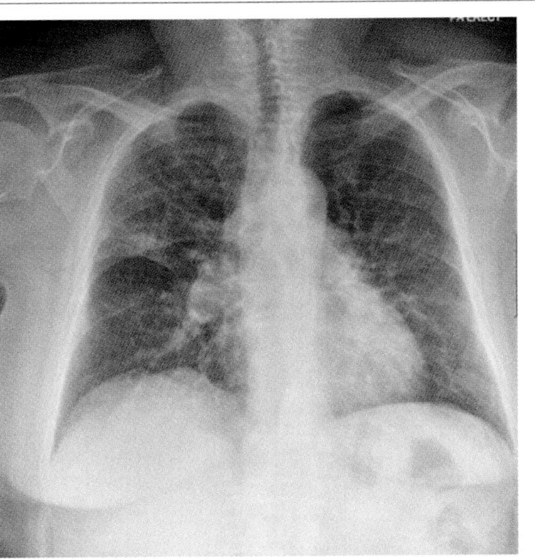

Figure 7.22 CXR of stage 3 pulmonary sarcoidosis showing pulmonary fibrosis.

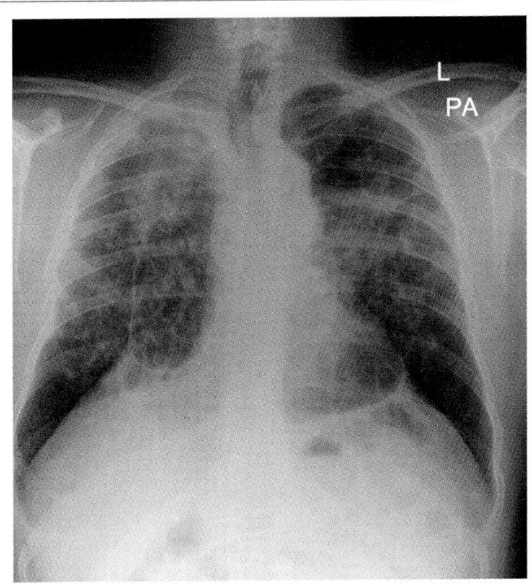

Figure 7.24 CXR of stage 4 pulmonary sarcoidosis showing extensive, chronic fibrosis.

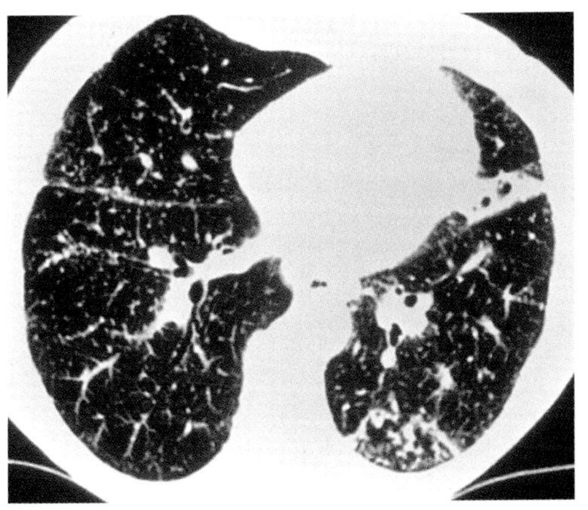

Figure 7.23 CT thorax of stage 3 pulmonary sarcoidosis showing pulmonary fibrosis.

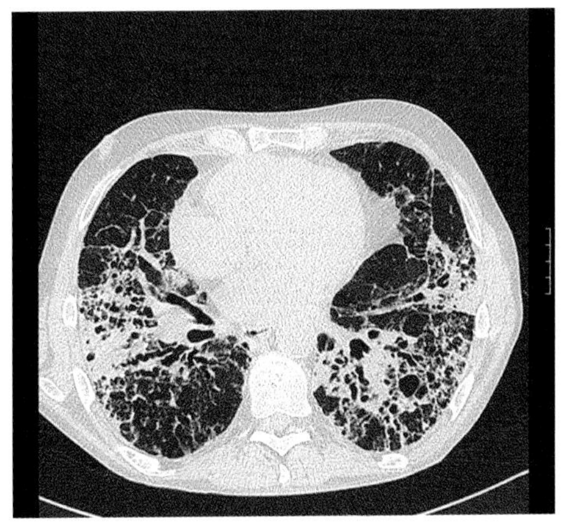

Figure 7.25 CT thorax of stage 4 pulmonary sarcoidosis showing extensive, chronic fibrosis.

elevation, architectural distortion, and traction bronchiectasis. A lymphocytic pleural effusion will occur in fewer than 5% of cases. Pneumothorax and chylothorax are very rare presentations of sarcoidosis.

A minority of patients may require further radiological investigations to confirm the extent of organ involvement. Gallium scanning is expensive and exposes the patient to significant radiation, but can be helpful in assessing disease activity, especially when an MRI scan is not possible. ^{67}Gallium, which is taken up preferentially by granulomas, can detect lesions not seen on a CT scan, particularly in the mediastinum, spleen, and salivary glands. Bilateral, symmetrical involvement of lymph nodes and salivary glands is typical of sarcoidosis with the characteristic 'lambda' sign where there is paratracheal and bilateral hilar uptake of ^{67}Ga and the 'panda' sign when there is uptake in the lacrimal and parotid glands. Magnetic resonance imaging (MRI) is required to investigate a patient suspected of neurosarcoidosis.

Blood tests

The serum ACE level is elevated in two-thirds of patients with active sarcoidosis, but lacks sensitivity and specificity so is of limited value in the diagnosis of sarcoidosis. Serum ACE levels do not correlate with the radiological stage of the disease and serial measurements are not recommended in the guidelines. Full blood count, corrected serum calcium, liver function tests, and 24-hour urine calcium levels should be measured in all patients with sarcoidosis. Mild leucopenia, mild anaemia, and a slight increase in transaminases can occur. C-reactive protein (CRP), the erythrocyte sedimentation rate (ESR), and serum immunoglobulin levels may be elevated in acute sarcoidosis, and immune complexes are often present. Hypercalcaemia can occur in 10–20% of patients with sarcoidosis due to dysregulation of the calcium metabolism. Macrophages within granulomas in lungs and lymph nodes synthesise calcitriol (1, 24 dihydroxy vitamin D) which results in increased calcium absorption from the gastrointestinal tract and increased bone resorption.

Some 30–50% of patients with sarcoidosis develop hypercalciuria which, if not treated, can progress to renal calculi, nephrocalcinosis, and renal failure.

Lung function test

The lung function test will be abnormal in 20% of patients with stage 1 sarcoidosis, and in the majority of those with stages 2, 3 and 4 sarcoidosis. The lung function test will show a restrictive defect, with reduction in FVC, TLC, and TLCO. There may be an obstructive element when there is significant endobronchial disease. The severity of the restrictive changes does not correlate well with the HRCT changes, and the baseline lung function does not predict the long term outcome. Serial lung function measurements can be used to monitor disease progression and response to treatment, with the vital capacity (VC) and TLCO being the most sensitive measures in predicting steroid-responsiveness.

Histological diagnosis of sarcoidosis

Histological confirmation is essential to rule out lymphoma, *Mycobacterium tuberculosis*, and other parenchymal lung diseases in those presenting with BHL. Biopsies should be obtained from the most accessible site. Most patients will have a bronchoscopy with a bronchoalveolar lavage (BAL) and a transbronchial lung biopsy (TBLB). The HRCT may be helpful in guiding which lobe to biopsy. Lymph nodes can be sampled through an endobronchial ultrasound-guided biopsy (EBUS). At bronchoscopy, endobronchial lesions may be seen which can be biopsied. A transbronchial biopsy is often diagnostic and is a relatively safe procedure with a < 10% risk of a pneumothorax. The BAL will show an increase in the CD4 and T-helper cells and raised CD4:CD8 T cell ratio. In all cases, bronchial fluid and biopsies should be sent for microscopy and culture to exclude infection, particularly mycobacterium tuberculosis infection.

Biopsies can also be taken from mediastinal lymph nodes via a mediastinoscopy, which is a surgical procedure requiring a general anaesthetic. A VATS lung biopsy or surgical open lung biopsy may be necessary in patients presenting with an atypical HRCT or those with pulmonary nodules where malignancy may be of concern. If other organ involvement is suspected, then biopsies can be obtained from these, for example, skin, liver, and bone.

Histology will show non-caseating granuloma but no acid-fast bacilli. Granulomas consist of a central area of macrophages that differentiate into epithelioid cells and fuse to form multi-nucleated giant cells surrounded by lymphocytes. The multi-nucleated cells have cytoplasmic inclusions, including asteroid bodies, Schaumann bodies, and birefringent crystalline particles. There is accumulation of CD4 T-helper cells within the granulomas with CD8 T cells around the periphery (Figure 7.26). The Kveim test, a diagnostic test used in the past, is no longer used because of the risk of infection.

Other investigations

Tuberculin skin testing, which is negative in sarcoidosis, can be useful in excluding *Mycobacterium tuberculosis*, except in patients who have HIV. Patients suspected of having cardiac involvement of sarcoidosis should have an ECG, an

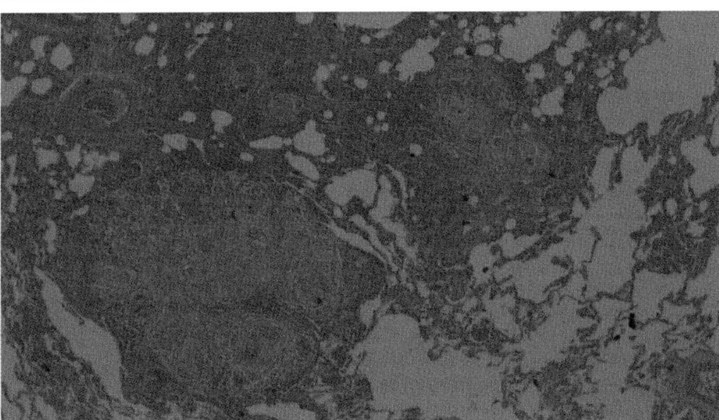

Figure 7.26 Histology of sarcoid lung showing granuloma with multinucleate giant cells, lymphocytes and histiocytes.

echocardiogram, and a cardiac MRI, before proceeding to a cardiac biopsy if necessary.

Management and prognosis of sarcoidosis

The natural history of sarcoidosis is variable and unpredictable, with spontaneous remissions and relapses. Acute sarcoidosis has a good prognosis: it is usually self-limiting with spontaneous resolution occurring in the majority, although relapses are common. For symptomatic patients (fatigue, fever, night sweat, and joint pains), a short course of oral corticosteroids (OCS) given for three and six months is recommended. Patients with eye symptoms should be referred to the ophthalmologist and are usually prescribed steroids eye drops.

The clinical course and prognosis in pulmonary sarcoidosis vary according to the radiological stage of the disease and the ethnicity of the patient. Overall, for all stages, two-thirds are in remission within 10 years but one-third progress, resulting in significant organ damage. Some 1–5% of patients die secondary to respiratory failure, cardiac arrhythmias, or neurosarcoidosis.

Spontaneous remission occurs in 55–90% of patients with stage 1 disease, 40–70% with stage 2 disease, and 10–20% with stage 3 disease, with most remissions occurring in the first six months of diagnosis. Treatment is not indicated for asymptomatic patients with stage 1 disease as the rate of spontaneous remission is so high. A "wait and watch" policy is recommended in this group.

Treatment with OCS for 6–24 months is indicated for symptomatic patients with stages 2 and 3 disease and abnormal lung function. A dose of 0.4 $mg\,kg^{-1}$ ideal body weight is recommended, usually 20–40 $mg\,day^{-1}$. The dose of OCS should be tapered according to clinical response and improvement in CXR and lung function. Most patients will improve with steroids, but 50% will relapse when the dose is reduced or stopped. There is little evidence for the use of inhaled corticosteroids in pulmonary sarcoidosis, although those with cough secondary to significant endobronchial disease and obstruction on lung function may benefit.

OCS treatment is indicated for patients with multisystem sarcoidosis and involvement of other organs. OCS are particularly effective in treating hypercalcaemia and hypercalciuria secondary to sarcoidosis.

In patients with refractory disease and in those who have significant side effects with corticosteroids, steroid-sparing agents, such as methotrexate, mycophenolate mofetil, and azathioprine should be considered. TNF-α inhibitors, such as infliximab and pentoxifylline, have not been shown in trials to be particularly effective in patients with chronic sarcoidosis and have significant side effects. Hydroxycholoroquine is often used for cutaneous sarcoid lesions and in chronic sarcoidosis. Low-dose thalidomide may also be beneficial in cutaneous sarcoidosis. In patients with refractory hypercalciuria, chloroquine, hydroxychloroquine, and ketoconazole can be used.

Multisystem sarcoidosis, particularly neurosarcoidosis and cardiac sarcoidosis, can be life-threatening and may require high doses of intravenous cyclophosphamide. There is some evidence that a combination of infliximab and mycophenolate mofetil is effective in neurosarcoidosis. Patients with multisystem sarcoidosis and those with significant organ involvement are often managed in specialist centres.

Many of these drugs are contraindicated in women of child-bearing age because of teratogenicity. These drugs can also cause significant side effects, particularly bone marrow suppression, so will need to be carefully monitored.

Patients with refractory pulmonary sarcoidosis and advanced fibrotic disease should be considered for lung transplantation before they develop respiratory failure, although there are reports of recurrence of disease in the transplanted organ. For those patients who do not respond to any treatment and develop pulmonary hypertension, cor pulmonale, and respiratory failure, long term oxygen therapy and palliative care should be offered.

Hypersensitivity pneumonitis (HP)

Hypersensitivity pneumonitis, also called extrinsic allergic alveolitis (EAA), can be classified as acute, sub-acute, or chronic depending on the frequency, length, and intensity of exposure and the duration of the illness. It is not a single disease but can be caused by exposure to microorganisms (fungal, bacterial, protozoan), animal or insect proteins, agricultural dusts, bio-aerosols, and certain reactive chemical species. The exact prevalence of HP is unknown because over 300 different aetiological agents have been identified and because there are no uniform diagnostic criteria. Prevalence and incidence vary depending on the intensity of exposure to inciting antigens, geographical conditions, and different methods of collecting data.

HP is an immunologically mediated type 3 hypersensitivity lung disease. It is postulated that both environmental and host factors are important in developing HP. The inhalation of antigens by an individual who has already been sensitised provokes a complex immune response involving antibody reactions, immune complex formation, complex activation, and cellular response, resulting in alveolitis. Only a small proportion of exposed individuals develop clinically significant HP.

Common causes of HP include thermophilic spores of saprophytic fungi and bird droppings. Farmer's lung, caused by thermophilic actinomycetes and saccharopolyspora rectivirgula, is one of the most common forms of HP, affecting 0.4–7% of the farming population. The prevalence varies by region, climate, and farming practices, being higher in humid areas (9%) and lower in drier climates (3%). When hay is harvested and stored in damp conditions, it becomes mouldy and generates heat that encourages the growth of fungi. Thermophilic actinomycetes are present in the atmosphere throughout the year and cause disease when individuals are exposed to large numbers of particles. The numbers of actinomycetes spores increase with temperature and humidity and can contaminate a wide variety of vegetables, wood bark, air-conditioning systems, and humidifiers.

Avian-related HP develops in pigeon fanciers and in those keeping budgerigars, parakeets, and chickens. The reported prevalence is 20–20 000/100 000 persons at risk. The prevalence of HP is higher among bird fanciers than farmers because contact with the inciting avian antigen is less limited by season or geographic location.

Table 7.2 lists some other known causes of HP. Cigarette smoking reduces antibody response to inhaled antigens so is associated with a decreased risk of developing HP, although once the disease is established, smoking does not appear to attenuate its severity and may predispose to a more chronic and severe course.

Acute hypersensitivity pneumonitis

Patients present with fever, rigors, chest pains, malaise, breathlessness, and cough which can occur within hours of exposure. The intensity of the reaction is proportional to the amount of inhaled antigen and the duration of exposure. Many patients with HP are misdiagnosed as suffering from viral illnesses or asthma as the CXR could be normal in the early stages and an occupational history is not taken by the doctor. Physical examination may reveal tachypnoea and diffuse fine crackles on auscultation of the lungs. In severe cases, the patient may become profoundly breathless and hypoxic and progress to type 1 respiratory failure.

HP is characterised by inflammation of the alveoli with a lymphocytic infiltration and minimal fibrosis. Blood tests will show a non-specific inflammatory picture with elevated ESR, CRP, and lactate dehydrogenase (LDH). If an occupational history is suspected, then serum-precipitating IgG antibodies against the causative

Table 7.2 Some causes of hypersensitivity pneumonitis.

Name of disease	Antigen	Source of antigen
Farmer's lung	Thermophilic actinomycetes Saccharaplyspora rectivirgula Micropolyspora faeni Aspergillus Species	Mouldy hay
Bird fancier's lung	Feather and bird droppings	Pigeon, budgerigars, parakeets, chicken
Malt worker's lung	*Aspergillus fumigatus, Aspergillus clavatus*	Mouldy barley
Coffee worker's lung	Coffee bean protein	Coffee bean
Detergent worker's lung	Bacillus subtilis enzymes	Detergent
Bagassosis	Thermoactinomyces vulgaris	Mouldy sugar cane
Humidifier lung	Thermoactinomyces vulgaris	Contaminated water in reservoirs or air conditioning systems
Hot tub lung	*Mycobacterium avium*	Mist from hot tubs
Cheese-washer's lung	*Aspergillus clavatus, Penicillium casei*	Mouldy cheese
Chemical worker's lung	Isocyanates	Spray paints, glues

antigen are usually detectable, but only indicate exposure as these are also present in 10–15% of exposed but asymptomatic individuals. False negative results can also occur. Bronchial washings are required to exclude infection. A differential cell count from the BAL will show an increase in CD8 T cells.

The CXR may show early interstitial changes in the middle and upper zones of the lungs. An HRCT is more sensitive and will reveal ground glass shadowing with areas of decreased attenuation and air trapping on expiratory scans. A lung function test will reveal a restrictive pattern. If histology is sought from a lung biopsy, it typically shows poorly formed, non-caseating, interstitial granulomas or mononuclear cell infiltration in a peribronchial distribution, often with prominent giant cells. The main differential diagnosis is sarcoidosis.

The symptoms and radiological changes of acute hypersensitivity pneumonitis can resolve rapidly when the antigen is removed. In those who are symptomatic and hypoxic, a course of oral corticosteroids can improve the symptoms and radiological changes. Steroids may be required for three to six months in a tapering course and relapse is common when the steroids are stopped. Re-exposure to the antigen will also cause a relapse.

Sub-acute hypersensitivity pneumonitis

The sub-acute form of HP is more insidious, developing over weeks and months. Patients present with progressively worsening dyspnoea, cough, anorexia, and weight loss. Clinical examination may reveal finger clubbing and inspiratory crackles.

The CXR may be normal, as in acute HP, or may show micronodular or reticular opacities, most prominent in the middle to upper lung zones. The HRCT will show diffuse micronodules, ground glass changes, focal air trapping, and mild fibrotic changes. A lung biopsy will show well-formed non-caseating granulomas in the interstitium, bronchiolitis with or without organising pneumonia, and interstitial fibrosis. The main clinical, radiological, and histological differential diagnosis of sub-acute HP is sarcoidosis.

Chronic hypersensitivity pneumonitis

The chronic form develops over months and can progress to pulmonary fibrosis and respiratory failure. Patients with advanced disease develop clubbing and will have clinical signs of volume loss, particularly in the upper zones, with fine crackles on auscultation. The CXR shows ground-glass changes and reticulation (Figure 7.27). The HRCT may show parenchymal micronodules, interstitial pneumonia, bronchiolitis obliterans, and fibrosis with honeycombing. It can be difficult to differentiate this from IPF and stage 4 sarcoidosis. A BAL will show an increase in neutrophils, which is a non-specific finding, but fluid should be sent for microbiology and culture to exclude infection, including pneumocystis jiroveci infection (Figure 7.28).

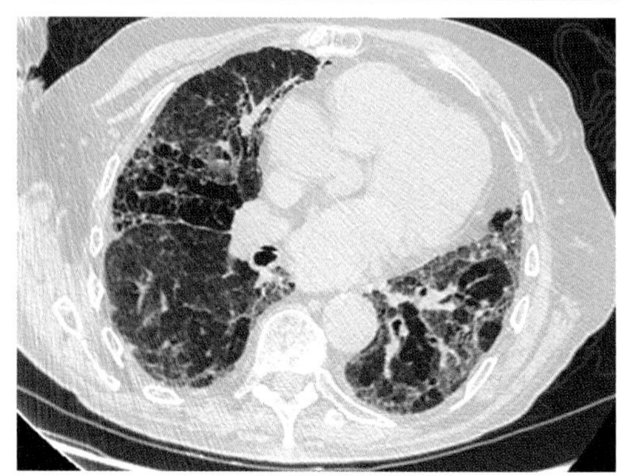

Figure 7.28 CT thorax of chronic hypersensitivity pneumonitis (HP) showing ground glass changes and fibrosis.

Management of HP

Antigen avoidance is the most important advice to give to patients diagnosed with HP. This will result in rapid resolution of symptoms over hours and days and avoid the need for corticosteroid treatment. This may be difficult for some if it is their hobby or occupation, in which case, measures to reduce antigen exposure, including wearing protective masks, head covering, and protective clothes should be advocated. Respirators can be used, although their efficacy in reducing exposure is unknown. Changes in the handling and storage of material, for example, hay, reducing the humidity of a building to below 60%, reducing stagnant water, and preventing the re-circulation of water in heating, ventilation, and air conditioning systems are essential measures. Wetting compost before handling it can reduce the dispersion of actinomycetes spores, and the use of antimicrobial solutions in sugar cane processing can reduce fungal growth and the development of bagassosis.

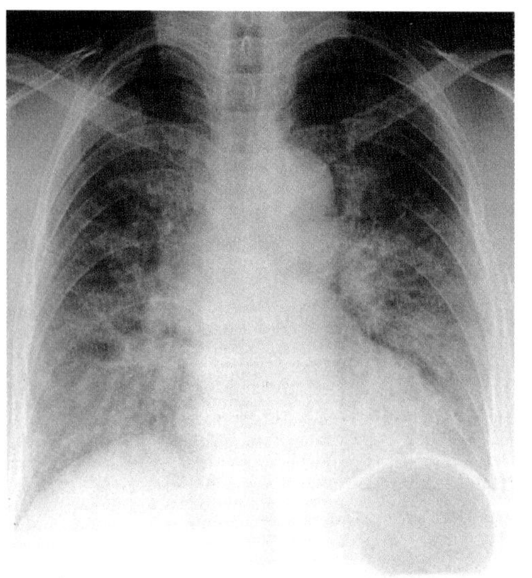

Figure 7.27 CXR of hypersensitivity pneumonitis (HP).

Corticosteroids are usually given to those with significant and persistent symptoms, those with hypoxaemia, those with reduced diffusing capacity on the lung function test and those with extensive radiological changes. Oral prednisolone given at a moderately high dose of 1 mg kg^{-1} day^{-1} (up to a maximum of 60 mg day^{-1}) for two weeks, with a reducing regime over the next two to four weeks, will improve the symptoms of fever, chest pain, and dyspnoea, and improve the radiological changes of acute and sub-acute hypersensitivity pneumonitis. Relapse can commonly occur when the dose of steroids is reduced or stopped.

However, there is no evidence of long term benefit with corticosteroids which are less effective in chronic hypersensitivity pneumonitis and established pulmonary fibrosis. Steroid-sparing agents, such as methotrexate, can be considered for those who require immunosuppression for a longer period or for those who have significant side effects with steroids.

Prognosis of HP

Most patients with acute and sub-acute hypersensitivity pneumonitis recover completely with antigen avoidance, although it may take up to two years for the lung function to recover completely. Those presenting acutely generally do better than those with a chronic presentation and established pulmonary fibrosis. Older age, digital clubbing at presentation, and honeycombing and traction bronchiectasis on HRCT confer a worse prognosis.

About 50% of patients with farmer's lung develop mild chronic lung impairment, usually obstructive in nature, often with emphysematous changes on HRCT. Bird fancier's lung carries a worse prognosis than farmer's lung, possibly due to the higher degree of exposure to antigens and the persistence of avian antigens at home despite attempts at decontamination. Mortality was 29% at five years in Mexican patients with chronic pigeon breeder's lung. Those with histological changes resembling NSIP or COP had a better prognosis than those with UIP-like changes. The prognosis of HP secondary to other aetiologies is less well described.

Lymphangioleiomyomatosis (LAM)

Pulmonary LAM is a rare condition occurring in women of child-bearing age. It is commoner in the Caucasian population, but the exact incidence and prevalence of LAM are unknown. Many cases of LAM are associated with germ line mutations in the tuberous sclerosis complex (TSC). Some 30% of women with TSC are affected by pulmonary LAM. Sporadic pulmonary LAM is associated with somatic mutations in the TSC1 or TSC2 genes in the lungs. LAM has been reported in men in association with the TSC complex. Oestrogen may be implicated in the development of clinically apparent LAM in genetically predisposed individuals.

LAM is a benign mesenchymal tumour characterised by the proliferation of atypical pulmonary smooth muscle and epithelioid cells, called LAM cells, around bronchovascular structures, resulting in the formation of multiple, small cysts in the distal airspaces. These cysts can vary in size from 0.1 cm to several centimetres in diameter. Rupture of the dilated and tortuous venules can result in haemosiderin deposition in the cysts. The thoracic duct can also be enlarged and thickened. Extra-pulmonary manifestations of LAM include renal angiomyolipomas and mediastinal, retroperitoneal, and pelvic lymphangioleiomyomas.

Although LAM is often classified as a DPLD, it has more similarities to asthma or emphysema clinically and radiologically, and can present with significant airflow obstruction. Patients present with progressive breathlessness, spontaneous pneumothorax, haemoptysis, and chylothorax. Patients presenting late may have evidence of pulmonary hypertension. Diagnosis is made on HRCT which shows multiple (usually between 2 and 10), small, thin-walled cysts (Figure 7.29, Figure 7.30). A chylous pleural effusion secondary to rupture of the thoracic duct can occur. If the radiological features are typical, then a tissue biopsy is not required. If a tissue biopsy is needed, then a lung biopsy can be obtained via TBLB, VATS or open

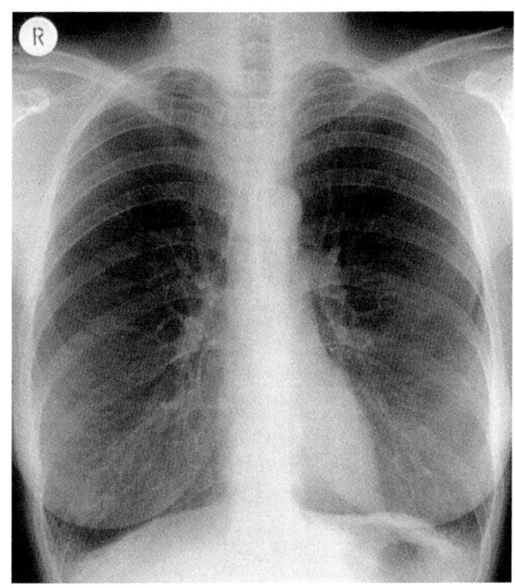

Figure 7.29 CXR of lymphangioleiomyomatosis (LAM) showing hyperinflation.

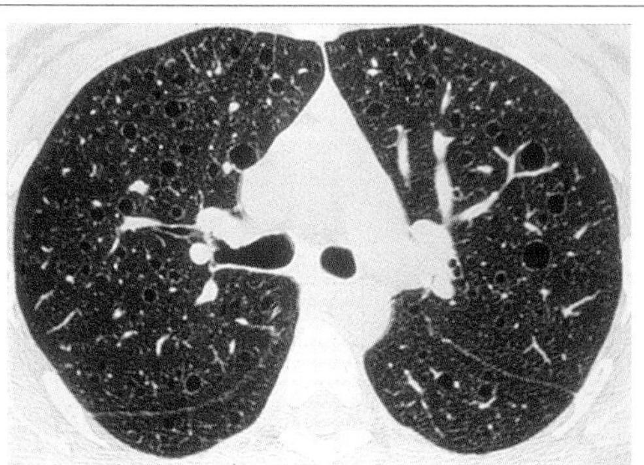

Figure 7.30 HRCT thorax of lymphangiomyomatosis (LAM) showing multiple cysts in both lungs.

lung biopsy, although an increased risk of pneumothorax must be taken into consideration.

A lung function test will be normal in 57% of cases but will show an obstructive picture, with an increase in TLC and RV compatible with hyperinflation, a marked reduction in TLCO, and reversibility to bronchodilators in the rest. A six-minute walk test will be abnormal in severe disease and is often used to monitor patients. The A-a gradient will be increased.

The differential diagnosis of LAM includes asthma, emphysema, and alpha-1 antitrypsin deficiency (see Chapter 6). Measurement of vascular endothelial growth factor (VEGF-D), which is elevated in LAM, may be helpful as a screening test if LAM is suspected, but is not commonly available.

There is no specific treatment for LAM, but the effectiveness of mTOR inhibitors sirolimus and everolimus is currently being evaluated in trials. Some studies have demonstrated disease stabilisation and modest improvement with progestational and anti-oestrogen agents, but it should be noted that long term treatment with progesterone increases the risk of venous thromboembolism and meningiomas. Symptomatic treatment of LAM includes the use of bronchodilators, oxygen therapy in those who are hypoxic, and pulmonary rehabilitation. Oestrogen therapy should be avoided. The prognosis is good, with survival of 29 years from the onset of symptoms. Patients who present with a spontaneous pneumothorax may require pleurodesis or pleurectomy. Patients who progress towards respiratory failure may be eligible for lung transplantation.

Pulmonary Langerhans cell histiocytosis (PLCH)

Pulmonary Langerhans cell histiocytosis (PLCH) is an uncommon interstitial lung disease that affects young adults, particularly cigarette smokers. The true incidence and prevalence are unknown, but it is commoner in men and was diagnosed in about 5% of lung biopsies in a study at the Mayo Clinic. Systemic LCH is commoner in young children between the ages of 1 and 3 where it can present with severe disseminated disease involving multiple organs, including bone, skin, lymph nodes, liver, spleen, lung, CNS, and oral mucosa.

The Langerhans cell is a differentiated cell of the macrophage-monocyte line which is usually found in the dermis, the reticulo-endothelial system, the lungs, and the pleura. The Langerhans cell has a pale-staining cytoplasm, a large nucleus, large nucleoli and Birbeck granules on electron microscopy. Langerhans cells have CD1 antigen on the cell surface and demonstrate positive immunohistochemical staining for S100 protein. An increase in Langerhans cells can be found in healthy smokers and in idiopathic pulmonary fibrosis. In PLCH, these cells are found in larger numbers in clusters, although there is no consensus as to the numbers of these cells required to make a diagnosis of PLCH.

Pulmonary involvement is seen in 10% of cases, and patients present with progressive breathlessness, dry cough, chest pain, and spontaneous pneumothorax, which can be recurrent in 15–25%. The HRCT will demonstrate characteristic cysts and nodules, predominantly in the upper zones (Figure 7.31, Figure 7.32). If the radiological picture is not typical, lung biopsy can be performed to make the diagnosis. Lung function tests demonstrate reduced lung volumes and diffusing capacity and, in advanced disease, patients develop airflow obstruction. Hypercalcaemia is a common finding in patients with PLCH due to increased production of calcitriol.

The emphasis in adults presenting with pulmonary LCH is smoking cessation and symptomatic treatment with bronchodilators and oxygen if

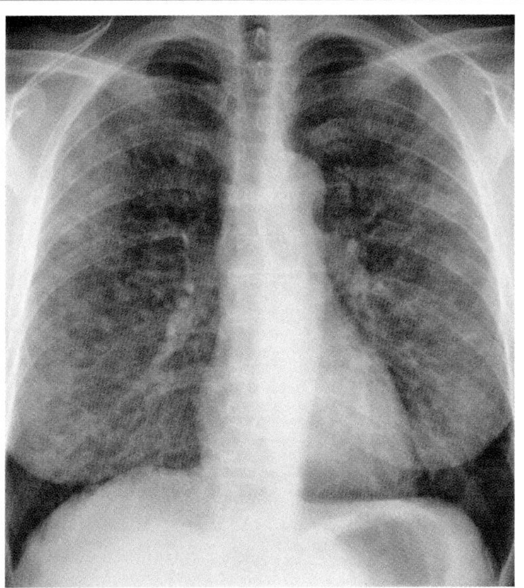

Figure 7.31 CXR of pulmonary Langerhans cell histiocytosis (PLCH).

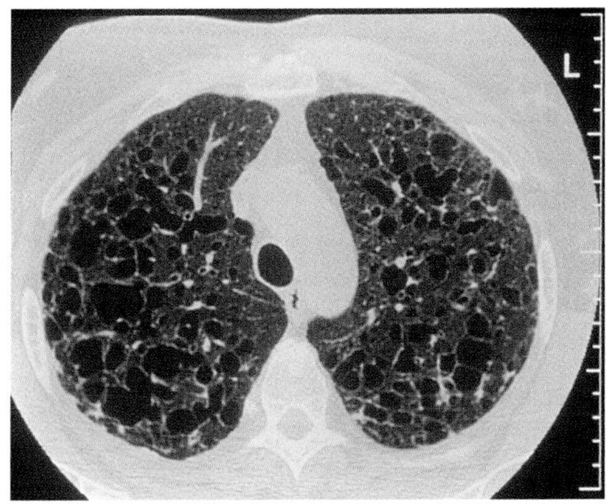

Figure 7.32 HRCT thorax of pulmonary Langerhans cell histiocytosis (PLCH) showing multiple cysts in both lungs.

required. Lung transplantation should be considered in young patients with progressive disease.

Pulmonary alveolar proteinosis (PAP)

PAP occurs due to accumulation of amorphous, periodic acid-Schiff (PAS)-positive lipoproteinaceous material composed of phospholipid surfactant and surfactant apoprotein in the distal air spaces of the lungs. There is no lung inflammation and the lung architecture is preserved. Congenital PAP occurs in neonates due to mutations in surfactant or mutations in the granulocyte macrophage-colony stimulating factor (GM-CSF) receptor, resulting in reduced or absent function of the GM-CSF receptor β-chain on mononuclear cells.

Secondary PAP can occur after inhalation of silica, aluminium dust, or titanium and after allogenic bone marrow transplantation for myeloid malignancy. It can be associated with haematological malignancies, haemolytic anaemia, polymyalgia rheumatica, ulcerative colitis, and granulomatosis with polyangiitis. Alveolar macrophage dysfunction due to altered GM-CSF function, impaired secretion of surfactant transport vesicles, impaired phagocytosis, and phagolysosome fusion results in an increased risk of opportunistic infections such as Nocardia, pneumocystis jiroveci, and mycobacterium tuberculosis.

The typical age of presentation for secondary PAP is 30–50 years, and it is twice as common in men as in women. PAP presents with insidious onset of dyspnoea in 55–80%, dry cough and expectoration of 'chunky' gelatinous material. Patients may also develop constitutional symptoms of fatigue, low grade fever, and weight loss. A third of affected patients are asymptomatic despite infiltration of the alveolar spaces. Physical examination is often normal, but 25% develop clubbing and cyanosis, and 50% develop crackles.

CXR of PAP shows bilateral, symmetric alveolar opacities located centrally in mid and lower zones, often in a bat-wing distribution (Figure 7.33). Segmental atelectasis can occur due to bronchiolar obstruction by thick, lipoproteinaceous material. In chronic cases, fibrosis can occur in foci or become extensive.

HRCT reveals ground-glass opacification in a homogeneous distribution, thickened intralobular structures and interlobular septa in typical polygonal shapes referred to as 'crazy paving' (Figure 7.34). The differential diagnosis for these radiological findings includes acute respiratory distress syndrome (ARDS), lipoid pneumonia, acute interstitial pneumonia (AIP), drug-related hypersensitivity reactions, and diffuse alveolar damage superimposed on usual interstitial pneumonia.

Lung function tests may show a restrictive ventilatory defect or an isolated decrease in

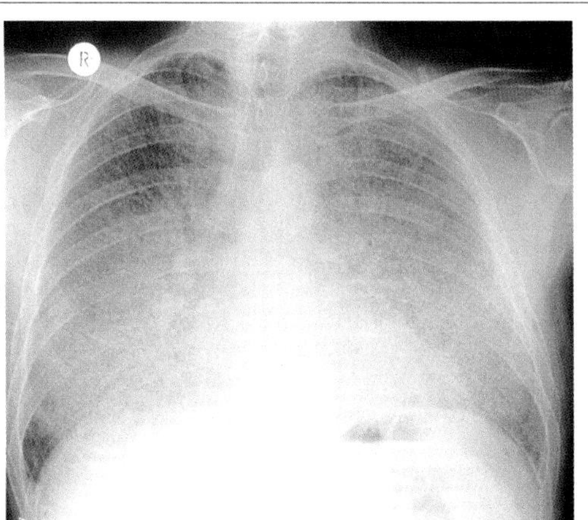

Figure 7.33 CXR of pulmonary alveolar proteinosis (PAP) showing extensive shadowing.

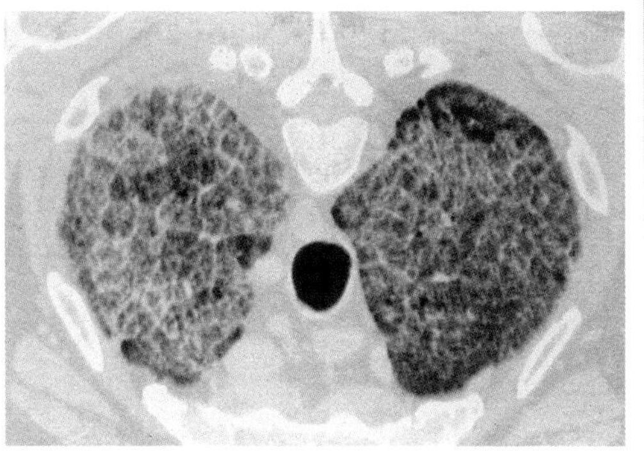

Figure 7.34 CT thorax in pulmonary alveolar proteinosis (PAP) showing extensive ground-glass changes.

diffusing capacity. Hypoxaemia and compensated respiratory alkalosis can worsen with exercise and suggest a right-to-left shunt.

The absolute diagnosis of PAP is made at bronchoscopy. A BAL will have a milky appearance due to lipoproteinaceous material which will settle on standing and contain lamellar bodies composed of phospholipids. which are derived from type 2 alveolar epithelial cells and contain high levels of anti-GM-CSF. Transbronchial and open lung biopsies will reveal terminal bronchioles and alveoli filled with macrophages that are engorged with PAS-positive material, large acellular eosinophilic bodies in a background of eosinophilic granules and cholesterol crystals. Transbronchial biopsy will show thickened alveolar septa due to type 2 epithelial cell hyperplasia with little or no inflammatory cell infiltration. Special stains to exclude infection, particularly fungal and protozoal, should always be done. Serum anti-GM-CSF level will be elevated, as will serum lactic dehydrogenase (LDH), which correlates with disease severity.

The treatment depends on the severity of symptoms and gas exchange abnormalities. Asymptomatic patients with minimal physiological impairment can be observed carefully, even if there are radiological changes. For those with mild symptoms, supplemental oxygen and close follow-up is recommended. For those with severe dyspnoea and hypoxaemia, whole lung lavage via a double-lumen endotracheal tube under general anaesthetic is indicated.

Administration of GM-CSF subcutaneously or by inhalation for idiopathic PAP is experimental, but is an option for adults who cannot undergo lung lavage or in those in whom lung lavage has failed. Glucocorticoids are contra-indicated in PAP. Other therapies include lung transplantation and plasmapheresis.

Pulmonary amyloidosis

Pulmonary amyloidosis results from the deposition of fibrils composed of low molecular weight subunits of 5–25 kD in the lungs. Amyloid deposits can infiltrate the trachea and the bronchial tree, causing hoarseness and airway obstruction. If severe, it can result in stridor and dysphagia from oesophageal compression. Some 1–2% of patients with systemic amyloidosis can develop persistent pleural effusions, caused either by pleural infiltration with amyloid deposits or secondary to amyloid-induced cardiomyopathy, and it can be difficult to differentiate between these. Parenchymal nodules (amyloidomas) can present as solitary pulmonary nodules. Rarely, pulmonary hypertension can occur due to amyloidosis.

A diagnosis of pulmonary amyloid is made with a lung biopsy which stains congo red and shows the typical apple-green birefringence with polarised microscopy. Management includes bronchoscopic laser resection or surgical resection of the areas involved. Management of amyloid-induced pleural effusions includes pleurodesis and bevacizumab, but persistent effusions confers a poor prognosis.

SUMMARY OF LEARNING POINTS

- Diffuse parenchymal lung diseases (DPLD) are a heterogenous group of more than 300 disorders.
- DPLD present with progressively worsening breathlessness, cough, and systemic symptoms.
- DPLD can occur due to a variety of lung insults; so a detailed history, including duration of symptoms, occupational, social, and travel history will need to be elicited.
- Patients presenting with a suspected DPLD will require HRCT, a BAL, and often a lung biopsy to make the diagnosis.
- The diagnosis is made by careful correlation of the clinical features with the radiological and histological findings.
- The management and prognosis of the individual DPLDs vary considerably, so it is essential to make the correct diagnosis.
- Idiopathic pulmonary fibrosis (IPF) has a poor prognosis with a median survival of 2.8 years.
- There is evidence that treatment of IPF with pirfenidone slows the rate of decline of the disease and stabilises it, but this drug has significant side effects.
- Nintedanib also slows disease progression of IPF but has significant side effects.
- NSIP is often secondary to CTD, but infection and HP need to be excluded.
- NSIP responds to immunosuppression, and has a better prognosis than IPF, with a median survival of 4.5 years.
- Sarcoidosis is the commonest DPLD worldwide and involves the lungs in 90% of cases.
- Sarcoidosis can present acutely, with chronic symptoms or as an incidental finding in an asymptomatic patient.
- Overall, pulmonary sarcoidosis has a good prognosis in stage 1 disease, with spontaneous resolution in most cases.
- Patients with multisystem sarcoidosis, who do not improve with corticosteroids, or those who have significant side effects, may require steroid-sparing agents such as methotrexate, azathioprine or mycophenalate mofetil.
- Hypersensitivity pneumonitis develops due to the inhalation of antigens and can present acutely or more insidiously.
- The management of HP includes removal of the antigen and, in some cases, immunosuppression with corticosteroids.
- There are several different types of eosinophilic pulmonary diseases, most of which respond to corticosteroids.
- Not all pulmonary eosinophilic diseases present with a peripheral eosinophilia.
- The commonest causes of peripheral eosinophilia in the UK include asthma, allergy, and drugs.
- LAM is a rare pulmonary disease that is associated with the tuberous sclerosis complex.
- LAM is more common in women, and oestrogen is implicated in its development.
- Patients with LAM often present with spontaneous pneumothorax.
- PLCH is commoner in men and in smokers.
- PLCH can present with spontaneous pneumothorax.
- Smoking cessation is the most important intervention in the management of PLCH.
- Pulmonary alveolar proteinosis is a rare condition which can be congenital or secondary to haematological malignancies and abnormalities of GM-CSF function.
- PAP can be treated with whole lung lavage and/or GM-CSF.
- Pulmonary amyloidosis is a rare cause of pulmonary nodules and can cause airway obstruction if it involves the main bronchi or trachea.
- Pulmonary amyloidosis affecting the main airways can be treated with laser or surgical resection.

MULTIPLE CHOICE QUESTIONS

7.1 Which of the following radiological features suggest a diagnosis of IPF?

A Bilateral patchy consolidation
B Ground glass opacification
C Middle and upper zone distribution
D Perivascular beading
E Subpleural honeycombing

Answer: E

IPF is characterised by bilateral, basal, subpleural areas of reticulation and honeycombing. Patchy consolidation is seen with cryptogenic organising pneumonia, ground glass changes are seen most commonly with NSIP or HP and perivascular beading is seen in sarcoidosis.

7.2 What treatments have been shown in multicentre trials to have some positive effects in IPF?

A Cyclophosphamide
B Etanercept
C Methylprednisolone
D N-acetyl cysteine
E Pirfenidone

Answer: E

Pirfenidone has been shown in trials to reduce decline in FVC with disease stabilisation.

7.3 Which of the following DPLDs, have the best prognosis without treatment?

A Alveolar proteinosis
B Hypersensitivity pneumonitis
C Idiopathic pulmonary fibrosis
D Non-specific interstitial pneumonia
E Sarcoidosis

Answer: E

Sarcoidosis has the best prognosis overall, with most patients showing spontaneous remission within 2 years. IPF has the worst prognosis with a median survival of 2.8 years.

7.4 A 35-year-old woman presenting with tiredness and Stage 1 pulmonary sarcoidosis should be managed as follows

A Inhaled corticosteroid therapy
B Methotrexate
C Oral corticosteroids for six months
D Oral corticosteroids for two years
E Wait and watch policy

Answer: E

Some 55–90% of patients with Stage 1 pulmonary sarcoidosis will have spontaneous remission of their disease, so immediate treatment is not indicated.

7.5 Which of the following statements about Hypersensitivity Pneumonitis (HP) is true?

A Acute HP has a good prognosis if the antigen is removed
B The presence of serum precipitins is diagnostic of HP
C Farmer's lung has a worse prognosis than pigeon fancier's lung
D Chronic HP responds well to immunosuppression
E HP mainly affects the lung bases

Answer: A

Removal of antigen results in rapid symptomatic and radiological improvement in acute HP. The presence of serum precipitins (IgG) is not diagnostic as it merely indicates exposure to the antigen. Bird fancier's lung has a worse prognosis than farmer's lung because there is greater exposure in the former. Chronic HP, which presents with pulmonary fibrosis, does not respond well to immunosuppression. HP affects the mid and upper zones of the lungs.

7.6 Which of the following statements about COP is true?

A Clubbing is present in the majority with COP
B There is Eosinophilia in bronchoalveolar lavage
C HRCT shows basal honeycombing
D Improvement is seen with oral corticosteroids
E Symptoms resolve with intravenous antibiotics

Answer: D

Clubbing is not a feature of COP and BAL will usually show a lymphocytosis. HRCT will show patchy areas of consolidation and basal honeycombing is seen with IPF. COP does not respond to antibiotics, but will improve with corticosteroids.

7.7 Which of the following statements regarding eosinophilic lung disease is true?

A Eosinophilic lung disease is always associated with a peripheral eosinophilia
B The commonest cause of peripheral eosinophilia in the UK is acute eosinophilic pneumonia
C The diagnosis can be made from characteristic radiological features in most cases
D Most pulmonary eosinophilic conditions respond to corticosteroids
E Chronic eosinophilic pneumonia affects the lungs, heart and gastrointestinal system

Answer: D

Not all eosinophilic lung diseases result in peripheral blood eosinophilia, so tissue biopsy or a BAL is necessary if lung involvement is suspected. The commonest causes of a peripheral blood eosinophilia in the UK are asthma, allergy, and certain drugs. The features on a CXR or HRCT are not specific. Most eosinophilic conditions respond well to oral corticosteroids, therefore investigations must be done prior to treating with corticosteroids. Chronic eosinophilic pneumonia only affects the lungs.

7.8 Which of the following statements about lymphangioleiomyomatosis (LAM) is true?

A LAM occurs most commonly in young men
B LAM is strongly associated with cigarette smoking
C LAM is characterised by the deposition of thick, lipoproteinaceous material in the alveoli
D LAM predisposes to spontaneous pneumothorax
E Lung function demonstrates a restrictive process with reduced TLC

Answer: D

LAM is commoner in young women. There is no association with cigarette smoking. It is characterised by the development of thin-walled cysts, which is made worse by oestrogen. This increases the risk of a spontaneous pneumothorax. Although classified as a DPLD, LAM is more like emphysema and lung function tests show hyperinflation with increased TLC and RV.

7.9 Which of the following statements about pulmonary Langherhans cell histiocytosis (PLCH) is true?

A PLCH is associated with smoking
B PLCH is characterised by Schaumann bodies
C PLCH is characterised by abnormal surfactant production
D PLCH can be effectively treated with oestrogen therapy
E The condition will progress despite smoking cessation

Answer: A

PLCH is strongly associated with smoking and will improve with smoking cessation. It is characterised by Birbeck granules. Schaumann bodies are found in sarcoidosis and abnormal surfactant is seen in pulmonary alveolar proteinosis.

7.10 The treatment of choice for a symptomatic patient with secondary pulmonary alveolar proteinosis who has a diffusion capacity of 30% predicted is

A Inhaled GM-CSF
B Intravenous cyclophosphamide
C Lung transplantation
D Oral corticosteroids
E Whole lung lavage

Answer: E

Immunosuppression is contra-indicated in patients with PAP and GM-CSF is as yet only experimental therapy. Although lung transplantation can be considered in patients who have not responded to other treatments, whole lung lavage is currently the treatment of choice.

Appendix 7.A Drugs that cause peripheral eosinophilia

- ACE inhibitors
- Aminosalicylates
- Amiodarone
- Ampicillin
- Anticonvulsants
- Antidepressants
- Antimalarial drugs
- Antituberculous medication
- Betablockers
- Bleomycin
- Cephalosporins
- Contrast given for radiology
- H2-receptor antagonists
- Methotrexate
- Minocycline
- Nitrofurantoin
- NSAID
- Proton pump inhibitor
- Sulphonamides
- Tetracycline

This lists some of the common drugs associated with a peripheral eosinophilia. See www.pneumotox.com for a comprehensive list of medications causing eosinophilia.

FURTHER READING

American Thoracic Society (ATS) (2017) ATS official documents: statements, guidelines and reports. [online] Available at: http://www.thoracic.org/about

American Thoracic Society American Thoracic Society/European (ATS) and European Respiratory Society (2002). Respiratory Society international multidisciplinary consensus classification of the idiopathic interstitial pneumonias. *American Journal of Respiratory and Critical Care Medicine* 165 (2): 277–304.

ATS/ERS/JRS/ALAT Committee on Idiopathic Pulmonary Fibrosis, Raghu, G., Collard, H.R. et al. (2011). An official ATS/ERS/JRS/ALAT statement: idiopathic pulmonary fibrosis: evidence-based guidelines for diagnosis and management. *American Journal of Respiratory and Critical Care Medicine* 183 (6): 788–824.

Barnard, J., Rose, C., Newman, L. et al. (2005). Job and industry classifications associated with sarcoidosis in A Case-Control Etiologic Study of Sarcoidosis (ACCESS). *Journal of Occupational and Environmental Medicine* 47 (3): 226–234.

Bradley, B., Branley, H., Egan, J. et al. (2008). Interstitial lung disease guideline: the British Thoracic Society in collaboration with the Thoracic Society of Australia and New Zealand and the Irish Thoracic Society. *Thorax* 63 (Supplement 5): v1–v58.

Collard, H.R., Moore, B.B., Flaherty, K.R. et al. (2007). Acute exacerbations of idiopathic pulmonary fibrosis. *American Journal of Respiratory and Critical Care Medicine* 176 (7): 636–643.

Gibson, G.J., Prescott, R.J., Muers, M.F. et al. (1996). British Thoracic Society Sarcoidosis study: effects of long-term corticosteroid treatment. *Thorax* 51 (3): 238–247.

Hunninghake, G.W., Costabel, U., Ando, M. et al. (1999). Statement on sarcoidosis: Joint Statement of the American Thoracic Society (ATS), the European Respiratory Society (ERS) and the World Association of Sarcoidosis and Other Granulomatous Disorders (WASOG) adopted by the ATS Board of Directors and by the ER. *American Journal of Respiratory and Critical Care Medicine* 160 (2): 736–755.

King, T.E. Jr. (2005). Clinical advances in the diagnosis and therapy of the interstitial lung diseases. *American Journal of Respiratory and Critical Care Medicine* 172 (3): 268–279.

King, T.E. Jr., Bradford, W.Z., Castro-Bernardini, S. et al. (2014). A phase 3 trial of pirfenidone in patients with idiopathic pulmonary fibrosis. *The New England Journal of Medicine* 370 (22): 2083–2092.

Liebow, A. (1975). Definition and classification of interstitial pneumonias in human pathology. *Progress in Respiratory Research* 8: 1–33.

Martinez, F.J., de Andrade, J.A., Anstrom, K.J. et al. (2014). Randomized trial of acetylcysteine in idiopathic pulmonary fibrosis. *The New England Journal of Medicine* 370 (22): 2093–2101.

Noble, P.W., Albera, C., Bradford, W.Z. et al. (2011). Pirfenidone in patients with idiopathic pulmonary fibrosis (CAPACITY): two randomised trials. *Lancet* 377 (9779): 1760–1769.

Paramothayan, S. and Jones, P. (2002). Corticosteroid therapy in pulmonary sarcoidosis: a systematic review. *Journal of the American Medical Association* 287 (10): 1301–1307.

Richeldi, L., du Bois, R.M., Raghu, G. et al. (2014). Efficacy and safety of Nintedanib in idiopathic pulmonary fibrosis. *New England Journal of Medicine* 370 (22): 2071–2082.

Schwartz, M.I., King, T.E. Jr., and Raghu, G. (2003). Approach to the evaluation and diagnosis of interstitial lung disease. In: *Interstitial Lung Disease*, 4e (ed. M.I. Schwartz and T.E. King), 1–30. USA, Shelton, CT: People's Medical House Publishing.

The Idiopathic Pulmonary Fibrosis Clinical Research Network, Raghu, G., Anstrom, K.J. et al. (2012). Prednisone, azathioprine and N-acetylcysteine for pulmonary fibrosis. *New England Journal of Medicine* 366 (21): 1968–1977.

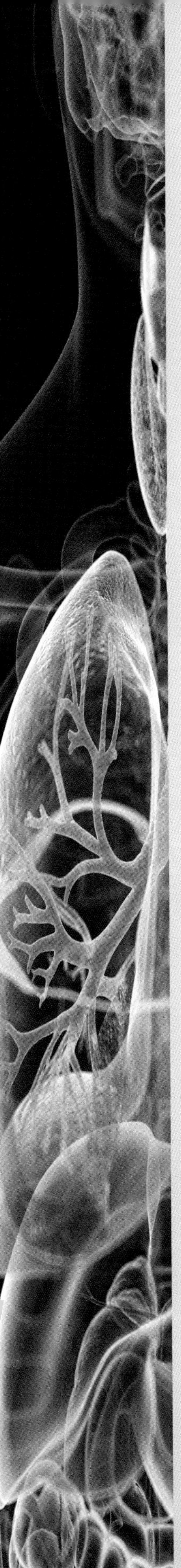

CHAPTER 8

Respiratory infections

Learning objectives

- To understand the common types of respiratory infections
- To appreciate the risk factors for developing respiratory infections
- To understand the aetiology and pathogenesis of community acquired pneumonia (CAP)
- To understand the presenting symptoms and signs of CAP
- To understand the investigations used to make a diagnosis of CAP
- To understand the management of CAP
- To understand the prognostic scores used in CAP
- To understand the aetiology and pathogenesis of hospital acquired pneumonia (HAP)
- To learn the management of HAP
- To recognise the prognosis in HAP
- To appreciate the diagnosis, management, and prognosis of ventilator-associated pneumonia
- To understand respiratory infections in the immune-incompetent host
- To understand the management of aspiration pneumonia
- To recognise the presentation, diagnosis, and management of *Mycobacterium tuberculosis*
- To understand the diagnosis and management of latent tuberculosis
- To learn the management of opportunistic mycobacterial infections

Essential Respiratory Medicine, First Edition. Shanthi Paramothayan.

Companion website: www.wiley.com/go/paramothayan/essential_respiratory_medicine

Abbreviations

AAFB	acid-alcohol-fast bacilli
ADA	adenosine deaminase
ALT	alanine transaminase
aMB	atypical mycobacterium
AST	aspartate aminotransferase
BAL	bronchoalveolar lavage
BCG	Bacille Calmette-Guérin
BOOP	bronchiolitis obliterans organising pneumonia
BTS	British Thoracic Society
CAP	community acquired pneumonia
CF	cystic fibrosis
CFT	complement fixation test
CMV	cytomegalovirus
CNS	central nervous system
CO_2	carbon dioxide
COPD	chronic obstructive pulmonary disease
CPAP	continuous positive airway pressure
CRPC	C-reactive protein
CT	computed tomography
DOT	directly observed therapy
GCS	Glasgow Coma Scale
GP	General Practitioner
HAP	hospital acquired pneumonia
Hib	*Haemophilus influenza* B
HIV	human immunodeficiency virus
HRCT	high-resolution computed tomography
ICU	intensive care unit
IGRA	interferon gamma release assay
INH	isoniazid
kPA	kilopascals
LFT	liver function test
LIP	lymphoid interstitial pneumonia
MAC	*Mycobacterium avium complex*
MAI	*Mycobacterium avium intracellulare*
MDRTB	multi-drug resistant tuberculosis
MRSA	methicillin-resistant *Staphylococcus aureus*
MTB	*Mycobacterium tuberculosis*
NICE	National Institute of Health and Care Excellence
NSIP	non-specific interstitial pneumonia
PCR	polymerase chain reaction
PCT	pro-calcitonin
PEG	percutaneous enterogastrostomy
PPD	purified protein derivative
PSI	pneumonia severity index
PYR	pyrazinamide
RIF	rifampicin
RSV	respiratory syncytial virus
SALT	speech and language therapy
SIADH	syndrome of inappropriate anti-diuretic hormone
SOL	space-occupying lesion
TB	tuberculosis
VAP	ventilator-associated pneumonia
WHO	World Health Organisation

Introduction

The respiratory tract communicates with the environment, allowing micro-organisms to directly enter the respiratory tract and lungs. Therefore, infections of the upper and lower respiratory tract are very common. The majority of these are self-limiting and do not require any treatment. These infections are more prevalent in the very young, the elderly, and in those who do not have a competent immune system.

Respiratory tract infections

The diagnosis of a respiratory tract infection is made on clinical grounds. Viruses are a common cause of respiratory tract infections. Individuals with viral infections of the respiratory tract will develop a cough, a sore throat, headaches, nasal symptoms, fever, and myalgia. Investigations are rarely required except during epidemics, for example, an influenza epidemic, or when the patient's symptoms are concerning. Most viral infections are self-limiting and those affected will recover without any treatment within a few days. They should be advised to rest, ensure adequate hydration, and take analgesia as required. Many will take over-the-counter cough medications to ease their symptoms. Box 8.1 lists the viruses that cause respiratory infections.

The common cold, caused by Rhinovirus, affects most of the population at least once every year. It does not require any treatment but is responsible for many days off work. Most adults would have had asymptomatic cytomegalovirus (CMV) infection during childhood. Only individuals who are immunosuppressed, especially those with HIV and those who have had solid organ transplants, develop symptoms when infected with CMV. Respiratory syncytial virus (RSV) infection results in seasonal outbreaks of respiratory illness,

Box 8.1 Viruses affecting the respiratory tract.

- Adenovirus
- Coronavirus
- Cytomegalovirus (CMV)
- Influenza
- Parainfluenza
- Respiratory syncytial virus (RSV)
- Rhinovirus

usually in the winter months and can cause complications in those with chronic lung and heart disease. RSV is the commonest cause of lower respiratory tract infection in infants and can be severe in premature babies who present with wheezing and apnoea; there is a risk of sudden death. Many of these viruses can cause pneumonia which will be discussed later in this chapter.

Sinusitis can occur due to a viral or bacterial infection of the maxillary sinus or, less commonly, the frontal and paranasal sinuses. Symptoms of sinusitis include headaches, periorbital and per nasal pain, fever, cough productive of purulent sputum, purulent nasal discharge, and post nasal drip. A CT scan of the sinus will show opacification of the maxillary sinus and mucosal oedema. Treatment of sinusitis is with antibiotics, nasal decongestants, and hydration. Rarely, surgical drainage may be required if medical therapy has failed.

Epiglottitis is a severe and potentially life-threatening infection of the epiglottis. It is common in young children and caused by haemophilus influenza type B (Hib) infection. Children will present with fever, sore throat, and cough, and the diagnosis must be made without delay. The treatment is with third generation cephalosporins, for example, cefotaxime. Epiglottitis can rapidly progress to respiratory distress and stridor caused by oedema of the epiglottis which can cause obstruction of the larynx. Children may require intubation and ventilation or an emergency tracheostomy. Children who are immunised with the Hib vaccine as protection against meningitis may also be protected against epiglottitis.

Laryngotracheobronchitis (croup) is most commonly caused by parainfluenza virus and is common in children in the winter months. It presents with a characteristic barking cough and fever, and can progress to respiratory distress and stridor. Treatment is with nebulised bronchodilators, nebulised steroids, and steam inhalation.

Acute bronchitis affects the lower respiratory tract and results in cough, breathlessness, pleuritic chest pain, and fever.

Pneumonia

Pneumonia is an infection of the lung parenchyma which can be viral or bacterial. Immunocompromised patients are also at risk of 'opportunistic' infections which do not normally affect healthy individuals. These opportunistic infections, which include fungal and protozoal infections, will be discussed in a later section. Aspiration of gastric content and lipoid material can also result in a chemical pneumonia.

Viral pneumonia

Common causes of a viral pneumonia include influenza, adenovirus, parainfluenza, respiratory syncytial virus (RSV) and human metapneumovirus. H1N1 and Avian influenza A (HSN1) occur in pandemics and result in significant morbidity and mortality, with patients often requiring admission to the intensive care unit (ICU).

Patients with a viral pneumonia present with symptoms of dry cough, breathlessness, fever, headache, and myalgia. Diagnosis is made on clinical history, examination, culture of appropriate respiratory samples (such as nasal secretions and bronchial lavage), and serological tests. Polymerase chain reaction (PCR)-based diagnostic panels are available that can detect several respiratory viruses simultaneously. Viral cultures can take several days to process and are less sensitive than PCR analysis of respiratory secretions.

Patients with viral pneumonia can develop a secondary bacterial infection. This should be suspected if there is clinical deterioration, increase in the volume of sputum, which may be purulent, worsening breathlessness, and systemic symptoms. Blood tests will show an elevated white cell count with a neutrophilia, a rise in CRP and infiltrates or consolidation on the chest X-ray (CXR). Secondary *Staphylococcus aureus* pneumonia can occur after an influenza infection.

Sputum samples are rarely recommended with a viral pneumonia as these can be difficult to analyse because many non-pathogenic micro-organisms colonise the respiratory tract. Therefore, any positive sputum culture result must be interpreted with the clinical presentation in mind. Certain organisms, such as coagulase-negative Staphylococci and Candida species, are rarely pathogens.

Bacterial pneumonia

Bacterial pneumonia is a common cause of morbidity in the community and a common presentation to hospital. It is important to distinguish community acquired pneumonia (CAP) from hospital acquired pneumonia (HAP) as the latter is associated with a higher morbidity and mortality. Box 8.2 lists the common symptoms and signs of pneumonia.

Community acquired pneumonia (CAP)

Community acquired pneumonia (CAP) is a common acute lung infection that affects individuals living in the community. The annual incidence of CAP is 5–11/1000 of the adult population, with a higher incidence in children and the elderly. Every year between 0.5 and 1% of adults are diagnosed with a CAP. Risk factors include chronic lung disease, chronic renal disease, diabetes, abnormal immune system, and a preceding viral infection, such as influenza.

In a young and otherwise fit patient, CAP has a good prognosis and can be managed with oral antibiotics in the community. However, the morbidity and mortality can be high in the elderly and in the immunocompromised individual. Overall, 22–42% will require hospital admission and 1–10% will require admission to the ICU. Mortality ranges from 5% in the ambulatory setting to 35% in those admitted to ICU. Most pneumonia-associated deaths occur in people over the age of 84 years.

Pathophysiology

Bacterial infection of the lung parenchyma results in an inflammatory response from the host, with an outpouring of neutrophils and exudate into the alveolar spaces, resulting in consolidation. This compromises the oxygen exchange because of the ventilation-perfusion mismatch and results in type 1 respiratory failure. Inflammation of the pleura results in pleuritic chest pain and the development of a parapneumonic pleural effusion in a third of those with CAP. An empyema may develop in a certain percentage as discussed in Chapters 10 and 12. Table 8.1 lists the causes, typical clinical and radiological features, and the treatment of the common pneumonias.

Box 8.2 Symptoms and signs of pneumonia in the young and the elderly.

Patient demographics	Symptoms	Signs
Young and immuno-competent	Productive cough (green/rusty brown) Fever (86%) Rigors (15%) Pleuritic chest pain (30%) Dyspnoea Haemoptysis Night sweats Headache Myalgia Nausea Vomiting Diarrhoea Lethargy	Coughing Temperature (86%) Tachypnoea Tachycardia Consolidation: decreased breath sounds, dullness on percussion, increased vocal resonance and tactile focal fremitus, coarse crackles, bronchial breathing
Elderly or immunocompromised	Symptoms above may be present or absent New confusion Anorexia Lethargy	As above Reduced mini mental test score (AMTS <8)

Table 8.1 Causes of pneumonia.

Type of organism	Organism	History	Investigations	Other features	Treatment
Virus	Influenza A or B	Acute viral symptoms	PCR: specificity >95%	Can develop secondary bacterial infections	Oseltamivir Vaccination of young, old, and susceptible
Virus	Parainfluenza	Acute viral symptoms	PCR	Usually self-limiting	Aciclovir
Virus	CMV	Asymptomatic in immunocompetent	PCR	Severe in immunocompromised patients, especially after transplant	Aciclovir Ganciclovir
Virus	Varicella	Acute viral symptoms Vesicular rash Pneumonia can be severe	PCR Serology	CXR shows multiple small nodules measuring 1–5 mm which coalesce Mortality without treatment 10%	Aciclovir Ganciclovir Immunisation of young, old, and susceptible individuals
Virus	Adenovirus	Common cold, sore throat, bronchitis, pneumonia	Usually none	Usually mild. Symptomatic treatment	Ribavirin if severe
Bacteria	*Streptococcus pneumonia*	Commonest pathogen (65%)	Pneumococcal urinary antigen positive in 54%, sputum culture positive in 17% and blood culture positive in 16%	Parapneumonic effusion in 30% Meningitis Sinusitis Otitis media Sinusitis Endocarditis Osteomyelitis	Amoxicillin Amoxicillin-clavulanate Ceftriaxone Vaccination of old and susceptible
Bacteria	*Haemophilus influenza*	Common cause of lower respiratory tract infection and pneumonia. In children, HiB can cause bacteraemia, epiglottitis, and acute bacterial meningitis	Bacterial culture on chocolate agar or latex particle agglutination from nasal or respiratory secretions	Opportunistic pathogen in the immunocompromised and in those with COPD	Cefotaxime Ceftriaxone Fluoroquinolones Hib vaccine

(*Continued*)

Table 8.1 *(Continued)*

Type of organism	Organism	History	Investigations	Other features	Treatment
Bacteria	*Legionella pneumophila*	Accounts for 2–9% of CAP Epidemics in areas with contaminated water source, such as hotels	Legionella urinary antigen	Jaundice Abnormal liver function tests	Macrolide Rifampicin
Bacteria	*Mycoplasma pneumophila*	Outbreaks occur in young adults. Cerebral symptoms	Culture, PCR, and serology of nasopharyngeal samples	Cold agglutinins Ground-glass changes on CXR	Macrolide Fluoroquinolone Tetracycline
Bacteria	Gram negative (proteus, *Escherichia coli*)	Usually gastroenteritis. Virulent strains can cause pneumonia and septic shock	Blood cultures Sputum	Can be severe in immunocompromised host	Fluoroquinolone Azithromycin Rifaximin
Bacteria	*Staphylococcus aureus*	Can be severe with high mortality Systemic infection causes shock secondary to sepsis MRSA common cause of morbidity and mortality	Sputum BAL Blood cultures Samples from lines, catheters Swabs from cannula sites, PEG sites, skin	Cavitating lesion in lung Lung abscess, parapneumonic effusion Empyema Osteomyelitis	Flucloxacillin Clindamycin Rifampin Fusidic acid Vancomycin for MRSA
Bacteria	*Klebsiella pneumonia*	Increased risk in alcoholics, malnourished individuals	Respiratory secretions BAL Blood cultures	Cavitating lesion on CXR. Lung abscess and empyema Nosocomial infections High mortality	Ampicillin Piperacillin/Tazobactam Ceftazidime Meropenem Ertapenem
Bacteria	*Pseudomonas aeruginosa*	Affects those with chronic lung disease (COPD, CF, bronchiectasis)	Respiratory secretions BAL Blood cultures	Common cause of HAP and ventilator-acquired pneumonia Often multi-drug-resistant	Aminoglycosides Quinolones Cephalosporins Carbapenems Polymyxins

Bacteria	Coxiella burnetti	Flu-like symptoms Non-productive cough Pneumonia	Increase in antibody titre	Usually mild but can progress rapidly to severe	Tetracycline Rifampin
Bacteria	Chlamydia psittaci	Transmitted by inhalation from poultry and farm animals Flu-like symptoms Rarely pneumonia	Complement fixation PCR	Usually not severe	Tetracycline Macrolide
Bacteria	Chlamydia pneumonia	Laryngitis Pharyngitis Fever, cough, and headache. Rarely severe pneumonia Myocarditis	Nasopharyngeal swabs to obtain samples, difficult diagnosis to make Sputum BAL	Usually asymptomatic or mild in immunocompetent	Macrolide Tetracycline
Fungus	Pneumocystis jiroveci	Occurs in immunocompromised: HIV positive with low CD4 count, solid organ transplant and haematological malignancies	Sputum BAL	Characteristic ground-glass changes on CT	Trimethoprim-sulfamethoxazole (septrin) Pentamidine Atovaquone Septrin prophylaxis in the susceptible
Fungus	*Aspergillus fumigatus*: invasive aspergillosis	Occurs in immunocompromised individuals: HIV, chemotherapy, haematological malignancies. SOB, cough, fever, haemoptysis	Blood cultures BAL Serological testing	Patchy shadowing on CXR and CT High mortality	Itraconazole Voriconazole Amphotericin B (Ambisome)

(*Continued*)

Table 8.1 *(Continued)*

Type of organism	Organism	History	Investigations	Other features	Treatment
Fungus	*Candida albicans*	Systemic infection (candidiasis) occurs in immunocompromised individuals, especially HIV Mortality high	Sputum BAL Blood cultures	Oral, pharyngeal, and vaginal infections common	Nystatin for oral infection Fluconazole Amphotericin B (Ambisome)
Fungus	*Histoplasmosis capsulatum*	Fever, joint pains, myalgia, dry cough, chest pain, SOB, and rash	CXR shows 'coin lesions' and calcification of lymph nodes Culture of blood and BAL Rise in antibody titre	Inhalation of spores from bird and bat droppings Endemic in North and Central USA Occurs in immunocompromised individuals	Itraconazole Fluconazole Amphotericin B (Ambisome)
Fungus	*Cryptococcus neoformans*	Cough, fever, SOB Can cause meningitis in immunocompromised		Occurs in immunocompromised individuals, individuals with diabetics	Amphotericin B Flucytosine
Fungus	*Nocardia asteroids*	Found in soil Opportunistic infection	Blood culture	Systemic infection in immunocompromised with nocardiosis and endocarditis	Trimethoprim-sulfamethoxazole Imipenem Amikacin Treatment for six months

As described in Box 8.2, CAP has a variety of presentations. Immunocompetent young adults present with a cough productive of green or rusty sputum, breathlessness, pleuritic chest pain, small volume haemoptysis, fever, rigors, night sweats, and myalgia. Patients with mycoplasma, chlamydia, and legionella pneumonias usually present with more systemic symptoms, for example, nausea, vomiting, diarrhoea, headaches, and myalgia. The elderly and the immunocompromised may not have these classic symptoms as they cannot mount an inflammatory response. They are more likely to present with anorexia, feeling generally unwell, with a new confusion, and a reduced mini-mental test score.

Diagnosis of CAP

The diagnosis of pneumonia is made on the clinical symptoms and signs, and a chest X-ray (CXR) confirming new parenchymal shadowing. Those presenting with symptoms suggestive of a CAP should have a comprehensive history, examination, and investigations to confirm the diagnosis of CAP and to determine the severity. Investigations should include blood tests, CXR, urinary pneumococcal and legionella antigens and sputum for microbiological analysis. A CURB-65 score should be calculated in every patient presenting with a CAP; this guides management and has prognostic implications. Box 8.3 describes how the CURB-65 score is calculated.

A full blood count will usually show an elevated white cell count, with a raised neutrophil count. Leukopenia, with a white cell count $<4 \times 10^9 l^{-1}$, is associated with a poorer outcome. Mycoplasma pneumonia can be associated with cold agglutinins and a haemolytic anaemia. An elevated eosinophil count should raise the possibility of an eosinophilic pneumonia and will warrant further investigations, such as a bronchoalveolar lavage (BAL), a lung biopsy, and a HRCT. Eosinophilic pneumonias are discussed in Chapter 7.

A raised urea signifies a worse prognosis. Hyponatraemia secondary to the syndrome of inappropriate anti-diuretic hormone (SIADH) can be associated with CAP, particularly legionella pneumonia. The CRP is always elevated in bacterial CAP, with a sensitivity of 73% and a specificity of 65%, although there is usually a lag, so it may not be raised at the onset of symptoms. Serial CRP measurements can be useful in monitoring response to treatment. Pro-calcitonin (PCT), a peptide precursor of calcitonin that is released by cells in response to bacterial toxins, can also be used to distinguish between bacterial and non-bacterial causes of pneumonia. PCT levels may also correlate with the severity of pneumonia.

Abnormal liver function tests (LFT), particularly a raised alanine transaminase (ALT) level, can occur with legionella or mycoplasma pneumonia. Deranged LFTs can also occur after treatment with intravenous antibiotics, particularly macrolides.

Box 8.3 CURB-65 score.

The CURB-65 score is calculated by giving one point for each of the following prognostic features:

1. Confusion (abbreviated Mental Test Score 8 or less, or new disorientation in person, place, or time)
2. Urea >7 mmol/L
3. Raised respiratory rate (30 breaths per minute or more)
4. Blood pressure low; diastolic of 60 mmHg or less, or systolic of 90 mmHg or less
5. Age over 65 years

Microbiological diagnosis of CAP

Patients with a low-severity CAP do not routinely require sputum analysis. However, sputum should be sent in those presenting with moderate or severe CAP and when there is cavitation on the CXR. If the patient has a productive cough, then a deep cough sputum sample should be sent for Gram staining, culture, and sensitivity prior to starting antibiotics. There is huge variation in getting a positive sputum result, ranging from 10–80%. Some infections, such as *Streptococcus aureus*, are easily cultured, whereas *Streptococcus pneumonia* and *Haemophilus influenzae* are more difficult to culture, so false negative results can occur. Culture results are reported according to the amount of growth, with moderate or heavy growth indicating a true pathogen, whereas a light growth may indicate colonisation.

Bronchoscopy and bronchoalveolar lavage (BAL) samples are not routinely required, but should be considered in the immunocompromised patient, those who have an abnormal CXR suggestive of malignancy, and in those not improving on empirical antibiotic therapy. BAL samples should have Gram staining, Ziehl-Neelsen staining for acid-fast bacilli (AFB), silver staining for pneumocystis jerovici, and stains for fungi. Cultures can take several days to weeks.

Blood cultures should be taken in those presenting with fever and other symptoms of sepsis, even in the absence of fever. Blood cultures are positive in 12% of hospitalised patients, with two-thirds growing *Streptococcus pneumonia*. Care should be taken when collecting blood for culture as there is a 10% rate of contamination with MRSA from the skin.

If *Streptococcus pneumonia* or legionella pneumophila infections are suspected, then urinary antigen testing is more sensitive and specific than blood cultures or sputum cultures, and gives a result more rapidly than cultures of sputum or blood. Urinary antigen testing has the advantage that the antigen will remain positive even after starting antibiotics, but as no pathogens are available, it is not possible to determine sensitivities. Therefore, it is recommended that sputum or BAL samples are also sent for microscopy, culture, and sensitivity.

Polymerase chain reaction (PCR) diagnostic kits are available to use on sputum samples which can give a result within a few hours for chlamydophila pneumoniae and mycoplasma pneumonia, although care must be taken to limit contamination from upper airway flora. If no sputum is available, then a throat swab for mycoplasma pneumonia PCR is recommended.

Complement fixation test (CFT), or paired serological test, can be used to diagnose legionella and mycoplasma infections, especially during outbreaks, and will show a fourfold rise in antibody titres. CFT is also recommended in any patient under 40 years presenting with pneumococcal pneumonia. The consultant microbiologist and public health consultant will usually be able to give advice about outbreaks and put in place public health safety measures, such as closure of infected hotels.

CMV serology can be requested if CMV pneumonia is suspected. Human immunodeficiency virus (HIV) test is recommended in any patient with an atypical presentation and an abnormal CXR.

Microbiological diagnosis is made in less than 40% of patients presenting with CAP. However, empiric antibiotic treatment results in outcomes as good as if the pathogen were detected, with only 1% treated in the community for CAP requiring hospitalisation because of treatment failure. The choice of initial antibiotic therapy is therefore made on the likelihood of the infecting organism.

Radiological diagnosis of CAP

The chest X-ray (CXR) is an essential investigation in making the diagnosis of CAP. NICE and British Thoracic Society (BTS) guidelines recommend that a CXR should be done in a timely way so that antibiotics can be prescribed within 4 hours of the patient presenting to hospital. The CXR may appear normal very early on or show interstitial infiltrates which are better seen on HRCT (Figure 8.1). In established CAP, the CXR will show consolidation in one or more lobes or show patchy consolidation of bronchopneumonia (Figure 8.2, Figure 8.3). Radiographic changes do not correlate with the pathogen,

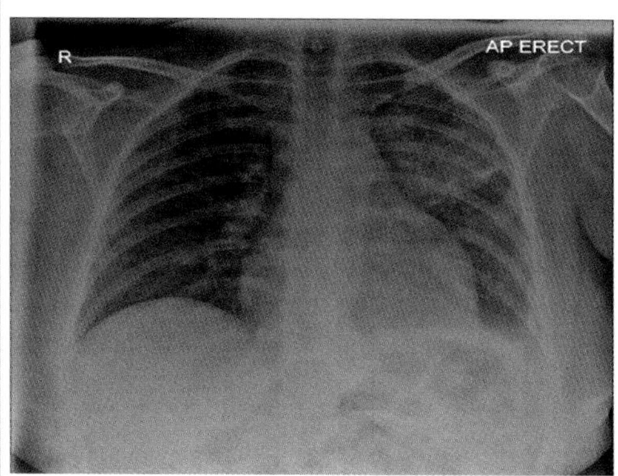

Figure 8.1 CXR showing left upper zone infiltration suggestive of early infection.

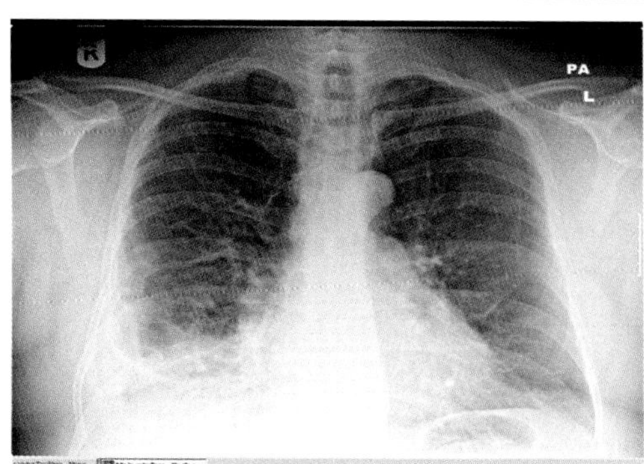

Figure 8.2 CXR showing right lower lobe consolidation.

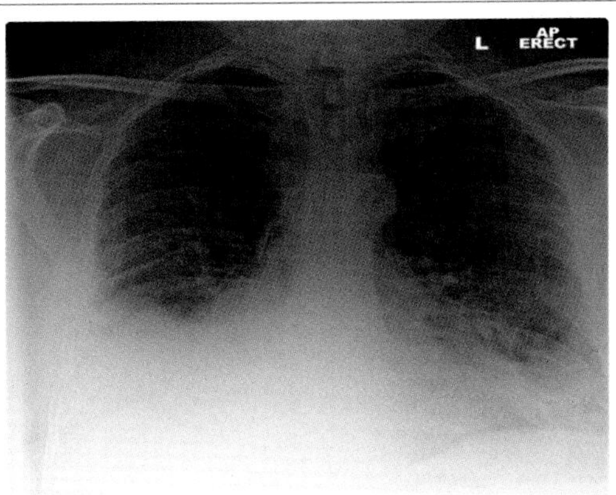

Figure 8.3 CXR showing right middle and right lower lobe consolidation.

although *Streptococcus aureus pneumonia* and *Klebsiella pneumonia* present with cavitating lesions, the differential diagnoses for which include *Mycobacterium tuberculosis* infection, lung cancer, and vasculitis.

The differential diagnosis of CAP includes an exacerbation of COPD, exacerbation of asthma, acute bronchitis, pulmonary oedema, pulmonary embolus, adenocarcinoma *in situ*, eosinophilic pneumonia, hypersensitivity pneumonia, cryptogenic organising pneumonia or diffuse parenchymal lung disease. If there is no clinical improvement with appropriate antibiotics, then further investigations will be required.

Management of CAP

Patients presenting to their General Practitioner (GP) with symptoms and signs of a CAP should have a CXR and blood tests, including CRP measurement, to guide management. Pulse oximetry may be helpful in determining whether a patient needs to be admitted to hospital.

NICE Guidelines recommend that a five-day course of a single antibiotic should be given to those with a CRP of greater than 100 $mg l^{-1}$ but with a CURB-65 score of less than 2. The choice of antibiotic will depend on local antibiotic prescribing guidelines and any antibiotic allergy that the patient may have. NICE recommends amoxicillin or tetracycline, and a macrolide or tetracycline for those with penicillin allergy. If symptoms do not resolve within three days, then the duration of antibiotic therapy should be increased. For those with a CRP between 20 and 100 $mg l^{-1}$, a delayed antibiotic prescription should be considered, and the patient should be instructed to take the antibiotic if symptoms worsen. Patients with a non-severe CAP should expect clinical improvement within a week and complete resolution of symptoms by 6 weeks, although many report feeling fatigued for up to three months.

Radiological resolution usually takes up to six weeks after antibiotic treatment is completed. It is recommended that a CXR is done after 6 weeks to ensure complete resolution of changes.

Patients seen in hospital with a CURB-65 score of 2 or less and with no other adverse prognostic features should be started on oral dual antibiotic therapy with amoxicillin and a macrolide for 7–10 days. Those who are allergic to penicillin should be given either a macrolide alone or a tetracycline. If there are no adverse features, they could be discharged home with follow-up by the GP. The patient should be advised to rest, have adequate hydration, and seek medical help if their symptoms do not improve.

Patients with a diagnosis of CAP who have a CURB-65 score > 2 and those who have adverse prognostic features should be hospitalised and receive intravenous antibiotics, intravenous fluids, oxygen, and thromboprophylaxis to prevent pulmonary emboli. Adverse features include fever, respiratory rate > 24 breaths per minute, tachycardia, systolic blood pressure < 90 mmHg, oxygen saturation < 90% on room air, and confusion.

The aim should be to maintain oxygen saturation in the range of 94–98%, ensuring that there is no evidence of CO_2 retention. Empirical intravenous antibiotic therapy should be started without delay once appropriate samples have been sent for microbiological analysis. These patients should be given nutritional support, a mucolytic agent, and physiotherapy for sputum clearance. Patients with COPD and asthma may benefit from regular nebulised bronchodilators.

The choice of empiric antibiotic therapy for CAP is based on the likelihood of a specific pathogen, and the local antibiotic prescribing guidelines which are based on resistance patterns. Microbiological classification prior to treatment is not practical as the organism is not always identified and waiting for identification may result in treatment delay.

As *Streptococcus pneumonia* is the commonest cause of CAP, it is recommended that intravenous amoxicillin or benzylpenicillin, together with a macrolide, is given. This combination has been shown to decrease mortality and length of hospital stay.

Patients who are allergic to penicillin should be commenced on a macrolide. Macrolides can cause prolongation of the QT interval and can interact with other drugs (discussed in Chapter 3). The prevalence of macrolide-resistant *Streptococcus pneumonia* is on the increase. Fluoroquinolones, such a levofloxacin and moxifloxacin, are also active against *Streptococcus pneumonia* so could be used as monotherapy. However, these drugs can also cause prolongation of the QT interval and ventricular arrhythmias in the elderly. Vancomycin and Teicoplanin are reasonable options in those who have travelled abroad where penicillin and macrolide resistance are high.

The antibiotic regime should be reviewed after 48 hours. If the patient is improving clinically, the fever has settled, and the CRP is coming down, then the intravenous antibiotics should be changed to oral antibiotics. There is no trial evidence regarding the optimal duration of antibiotic therapy, but treatment for 5–10 days is usually given as this results in improvement while minimising the risk of antibiotic-associated clostridium difficile infection.

Patients with a CURB-65 score of 3 or 4 with evidence of sepsis may develop hypotension and severe hypoxaemia requiring inotropic support, intubation, and ventilation on ICU.

A parapneumonic effusion occurs in 30–50% of patients with a CAP and will usually resolve without any intervention (Figure 8.4). In some cases, the effusion can progress to an empyema, the diagnosis and management of which are discussed in Chapter 12. Certain organisms, such as *Staphylococcus aureus* and *Klebsiella pneumonia*, can predispose to the development of a lung abscess, which is discussed in Chapter 12.

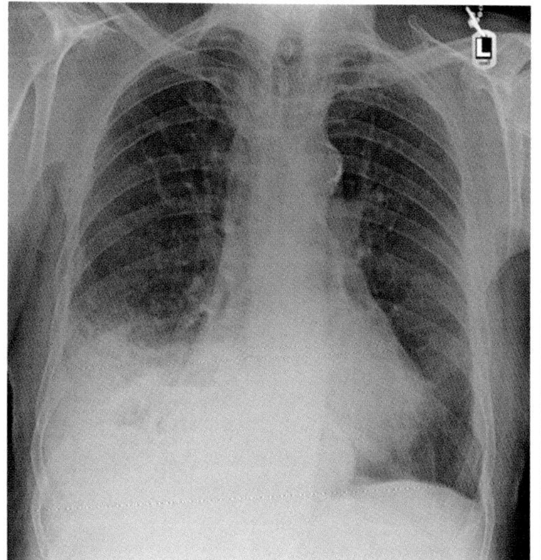

Figure 8.4 CXR showing right lower lobe consolidation with cavitation and a parapneumonic effusion.

Prognosis with CAP

Predictors of mortality include the CURB-65 score and the Pneumonia Severity Index (PSI) which is based on the patient's gender, age, co-morbidities (diabetes, cardiac failure, renal failure), results of clinical examination, blood test results, and CXR findings. Additional adverse features include hypoxaemia (SaO_2 <92% or PaO_2 <8 kPA), white cell count >20×10 $9 l^{-1}$ or <4×10 $9 l^{-1}$, multilobe involvement and positive blood culture. Leukopenia, thrombocytopenia, and a raised serum glucose concentration in a non-diabetic patient, are also predictors of mortality.

A CT thorax should be considered when the CXR shows no improvement in the radiological changes, when there is a cavitating lesion, possible adenopathy, or clinical features of malignancy. These patients may also require a bronchoscopy to see if there is an obstructing lesion.

Mortality from CAP ranges from 5.1–13.6% (for all CURB-65 scores) in the community, but increases to 36% in patients who require admission to ICU. Young patients with a CURB-65 score of 0 have a good prognosis with a mortality of <1%. The majority will return to full health within a few weeks. The morbidity and mortality are greater in those over the age of 65 and those with co-morbidities, such as diabetes and COPD. Patients with a CURB-65 of 2 have a ninefold increase in risk of death. Those who survive complain of persistent fatigue, cough, and breathlessness. There is an increased risk of death in survivors over the next three years, with a one-year mortality of 27%, as hypoxia and the acute inflammatory response due to CAP are associated with death due to acute cardiac events. Box 8.4 lists the mortality associated with CURB-65 score.

Annual influenza vaccination is offered to the elderly and those with co-morbidities as this reduces the risk of ICU admission and the risk of death by 30%. Vaccination against pneumonia also offers protection against *Streptococcus pneumonia*.

Box 8.4 CURB-65 score and mortality.

CURB-65 score	Mortality (%)	Management
0	0.7	Oral antibiotics in community
1	2.1	Oral antibiotics in the community
2	9.2	Admit to hospital for intravenous antibiotics and close monitoring
3	14.5	Admit to hospital for intravenous antibiotics and close monitoring. May require ICU
4	40	Admit to ICU

Hospital acquired pneumonia (HAP)

Hospital acquired (nosocomial) pneumonia (HAP) is defined as a pneumonia that develops more than 48 hours after admission to hospital in a patient who did not have any symptoms or signs of pneumonia on admission. HAP accounts for 1.5% of all infections acquired in hospital and for most infection-associated deaths in hospitals. HAP increases the length of hospital stay by eight days and has a mortality of between 30 and 70%. HAP has a worse prognosis than CAP because the patient is older, has co-morbidities, and is infected with more virulent organisms. Elderly patients, those with diabetes, heart failure, and those who are immunocompromised are more likely to succumb to a HAP. The highest mortality is associated with *Pseudomonas aeruginosa*, *Klebsiella pneumoniae*, *Escherichia coli* (41%) and methicillin-resistant *Staphylococcus aureus* (MRSA) at 32%. Anaerobic organisms are rarely implicated in a HAP.

Patients who develop HAP may not always have the usual symptoms and signs of pneumonia, such as fever and cough. They may appear non-specifically unwell, become confused, refuse to eat and drink, become hypoxic, and develop signs of consolidation. Doctors looking after hospitalised patients should be alert to the possibility of HAP, and ensure that appropriate samples (sputum and blood cultures) are taken from these patients. A CXR may show a new area of consolidation, and blood tests may reveal a rising CRP and neutrophilia. Empirical intravenous antibiotic therapy, in accordance with local hospital policy, should be commenced while waiting for the results of cultures and sensitivities. As multi-drug resistance is common in this group of patients, a combination of antibiotics is often given with careful monitoring of the patient's clinical state and the inflammatory markers. Usual antibiotics include Tazocin or Meropenem together with a macrolide.

Patients with HAP are likely to require intravenous fluids, nutritional supplements, and oxygen. Patients with a severe HAP often develop type 1 respiratory failure requiring continuous positive airways pressure (CPAP) or intubation and ventilation in the ICU. Deep vein thrombosis prophylaxis is essential.

Outpatients who have extensive contact with hospitals, including those on renal dialysis and those receiving chemotherapy, have an increased risk of developing multi-drug resistant infections, including MRSA. Other groups at risk include residents of nursing homes and other institutes. Healthcare workers are also more susceptible to developing these infections.

Ventilator-associated pneumonia

Ventilator-associated pneumonia (VAP) is a type of HAP that develops after a patient is intubated and ventilated on the ICU. Some 50% of those who are intubated and ventilated in the ICU will develop pneumonia, either through micro-aspiration or through contamination of the ventilator equipment. The routine use of proton pump inhibitors increases gastric pH, allowing bacteria to flourish. The organisms that cause VAP are the same as those causing HAP. Other organisms include Acinetobacter species and Stenotrophomonas maltophilia.

VAP is managed according to local antibiotic policies and the advice of the consultant microbiologist. Risk factors for developing multidrug resistance include hospitalisation for more than 48 hours, antibiotic therapy in the past 6 months, immunosuppression, and significant other co-morbidities.

Aspiration pneumonia

Aspiration pneumonia is common in patients with impaired swallowing which includes elderly patients, those with dementia, after a stroke, and those with neurological disease, for example, Parkinson's disease and multiple sclerosis. Aspiration of gastric contents can also occur after a seizure when the airway is not protected and is commoner in alcoholics. Gastric contents are aspirated into the respiratory tract, resulting in a chemical pneumonia and anaerobic bacterial infection with organisms such as Bacteroides species. CXR will often show a right middle lobe consolidation as the right main bronchus leads directly from the trachea.

Management includes antibiotics with anaerobic cover, such as metronidazole, chest physiotherapy, and oxygen therapy. Any patient suspected of an aspiration pneumonia should be kept 'nil by mouth' until a speech and language therapy (SALT) assessment is made. If it is not safe for the patient to swallow, then nasogastric tube feeding may be necessary until the patient recovers. Recurrent aspiration pneumonia may warrant a percutaneous enterogastrostomy (PEG) tube in selected cases.

Micro-aspiration is also prevalent in hospitalised patients, especially in intubated and ventilated patients. Common organisms include gram-negative bacilli, such as *Escherichia coli*, *Klebsiella pneumoniae*, *Pseudomonas aeruginosa*, and *Enterobacter* spp. Gram-positive cocci include *Staphylococcus aureus*, MRSA, and Streptococcus species.

Lipoid pneumonia

Lipoid pneumonia is caused by the aspiration of exogenous lipid material into the lungs. This can occur in those taking laxatives and those taking nasal decongestants.

Pulmonary infections in the immunocompromised

Patients with an abnormal immune system are predisposed to developing viral, bacterial, fungal, and parasitic respiratory infections that rarely affect those with a normal immune system. Box 8.5 lists some conditions that increase the risk of opportunistic infections. Opportunistic viral infections include cytomegalovirus (CMV), varicella zoster, and herpes simplex infections. These patients are

Box 8.5 Patients at increased risk of respiratory infections.

Infection	Opportunistic infection
HIV infection	See Box 8.6
Immunosuppressive drugs	Bacterial, viral, fungal
Cytotoxic drugs for cancer	Bacterial, viral, fungal
Post bone marrow transplant	Invasive aspergillosis
Lymphoma	Bacterial, viral, fungal
Myeloma	Bacterial, viral, fungal
Splenectomy	*Streptococcus pneumonia*
Sickle cell disease	*Streptococcus pneumonia*
Renal transplant	CMV pneumonia

also more likely to develop bacterial pneumonia, often with more virulent organisms. Immunocompromised patients also succumb to fungal infection, such as pneumocystis jiroveci (previously known as pneumocystis carinii and still referred to as PCP), *Cryptococcus neoformans*, *Aspergillus fumigatus*, *Aspergillus niger*, *Histoplasmosis*, and *Candida albicans*. Immunocompromised patients can be infected with parasites, such as toxoplasma, cryptosporidium, microsporidium and *Strongyloides stercoralis*. Immunocompromised hosts are more likely to be infected with *Mycobacterium tuberculosis* (MTB) and atypical mycobacteria, especially *Mycobacterium avium intracellulare* (MAI).

The immunocompromised host, when infected, may not present with the symptoms associated with infection, such as fever, as they are unable to mount an inflammatory response: they present with vague, non-specific symptoms.

Patients with lymphoma or myeloma have an immune paresis so that their white blood cells do no function properly. Patients who have had a splenectomy are at an increased risk of Gram positive cocci, for example, *Streptococcus pneumonia*, as are individuals with sickle cell disease. These individuals should be vaccinated against this organism and take penicillin V prophylaxis. Invasive pulmonary aspergillosis can occur after bone marrow transplant or in patients with lymphoma and has an extremely high mortality, even with intravenous antifungal treatment.

Patients with T-cell suppression, for example, after renal transplant, are at an increased risk of developing cytomegalovirus (CMV) pneumonia. The risk of this is increased if a seronegative patient receives an organ from a seropositive donor. The patients will develop non-specific symptoms, including cough, and the radiological features are also non-specific. A BAL or lung biopsy will reveal the characteristic '*owl eye*' intranuclear inclusion bodies. Blood tests will show an increase in CMV IgM. Treatment is with Ganciclovir, foscarnet, or ribavarin.

Patients with HIV and a low CD4 count are at risk of being infected with a variety of opportunistic pathogens which are listed in Box 8.6.

Pneumocystis jiroveci infection can affect patients with HIV and a CD 4 count of $<200\ mm^{-3}$. The affected individual will present with a cough, severe breathlessness, and hypoxia. CXR will show bilateral, interstitial ground glass shadowing in a *bat's wing* appearance (Figure 8.5, Figure 8.6).

Box 8.6 Pulmonary infections associated with HIV.

- **Bacteria:** *Mycobacterium tuberculosis*, *Streptococcus pneumonia*, *Staphylococcus aureus*, *Cryptosporidium neoformans*, *Histoplasma capsulatum*, *Mycobacterium* avium intracellulare (MAI).
- **Virus:** Pneumocystis jiroveci (PCP), cytomegalovirus (CMV), herpes simplex virus (HSV), varicella zoster (HVZ).
- **Fungi:** *Aspergillus fumigatus*, *Candida albicans*.
- **Parasites:** *Toxoplasma gondii*, *Cryptosporidium*, Microsporidium, *Strongyloides stercoralis*

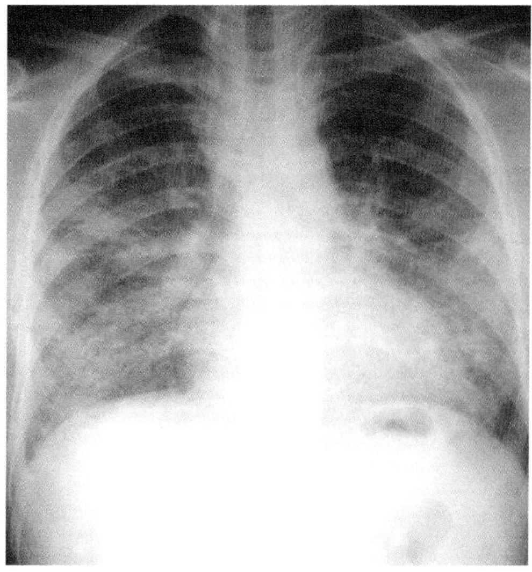

Figure 8.5 CXR showing ground-glass shadowing of pneumocystic jiroveci.

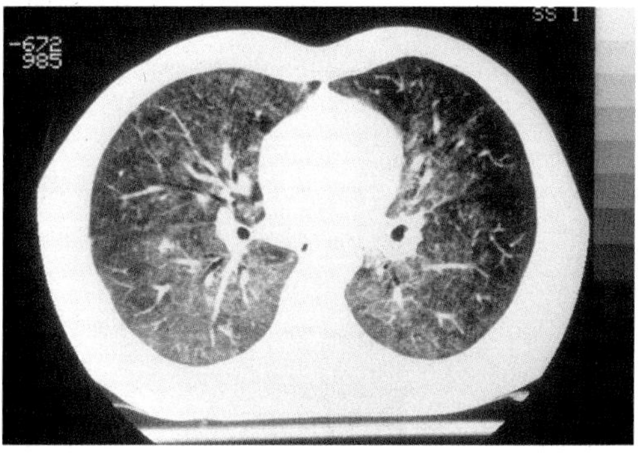

Figure 8.6 HR CT thorax showing ground-glass shadowing of pneumocystis jiroveci.

Bronchial washings or a transbronchial biopsy will show organisms that stain positive with silver stains. Treatment for pneumocystis jiroveci is with high dose co-trimoxazole. Patients with HIV and a low CD 4 count should have prophylaxis with oral co-trimoxazole or nebulised pentamidine.

HIV can also result in a lymphoid interstitial pneumonia (LIP), non-specific interstitial pneumonia (NSIP) and bronchiolitis obliterans organising pneumonia (BOOP). HIV also predisposes to the development of pulmonary hypertension, Kaposis's sarcoma, non-Hodgkin's lymphoma, and Hodgkin's lymphoma.

Mycobacterium tuberculosis

Tuberculosis (TB) is caused by the organism *Mycobacterium* tuberculosis (MTB). Mycobacterium bovis, which was endemic in cattle, was a cause of tuberculosis in humans in the past when milk was not pasteurised.

Epidemiology

Incidence: Worldwide, there are approximately nine million new cases of MTB every year, most occurring in the developing world, particularly Africa and Asia. Three million deaths/year are attributed to this infection worldwide. The World Health Organisation (WHO) has declared TB to be a global emergency.

In the UK, 12/100 000 of the population is affected. Immigrants from the Indian subcontinent are 40 times more likely to develop MTB than the Caucasian population (120/100 000) and those from Africa are 50 times more likely to develop MTB (211/100 000). Most new cases in the UK occur in inner cities, particularly London. There are approximately 8500 new cases in England and Wales every year and 73% of these occur in those born outside the UK.

Prevalence: A third of the world's population, approximately 2 billion, are infected with latent TB and 15–20 million people have active TB.

Pathogenesis of primary pulmonary tuberculosis

Active pulmonary tuberculosis accounts for 52% of TB cases in the UK. MTB is spread from one individual to another through the respiratory tract by inhalation of a droplet containing the organism, and the formation of a **Ghon focus** in the upper lobes of the lung. MTB is an obligate aerobe and therefore has a predilection for the periphery of the upper lobes of the lungs which are relatively poorly perfused but well ventilated. The Ghon focus, together with mediastinal or hilar lymph node enlargement, is called the **Primary Complex** which forms within eight weeks of inhalation of the organism (Figure 8.7). In 90% of immunocompetent individuals the organism is contained, remains dormant, and does not cause clinical disease other than a mild febrile illness and in some cases erythema nodosum.

Over time, fibrosis of the upper zones can occur with calcification of the Ghon focus, resulting in the characteristic granuloma (Figure 8.8, Figure 8.9). Before it is calcified, it can be suspicious of an early lung cancer and, if in doubt, should be treated as a solitary pulmonary nodule (see Chapter 9).

Factors that predispose to the development of MTB include poor and overcrowded housing, overcrowded institutions, such as prisons, homelessness, poor nutrition, vitamin D deficiency (< 50 nmol l^{-1} of 25 hydroxycholecalciferol), alcoholism, and social deprivation. Individuals who are immunocompromised, the elderly, and those with chronic diseases, such as diabetes mellitus and chronic kidney disease, are also more susceptible to developing active TB.

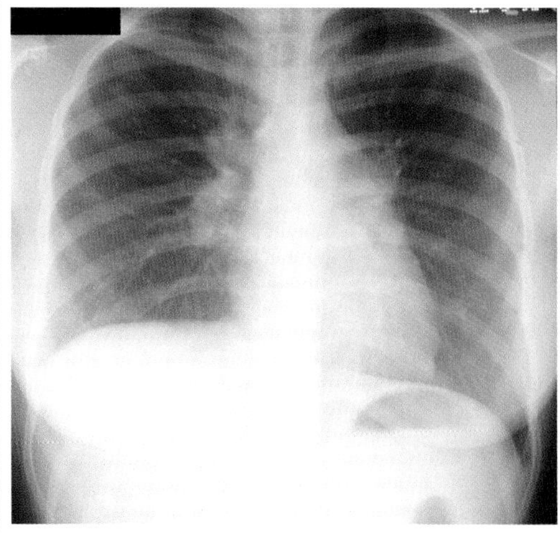

Figure 8.7 CXR showing primary *Mycobacterium tuberculosis* infection.

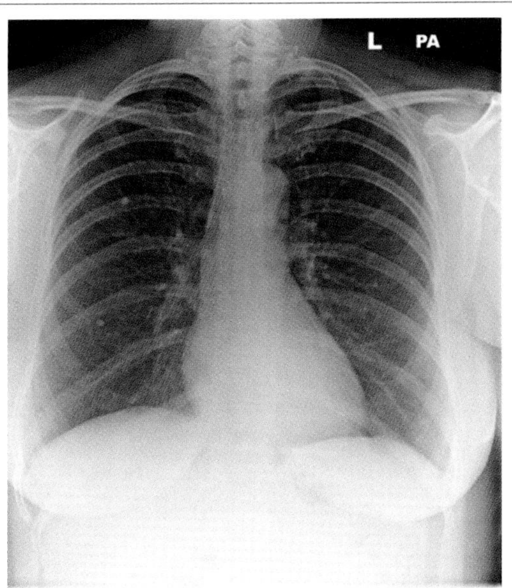

Figure 8.8 CXR showing granulomas in the right lung.

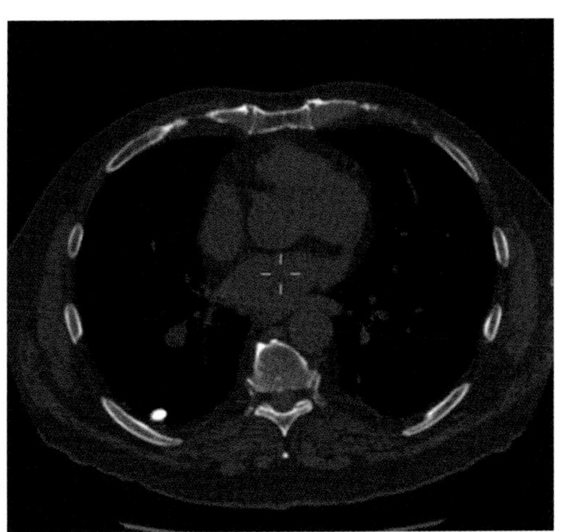

Figure 8.9 CT thorax showing a calcified granuloma in the right lung.

In the UK, almost half of new cases are due to reactivation of MTB, which can occur decades after the original asymptomatic infection. Those with HIV with a CD4 count of less than 200 mm^{-3} are at risk of reactivation of MTB infection. Once reactivated, the organism can spread from the lungs to other parts of the body through the bloodstream.

Post-primary tuberculosis

In fewer than 10% of cases, the individual will develop the active disease after exposure, presenting with fever, malaise, poor appetite, and weight loss. This is called *post-primary pulmonary TB* and occurs in those who have some immune dysfunction, for example, HIV. The infection will spread through the lungs and present with radiological changes. The organism can spread to other organs and cause active disease, or lie dormant until it is reactivated. Tuberculin testing will be strongly positive in those who have a normal immune system.

Immunology

The host's defence system recognises mycobacterial infections through toll-like receptors and destroys these organisms through the release of cytokines, including interferon-gamma. The formation of a granuloma by the human host 'contains' the organism in its dormant state. The lipids in the cell wall play an important role in the way the organism interacts with the host's immune response.

Diagnosis

A diagnosis of MTB is made with careful clinical evaluation, a high level of suspicion and the appropriate investigations. Most of the symptoms are non-specific and in 25% of cases, they are absent. Box 8.7 lists the common clinical symptoms and signs of pulmonary tuberculosis.

Delay in making the diagnosis is common, resulting in transmission of the infection to others.

Box 8.7 Clinical symptoms and signs of *Mycobacterium tuberculosis.*

Symptoms	Signs
Productive cough	Cachexia
Haemoptysis	Lymphadenopathy
Fever	Fever
Malaise	
Night sweats	
Weight loss	

The median time between the onset of symptoms and diagnosis is 10 weeks, although in 42% of cases it takes more than three months for the diagnosis to be made. Many of these patients are treated with multiple courses of antibiotics without sputum samples being sent for culture. Individuals with HIV may present with atypical symptoms and signs, and all patients diagnosed with MTB should have an HIV test. MTB is a notifiable disease and information should be sent to Public Health England.

Radiological diagnosis

Patients who present with symptoms suggestive of TB should have a CXR. In acute pulmonary TB this may show as an area of consolidation, as a cavitating lesion in the upper lobes of the lung (Figure 8.10) and lymph node enlargement in any of the lymph nodes in the mediastinum. Rarely, widespread disease affecting the lung parenchyma can result in what is called **miliary TB** as the nodules, measuring less than 5 mm in size, resemble millet seeds (Figure 8.11). Chickenpox pneumonia resembles miliary tuberculosis (Figure 8.12).

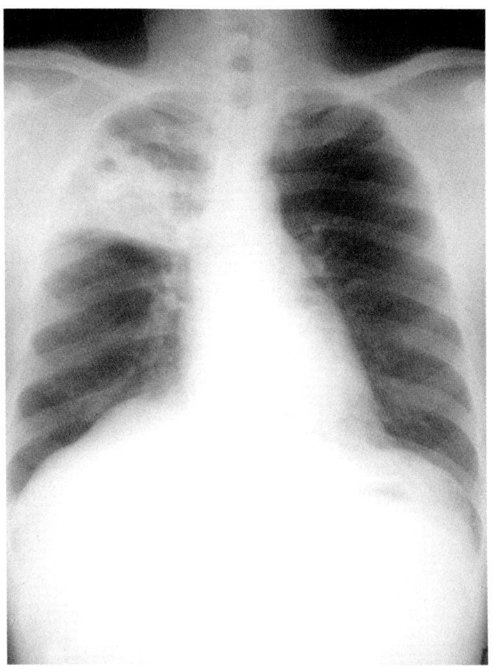

Figure 8.10 CXR showing right upper lobe consolidation in active mycobacterium infection.

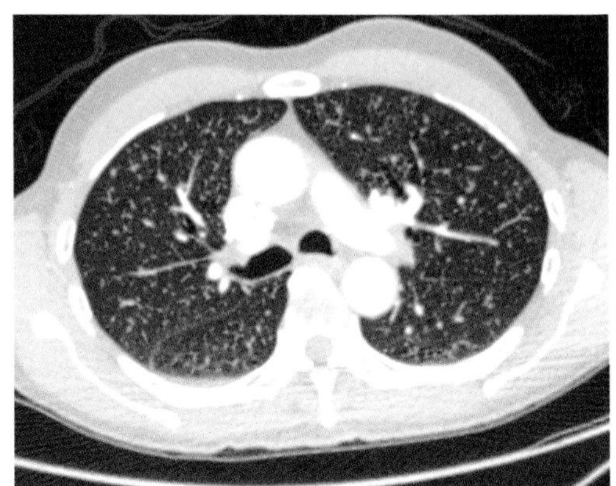

Figure 8.11 CT thorax showing miliary tuberculosis.

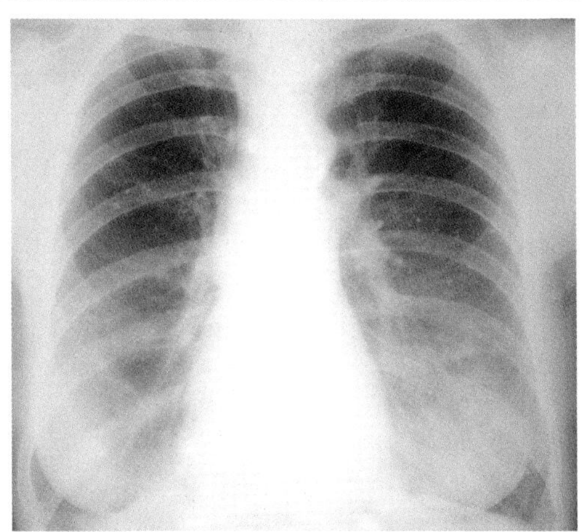

Figure 8.12 CXR of previous chickenpox pneumonia.

A unilateral pleural effusion is a common presentation. Some 5% of patients with pulmonary TB will have a normal CXR. Chronic lung changes from previous MTB infection include upper zone fibrosis, traction bronchiectasis, and signs of volume loss (Figure 8.13, Figure 8.14).

Microbiological and histological diagnosis

It is important to culture samples from the area that is affected to make a definite diagnosis of MTB and to find out the sensitivities to anti-tuberculous medication. Samples that could be sent include sputum, bronchial lavage, pleural fluid,

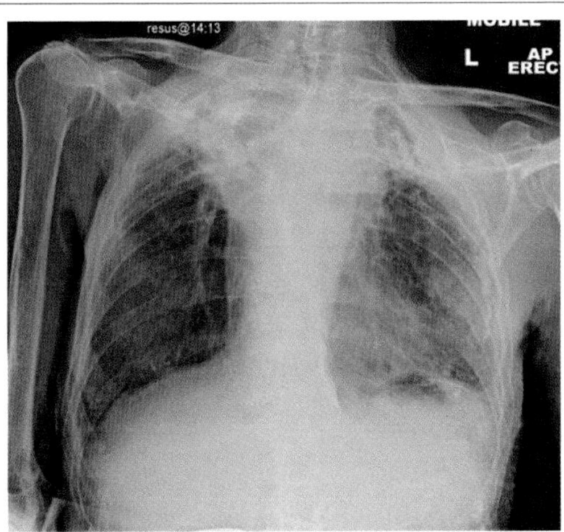

Figure 8.13 CXR showing changes of chronic mycobacterium tuberculosis infection.

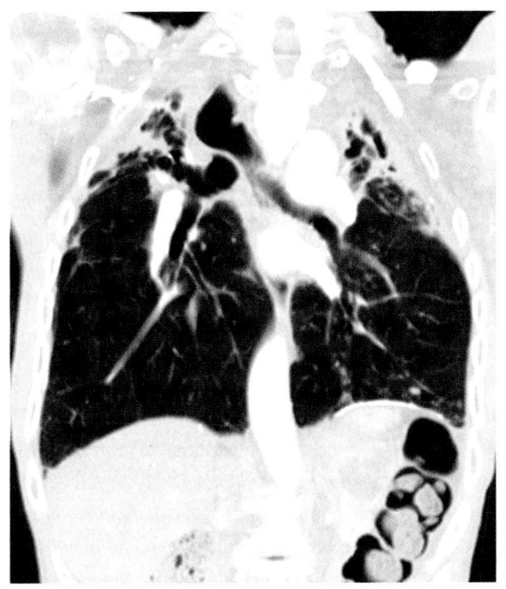

Figure 8.14 CT thorax showing changes of chronic tuberculosis.

pleural biopsy, or lymph node biopsy. It is recommended that samples are taken before starting treatment, but treatment should be initiated while waiting for cultures if the patient is symptomatic.

Sputum, if possible three early morning samples, should be sent for microbiological analysis and culture as the bacterial load is greater in these early samples. If the patient is unable to produce a sputum sample, then an induced sputum sample or bronchoalveolar lavage can be taken. In children, gastric washings can be helpful.

If viable mycobacteria are seen in the sputum, then it is called a '*smear-positive*' case. Sputum microscopy will detect acid-fast bacilli (smear-positive result) within 24 hours but will not differentiate between different strains of mycobacteria or whether the organism is alive or dead. Cultures are required for that which takes several weeks as the organism is a slowly growing one.

Samples of urine, cerebrospinal fluid (CSF), or tissue from any affected site can be cultured if extra-pulmonary MTB is suspected. Samples for histology should be stained using the Ziehl-Neelsen stain which uses the Carbol-fuschin red dye which is acid and alcohol fast; the report will say '*acid-alcohol-fast bacilli*' (AAFB).

The characteristic histological appearance of TB is a **caseating granuloma**. This is composed of an area of central necrosis surrounded by epithelioid giant cells, macrophages, and lymphocytes.

Specimens should not only be stained but should be cultured in a Lowenstein-Jensen medium which takes six weeks. There are newer culture techniques which can give the result of drug sensitivities within three weeks, although these are not in routine use yet.

Polymerase chain reaction (PCR) techniques can be useful when clinical suspicion is high but only small amount of material is available. DNA probes can be used for detecting certain multi-drug-resistant strains of TB which can also help trace the spread of the drug-resistant TB. Adenosine deaminase levels $>50\,U\,l^{-1}$ in pleural fluid are strongly suggestive of pleural TB, even if organisms themselves are not cultured from the pleural fluid, with a sensitivity of 90% and specificity of 89%.

Immunological diagnosis

The host responds to MTB infection by a delayed Type 1V hypersensitivity reaction to the tubercle bacilli. Diagnostic tools that are based on this cellular immunity have been developed.

The cutaneous immune response to an intradermal injection of purified protein derivative (PPD) from the bacterium is used to determine whether there is an active infection, especially when it is not possible to culture the organism.

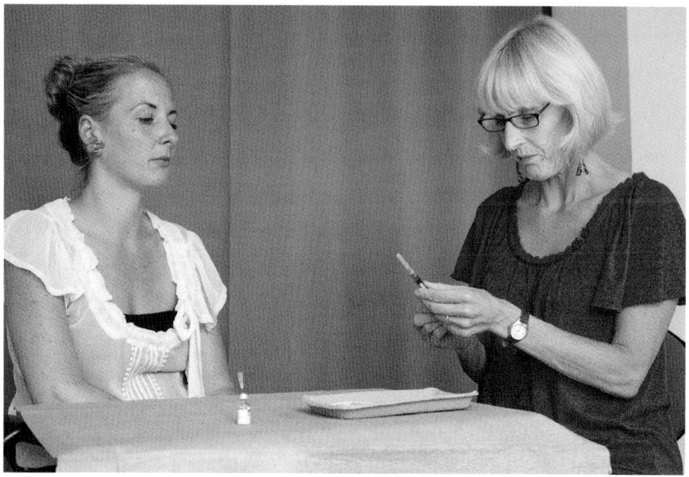

Figure 8.15 Preparation for a Mantoux test.

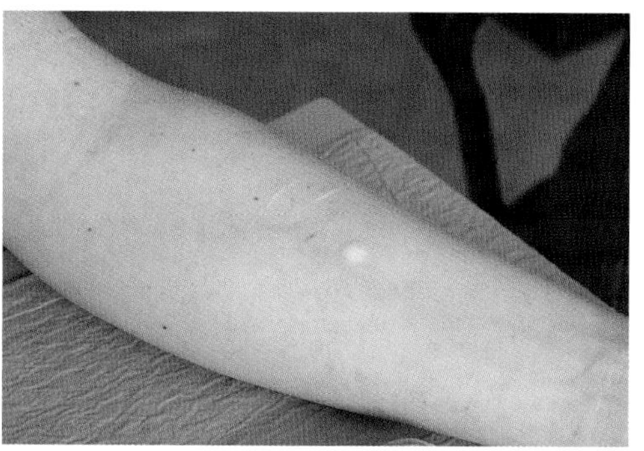

Figure 8.16 Forearm with purified protein derivative instilled intra-dermally.

In the Mantoux Test, 10 units (0.1 ml) of PPD is injected intra-dermally and the size of the induration is measured after 48–72 hours (Figure 8.15, Figure 8.16). In the Heaf Test, a fixed amount of the PPD is injected intra-dermally using a spring-loaded gun and the size of the induration is measured.

The size of the reaction from either of these methods is read after 48–72 hours and graded according to the size of the induration as 1–4. Skin induration greater than 5 mm is considered positive and induration greater than 15 mm strongly positive. The response will be affected by the BCG vaccination status of the individual, as those who have had the BCG vaccine will show a mild response, even when they are not infected with MTB. This delayed Type 1V hypersensitivity test is not useful in individuals over the age of 35, those who have previously had active TB, in those who are immunocompromised, and those with miliary tuberculosis. Supplementary material demonstrates how a Mantoux test is carried out (www.wiley.com/go/Paramothayan/Essential_Respiratory_Medicine). A strongly positive tuberculin response (Grade 3 or 4) should be investigated further with clinical assessment, chest X ray, and samples for culture as appropriate.

The interferon gamma release assay (IGRA) is an *in vitro* test that measures T-cell activation by MTB antigens. The Quantiferon Gold assay and the T-spot TB assay are available in the UK. Blood taken must be analysed within a few hours. The results of these investigations must be interpreted carefully together with all the other information available as a positive test on its own does not necessarily mean that the patient has MTB (Figure 8.17).

The differential diagnosis of MTB always includes sarcoidosis. Sarcoidosis (discussed in Chapter 7) presents with similar clinical symptoms and signs, similar radiological appearances, for example, hilar lymphadenopathy, and granuloma on biopsy samples. However, caseation is not seen with sarcoidosis and the immunological tests will be negative.

Management of MTB

Prior to the availability of anti-tuberculous drugs, patients with mycobacterium tuberculosis infection were treated with a variety of procedures

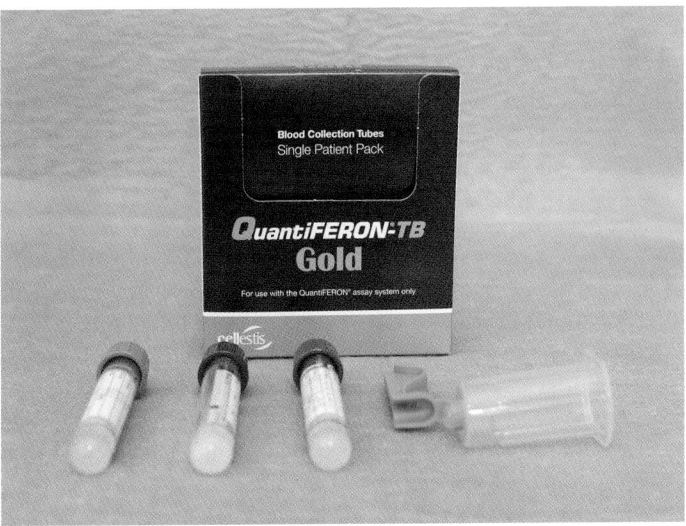

Figure 8.17 Quantiferon testing kit.

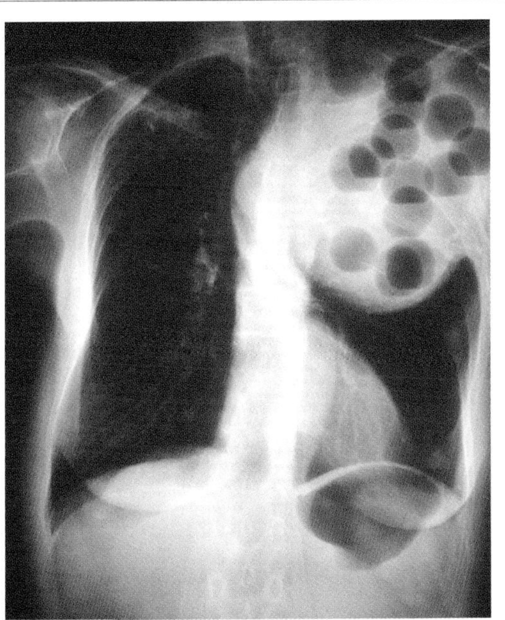

Figure 8.18 CXR showing plombage left lung.

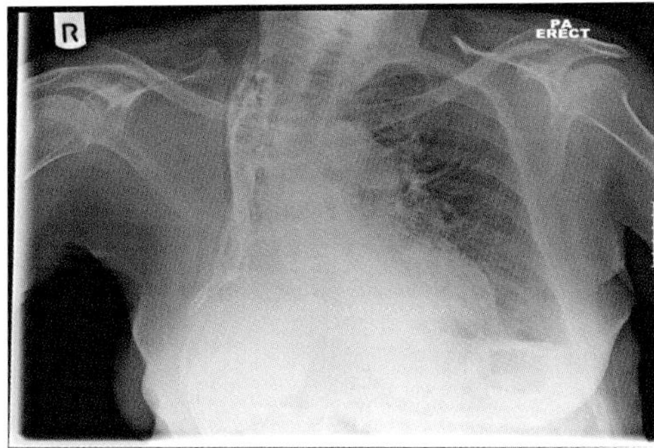

Figure 8.19 CXR showing right-sided thoracoplasty.

which were aimed at containing the infection by preventing ventilation of the lung. This included plombage whereby several plastic balls were placed in the pleural space to prevent ventilation (Figure 8.18) or by thoracoplasty and rib resection (Figure 8.19) to remove the infected lung. Patients were also given an artificial pneumothorax.

The standard treatment regime is a combination of Isoniazid (INH), Rifampicin (RIF), Pyrazinamide (PYR), and ethambutol for two months, followed by rifampicin and isoniazid for a further four months. If the organism is sensitive to these drugs and the drugs are taken as advised, this regime is very effective with a <3% risk of relapse. The dose is calculated according to the weight of the patient and given once a day on an empty stomach. Combinations of drugs, for example, Rifinah, which contains rifampicin and isoniazid and Rifater which contains rifampicin, isoniazid, and pyrazinamide, reduce the number of tablets that the individual needs to take, making compliance easier. Pyridoxine, 10 mg, is always given to prevent INH-induced peripheral neuropathy.

Although the standard treatment is with four drugs, three drugs (RIF, INH, and PYR) can be used if the patient is a close contact of an index case who has a fully sensitive organism.

MTB is usually managed in secondary care by respiratory physicians and TB nurses. To ensure compliance, some patients may need directly observed therapy (DOT), when a healthcare professional observes the patient swallowing the tablets. DOT is recommended in immigrants with poor language skills, those in whom compliance is suspect and those with possible MDRTB. The WHO recommends DOT as a standard procedure for eradicating MTB worldwide as it has a success rate of around 95%.

Compliance can also be checked by looking at a urine sample which will turn an orange/red color if the patient is taking rifampicin.

In most cases (85%) of smear-positive TB which is fully sensitive, the sputum sample will be clear after two weeks of treatment. In cases where there is extensive cavitation on the CXR and a large burden of disease, several weeks or months of treatment may be required before the sputum is smear-negative.

These drugs are safe to take during pregnancy and while breast feeding. Standard treatment is for six months. The recommended regime should be continued even if the culture results are subsequently negative.

Box 8.8 lists the main side effects of the first line anti-tuberculous drugs. All of them can cause nausea, especially if taken on an empty stomach. Approximately 9% of patients on these drugs develop significant side-effects requiring all medication to be stopped and then reintroduced carefully, one at a time, to see which one has caused the problem. Patients who are older, female, and HIV positive are more likely to develop serious side effects to anti-tuberculous drugs. Patients with liver disease are at increased risk of hepatotoxicity, so should be monitored more closely. These patients may require second-line drugs. Patients with chronic renal failure will require a lower dose of ethambutol.

Hepatitis is the commonest side-effect, resulting in the medications having to be stopped. The liver function tests should be checked before

Box 8.8 Common side effects of anti-tuberculous drugs.

Drug	Dose and duration	Prior testing and monitoring	Common side effects
Isoniazid (INH)	300 mg for 6 months	Liver function test	Hepatitis Peripheral sensory neuropathy Rash Fever
Rifampicin (RIF)	450 mg if <50 kg 600 mg if >50 kg for 6 months	Liver function tests	Hepatitis Thrombocytopaenia Itching Fever Red urine and secretions Enzyme inducer of cytochrome P450 so interaction with many drugs
Pyrazinamide	1.5 g if <50 kg 2.0 g if >50 kg for initial 2 months	Liver function tests	Hepatitis Rash Elevated uric acid level Rash
Ethambutol	15 mg kg^{-1} for initial 2 months	Visual acuity	Optic neuritis

commencing treatment, two weeks after starting treatment, and then at two months. Rifampicin blocks the excretion of bilirubin and results in an isolated increase in bilirubin which is not of concern. This will usually return to normal after two weeks. A rise in alanine transaminase (ALT) and aspartate transaminase (AST) are common in the first two to three months of treatment. It is only of concern if the levels rise to greater than four times the baseline and if the patient becomes symptomatic.

Although there is *in vitro* evidence that vitamin D enables monocytes and macrophages to kill MTB, there is no clinical trial evidence that treating vitamin D deficiency prevents infection with MTB or that giving vitamin D to patients with TB is beneficial.

A paradoxical reaction can occur in 6–30% of patients approximately 60 days after starting anti-tuberculous treatment when it appears that there is clinical and/or radiological worsening of the condition in a patient who initially appears to be improving.

HIV and MTB

Approximately 10% of patients with HIV are co-infected with MTB, therefore a high index of suspicion is required in this group, especially as these patients may not manifest the usual symptoms. Tuberculin testing will be negative because they are unable to mount an immunological reaction as their T lymphocytes are not functioning. These patients may present with lower lobe disease or disseminated disease if their CD4 count is less than 200 mm^{-3}. Anti-retroviral treatment may worsen the condition, so anti-tuberculous treatment should be initiated before commencing antiretroviral treatment, so long as the CD4 count is >200 mm^{-3}. For patients with HIV with a CD4 count of between 100 and 200 mm^{-3} and MTB, there is conflicting guidance as to when to start the TB treatment and anti-retroviral treatment, so specialist input from the genitourinary physician will be required.

Information to patients with TB

An individual who has been diagnosed with MTB should be given clear, written information about the disease, the medication required and the fact that six months of treatment is required to cure them of the disease. The side effects of the medication should be explained, and they should be advised to stop the medication if they develop symptoms, such as fever, vomiting, or severe rash. If they are on medication that may interact with rifampicin, for example, anticoagulants, anticonvulsants, steroids, or oestrogens, including the oral contraceptive pill, they need to understand the consequences. It is essential that they understand that the tablets must be taken daily to prevent relapse and the development of MDRTB. Contracting TB is still a stigma in many societies and this will need to be addressed.

Infectivity of tuberculosis

Active TB will, if untreated, infect 10–15 people every year, so is a major public health concern. Those with pulmonary tuberculosis who are found to have AAFB in their sputum or BAL are considered infectious and called '*smear-positive*'. These patients are usually admitted to a negative pressure isolation room on the ward, commenced on anti-tuberculous treatment and kept in isolation for two weeks. After this time, in most cases, they will no longer be considered infectious, although when the bacterial load is large, a longer period of isolation may be required. If there is any doubt about multi-drug resistance, then the individual should be kept in isolation until the sensitivities are confirmed. Healthcare workers should wear a proper protective mask as should the patient if he or she were to go outside the room for any reason. Extra-pulmonary tuberculosis cannot be caught, even by close contacts.

Contact tracing

Approximately 1–3% of close contacts of a smear-positive patient will be found to have the active disease. It is important, therefore, to assess the close contacts of the index case to see if they might have contracted tuberculosis. This includes close family members and work colleagues. This is important because contacts who might have been infected may not show any clinical symptoms which may later become activated. These individuals are considered to have latent tuberculosis. Contact tracing involves clinical assessment of symptoms, CXR, tuberculin testing, Quanteferon testing, and BCG status.

MTB is a notifiable disease and should be reported to Public Health England. The Public

Health consultant will be involved in any case of outbreak in the community. The Occupational Health Department will be involved in identifying and managing healthcare workers in any setting, for example, hospital or nursing home.

Screening of immigrants

All individuals arriving in the UK from areas of high prevalence of MTB are screened with a health status interview, evidence of BCG vaccination and a CXR, usually done at their country of origin. A tuberculin test is carried out in those younger than 35 years.

Latent tuberculosis

Individuals who are exposed to the organism but do not develop active disease are considered to have latent tuberculosis. The organism lies dormant because the host's immune system contains it. These individuals are asymptomatic, are not infectious and will have a normal CXR, but will have a strongly positive tuberculin reaction.

These individuals are at risk of reactivation of tuberculosis at a later stage, for example, when they are older or become immunocompromised. Identifying and treating individuals with latent TB infection reduces the risk of reactivation which is 5–10%. The risk is greatest within the first two years of acquiring the infection.

Individuals with latent tuberculosis should be offered chemoprophylaxis, usually with INH for six months or INH and RIF for three months. As discussed earlier, there is a risk of a rise in liver enzymes, therefore liver function tests should be checked prior to starting treatment and one week later. Individuals who are candidates for biological therapy, such as anti-TNF-α treatment, which is commonly given for a variety of rheumatological, dermatological, and gastroenterological conditions, or those who are going to have chemotherapy or organ transplant, should also receive chemoprophylaxis.

In London, the 'Find and Treat' initiative screens patients at high risk of developing TB by CXR and symptom enquiry as there is evidence that reactivation of latent disease accounts for more new cases than new infections from transmission.

Prevention of *Mycobacterium tuberculosis* (MTB)

The BCG vaccination, containing a live attenuated strain of mycobacterium bovis, is offered to the children of high risk groups, such as immigrants, ethnic minorities, and healthcare workers who may be exposed to TB. Neonates and infants up to the age of three months can be given the BCG vaccination without tuberculin testing. Older children need Heaf testing to demonstrate a negative response before immunisation. The BCG provides 75% protection against the disease for a period of 15 years. The protective effect is stronger for TB meningitis than for pulmonary disease. There is little evidence that BCG offers protection when given to adults.

Treatment of multi-drug-resistant tuberculosis (MDRTB)

Multi-drug-resistant TB (MDRTB) occurs in those who have had a failure of treatment with anti-tuberculous drugs, usually in those who did not complete the treatment regime. The majority of these are from Africa or the Indian sub-continent, and rates of MDRTB have doubled in the UK in the past decade due to immigration. The rate of resistance is 8% for isoniazid, 1.7% for rifampicin and 1.2% for both. MDRTB causes approximately 10% of all TB deaths worldwide.

Patients with MDRTB must be isolated as they pose a huge public health risk. Outbreaks occurring in hospitals and prisons result in high mortality. MDRTB is managed in centres with expertise and experience. A prolonged course of second line drugs, for up to 24 months, may be required. Box 8.9 lists the second and third line drugs used for MDRTB. There is less evidence for the efficacy of the third line drugs.

In cases of MDRTB where drugs appear ineffective or when there are serious side effects from drug therapy, a lobectomy or pneumonectomy could be considered to remove the infected lung.

Box 8.9 Drugs used to treat MDRTB.

Second line drugs
- Aminoglycosides: amikacin, kanamycin
- Polypeptides: Capreomycin, viomycin, enviomycin
- Fluroquinolones: ciprofloxacin, levofloxacin, moxifloxacin
- Thioamides: ethionamide, prothionamide
- Cycloserine
- Terizidone

Third line drugs
- Rifabutin
- Macrolides
- Linezolid
- Thioacetazone
- Thionidazine
- Arginine
- Bedaquiline

Pulmonary complications of mycobacterium tuberculosis

Box 8.10 lists some of the pulmonary complications of MTB.

Box 8.10 Pulmonary complications of MTB.

1. Cavities
2. *Aspergillus fumigatus* or *Aspergillus niger*
3. Pneumothorax
4. Lobar collapse
5. Pleural effusion

Extra-pulmonary tuberculosis

MTB can disseminate and spread haematogenously to other organs. Approximately 20% of patients with pulmonary TB will have extra-pulmonary disease in an additional site. The very young, the elderly, and those who are malnourished and immunocompromised are most likely to develop extra-pulmonary TB. Extrapulmonary TB is more common in those from high prevalence nations.

Table 8.2 lists the other organs involved, the frequency of this involvement, the clinical presentation and what kind of specimen is used to make the diagnosis.

The diagnosis is confirmed by observing the acid-fast bacilli and culturing the organism from the samples. PCR analysis can be diagnostic if only a small amount of sample is available. Samples from pleura, the liver, the lymph nodes, and bone marrow generally have a good yield but CSF and pleural fluid less so. Samples should be sent to the laboratory in a sterile pot with no additives. Histopathology will show granuloma containing epithelioid macrophages, Langerhans giant cells and lymphocytes, with caseation in the centre.

Some 25% of patients with TB lymphadenitis may develop pain and increased swelling of the lymph nodes with treatment. This is a well-recognised phenomenon and does not indicate treatment failure. Oral corticosteroids are often given in this situation. The lymph nodes will start to shrink two to three months after treatment is started. Surgical removal of very large lymph nodes could be considered.

TB can affect the central nervous system (CNS) resulting in TB meningitis or a tuberculoma, which can present as a space-occupying lesion. In TB meningitis, cerebrospinal fluid (CSF) will have a high protein level, high lymphocyte count, and a low glucose level, and become culture positive in 50% of cases. CNS TB will require 12 months of treatment. Dexamethasone, 8–12 mg daily, reducing over six weeks, is usually given for TB meningitis. There is some evidence that thalidomide may be of benefit in TB meningitis.

TB of the spinal cord can result in TB myelitis and progress to involve the spinal cord with cord compression. Surgical decompression may be required. Surgery may also be required for the drainage of any tuberculous abscess.

Miliary tuberculosis results from the haematogenous dissemination of mycobacterium tuberculosis to many organs. The CXR will show multiple, small nodules throughout the lung fields which is more obvious on a CT scan of the thorax. In patients who present with miliary tuberculosis, evidence of involvement of other

Table 8.2 Non-pulmonary tuberculosis.

Organ and frequency of involvement	Symptoms	Signs	Investigation and diagnosis
CNS (5%)	Headaches Confusion Decreased consciousness Seizures Vomiting Malaise Cranial nerve palsies	Consistent with a space occupying lesion Decreased GCS Fever Cranial nerve palsies	Lumbar puncture: CSF may show organism, high protein, low glucose, and lymphocytes. MTB seen in 25% and culture positive in 60% CT head: SOL, tuberculoma
Lymph nodes (25%)	Painful or painless swelling in cervical and supraclavicular lymph nodes	Lymphadenopathy	Lymphadenopathy on ultrasound neck, mediastinal lymphadenopathy on CT thorax. Biopsy of lymph node shows caseating granuloma
Gastrointestinal tract (peritoneal, ileocaecal and appendix)	Abdominal pain Bowel Obstruction	Peritonitis Bowel obstruction	CT abdomen may show an 'appendix mass'. Histology of peritoneum, ascitic fluid or biopsy of appendix mass will show caseating granuloma. Can resemble Crohn's disease
Heart (TB pericarditis)	Systemic symptoms Chest pain Dyspnoea	Signs of pericardial effusion	Pericardial fluid: low glucose, high protein, lymphocytic, organism may be seen
Bone, joints, and vertebrae (Potts disease):10–35%	Pain Symptoms of spinal cord compression Chronic osteomyelitis	Paraplegia Chronic sinus formation Cold abscess	Bone X-ray shows lesions CT abdomen may show cold abscess which can track from the psoas muscle to the abdomen. Aspiration or biopsy of infected tissue
Genitourinary tract: 15% kidneys bladder epididymis prostate	Systemic features Dysuria Hematuria Prostatitis Epididymitis	Caseating granuloma in glomeruli, damage to medulla, destruction of renal papilla, fibrosis, and stenosis of collecting ducts	Sterile pyuria Microscopic haematuria (in 90%) Scarring of bladder and thimble bladder causing obstruction seen on X-ray and IV pyelogram Organism seen in three early morning urine samples. PCR 93% sensitivity and 95% specificity
Skin	Painful nodular lesion on face Hypersensitivity Painful rash on legs	Lupus vulgaris Erythema nodosum Erythema induratum	Granuloma seen on skin biopsy

organs should be actively sought. A CT head and lumbar puncture for analysis of CSF should be done urgently.

Opportunistic (atypical) mycobacterium

Opportunistic mycobacteria, often called atypical mycobacteria, are saprophytes that are found in the environment; in soil and water. These organisms only cause disease in those who are immunocompromised or those with chronic lung disease. *Mycobacterium avium* complex (MAC) is a common cause of pulmonary disease worldwide.

Box 8.11 lists some of the opportunistic mycobacteria. Box 8.12 lists some of the common conditions that predispose to infection with these organisms.

Individuals with opportunistic mycobacteria infections present with cough, haemoptysis, malaise, and weight loss, but generally with less systemic symptoms than MTB. These organisms are not infectious and therefore cannot be caught by close contacts. These infections do not require contact tracing and are not notifiable. Disseminated MAI infections can occur in HIV patients, especially those with a low CD count of less than 200 mm^{-3}.

Diagnosis of opportunistic mycobacteria is made with a history of respiratory symptoms, CXR, and HRCT thorax showing the characteristic 'tree in bud' appearance (Figure 8.20). Sputum and BAL samples will stain positive with Ziehl-Neelsen stain, raising the possibility of MTB. Cultures will exclude MTB and identify the correct species.

Treatment is required if the patient is systemically unwell. Treatment is with a combination of macrolides (clarithromycin or azithromycin), rifamycins (rifampicin or rifabutin) and ethambutol for 18–24 months. Other drugs that are used include fluroquinolones and aminoglycosides. Complete eradication is difficult, especially in those with chronic lung disease. Surgery in the form of lobectomy or pneumonectomy may be an option in those with heterogeneous disease, who are fit for major surgery.

Box 8.11 Opportunistic mycobacteria.

1. *Mycobacterium* kansasii
2. *Mycobacterium* avium intracellular intracellulare (MAI): also called *Mycobacterium* avium intracellular complex (MAC)
3. *Mycobacterium* xenopii
4. *Mycobacterium* malmoense
5. *Mycobacterium* chelonae
6. *Mycobacterium* marinarum
7. *Mycobacterium* gordonae
8. *Mycobacterium* abscessus

Box 8.12 Conditions that predispose to opportunistic mycobacterial infection.

1. Bronchiectasis
2. Pulmonary fibrosis
3. Cavitating lung diseases
4. Human immunodeficiency virus (HIV) infection

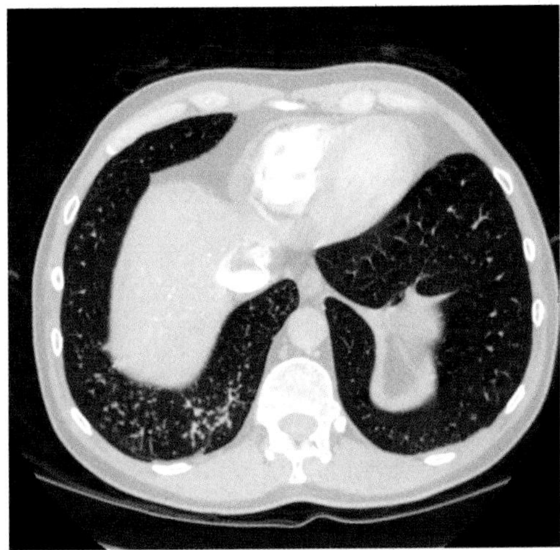

Figure 8.20 CT thorax showing 'tree in bud' appearance of atypical mycobacterial infection.

SUMMARY OF LEARNING POINTS

- Infections of the respiratory tract are very common and are mostly self-limiting.
- Viral infections of the upper respiratory tract are responsible for the common cold, laryngitis, and tracheobronchitis; these can be troublesome in infants and young children.
- Community acquired pneumonia is a common presentation to general practice and to hospitals and is caused by a variety of bacteria.
- The management and prognosis of CAP depend on whether the individual is immunocompetent, the CURB-65 score, and the causative organism.
- Patients with a CURB-65 score of 0 or 1 can be managed in the community with oral antibiotics and their prognosis is excellent.
- Patients with a CURB-65 score of 2 or more should be managed in hospital with intravenous antibiotics and supportive treatment, such as intravenous fluids, oxygen, and mucolytics.
- Investigations for CAP include CXR, blood cultures, sputum cultures, and urinary antigens for legionella and pneumococcus.
- The mortality of patients with a CURB-65 score of 3 or 4 is significant, and is greater in those who are over 85 years of age.
- The commonest organism causing CAP is *Streptococcus pneumonia*.
- The differential diagnosis for a cavitating lesion on CXR includes *Staphycoccus aureus*, *Klebsiella pneumonia*, *Mycobacterium tuberculosis*, vasculitic lesions, and lung cancer.
- HAP is a new infection which occurs in an individual who has been in hospital for at least 48 hours. The infecting organisms include Gram negative organisms such as Pseudomonas, Klebsiella and MRSA. HAP has a worse prognosis than CAP.
- VAP occurs in 50% of patients who are ventilated on the ICU. The risk of multi-drug-resistant organisms is high and VAP has a high morbidity and mortality.
- Immunocompromised individuals are at high risk of respiratory infections with opportunistic organisms: CMV, bacteria, fungi, and parasites.
- Patients with HIV and a CD4 count of less than 200 cells mm^{-3} are at risk of contracting a variety of infections, including CMV, HSV, HVZ, PCP, MTB, aspergillosis, cryptosporidium, and MAI.
- MTB is an enormous health problem worldwide; 15–20 million with active TB, 9 million new cases every year and 3 million TB-related deaths every year.
- Factors that predispose to the development of MTB include malnutrition, deprivation, poverty, and overcrowding.
- Most patients who develop MTB in the UK are individuals from the African and Indian sub-continents.
- MTB is a notifiable disease. Contact tracing of the index case is required.
- The diagnosis of MTB is made based on clinical history, suspicious radiology and organisms being detected in appropriate samples; sputum, BAL, urine, pleural fluid.
- All those with a diagnosis of MTB should have an HIV test as the prevalence of HIV is 10% in this group.
- Treatment of pulmonary TB is usually with four drugs for 6 months. It is essential for individuals to complete treatment as otherwise there is a risk of multi-drug resistance and poorer outcomes.
- The WHO advocates DOT for individuals at risk and those who may not be compliant.
- Anti-tuberculous medications have side-effects, including hepatitis, so monitoring is required.
- Anti-tuberculous medications interact with many other drugs through the cytochrome P450 enzyme system.
- Patients who are immunosuppressed and those who are eligible for biological therapy (TNF-α) are at a risk of reactivation of latent TB and should have chemoprophylaxis.
- The results of the Mantoux test and Quanteferon should be interpreted carefully and will be affected by the age, ethnicity, and the BCG status of the individual.

- Extra-pulmonary TB can affect the lymph nodes, CNS, bone, the genito-urinary system, the gastrointestinal system, and skin.
- Tuberculous meningitis has significant morbidity and mortality. Diagnosis must be made promptly and treatment may be required for 9–12 months.
- Atypical mycobacteria are only pathogenic in immunocompromised individuals and those with chronic lung diseases. Treatment may be required for 18–24 months.

MULTIPLE CHOICE QUESTIONS

8.1 Which of the following statements about CAP is true?

A Antibiotic treatment should be delayed until positive cultures and sensitivities are available
B CAP should always be managed in hospital
C CAP should be suspected in a patient who becomes unwell after several days in hospital
D CURB-65 score is of prognostic value and should be always calculated
E Diagnosis of a CAP is made from the presenting symptoms

Answer: D

The diagnosis of CAP is made after assessing the clinical symptoms, signs, and radiological changes on a CXR in a patient who presents from the community. Once confirmed, antibiotic treatment should be started without delay. Patients who are young, have no serious co-morbidities, and a CURB-65 score of 0 or 1 should be managed in the community with oral antibiotics. If a patient who has been in hospital for more than 48 hours develops pneumonia, then that is called a HAP.

8.2 Which of the following statements about CAP is true?

A Annual incidence of CAP is 50/1000 of adult population
B The commonest pathogen causing CAP is *Staphylococcus aureus*
C Mortality from severe CAP with a CURB-65 of 4 is 10%
D Patients with CAP always present with productive cough and fever
E Urinary antigens for pneumococcus have a high sensitivity and specificity

Answer: E

The annual incidence of CAP is 5–11/1000 of the adult population. The commonest pathogen is *Streptococcus pneumonia*. Mortality of severe CAP with a CURB-65 score of 4 is very high at 40%. These patients should be admitted to the ICU. Elderly and immunocompromised patients may not present with cough and fever as they are unable to mount an immune response. They often present with generalised malaise, confusion, and reduced appetite. Urinary pneumococcal antigen has a high sensitivity and specificity.

8.3 Which of the following statements about HAP is true?

A It accounts for 10% of all infections in hospital
B Mortality from HAP is 10%
C Pseudomonas aeruginosa is a common organism in HAP
D It is less common in ventilated patients on ICU
E Patients with HAP always present with fever and cough

Answer: C

Pseudomonas aeruginosa and other Gram-negative bacteria are common causes of a HAP which is more likely to occur in those who are immunocompromised, have co-morbidities, and chronic lung disease. HAP accounts for 1.5% of all infections in hospital and mortality is 30–70%. HAP (or VAP) is more common in intubated patients due to micro-aspiration. Patients who are immunocompromised do not always present with the classic symptoms of an infection.

8.4 Which of the following statements about respiratory infections in the immunocompromised host is true?

A Pneumocystis jiroveci pneumonia only occurs in those with HIV
B Patients with HIV and MTB should not have anti-tuberculous treatment until they receive anti-retroviral drugs first
C Patients who have sickle cell disease are likely to develop fungal infections
D Patients with T cell suppression are at risk of developing CMV pneumonia
E Aspergilloma occurs in patients with HIV

Answer: D

PCP can occur in any patient who is immunocompromised, those with bone marrow or solid organ transplant, on chemotherapy, or immunosuppressed with drugs. Patients with HIV who develop TB should have treatment for TB. Patients with sickle cell disease are at risk of developing *Streptococcus pneumonia* infection so should have the vaccine against this organism and take prophylactic penicillin V.

8.5 Which of the following statements about MTB is true?

A Worldwide more people have active TB than latent TB
B 10% of individuals with HIV get TB
C 90% of individuals exposed to MTB will develop the active disease
D 25% of new cases of TB occur in those born outside the UK
E A granuloma is highly infectious

Answer: B

Approximately one-third of the world's population has latent TB and 15–20 million have active TB. Fewer than 10% of those exposed to the organism develop the active disease. Some 73% of the new cases in the UK develop in those born outside the UK, predominantly from Africa and the Indian subcontinent. A granuloma is a calcified Ghon focus seen on a CXR and is not infectious.

8.6 Which of the following statements about MTB is true?

A Patients with TB and a cough are always infectious to others and should be kept in isolation
B Negative sputum samples rules out TB
C A Mantoux test is a specific and sensitive test in diagnosing TB
D Patients with CNS TB should be treated for 12 months
E Tuberculous pleural effusion is neutrophilic

Answer: D

Only patients with live mycobacterium in their sputum (smear-positive) are infectious and should be kept away from others at least until two weeks of treatment is complete. Negative sputum samples do not rule out TB which is made with a combination of clinical, radiological, microbiological, and immunological tests. A Mantoux test is not sensitive or specific as it is affected by previous BCG, the age of the patient, and conditions that affect the T-lymphocytes, such as HIV, when it will be negative. CNS TB requires 12 months of treatment with anti-tuberculous drugs and often dexamethasone. Tuberculous pleural effusions are lymphocytic.

8.7 Which of the following statements about anti tuberculous therapy is true?

A Pyrazinamide is the drug which is most likely to cause hepatitis
B The drugs should be stopped if there is any rise in liver enzymes
C Visual acuity should be checked before starting ethambutol
D Multi-drug-resistant TB is responsible for 50% of TB deaths.
E Fast acetylators are more likely to develop hepatitis than slow acetylators

Answer: C

Isoniazid is the drug most likely to cause hepatitis but adding in rifampicin increases the risk. Liver enzymes should be measured before starting the drugs and again two weeks after starting treatment. A small rise in the levels should be noted and monitored, but the drug should only be stopped if the patient becomes unwell and the enzymes (ALT and AST) rise four times greater than baseline. MDRTB is responsible for 10% of deaths worldwide. Genetic polymorphism means that low acetylators are more likely to develop liver failure than fast acetylators.

8.8 Which one of the following statements is true?

A 1–3% of close contacts of smear-positive patients will develop the active disease
B Latent TB is diagnosed with positive organisms on culture
C Those with latent TB will require four anti-tuberculous drugs for six months
D Risk of reactivation of latent TB is 25%
E The BCG vaccination should be offered to all university students

Answer: A

Latent TB implies that there are no organisms as there is no active disease and so treatment is with isoniazid for six months or isoniazid and rifampicin for three months. The risk of reactivation is 5–10% and is greatest in the first two years after infection. The BCG vaccination is usually given to babies and young children at high risk, such as immigrants and ethnic minorities. Although there is little evidence that it offers protection to adults, it is often offered to healthcare workers.

8.9 Which of the statements regarding opportunistic mycobacteria is true?

A Infections with opportunistic mycobacteria always need treating
B Treatment may be required for up to five years
C The characteristic radiological appearance is 'tree in bud'
D Opportunistic mycobacteria are highly infectious
E Opportunistic mycobacteria infections should be notified

Answer: C

Opportunistic or atypical mycobacteria affect those with chronic lung disease and those who are immunocompromised and only need to be treated if the patient is symptomatic. Up to two years of treatment may be required. These saprophytes are not infectious and cannot be 'caught' and therefore not notifiable.

8.10 Which of the following statements regarding pneumocystis jiroveci (PCP) is true?

A Pneumocystis jiroveci is a parasite
B Pneumocystis jiroveci may be asymptomatic in the immunocompromised patient
C Diagnosis is made after culture of the organism for eight weeks
D Treatment is with macrolide antibiotics for six months
E CXR will show bilateral pleural effusions

Answer: B

PCP is a fungus which affects those who are immunocompromised. Patients can be asymptomatic in the early stages. Diagnosis is made on silver staining or florescent staining but it cannot be cultured. CXR usually shows bilateral ground glass infiltrates. Treatment is with co-trimoxazole or pentamidine.

FURTHER READING

American Thoracic Society (2005). Guidelines for the management of adults with hospital-acquired, ventilator-associated, and healthcare-associated pneumonia. *American Journal of Respiratory and Critical Care Medicine* 171 (4): 388–416.

American Thoracic Society and Centers for Disease Control and Prevention of Infectious Diseases (CDC) (2000). Targeted tuberculin testing and treatment of latent tuberculosis infection. *American Thoracic Society, American Journal of Respiratory and Critical Care Medicine* 161: S221–S223.

Fine, M.J., Smith, M.A., Carson, C.A. et al. (1996). Prognosis and outcomes of patients with community-acquired pneumonia: a meta-analysis. *Journal of the American Medical Association* 275 (2): 134–141.

Fine, M.J., Stone, R.A., Singer, D.E. et al. (1999). Processes and outcomes of care for patients with community-acquired pneumonia results from the Pneumonia Patient Outcomes Research Team (PORT) cohort Study. *Archives of Internal Medicine* 159 (9): 970–980.

Lim, W., Baudouin, S., George, R.C. et al. (2009). BTS guidelines for the management of community acquired pneumonia in adults: update 2009. *Thorax* 64 (Suppl 3): iii1–iii55.

Lim, W.S., van der Eerden, M.M., Laing, R. et al. (2003). Defining community acquired pneumonia severity on presentation to hospital: an international derivation and validation study. *Thorax* 58 (5): 377–382.

Menéndez, R., Torres, A., Zalacaín, R. et al. (2005). Guidelines for the treatment of community-acquired pneumonia: predictors of adherence and outcome. *American Journal of Respiratory and Critical Care Medicine* 172 (6): 757–762.

National Institute for Health and Care Excellence (2011). Tuberculosis: clinical diagnosis and management of tuberculosis, and measures for its prevention and control. NICE Guidelines (CG117). Available at: www.nice.org.uk/

National Institute for Health and Care Excellence (2014) Pneumonia in adults: diagnosis and management management. NICE \guidelines (CG191), (December). Available at: www.nice.org.uk/

National Institute for Health and Care Excellence (2016) Tuberculosis. NICE Guideline (NG33). [online] Available at: www.nice.org.uk/guidance/ng33/resources/tuberculosis-1837390683589.

Stagg, H.R., Zenner, D., Harris, R.J. et al. (2014). Treatment of latent tuberculosis infection a network meta-analysis. *Annals of Internal Medicine* 161 (6): 419–428.

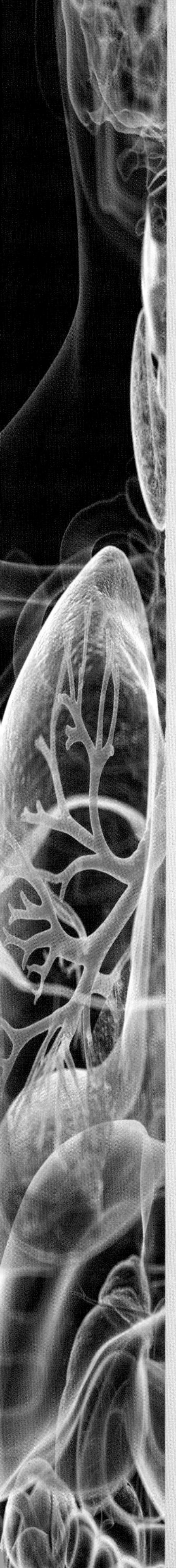

CHAPTER 9
Lung cancer

Learning objectives

- To understand the epidemiology and risk factors for lung cancer
- To appreciate the importance of prevention and early detection
- To recognise the symptoms and signs of lung cancer
- To understand the investigations used to make a diagnosis of lung cancer
- To learn the classification of lung cancers
- To understand the radical and palliative management of lung cancer
- To appreciate the importance of a multidisciplinary approach in the management of lung cancer
- To understand the differential diagnoses and management of benign lung lesions
- To understand the differential diagnoses and management of solitary pulmonary nodules

Essential Respiratory Medicine, First Edition. Shanthi Paramothayan.

Companion website: www.wiley.com/go/paramothayan/essential_respiratory_medicine

Abbreviations

ALK	anaplastic lymphoma kinase
APUD	amine uptake and decarboxylation
AVM	arterio-venous malformation
CEA	carcinoembryonic antigen
CHART	continuous hyper-fractionated accelerated radiotherapy
COPD	chronic obstructive pulmonary disease
CT	computed tomography
CXR	chest X-ray
EBUS	endobronchial ultrasound
EGF	epidermal growth factor
EGFR	epidermal growth factor receptor
EMLA	echinoderm microtubule-associated protein-like 4
ENT	ear, nose and throat
EUS	endoscopic ultrasound
FDG	^{18F}-Fluorodeoxy glucose
FEV_1	forced expiratory volume in 1 second
FNA	fine-needle aspiration
FVC	forced vital capacity
Gy	Grey is a derived SI unit for ionising radiation
HPOA	hypertrophic pulmonary osteoarthropy
LCNS	lung cancer nurse specialist
MDT	multidisciplinary team
MRI	magnetic resonance imaging
NICE	National Institute of Health and Care Excellence
NSCLC	non-small cell lung cancer
PD-L1	programmed death ligand 1
PD-L1R	programmed death ligand 1 receptor
PET-CT	positron emission tomography with computed tomography
PORT	post-operative radiation therapy
PSA	prostate specific antigen
PTH	parathyroid hormone
RCT	randomised controlled trial
SABR	stereotactic ablative radiotherapy
SCLC	small cell lung cancer
SIADH	syndrome of inappropriate anti-diuretic hormone
SPN	solitary pulmonary nodule
SUV	standardised uptake value
SVCO	superior vena cava obstruction
TBNA	transbronchial needle aspiration
TLCO	diffusion capacity/transfer factor for CO
TWR	two-week rule
UK	United Kingdom
VATS	video-assisted thoracoscopic surgery
VEGF	vascular endothelial growth factor
WHO	World Health Organisation

Introduction

The majority (95%) of primary lung cancers are bronchogenic carcinomas which arise from the epithelial cells of the bronchial mucosa. These can be subdivided into non-small cell lung cancer (NSCLC), which arises from the epithelial and glandular cells, and small cell lung cancer (SCLC), which arises from the neuroendocrine cells. Adenocarcinoma in situ, previously known as bronchoalveolar cell carcinoma (5%), arises from the alveolar cells. Mesothelioma, a malignant tumour of the pleura, is discussed in Chapter 12. Metastases to the lungs from other primary tumours, such as breast, colon, prostate, kidneys, ovary, and thyroid can also occur. In this chapter we will discuss primary lung tumours.

Lung cancer is the commonest fatal malignancy for both men and women in the UK and the third commonest cause of death in the UK. Worldwide, it accounts for one million deaths each year. Lung cancer has a poor prognosis because many types are rapidly growing, aggressive, and have usually metastasized at the time of presentation. In addition, lung cancer often presents late because many of the symptoms, such as cough and breathlessness, are non-specific and common in smokers. There is no screening programme for lung cancer in the UK. Current studies are evaluating whether screening is feasible, cost-effective, and likely to reduce mortality.

Epidemiology of lung cancer

- **Incidence:** 40 000/year in UK.
- **Mortality:** 34 000 deaths/year in UK.
- **Male: Female ratio** is 1.5 : 1, largely reflecting previous smoking habits in men and women (Figure 9.1).
- The **prevalence of lung cancer in women** is still increasing as there is a 30-year lag between smoking and developing lung cancer (Figure 9.2). Lung cancer has overtaken breast cancer as the leading cause of cancer deaths in women.

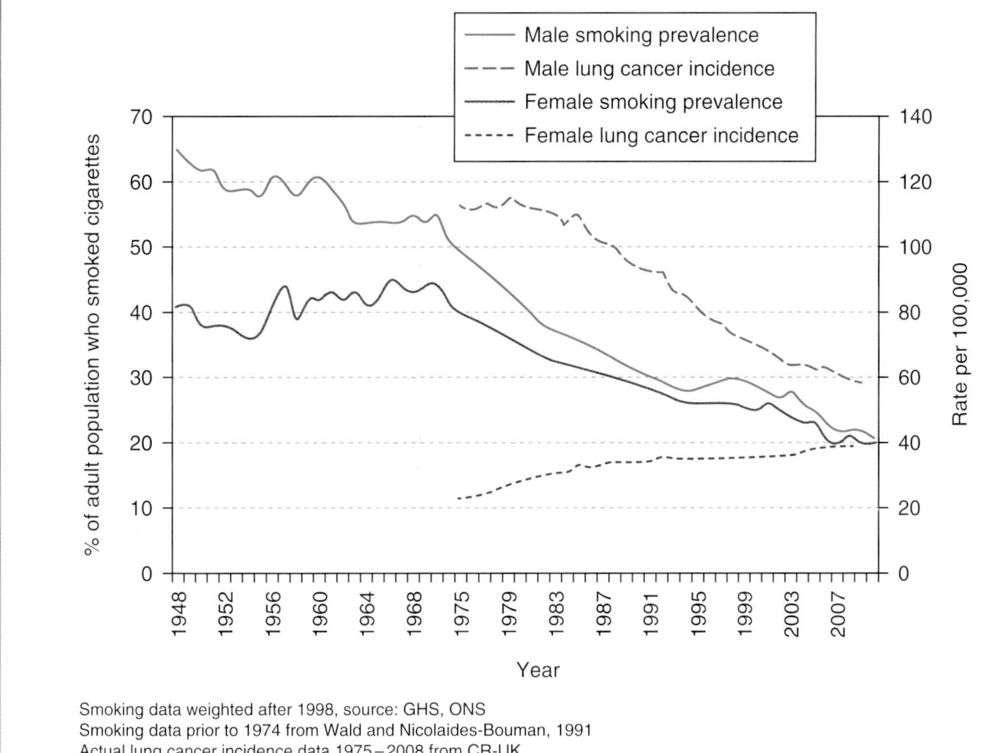

Figure 9.1 Lung cancer incidence and smoking trends for adults by sex, 1948–2010 in Great Britain, from Cancer Research UK.

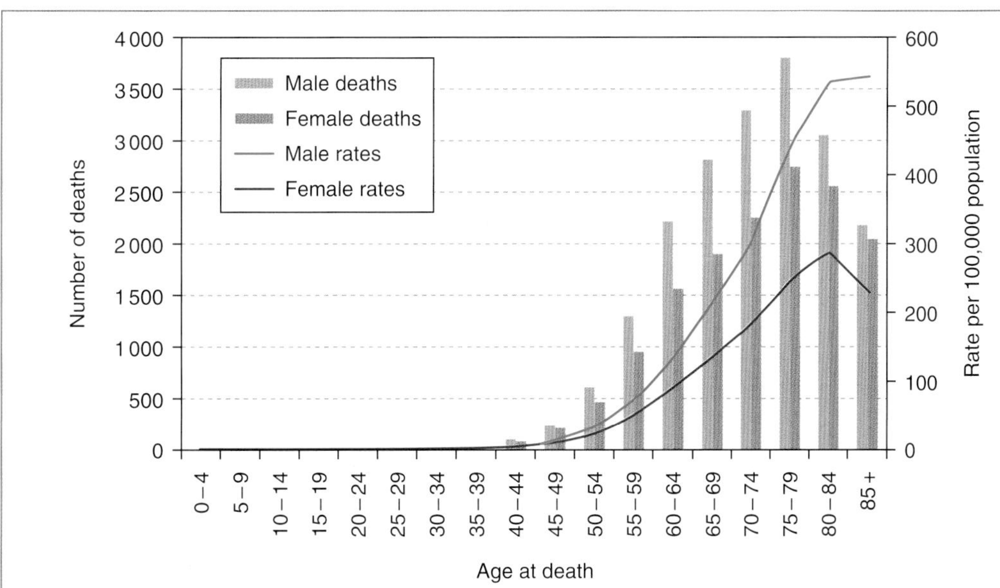

Figure 9.2 Number of deaths and age-specific mortality rates for lung cancer in UK, 2007, from Cancer Research UK.

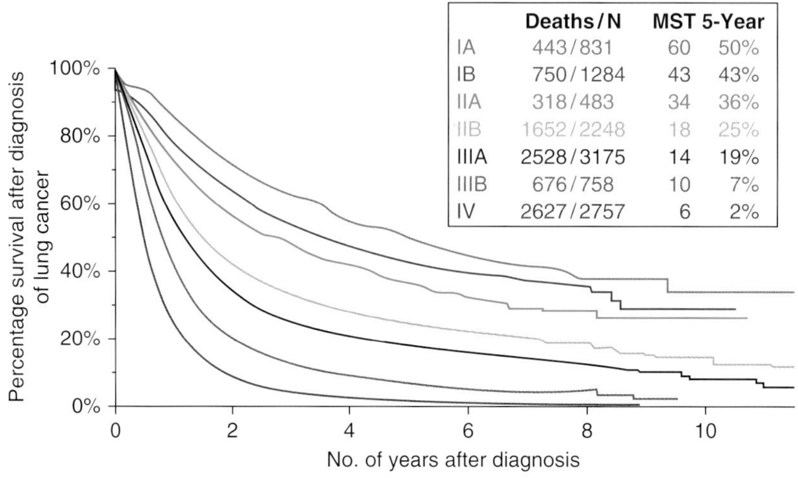

Figure 9.3 Survival in lung cancer according to stage at diagnosis. *Source:* from Staging at http://Cancer.org.

- There is a higher prevalence of lung cancer in the North of England and Scotland compared to the South of England reflecting the higher prevalence of smoking in those areas. Lung cancer is also commoner in the lower socio-economic groups: this may be due to smoking habits as well as poor nutrition.
- **Survival:** the overall 1-year survival for lung cancer is still only 30% in men and 35% in women with a 5-year survival of only 9.5% (Figure 9.3). There has been no convincing reduction in mortality despite some advances in diagnosis and treatment and the introduction of guidelines, pathways, and multidisciplinary working. This highlights the importance of prevention and early diagnosis.

Box 9.1 Aetiology of lung cancer.

- Cigarette smoking (active)
- Cigarette smoking (passive)
- Asbestos exposure
- Ionising radiation (radon gas): background radiation from the ground and rocks
- Polycyclic aromatic hydrocarbons
- Arsenic
- Genetic predisposition (family history): variation in ability to metabolise carcinogens
- Idiopathic pulmonary fibrosis
- Scar carcinoma: tumours can arise from areas of chronic fibrosis

Aetiology of lung cancer

Several factors are implicated in the development of lung cancer. These are listed in Box 9.1.

Some 90% of lung cancers are related to smoking, which is the main risk factor. Before smoking became popular in the twentieth century, lung cancer was rare. The probability of developing lung cancer correlates to the number and duration of cigarettes smoked, quantified as the number of pack years. The earlier the onset of smoking, the higher the risk of developing lung cancer, as there is a 30-year latent period.

A smoker of 20/day has 20× the risk of dying from lung cancer compared to a non-smoker. The risk of developing lung cancer is halved every 5 years after smoking cessation but remains higher than for a non-smoker. The prevalence of smoking is slowly reducing in the UK, with 17.7% of men smoking on average 12 cigarettes daily and 15.8% women smoking approximately 11 cigarettes every day. However, rates of smoking and lung cancer are increasing in China, India, and other developing countries.

In the past decade, evidence has accumulated that passive smoking, caused by exposure to the cigarette smoke from others, increases the risk of lung cancer 1.5 x. This evidence has resulted in a ban in smoking in public places in the UK. Children are particularly vulnerable to the effects of smoking, especially in places with little ventilation, such as cars. It is likely that there will be further legislation to protect children.

Chapter 15 discusses the carcinogenic properties of cigarette smoke and the seminal studies by Hill and Doll establishing the link between lung cancer and smoking. In Chapter 3 the NICE guidelines for smoking cessation are discussed.

Asbestos exposure is a risk factor for developing lung cancer. Asbestos exposure and smoking act synergistically and increase the risk of lung cancer 100 times compared to a non-smoker. There is a latent period of 30–40 years from asbestos exposure to developing lung cancer. Asbestos exposure is also a risk factor for mesothelioma, a malignant tumour of the pleura, which is discussed in Chapter 10.

Pathophysiology of lung cancer

Damage to the bronchial mucosa by carcinogens causes squamous metaplasia which can progress to dysplasia, often in many separate areas. Some dysplastic cells then progress to become malignant. Areas of dysplasia can be visualised at bronchoscopy using fluoroscopy, but this is still largely a research tool.

The cancer initially invades local tissues, spreading to the parenchyma, pleura, pericardium, oesophagus, ribs, and muscle. This can result in cough, pain, breathlessness, dysphagia and pleural and pericardial effusions. Invasion of local nerves can cause vocal cord palsy (left recurrent laryngeal nerve), raised hemidiaphragm (phrenic nerve), and brachial plexus symptoms. The tumour can also spread to lymph nodes via the lymphatics and metastases to distant sites occurs haematogenously.

Clinical presentation of lung cancer

Lung cancer is a common condition, so all healthcare professionals should be alert to the possibility that patients with risk factors for lung cancer or a family history of malignancy, and who present with certain symptoms, may have lung cancer. Lung cancer can present with local or systemic symptoms, some of which are non-specific. As most patients with lung cancer are smokers and likely to have chronic obstructive pulmonary disease (COPD), many of the symptoms, such as cough (which is the commonest symptom of lung cancer) and worsening breathlessness may be overlooked by the patient and the doctor (Box 9.2). A detailed clinical history and thorough examination should be conducted. Basic investigations, such as a chest X-ray, should be conducted without delay and the

Box 9.2 Symptoms of lung cancer.

Respiratory symptoms

- Cough, persistent and longer than 3 weeks' duration in 80% of cases
- Breathlessness, progressively worsening in 60% of cases
- Chest pain (from local invasion) in 50% of cases
- Haemoptysis in 30% of cases
- Monophonic wheeze
- Stridor
- Shoulder pain secondary to Pancoast's tumour with invasion of the brachial plexus: this can result in weakness of the small muscles of the hand
- Hoarse voice suggests vocal cord palsy secondary to recurrent laryngeal nerve involvement
- Raised hemidiaphragm secondary to phrenic nerve palsy
- Superior vena cava obstruction (SVCO) can occur in 20% and is commoner with SCLC.
- Cervical or supraclavicular lymphadenopathy

Systemic symptoms

- Weight loss
- Lethargy
- Pain suggestive of metastases to other organs, for example, bone pain
- Neurological symptoms secondary to brain metastases
- Spinal cord compression
- Paraneoplastic symptoms result from the secretion of hormones or cytokines by the tumour. Lambert-Eaton myasthenic syndrome is associated with SCLC and results from autoantibodies to the presynaptic membrane
- Peripheral neuropathy
- Dermatomyositis
- Thrombophlebitis migrans
- Cerebellar degeneration

patient referred to a specialist via the Two-Week Rule Pathway if there is any concern. Some 15% of lung cancers are found incidentally in patients who have had a chest X-ray (CXR) or computed tomography of the thorax (CT thorax) for other reasons, for example, during pre-assessment for surgery.

Clinical signs of lung cancer

Patients with early, asymptomatic lung cancer may not have any abnormal signs and clinical examination will be normal. Box 9.3 details some possible signs in patients with lung cancer.

Ectopic secretion of hormones in lung cancer

Small cell lung cancers, which originate from the Kutchinsky neuroendocrine cells of the amine uptake and decarboxylation (APUD) system, can secrete ectopic hormones, so patients with hyponatraemia or hypercalcaemia may have an underlying malignancy.

Ectopic secretion of anti-diuretic hormone (ADH) can occur in 15% of patients with SCLC

Box 9.3 Clinical signs of lung cancer.

- Cachexia
- Clubbing in 20% with NSCLC (Figure 9.4)
- Hypertrophic pulmonary osteopathy (HPOA) is commoner with adenocarcinoma and regresses with treatment of the primary cancer (Figure 9.5)
- Hoarse voice or bovine cough secondary to invasion of the left recurrent laryngeal nerve by tumour as it passes around the aortic arch to the superior mediastinum
- Tachypnoea
- Horner's syndrome (meiosis, ptosis, enophthalmos, and anhydrosis) from invasion of the lower cervical sympathetic ganglion (Figure 9.6)
- Cervical lymphadenopathy
- Tracheal deviation (secondary to upper lobe collapse)
- Superior vena cava obstruction (SVCO).
- Clinical signs of lobar collapse (Figure 9.8)
- Clinical signs of pleural effusion
- Pathological fracture of bone
- Unexplained pulmonary emboli
- Unexplained hyponatraemia
- Unexplained hypercalcaemia

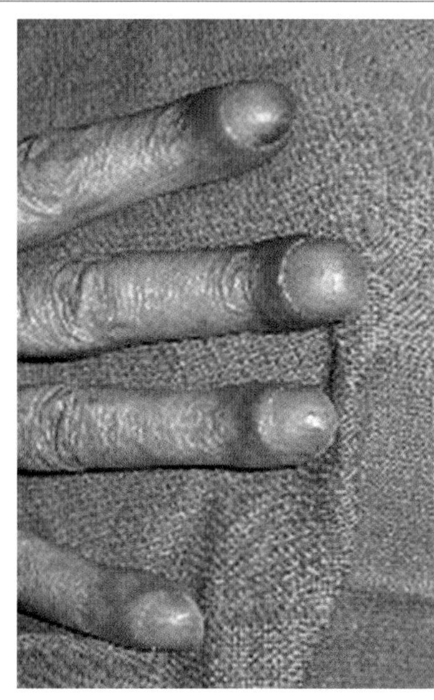

Figure 9.4 Photograph showing clubbing of finger nails. *Source: ABC of COPD*, 3rd Edition, Figure 3.3.

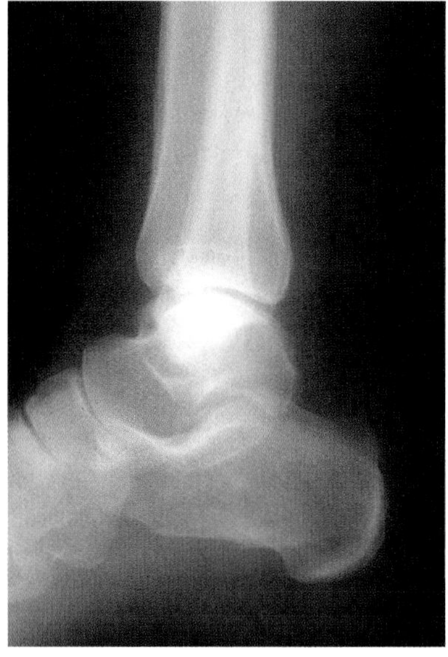

Figure 9.5 X ray showing hypertrophic pulmonary osteoarthropathy (HPOA).

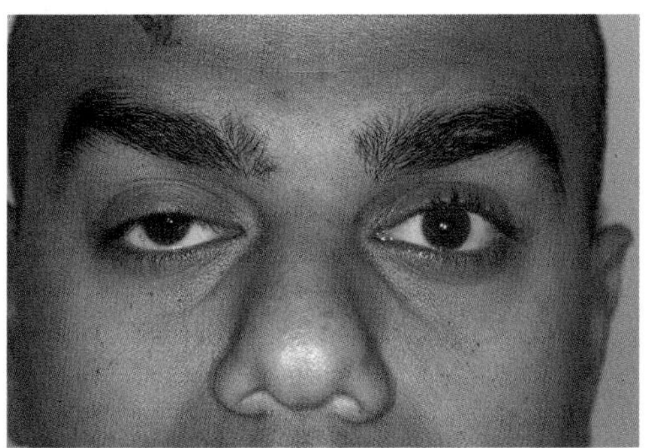

Figure 9.6 Photograph showing Horner's syndrome. *Source:* Medical Photography, Epsom and St. Helier NHS Trust.

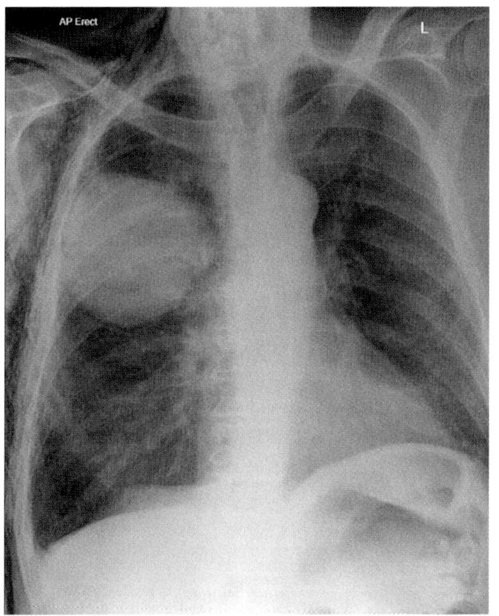

Figure 9.7 CXR showing a right-sided lung mass suspicious for lung cancer.

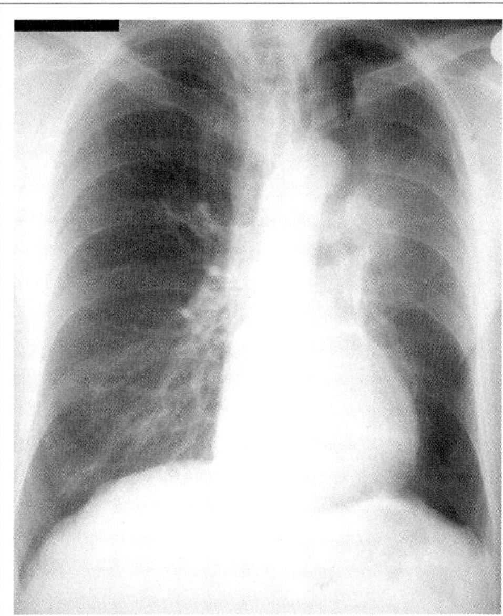

Figure 9.8 CXR showing lobar (left upper lobe) collapse.

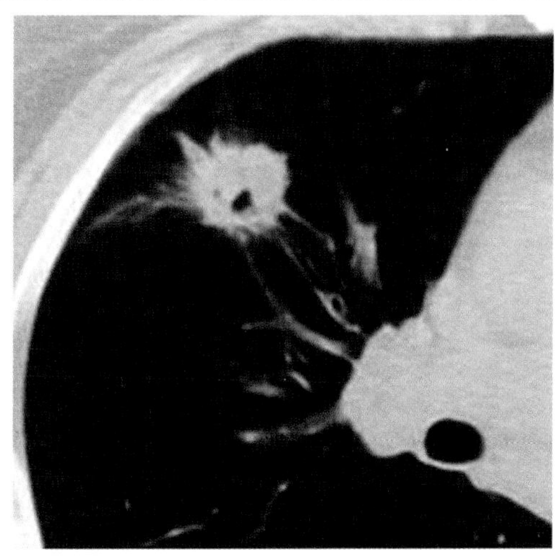

Figure 9.9 CXR showing a cavitating solitary pulmonary nodule.

resulting in hyponatraemia (serum sodium <139mmol/L). The patient can present with confusion and weakness. To make a diagnosis of syndrome of inappropriate ADH (SIADH) the serum osmolality must be <280 mosmol l^{-1} and the urine osmolality >500 mosmol l^{-1}. Hyponatraemia due to SIADH can be managed by fluid restriction (1–1.5 l). If this fails, then pharmacological agents, such as demeclocycline, a vasopressin inhibitor or tolvaptan, a selective V2 receptor antagonist can be used.

Hypercalcaemia (serum corrected calcium >2.8mmol/L) in lung cancer can be due to the secretion of parathyroid hormone-related (PTH-related) peptide by squamous cell carcinoma which binds to the PTH receptors and increases bone and tubular resorption and decreases bone formation. Hypercalcaemia can also occur when there are bone metastases. Hypercalcaemia secondary to malignancy responds well to intravenous fluids, intravenous diuretics, steroids (prednisolone or dexamathasone), and intravenous bisphosphonate, such as pamidronate.

Ectopic ACTH secretion is rare (2–5% with SCLC), but presents with raised cortisol and Cushing's syndrome.

Management of superior vena cava obstruction (SVCO)

Patients with SVCO present with headaches, distended, engorged, pulseless neck veins, collateral veins on the chest and arms, and facial oedema. The CXR may show a mass on the right side of the thorax and a widened mediastinum. The diagnosis can be confirmed with a contrast CT thorax which can identify the anatomical structures and collateral circulation. Invasive contrast venography and Doppler scanning may be helpful in assessing the extent of the obstruction. Severe SVCO can present as an emergency and must be discussed with the respiratory and radiology consultants. Management depends on the patient and the imaging, but includes commencing dexamethasone (up to 8 mg twice a day), after tissue biopsy if possible. Insertion of a metallic stent by an interventional radiologist can be considered in an emergency, and anticoagulation must be considered if there is thrombus present. Radiotherapy for NSCLC and chemotherapy for SCLC can reduce the obstruction but may take weeks to be effective.

Management of a patient suspected of having a lung malignancy

Lung cancer has a poor prognosis because patients often present late with evidence of local or distant metastases. This may be because neither the patient nor the doctor is alert to the common symptoms of lung cancer, which are often non-specific. Currently there is no screening programme to detect lung cancer early. Other factors resulting in low survival rates for lung cancer in the UK include poor surgical rates of only 15% compared to at least 20% in the USA and in Europe. Patients with lung cancer also have significant co-morbidities which often preclude radical treatment.

To improve early referral, diagnosis, and treatment, patients with symptoms or signs suggestive of lung cancer must be referred as a two-week rule (TWR) to the respiratory team. The patient must be seen by a consultant respiratory physician within 14 days of referral, have all investigations completed within 28 days of referral, be discussed at the lung cancer multidisciplinary team (MDT) meeting and have treatment within 62 days of the original referral. These timeframes are likely to reduce in the next few years.

Clinical assessment of patient with suspected lung cancer

Patients should have a detailed history and examination (see Box 9.2, Box 9.3). In addition, the World Health Organisation (WHO) performance status, oxygen saturation, and spirometry must be noted (Box 9.4).

Investigations for patients suspected of having lung cancer

Blood tests should include full blood count to exclude anaemia and infection, urea and electrolytes, liver function test, clotting, corrected calcium and plasma and urine osmolalities if there is hyponatraemia.

Radiological investigations includes a plain chest X-ray followed by a contrast staging CT scan of thorax and abdomen. Box 9.5 details chest X-ray changes that need to be investigated further. Rarely, with central tumours or with small tumours, the chest X-ray may appear normal. If the patient has unexplained symptoms or signs, which includes haemoptysis, a staging CT scan is indicated even if the chest X-ray appears normal.

A **staging CT scan of thorax and abdomen** with contrast will show the primary tumour, lymph node enlargement within the thorax, local lung metastases and distant metastases to liver, adrenal glands and bone (Figure 9.12).

A **CT-PET scan** is required for accurate staging and is essential if radical treatment is being considered. A CT-PET scan is done in a specialist centre

Box 9.4 WHO performance status.

1. able to carry out normal activity
2. symptomatic but ambulatory and able to carry out light work
3. in bed 50% of the day, unable to work but capable of self-care
4. in bed >50% of the day, limited self-care
5. bedridden, unable to self-care

Box 9.5 CXR appearances of concern.

- Mass (Figure 9.7)
- Lobar collapse (Figure 9.8)
- Solitary pulmonary nodule (SPN) (Figure 9.9)
- Lymphadenopathy
- Pleural effusion
- Unilateral raised hemidiaphragm (Figure 9.10)
- Persistent consolidation
- Lymphangitis carcinomatosis: there is infiltration of the pulmonary lymphatics by tumour (Figure 9.11). The appearances can resemble pulmonary oedema

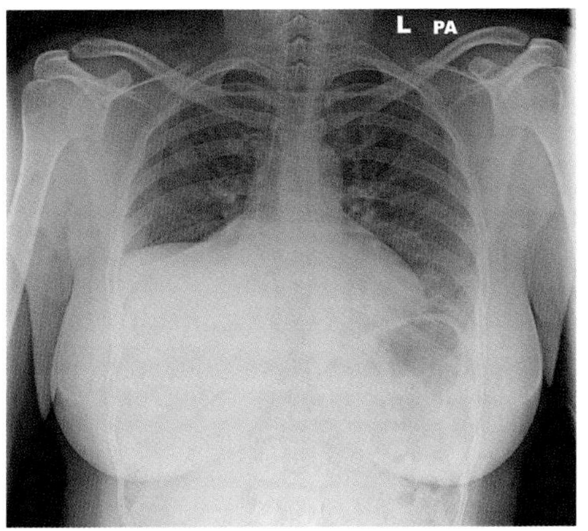

Figure 9.10 CXR showing elevation of the right hemidiaphragm.

and can 'up' or 'down' stage the CT staging. A CT-PET has a sensitivity of 95% and a specificity of 83% for lung cancer.

A CT-PET is poor at detecting slow-growing tumours, such as adenocarcinoma in situ and carcinoid tumours, and poor at detecting brain metastases. False positive CT-PET scans can also be found with infective and inflammatory processes. The standardised uptake value (SUV max) is used to calculate the FDG uptake (Figure 9.13). An SUV max <2.5 suggests a benign lesion (Figure 9.14).

A **bone scan** may be indicated if the patient has bone pain or hypercalcaemia to see if there are bony metastases, although this can also be detected with a CT-PET scan.

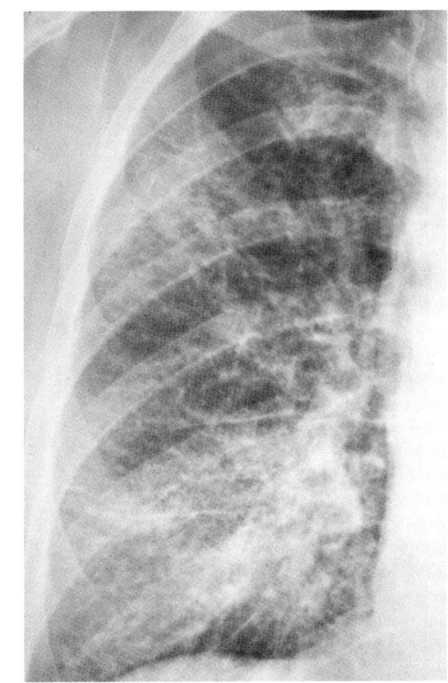

Figure 9.11 CXR showing lymphangitis carcinomatosis.

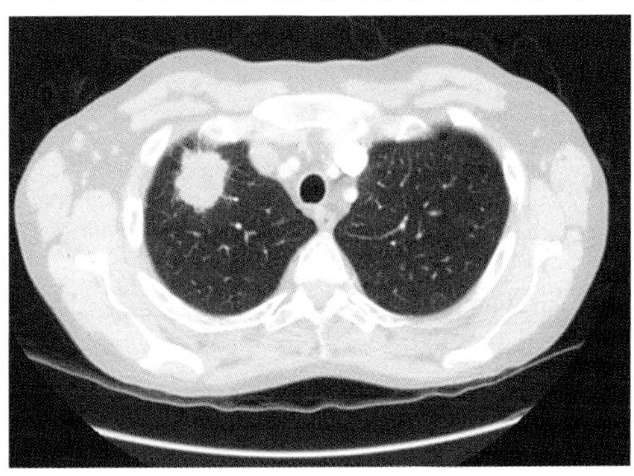

Figure 9.12 CT thorax showing a suspicious, spiculate mass in the right upper lobe.

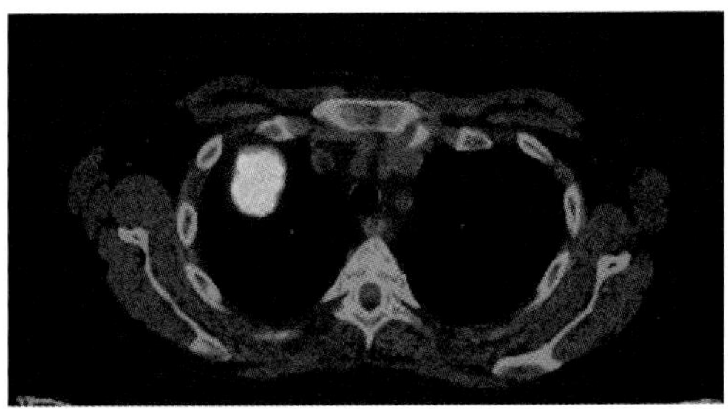

Figure 9.13 PET scan showing an FDG-avid lesion in the right upper lobe suspicious of lung cancer.

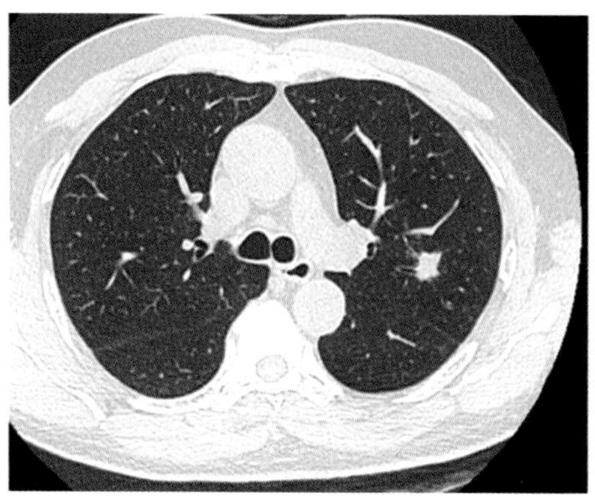
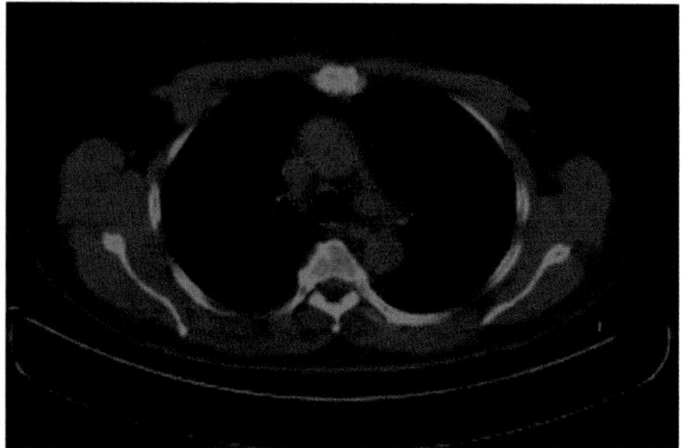

Figure 9.14 CT and PET scans showing a non-FDG-avid nodule in the left lung.

An **MRI scan of the thorax** can determine if the tumour involves the chest wall and may be required if resection of the chest wall is being considered. It is also useful for assessing the extent of the disease in superior sulcus tumours. An urgent MRI scan is indicated for spinal cord compression. An MRI brain may be required if there is indication of an operable brain metastasis.

A **CT brain scan** is required if the patient has neurological symptoms or signs suggestive of brain metastases. It is also done routinely in patients who are being considered for radical treatment.

Histological diagnosis

The NICE guidelines (2011) stipulate that histological diagnosis should be obtained in at least 85% of patients presenting with lung cancer. However, an invasive procedure carries a risk of morbidity and even mortality. The patient must be fully informed of the potential risks and benefits of any invasive procedures and must be prepared to accept these risks.

The investigation that gives the most information about the diagnosis and staging with the least risk to the patient should be chosen. For example, if there are enlarged lymph nodes of more than 10 mm maximum short axis on CT, then these should be sampled by endobronchial ultrasound (EBUS)-guided biopsy or transbronchial needle aspiration (TBNA). Neck ultrasound and sampling of visible lymph nodes is also advised. Several samples may need to be taken to get sufficient tissue to identify the mutational status of the tumour which can guide treatment. While it is important to take adequate samples, the patient should not be put at any risk. Histology obtained from a biopsy is preferred to cells obtained from brushings and washing alone, although often, as the case with a pleural effusion, a cytological diagnosis may be sufficient.

Sputum cytology can be helpful in 40% of cases and more likely to be diagnostic with central tumours. This may be the only way to get cytological confirmation if the patient is too unfit for an invasive procedure such as a bronchoscopy.

A flexible fibre-optic bronchoscopy is often the first investigation used to obtain tissue if the tumour is endobronchial and central. The tumour can be directly visualised and the distance of the tumour from the carina and the extent of obstruction of the bronchus can be noted. Bronchoscopy can also identify vocal cord palsy.

Biopsies, brushings and washings (bronchoalveolar lavage) can be taken directly from the tumour site through the bronchoscope for histological diagnosis. Sometimes, although no definite endobronchial lesions are seen, mucosal abnormalities may be visible which can be biopsied. The centre of a large tumour mass is often necrotic, so samples may not be diagnostic, even when large pieces of tissue are obtained. Other limitations to obtaining an adequate sample include poor patient tolerance of the procedure and vascular tumours that bleed easily. A rigid bronchoscopy, which is done under general anaesthetic, gives the operator more control, and may increase the diagnostic yield with difficult cases and when the tumour is near the carina.

If the tumour is peripheral, then a CT-guided fine needle aspiration (FNA) conducted by the radiologist is diagnostic in 90–95% of cases when the lesion is >2 cm. It is not possible to undertake an FNA on a

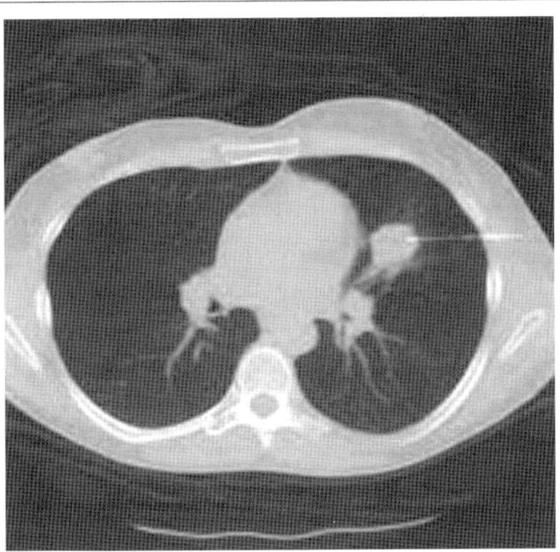

Figure 9.15 CT-guided FNA of lung mass showing needle in the lung mass.

lesion <1 cm (Figure 9.15). Patients referred for this must have reasonable spirometry, normal oxygen saturation, be able to hold their breath and able to lie down flat. CT-guided FNA is usually contraindicated in patients with an FEV_1 of less than 1 L and with severe emphysematous lung disease on CT scan as their risk of pneumothorax is high and they will not be able to safely tolerate it. The overall pneumothorax risk of a CT-guided FNA is 20%.

The other risk of lung biopsy is bleeding, with 8% experiencing haemoptysis post-procedure. If the patient is on an anticoagulant, then this must be stopped several days prior to the procedure and clotting checked. The patient may need to be treated with low molecular weight heparin in the interim if necessary. Patients on aspirin should be informed not to take aspirin on the day of the procedure.

Sampling of enlarged, PET positive lymph nodes will ensure accurate staging which can determine whether the patient should receive radical or palliative treatment. Transbronchial needle aspiration (TBNA), endobronchial ultrasound (EBUS), and endoscopic ultrasound (EUS) can be used to biopsy paratracheal and peribronchial nodes. A mediastinoscopy can be done under general anaesthetic by a thoracic surgeon to sample mediastinal lymph nodes.

Cytology obtained by pleural aspiration of a pleural effusion can be diagnostic of lung cancer, but histology is preferable as tissue is required for molecular testing. A video-assisted thoracoscopic (VATS) pleural biopsy done under general anaesthetic can be diagnostic when there is pleural involvement. Histological diagnosis of lung cancer can also be made by taking a biopsy from an extra-thoracic site, such as a cervical or supraclavicular lymph node, the liver, adrenal, skin or bone (Figure 9.16). This may be necessary when CT-guided FNA of the primary lung lesion is not possible.

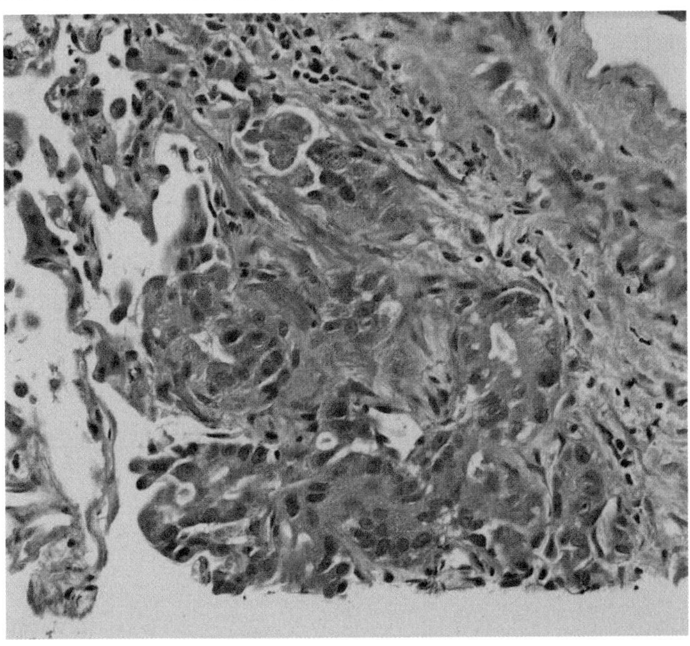

Figure 9.16 Histology of adenocarcinoma from a CT-guided biopsy of lung mass.

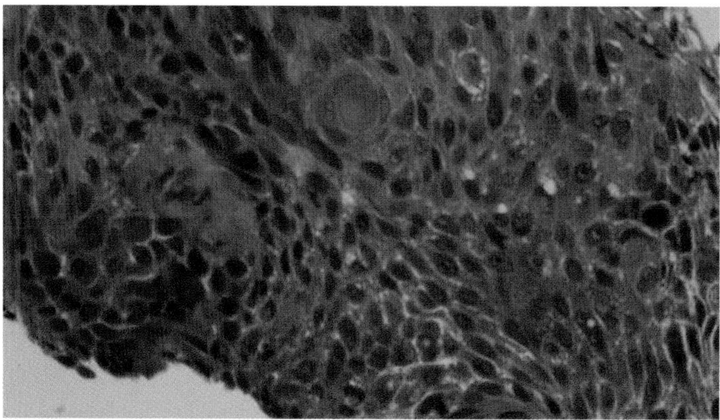

Figure 9.17 Histology of squamous cell carcinoma from a CT-guided biopsy of lung mass.

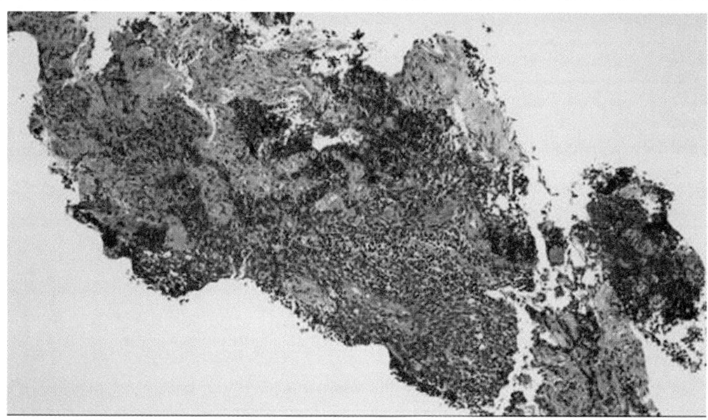

Figure 9.18 Histology of small cell carcinoma from an endobronchial biopsy.

While every attempt should be made to obtain a histological diagnosis, this is often limited by the patient's poor performance status (WHO performance status 3 or 4) and co-morbidities (Figure 9.17, Figure 9.18). The decision not to pursue a histological diagnosis should be made at the lung cancer MDT after discussion with the patient and family. Pursuing a histological diagnosis may not be recommended in frail patients with a poor performance status, and in patients with extensive disease who are only suitable for palliation. Some patients may choose not to pursue further investigations for a variety of reasons and their wishes must be respected, so long as all the information has been given in a clear way. Good and empathetic communication is essential when dealing with patients with lung cancer.

Other investigations required in a patient with suspected lung cancer includes spirometry to assess the patient's fitness for a procedure, such as a CT-guided biopsy. If this suggests an airways obstruction, then the patient should be given optimal treatment to improve symptoms. A full lung function with transfer factor is required when planning radical treatment, such as surgery or radiotherapy. An ECG and echocardiogram may be necessary prior to radical treatment if the patient has a cardiac history.

Classification of lung cancer

Non-small cell lung cancer (NSCLC) accounts for 80% of lung cancers. Small cell lung cancer (SCLC), previously called oat-cell cancer, is more aggressive and accounts for 20% of lung cancers.

Histological diagnosis is made from the morphological characteristics of the cells and the immunophenotyping. The biopsy is first processed and assessed by routine haematoxylin and eosin (H + E) stained sections. In most cases, a reliable diagnosis of NSCLC or SCLC can be made, although when the tumour is very poorly differentiated, this can be difficult. With advances in chemotherapy and immunotherapy, it is no longer acceptable to classify tumours simply as NSCLC.

Immunocytochemistry is required to classify NSCLC as squamous cell carcinoma or adenocarcinoma. Immunocytochemistry is a technique in which antigens in the tumour cells are bound to antibodies with attached chemical markers that allow them to be visualised in tissue sections. Many antibodies are available and their affinity to the different tumour markers has often been found empirically. The sensitivity and specificity are therefore variable, and it is normal to use a panel of antibodies. It can be difficult to differentiate between a primary lung adenocarcinoma and metastases from prostate, breast, and colon. Other markers may be helpful in differentiating between lung and metastases from other organs. By using these methods, over 90% of tumours can be classified accurately.

Tissue should be conserved for molecular mutation testing, such as for Epidermal Growth Factor Receptor (EGFR,) programmed death ligand 1 and its receptor (PD-L1), and anaplastic lymphoma kinase (ALK). NICE guidelines recommend that the majority of NSCLC should have testing for EGFR. EGFR inhibitors are discussed later in this chapter.

There has been a change in the type of lung cancer over the last decade, with a decrease in squamous cell carcinoma and an increase in adenocarcinoma. This may be due to an increase in the low-yield brands of cigarettes with filters which result in more peripheral deposition of carcinogens.

Staging of NSCLC

The TNM classification is used to stage NSCLC (Tables 9.1 and 9.2). The TNM classification was revised by the International Staging Committee of the International Association for the study of Lung Cancer. Data was collected on 68 463 patients with NSCLC and 13 032 patients with SCLC between 1990 and 2000. The modifications were recommended because of differences in survival and prognosis. Although it is not used in routine practice, staging that includes size of tumour, the histological type, late recurrence risk, and the age of the patient is more accurate. Accurate staging guides management and enables a more accurate prognosis to be made. Table 9.3 details the overall survival of patients with NSCLC according to the stage of the disease.

Staging of SCLC

The majority of SCLC present with evidence of metastases. If the disease is confined to the thorax, then it is staged as "limited", and if there is evidence of spreading outside the thorax, then it is staged as "extensive".

Management of lung cancer

Treatment decisions are made by the lung cancer multidisciplinary team (MDT) after consideration of the histological cell type (including immunocytochemistry), radiological stage, performance status of patient, lung function, co-morbidities, and the wishes of the patient.

The key decision is whether the patient is suitable for radical, potentially curative treatment: surgery or radiotherapy. This can be followed by adjuvant treatment, either chemotherapy, radiotherapy, or both.

If the cancer is too advanced for radical treatment or the patient is unfit for radical treatment, then palliative options, which include chemotherapy and radiotherapy, can be considered. Palliation also includes procedures such as insertion of an endobronchial stent and draining of a pleural effusion with pleurodesis to relieve breathlessness. When patients have advanced disease and a poor performance status, then symptom control may be the best option. In the next section the various treatment options are discussed.

Surgery

The aim of surgery in lung cancer is to remove the tumour completely and it offers the only real chance of a cure. The latest figures from the National Lung Cancer Audit show that only 15% of patients with lung cancer in the UK have surgical resection. Although this is an improvement from previous years, it is poor compared to figures in Europe and USA, where over 20% of patients had surgical resection.

This low resection rate may be because patients with lung cancer present late with locally advanced or widely disseminated disease. However, there is evidence that not every patient who is suitable for surgery is referred for a surgical opinion.

Table 9.1 Eighth edition of TNM classification of NSCLC.
T = Size of tumour in CM.
TX: primary tumour cannot be assessed, or tumour cells in sputum or bronchial cells, but not visualised at bronchoscopy.
T0: No evidence of primary tumour.
Tis: Carcinoma in situ.
T1: Tumour ≤3 cm in greater dimension, surrounded by lung or visceral pleura, without bronchoscopic evidence of invasion more proximal than the lobar bronchus (not in main bronchus).
T1mi: minimally invasive adenocarcinoma.
T1a: tumour ≤1 cm or less in greatest dimension.
T1b: tumour >1 cm and <2 cm in greatest dimension.
T1c: tumour >2 cm but <3 cm in greatest dimension.
T2: tumour >3 cm but <5 cm or with any of the following features: involves main bronchus regardless of distance to the carina, but not involving the carina, invades visceral pleura, associated with atelectasis or obstructive pneumonia that extends to the hilar region either involving part or the entire lung.
T2a: tumour >3 cm but <4 cm in greatest dimension.
T2b: tumour >4 cm but <5 cm in greatest dimension.
T3: tumour >5 cm but <7 cm in greatest dimension or one that directly invades any of the following: parietal pleura, chest wall (including superior sulcus tumours), phrenic nerve, parietal pericardium: or separate tumour nodule (s) in the same lobe as the primary.
T4: tumour >7 cm or of any size that invades any of the following: diaphragm, mediastinum, heart, great vessels, trachea, recurrent laryngeal nerve, oesophagus, vertebral body, carina; separate tumour nodule(s) in a different ipsilateral lobe to that of the primary.
N = regional lymph node involvement
NX: Regional lymph nodes cannot be assessed.
N0: No regional evidence of metastasis.
N1: Metastasis in ipsilateral peribronchial and/or ipsilateral hilar lymph nodes and intrapulmonary nodes, including involvement by direct extension.
N2: Metastasis in ipsilateral mediastinal and/or subcarinal lymph node(s).
N3: Metastasis in contralateral mediastinal, contralateral hilar, ipsilateral, or contralateral scalene, or supraclavicular lymph node(s).
M = distant metastasis
M0: No evidence of distant metastasis.
M1: Distant metastasis.
M1a: Separate tumour nodule(s) in a contralateral lobe; tumour with pleural or pericardial nodules or malignant pleural or pericardial effusion.
M1b: Single extrathoracic metastasis in a single organ.
M1c: Multiple extrathoracic metastases in a single, or multiple organs.

Table 9.2 Staging using the TNM classification for NSCLC eighth edition.

Stage	T	N	M
Occult	Tx	N0	M0
0	Tis	N0	M0
IA	T1	N0	M0
IA1	T1mi T1a	N0 N0	M0 M0
IA2	T1b	N0	M0
IA3	T1c	N0	M0
IB	T2a	N0	M0
IIA	T2b	N0	M0
IIB	T1a-c, T2a, b IIIA T3	N1 N0	M0 M0
IIB	T1a-c, T2a, b T3, T4	N3 N2	M0 M0
IIIC	T3, T4	N3	M0
IV	Any T	Any N	M1
IVA	Any T	Any N	M1a, M1b
IVB	Any T	Any N	M1c

Table 9.3 Overall 5-year survival for NSCLC.

Stage	5-year survival rate (%)
IA	49
IB	45
IIA	30
IIB	31
IIIA	14
IIIB	5
IV	1

Source: http://www.cancer.org/cancer.

Of those undergoing resection, only 30% will be alive in 5 years. The prognosis depends on the final pathological stage of the cancer.

Surgery with curative intent should be considered in patients who are medically fit (WHO performance status 0 or 1), who have a reasonable lung function, and who have no significant co-morbidities. This includes NSCLC Stages Ia to Stage IIIa (up to T3N1M0).

Surgery includes the removal of a lobe (lobectomy) or the entire lung (pneumonectomy). A pneumonectomy would be indicated if hilar nodes are found to be involved. The aim is to ensure that the resection margins are macroscopically free of tumour. The local lymph nodes are removed at surgery for pathological staging.

If the patient's lung function and performance status are poor, then a wedge resection or segmentectomy can be considered for peripheral tumours. The tumour, with a small amount of surrounding lung tissue, is removed. Where appropriate, bronchoangioplastic or sleeve resections may sometimes be possible to preserve the lung function. The mortality for this procedure is 1–3.5% and the tumour recurrence rate is about 23%.

Those who have had a lobectomy have better survival rates than segmentectomy for tumours >3 cm. Local recurrence after lobectomy is less compared to segmentectomy regardless of the size of the tumour. A Cochrane meta-analysis of 11 RCTs showed that 4-year survival was increased in patients with Stage I, II and IIIA NSCLC who underwent lobectomy and complete mediastinal lymph node dissection compared to those who had complete resection and lymph node sampling. There were differences in operative mortality between the groups, with more complications in the lymph node dissection group.

Surgery is occasionally considered for selected patients with Stage IIIA NSCLC (T4N0M0, T4N1M0, T1-3N2M0) as part of radical multimodality management with neoadjuvant chemotherapy and/or radiotherapy which may reduce the tumour size. Restaging may confirm operability. Stage IIIB NSCLC and Stage IV NSCLC are considered inoperable.

Neurosurgical resection can be considered for a solitary brain metastasis. The staging described in the section refers to the TNM classification version 7.

Essential investigations prior to surgery

A staging CT scan with contrast of the thorax and upper abdomen, which is an essential investigation for all patients with lung cancer, will demonstrate tumour anatomy, location, and size, with an accurate measurement of the T-stage. CT also demonstrates abnormal enlargement of loco-regional lymph nodes based on the size in the short axis and gives information about other diseases, such as emphysema. A PET-CT will clarify lymph node involvement and detect occult metastases and is essential prior to surgery.

Fitness for surgery

The average mortality risk for lobectomy in the UK is 2–3%. In assessing fitness for surgery, the operative mortality, the risk of peri-operative myocardial events and the risk of post-operative dyspnoea should be considered. Patients should also be counselled regarding commonly occurring complications associated with lung resection.

Although **age** is not an absolute contraindication, patients aged over 80 do have an increased morbidity and mortality. Patients over 80 who have a lobectomy have a 7% mortality compared to 2–3% in younger patients. Those over 80 undergoing a pneumonectomy have a 14% mortality compared to 5–6% in younger patients. Despite this, the increased resection rates seen in recent years have been most marked in the older age group, probably reflecting a longer life expectancy.

Lung function is used in the pre-operative assessment to estimate the risk of operative mortality and the impact of lung resection on quality of life, especially in relation to post-resection dyspnoea. Although often regarded as being very important in assessing patients for surgery, forced expiratory volume in 1 second (FEV_1) has not been shown to be an independent predictive factor for perioperative death and best serves as a useful predictor of postoperative dyspnoea. Diffusion capacity (TLCO) is an important predictor of post-operative morbidity and should be performed in all patients regardless of spirometric values. A TLCO of greater than 40% predicted is required for surgery to be considered.

Although values of $FEV_1 > 1.5$ L for a lobectomy and $FEV_1 > 2$ L for a pneumonectomy were previously used in recommending surgery, surgical resection should still be offered to patients at moderate to high risk of post-operative dyspnoea and associated complications if it is felt that this is the better treatment option and the patient is willing to accept the higher risk.

Several other investigations can be useful for assessing the fitness of patients with moderate to high risk of post-operative dyspnoea and borderline lung function: ventilation and perfusion scintigraphy (VQ scan), quantitative CT or MRI, cardiopulmonary exercise testing and shuttle walk testing.

Patients should be informed that smoking increases the risk of pulmonary complications. They should be strongly advised to stop smoking, prescribed medication to aid smoking cessation, and referred to a smoking cessation clinic. Smoking cessation is discussed in Chapter 3.

Patients with **co-morbidities** will require appropriate investigations prior to referral for surgery. Cardiac problems are common, so patients may require an ECG, echocardiogram, and a cardiac opinion. Surgery should be avoided within 30 days of a myocardial infarction. Patients with coronary artery disease should have their medical treatment and secondary prophylaxis optimised as soon as possible.

It is essential to rule out metastases prior to referral for surgery. Although a CT-PET scan can detect most metastases, it is not good at detecting brain metastases, so a CT brain should be done.

Post-operative complications

Complications of lung resection can be divided into three categories. Pulmonary complications include atelectasis, pneumonia, empyema, prolonged air leak, basal collapse, hypoxaemia, and respiratory failure. Post-operative air leaks often occur from a breach in the visceral pleura, so drains are placed at the time of surgery to deal with this. In most cases, prolonged drainage is sufficient and rarely is re-operation necessary to seal the leak. Bronchopleural fistula is a serious complication after pneumonectomy, with a high morbidity and mortality. The bronchial stump dehisces, and the pneumonectomy space inevitably becomes infected. Early mobilisation and physiotherapy are vital to reduce some of these complications. Cardiovascular complications include arrhythmia and myocardial infarction. Other common complications include bleeding, wound infection, and chronic chest wall pain.

Table 9.4 Differences in 5-year survival rates with CT staging and pathological staging.

CT staging	5 year survival (%)	Pathological staging	5 year survival (%)
CNO without surgery CNO with surgery	42 50	pNO	56
CN1 without surgery CN1 with surgery	29 39	pN1	38
CN2 without surgery CN2 with surgery	18 31	pN2	22
CN3 without surgery CN3 with surgery	7 21	pN3	6
M1a (nodules in another ipsilateral lobe)	16		
M1a (pleural metastases)	6		
M1b (contralateral lung nodule	3		
M1b (distant metastases)	1		

Follow-up post-surgery

All patients who have had surgery for lung cancer should be discussed at the Lung MDT with the full surgical and pathological report where decisions regarding the need for adjuvant chemotherapy or radiotherapy can be made. Patients who have had surgery for lung cancer require careful and regular follow-up for 5 years, with regular CXR and CT thorax at 12 months. The patient should be advised to report any symptoms of concern.

If the resection margins are not clear or nodal disease is found at surgery, then radiotherapy can reduce the chance of local recurrence, although it does not improve survival. There is no evidence that patients with Stage IA NSCL who have clear resection margins benefit from adjuvant chemotherapy or radiotherapy, although a significant number will eventually develop local or distant metastases. For Stage IB disease, chemotherapy may offer survival benefits if the tumour is >4 cm. Chemotherapy may be effective in patients with Stage II and Stage IIIA NSCLC after surgery.

Post-operative radiation therapy (PORT) does not improve the outcome of patients with completely resected Stage I NSCLC.

Table 9.5 5-year survival after surgery for NSCLC.

Stage IA (T1N0M0): 70%
Stage IB (T2N0M0): 40%
Stage II (T1-2N1M0): 25%

Table 9.4 compares the differences in 5-year survival rates with CT and pathological staging. Table 9.5 describes the 5-year survival after surgery for NSCLC.

Radiotherapy

Radical radiotherapy

Radical radiotherapy with curative intent can be given either alone or as part of a multi-modal treatment approach with chemotherapy and/or surgery. Radical radiotherapy can be considered for patients with early stage NSCLC (Stages I, II, IIIA) who are not suitable for surgery due to co-morbidities or those who decline surgery. Squamous cell carcinomas are more radiosensitive than adenocarcinomas. One-year survival after radical radiotherapy is 60% for Stage IA and 32% for Stage IB NSCLC.

A sub-group of patients with small peripheral tumours are suitable for complex highly focused stereotactic ablative radiotherapy (SABR) which is associated with excellent local disease control. Radical radiotherapy is also the mainstay of treatment for patients with locally advanced inoperable disease, either as single modality treatment or combined with chemotherapy. This can be given either concomitantly or sequentially and is associated with improved outcomes. Patients need to have a good WHO performance status of 0–1 and have FEV_1, FVC and TLCO>40% predicted. Stereotactic treatment could be considered in patients with worse lung function.

Modern radiotherapy planning and delivery techniques ensure adequate doses are delivered to the tumour with limited damage to the surrounding normal tissues. Standard radical fractionation schedules comprise of 60–66 Gy given in 30–34 daily fractions over 6–7 weeks. There is evidence to suggest that accelerating the course of treatment and completing it over a shorter time is associated with improved outcomes. This can be done either by increasing the number of fractions given per day (hyper-fractionation), for example, using the continuous hyper-fractionated accelerated radiotherapy (CHART) schedule, or by increasing the dose given per fraction (hypo-fractionation), for example, 55 Gy given in 20 daily fractions over 4 weeks.

Side effects of thoracic radiotherapy include breathlessness, cough, tiredness, nausea, skin reaction, and dysphagia. Post-radiation pulmonary fibrosis can also occur, causing breathlessness.

Palliative radiotherapy

Palliative radiotherapy can improve symptoms of pain and haemoptysis in patients with lung cancer. It can also be effective in treating bone and brain metastases. Radiotherapy can also relieve breathlessness secondary to lobar collapse caused by tumour obstruction.

Radiotherapy may be indicated as emergency treatment in patients with spinal cord compression who are not suitable for neurosurgical intervention. It can be considered for mediastinal compressive symptoms, such as SVCO, stridor, and dysphagia. Palliative radiotherapy schedules include 36 Gy in 12 daily fractions, 20 Gy in 5 daily fractions and single fractions of 8–10 Gy, depending on treatment intent and the patient's performance status. Endobronchial brachytherapy may also be considered for local disease control.

Chemotherapy

Chemotherapy forms part of the potential treatment modality for most patients diagnosed with lung cancer. It is rarely curative but is the only option for most patients with SCLC and in many patients with NSCLC. Most lung cancers are disseminated at presentation and chemotherapy offers systemic treatment. It can also be given as adjuvant treatment to increase survival after surgery. It is often given in combination with radiotherapy to increase treatment response and survival. Neo-adjuvant chemotherapy can be given to downstage a tumour in the hope that this will make it radically treatable. There is usually a good initial response to chemotherapy with a reduction in tumour size and an improvement in symptoms in 70% of patients. Patients who are unfit for radical treatment may benefit from palliative chemotherapy.

Assessing fitness for chemotherapy

The toxicity of chemotherapy needs to be considered when offering patients systemic treatment. Underlying coronary artery disease, renal impairment, tinnitus, and peripheral neuropathy are particularly relevant. The functional status of the patient should be assessed using either the WHO performance status or the Karnofsky scoring system. The potential benefits and side effects of treatment should be discussed with the patient.

Chemotherapy for NSCLC

NICE guidelines (2011) recommend that chemotherapy is considered for patients with Stage III and IV NSCLC with a performance status of 0 or 1. Treatment can prolong life by two months and increase one-year survival from 5% to 25%. There are many clinical trials recruiting patients who should be offered the chance to participate.

Combinations of drugs are given at intervals of four weeks, up to six cycles of treatment, with careful monitoring of clinical and radiological response. Third-generation drugs, which include docetaxel, gemcitabine, paclitaxel, vinorelbine, and pemetrexed are given together with platinum drugs, carboplatin, or cisplatin. It is not within the scope of this book to discuss the details of chemotherapy drugs.

Adjuvant chemotherapy can be given after radical treatment, either radiotherapy or surgery. It is given after surgery for Stage IB disease when the tumour is >4 cm and for Stage II and Stage III lung cancer. A platinum-agent or a third-generation drug except pemetrexed can be given.

Neo-adjuvant chemotherapy should be considered is patients who are not radically treatable. Chemotherapy could downstage the tumour, making it suitable either for radical radiotherapy or surgery.

Chemotherapy for SCLC

NICE guidelines recommend that patients with SCLC should be seen by a medical oncologist within a week of diagnosis. Surgery should be considered for patients with early-stage SCLC (T1-2aN0M0) with a good WHO performance status of 0 or 1. Patients with SCLC undergoing surgery will require adjuvant chemotherapy. Radiotherapy may also be an option for early stage SCLC.

Chemotherapy can improve survival from 3 months to 12 months in limited SCLC and from 6 weeks to 12 weeks in extensive SCLC. Drugs used to treat SCLC include Topisomerase 1 poison (Topotecan), Topisomerase 11 poison (Etoposide) and the platinum drugs, carboplatin and cisplatin.

Palliative chemotherapy

A combination of a third-generation drug and a platinum drug is given if the patient can tolerate it without toxicity and the renal function is reasonable. Combinations of drugs given at intervals of 3 weeks, up to a maximum of six cycles, can improve symptoms.

Side effects of chemotherapy

The side effects of chemotherapy include systemic symptoms, such as nausea, vomiting, and diarrhoea which can be managed with antiemetics and fluids. Bone marrow suppression a few days after chemotherapy can result in anaemia, neutropenia, and thrombocytopaenia. Neutropenic sepsis is a real concern and must be considered in all patients who present feeling unwell. Neutropenic sepsis should be managed according to the NICE guidelines. It includes careful clinical assessment, septic screen (blood culture, urine culture, and chest X-ray), barrier nursing, and immediate intravenous antibiotics, usually tazocin and gentamicin.

> **Box 9.6 Radiological assessment of treatment response.**
>
> - **Disease progression:** the development of new lesions or an increase in tumour measurement by at least 20%
> - **Partial response:** at least a 30% decrease in tumour measurements
> - **Stable disease:** up to a 19% increase or 29% decrease in tumour measurements
> - **Complete response:** resolution of all previously visible tumour and tumour markers

Treatment response

Response to treatment is assessed according to an improvement in symptoms and radiological improvement. Radiological treatment response is classified as defined in Box 9.6.

Targeted molecular therapy

Cancer cells have been found to have an over-expression of certain receptors. The ability to target specific proteins has been a major development in the treatment of patients with incurable lung cancer. Inhibitors which target several receptors have been developed, tested in trials, and have a licence for use in patients.

Epithelial growth factor receptor (EGFR) has been found to be over-expressed in non-smokers with adenocarcinoma, particularly women. EGFR inhibitors, such as Geftinib (Iressa) and Erlotinib (Tarceva), are particularly active in patients whose tumours contain an EGFR-activating mutation. Erlotinib has also demonstrated efficacy in patients who have relapsed after first line chemotherapy.

Bevacizumab is a monoclonal antibody that binds vascular endothelial growth factor (VEGF) and can be used in combination with chemotherapy. Crizotinib targets a constitutively active kinase formed by a chromosomal rearrangement between the EMLA (echinoderm microtubule-associated protein-like 4) and anaplastic lymphoma kinase (ALK) genes. Expression of programmed death ligand 1 protein on the surface of cancer cells increases the responsiveness to immunotherapy. Immunotherapies that target the programmed death ligand 1 (PD-L1) and its receptor (PD-L1R) have been shown to increase survival in a subgroup of patients with advanced NSCLC.

The systemic treatment of lung cancer is rapidly changing. There are new and exciting developments in immunotherapy. It is beyond the scope of this book to discuss these in detail.

Palliative treatment

Palliative treatment, which focuses on the relief of symptoms, is the only option for most patients with SCLC and many with NSCLC. Patients should be referred to the palliative care team of doctors and nurses who specialise in symptom control. Patients can be seen in the hospital, in the hospice, or in the community. Symptoms that can be managed effectively include pain, breathlessness, nausea, constipation, anxiety, and insomnia.

The palliative care team can also offer psychological and emotional support to the patient and their family. They can refer the patient to the occupational therapist, physiotherapist, and social services. They can offer support and discussion about where the patient wishes to spend the last days of their life and where they wish to die, whether in a hospital, hospice or at home with appropriate support (hospice at home). Decisions about end-of-life care and the ceiling of treatment should be fully discussed with the patient and his/her family and should also be shared with all healthcare practitioners. Documentation and entry into a register, such as Co-ordinate My Care, will enable this to happen.

Palliative procedures

An endobronchial stent, inserted through a rigid bronchoscope, can aerate a part of the lung that has collapsed secondary to endobronchial obstruction caused by the tumour. This is most successful if the narrowing caused by the tumour is in one specific area. The patient will need to be fit enough for a general anaesthetic and have a prognosis of at least a few months. An endobronchial laser through a rigid bronchoscope can also open-up a bronchus narrowed by tumour. Endobronchial radiotherapy can cause shrinkage of an endobronchial tumour and reduce haemoptysis.

A **malignant pleural effusion** can be drained, followed by either a medical or surgical pleurodesis. A surgical pleurodesis using talc is generally preferable and more successful but requires that the patient is fit enough for general anaesthetic. A pleurax catheter can also be inserted for a recurring malignant pleural effusion. This may be an option in a patient who is still undergoing chemotherapy. The management of a malignant pleural effusion is discussed fully in Chapter 10.

Communicating the diagnosis of lung cancer

It can be difficult to inform a patient and his/her family the diagnosis of lung cancer, particularly if the disease is advanced and there is no curative treatment. Patients will be distressed and will go through the various stages of grief. They may become angry, and may blame themselves or the healthcare professionals if there has been any delay in obtaining the diagnosis. They may ask many questions, some of which can be difficult to answer. Most commonly, patients ask about their prognosis. This can be difficult to determine so should be discussed by a senior doctor who has all the information to hand. All patients with lung cancer should be discussed in the lung cancer MDT. All conversations should be recorded in the notes so that other healthcare professionals reading them are aware of what has been discussed and the completed proforma should be sent to the GP.

The lung multidisciplinary meeting

All patients with lung cancer must be discussed at the multidisciplinary meeting in a timely way. The MDT comprises of a respiratory physician, radiologist, histopathologist, medical oncologist, clinical oncologist, thoracic surgeon, palliative care consultant, and a lung cancer nurse specialist (LCNS). The LCNS should ideally be present when the patient receives the diagnosis of lung cancer and at discussions regarding management. The LCNS will offer additional information, for example, about benefits, offer support to the patient and family, and liaise with other members of the team. The lung MDT co-ordinator prepares the list and notes for the MDT and enters the data into a National Database.

The documentation must include information about the staging of the cancer, the WHO performance status of the patient (see Box 9.4) and the management plan which must be communicated to the patient, the GP, and other relevant people, such as the palliative care team.

Tracheal and laryngeal tumours

Tracheal and laryngeal tumours have a similar aetiology to primary lung cancers, with smoking being the main risk factor. Tracheal tumours may present with breathlessness, wheeze, and stridor. A CXR may appear misleadingly normal. An urgent CT scan of the upper thorax and neck may show the tumour. Bronchoscopy and biopsy should be carried out with caution as there is a possibility of causing complete obstruction of the airway if the tumour is large or if there is bleeding post-biopsy. It may be safer to carry out a rigid bronchoscopy under general anaesthetic with ENT support if necessary. Carcinoma of the larynx usually presents with a hoarse voice secondary to vocal cord paralysis. The diagnosis is made by bronchoscopy or nasendoscopy and is managed by the ENT surgeons.

Benign lung masses and solitary pulmonary nodules (SPN)

With improvements in CT scanning techniques and the increased frequency of scanning, there has been an increase in the detection of lung nodules and masses. A lesion <3 cm is considered a solitary pulmonary nodule (SPN) and one >3 cm as a pulmonary mass. It must be assumed that any mass or nodule in the lung is malignant unless radiological features or a biopsy prove otherwise. If a patient is referred with an abnormal CXR, it is useful, if possible, to look at previous imaging to see if this is a new nodule or if there has been any changes in the size or shape of the nodule. Benign pulmonary masses or nodules, which are often congenital, will appear stable in appearance on serial imaging.

Table 9.6 Features of malignant and benign lung lesions.

Malignant	Benign
Older age	Younger age (<40 years)
Smoker	Non-smoker
Size >1 cm	Size <1 cm
Increase in size on interval CT scan	Stable or decrease in size on interval CT scan
Irregular or spiculated margin	Smooth, well-defined margins
Distortion of adjacent vessels ('corona radiata' sign)	Benign pattern of calcification
Cavitation with thick irregular walls	Cavitation with thick, smooth walls
Increased enhancement with contrast	Lack of contrast enhancement
Increased FDG uptake on CT-PET	Low FDG uptake on CT-PET

Table 9.6 lists the radiological features of benign and malignant lung lesions.

Solitary pulmonary nodules are common, and approximately 150 000 per year are found with imaging. A SPN is a discrete, well-marginated, rounded opacity, less than or equal to 3 cm in diameter which is surrounded by lung parenchyma, does not touch the hilum or mediastinum, and has no associated atelectasis or pleural effusion.

The majority of SPNs are asymptomatic, detected incidentally and are benign, but this can only be determined after investigations as 20–30% of lung cancers present as SPNs. Solitary lung metastasis from other primary tumours can also occur. Carcinoid tumour of the lung can also present as a SPN and is discussed later in this chapter.

A SPN should be investigated according to the clinical symptoms, signs, and appearance on CT scan. In smokers with a risk of lung cancer, a SPN should be considered as malignant unless otherwise proven and patients should have a full staging CT scan of thorax, abdomen and pelvis, CT-PET scan,

Table 9.7 Risk factors for malignancy.

Low (<5%)	Intermediate (5–65%)	High (>65%)
Young patient	Mixture of low and high probability features	Older patient
Minimal smoking history		Heavy smoking history
No history of malignancy		Previous malignancy
Small nodule size		Larger nodule size
Regular margin		Irregular margin
Non-upper lobe		Upper lobe location

and a CT-guided biopsy. Measurement of tumour markers, such as PSA, CA 125, CEA and Ca99, may be indicated if metastases from other tumours is suspected. Table 9.7 outlines the risk of a SPN being malignant or benign.

The **Fleischner Society Guidelines** for the management of SPNs <1 cm in diameter are applied to SPNs according to whether the patient has a high or low risk for lung cancer. Table 9.8 outlines the guidelines. The WHO performance status of the patient, lung function, and extent of emphysema on CT should be taken into consideration before attempting a CT-guided biopsy. It should also be remembered that CT and CT-PET constitute a lot of radiation, and the pros and cons of following nodules up with repeated imaging should be discussed clearly with the patient.

Common causes of SPN and benign lung mass

A hamartoma is the commonest benign tumour of the lung, usually measuring <4 cm and asymptomatic. It is composed of epithelial tissue, fibrous tissue, cartilage, and fat and is described as having '*popcorn calcification*' on a chest X-ray (Figure 9.19).

A tuberculous granuloma is a small, usually calcified nodule, often in the lung apex (Figure 9.20, Figure 9.21). There may be radiological changes suggestive of previous tuberculosis, such as apical fibrosis.

A non-tuberculous granuloma is usually an incidental finding in patients with sarcoidosis and other granulomatous disease,

An arterio-venous malformation (AVM) can look like a SPN on imaging and can present with haemoptysis. A pulmonary angiogram may be required to make the diagnosis. See Chapter 11 for the diagnosis and management of AVM.

Lung sequestration, or rounded atelectasis, can present as a pleurally-based mass associated with pleural thickening and with characteristic radiological features.

Other causes of SPN include pulmonary infarction, mucoid impaction in patients with asthma or bronchiectasis and rheumatoid nodules.

Cavitating lung lesions

There are many causes of a cavitating lung lesion. Malignant lesions, especially squamous cell carcinoma of the lung, can cavitate. Infective causes include lung abscess, fungal infections (aspergilloma, histoplasmosis, actinomycosis), bacterial infections (*Klebsiella pneumonia*, *Staphylococcus aureus*, and *Mycobacterium tuberculosis*), and parasitic infections (hydatid) are discussed in Chapter 8. Granulomatosis with polyangiitis is discussed in Chapter 11.

Carcinoid tumour

Carcinoid tumours are rare tumours arising from neuroendocrine cells (Figure 9.22). The majority are non-malignant, grow slowly and rarely spread to other parts of the body. Some 85% of carcinoid tumours occur in the gastrointestinal tract, 10% in the lung, 3% in the pancreas and 2% in the kidney, ovary, and testis (Figure 9).

Carcinoid tumours of the lung account for 1–2% of all lung malignancies and occur equally in men and women, mainly in 40–50-year-olds. The majority are endobronchial and present with symptoms of cough, haemoptysis, wheeze, and breathlessness. Some 25% are found incidentally as

Table 9.8 Fleischner Society Guidelines for management of SPN, 2017.

Type of nodule	Size (mm)	Number of nodules	Risk of malignancy	Follow-up interval for CT
Solid	<6	Single	Low	No routine follow-up
Solid	<6	Single	High	Optional CT at 12 months
Solid	<6	Multiple	Low risk	No routine follow-up
Solid	<6	Multiple	High risk	Optional CT at 12 months
Solid	6–8	Single	Low risk	6–12 months, then consider CT at 18–24 months
Solid	6–8	Single	High risk	6–12 months, then consider CT at 18–24 months
Solid	6–8	Multiple	Low risk	3–6 months, then consider CT at 18–24 months
Solid	6–8	Multiple	High risk	3–6 months, then CT at 18–24 months
Solid	>8	Single	All	CT in 3 months or PET/CT or biopsy
Solid	>8	Multiple	Low risk	CT at 3–6 months, then consider CT at 18–24 months
Solid	>8	Multiple	High risk	CT at 3–6 months, then CT at 18–24 months
Subsolid: Ground-glass	< 6	Single	All risk	No follow-up needed
Subsolid: Ground-glass	>6	Single	All risk	CT 6–12 months to confirm presence then at 3 years and 5 years
Part-solid	<6	Single	All risk	No follow-up indicated
Pat-solid	>6	Single	All risk	CT 3–6 months to confirm presence then annual for 5 years
Subsolid: Multiple	<6	Multiple	All risk	CT at 3–6 months, If stable CT at 2 and 4 years
Subsolid: Multiple	>6	Multiple	All risk	CT at 3–6 months. Subsequent management based on most suspicious nodule

a SPN in the peripheral parenchyma. A CT scan will confirm a nodule or mass in the thorax (Figure 9.23). A CT-PET is not very sensitive for detecting carcinoid, with only 75% sensitivity (Figure 9.24). At bronchoscopy the carcinoid tumour appears smooth and red. There is an increased risk of bleeding if biopsied. Typical carcinoids (5–15%) can metastasize to local lymph nodes, have a 5-year survival of 100% and a 10-year survival of 87%.

Some 1% of patients with carcinoid tumour of the lung develop the carcinoid syndrome due to the release of large amounts of serotonin, resulting

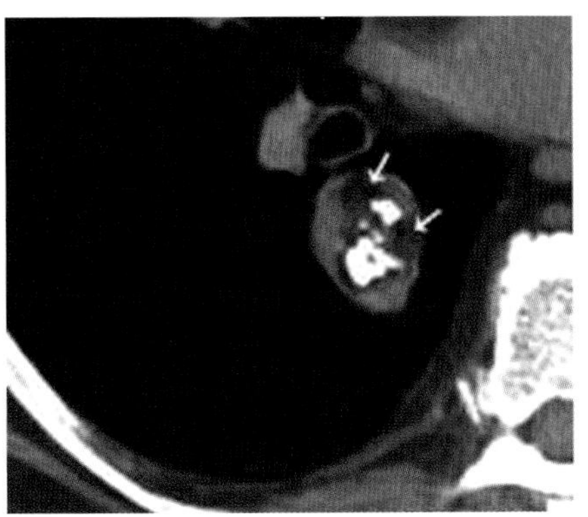

Figure 9.19 CT thorax showing a hamartoma with the typical popcorn calcification.

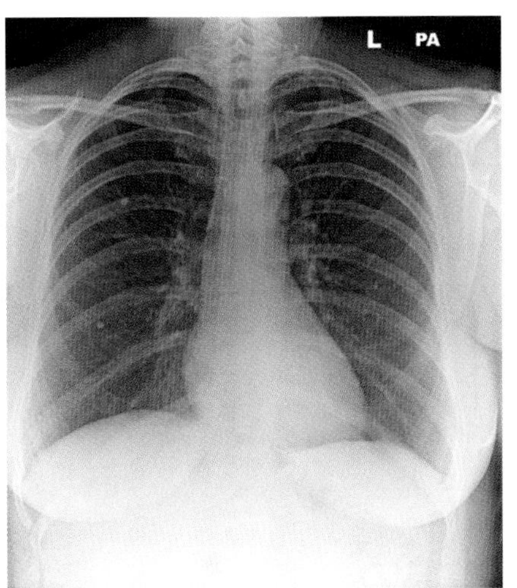

Figure 9.20 CXR showing granulomas in the right lung.

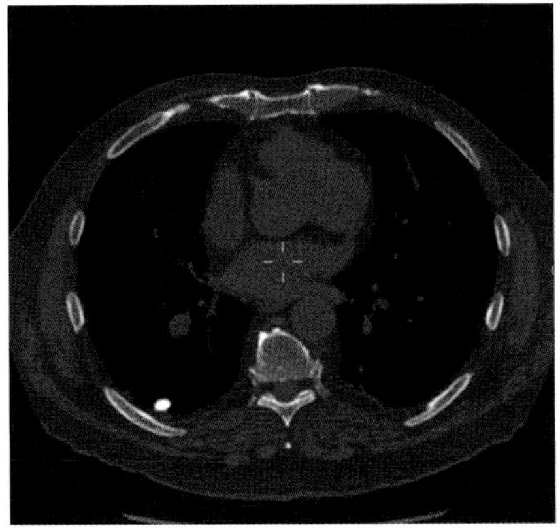

Figure 9.21 CT thorax showing a calcified granuloma in the right lung.

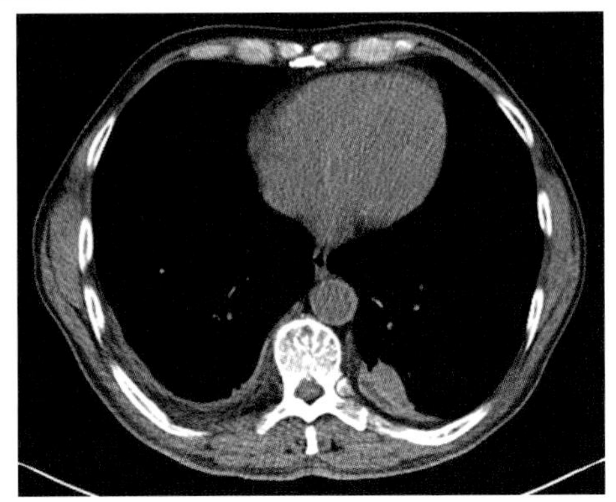

Figure 9.22 CT showing round atelectasis which looks like a solitary pulmonary nodule.

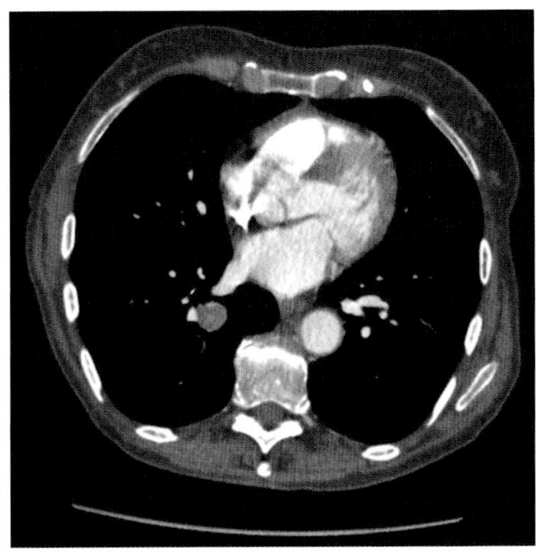

Figure 9.23 CT thorax of carcinoid tumour of the lung.

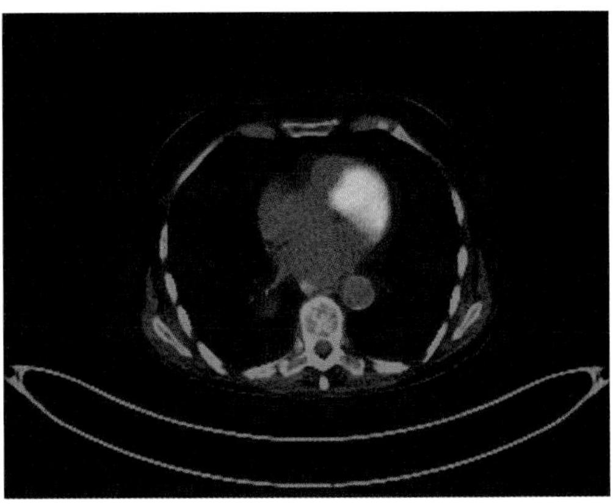

Figure 9.24 PET scan of carcinoid tumour showing low FDG uptake.

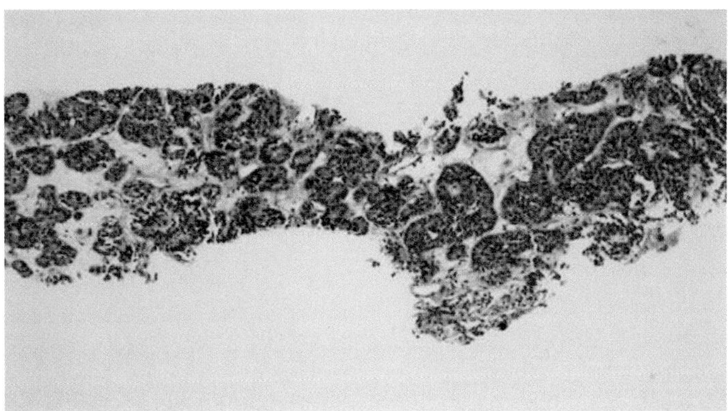

Figure 9.25 Histology of carcinoid tumour.

in flushing of the skin, abdominal cramps, diarrhoea, wheeziness, palpitations, and hypotension (Figure 9.25). The carcinoid syndrome is more likely if the tumour has spread to the liver. A diagnosis of carcinoid syndrome can be made by an octreotide scan or somatostatin receptor scintigraphy. High levels of serotonin and chromogranin A can be measured in the blood, and high levels of 5 hydroxy-indole acetic acid (the product of serotonin metabolism) can be measured in a 24-hour urine collection.

Carcinoid tumour presenting as a SPN in the lung can be resected if there is no evidence of spread. Somatostatin analogues, octreotide, and lanreotide, can control the symptoms of carcinoid syndrome.

Malignant carcinoid tumours show areas of focal necrosis, with 48% metastasising to lymph nodes and 20% metastasising to distant sites. These have a 5-year survival of 69% and a 10-year survival of 52%. Somatostatin analogues, either alone or in combination with chemotherapy, can be considered for malignant lesions. Targeted radiotherapy and interferon can be effective in a significant number of patients with symptoms.

Future developments

Lung cancer remains a fatal disease in most patients. Lung cancer screening using low dose CT scanning in patients at risk may improve early detection. Studies are underway to see of this is safe and cost-effective. Much research is being done on targeted molecular therapies and gene expression profiling to determine response to treatment. This may translate into more individualised treatment for patients.

SUMMARY OF LEARNING POINTS

- Lung cancer is the commonest fatal malignancy in men and women in the UK, responsible for 40 000 deaths each year.
- The symptoms and signs of lung cancer may be non-specific, so patients and all healthcare professionals should be educated about these.
- Emphasis should be placed on smoking avoidance and smoking cessation as these are the only measures that will significantly reduce the incidence of lung cancer.
- The diagnosis of lung cancer is made with CT and CT-PET imaging for staging, and histological diagnosis.
- An assessment of the patient's fitness for treatment includes lung function testing, cardiac testing, and calculation of the WHO performance status.
- Early detection of lung cancer can improve survival as these patients can be offered radical treatment.
- Patients with lung cancer should be discussed in a lung MDT and the diagnosis communicated sensitively to the patient and family.
- Surgical resection offers the best chance of survival in a patient with NSCLC.
- Multimodality treatments are available for all stages of lung cancers in both SCLC and NSCLC, which in trials have resulted in symptom relief and prolonged survival.
- New inhibitors for NSCLC have shown benefit in patients with Stage IV NSCLC and approved by NICE.
- Solitary pulmonary nodules have a wide differential and should be managed with careful history, examination, imaging, and biopsy if indicated.

MULTIPLE CHOICE QUESTIONS

9.1 What is the commonest histological type of lung cancer?

A Adenocarcinoma
B Bronchoalveolar cell carcinoma
C Large cell carcinoma
D Small cell carcinoma
E Squamous cell carcinoma

Answer: E

Squamous cell lung cancer is still the commonest lung cancer, although adenocarcinoma is now increasing in frequency, possibly reflecting the type of filters used in cigarettes.

9.2 Passive smoking increases the risk of lung cancer by how many times?

A 1×
B 1.5×
C 2×
D 4×
E 10×

Answer: B

Passive smoking increases the risk of lung cancer by 1.5×. This evidence has led to the banning of smoking in public places. A history of significant passive smoking should be elicited from all patients.

9.3 What is the overall 5-year survival for Stage IA NSCLC?
A 10%
B 20%
C 35%
D 50%
E 70%

Answer: D

The latest figures from Cancer Research UK suggest that the overall 5-year survival for Stage IA NSCLC is only 50%.

9.4 What is the 5-year survival after surgery for Stage IA NSCLC?
A 20%
B 30%
C 50%
D 70%
E 90%

Answer: D

Patients who have surgery for Stage IA NSCLC have a better outcome, with 70% surviving five years. These patients are not currently offered adjuvant chemotherapy.

9.5 Testing for EGFR mutational status is recommended for patients with which condition?
A Adenocarcinoma
B Carcinoid tumour
C Non-small cell lung cancer
D Small cell lung cancer
E Squamous cell carcinoma

Answer: A

All patients with an adenocarcinoma should have EGFR testing. EGFR is over-expressed in non-smokers with adenocarcinoma and particularly in women. These patients may respond to EGFR inhibitors.

9.6 Which feature of a solitary pulmonary nodule suggests that it might be malignant?
A Calcification
B Less than 1 cm in diameter
C Low FDG uptake on PET scan
D Smooth margins
E Thick-walled cavity

Answer: E

The other features suggest a benign aetiology.

9.7 Which is the commonest benign lung mass?
A Arteriovenous malformation
B Bronchogenic cyst
C Carcinoid tumour
D Granuloma
E Hamartoma

Answer E

A hamartoma is the commonest benign lung mass. It is described as having 'popcorn calcification' on the chest X-ray.

9.8 Pulmonary carcinoid tumours are associated with the carcinoid syndrome in what percentage of cases?
A 1%
B 5%
C 10%
D 25%
E 50%

Answer: A

Pulmonary carcinoids are usually benign and only 1% are associated with the carcinoid syndrome.

9.9 A 52-year-old man with a 30-pack year history of smoking goes to his GP with a one-month history of a persistent, dry cough. He has no other symptoms of concern. Clinical examination is normal. What should his GP do?
A Reassure him and advise him to stop smoking
B Prescribe oral antibiotics for 7 days
C Refer him to smoking cessation clinic and organise a chest X-ray
D Organise a CT thorax
E Refer urgently to a respiratory physician

Answer: C

All smokers with a persistent cough require a chest X-ray as cough is the commonest symptom of lung cancer. These patients should be strongly advised to stop smoking and referred to a smoking cessation clinic.

9.10 A 52-year-old woman is referred to the respiratory outpatient clinic with a 6-week history of a cough productive of a copious amount of white sputum, chest discomfort, breathlessness, and a weight loss of 5 kg. She had been a smoker of five cigarettes per day from the age of 17 until 20 years. Her GP had given her oral amoxicillin for 2 weeks followed by oral clarithromycin and prednisolone, 30 mg for 2 weeks without any improvement in her symptoms. Sputum samples have not grown any organisms. Her chest X-ray shows persistent consolidation in the left lower lobe. What would you be concerned about?

A Adenocarcinoma in situ
B Atypical pneumonia
C Mesothelioma
D Organising pneumonia
E *Mycobacterium tuberculosis*

Answer: A

This presentation and imaging mean that adenocarcinoma in situ is a possibility and should be actively excluded by obtaining histology.

9.11 A 55-year-old man with a 60-pack year history of smoking is admitted through Accident and Emergency Department with weakness, confusion, and after he had collapsed at home. His wife reported that he had been unwell for several months, unable to work, and complained of lethargy, weakness, and a cough. He had lost 10 kg in weight and appeared cachectic. A CT head was normal. Chest X-ray was not normal. Blood results were as follows: Hb 9.9 g dl^{-1}, WCC 4.3, platelets 199, Na + 122, K+ 4.1, Urea 8.1, creatinine 100, EGFR >60. What is the most likely diagnosis?

A Adenocarcinoma of lung
B Carcinoid tumour
C Large cell poorly differentiated tumour
D Small cell carcinoma
E Squamous cell carcinoma of lung

Answer: D

This patient has presented with a SIADH. SCLC is associated with ectopic secretion of ADH.

9.12 A 70-year-old woman is found to have a nodule on a chest X-ray which was performed routinely prior to a left hip replacement. She has smoked 10 cigarettes per day for 20 years but had stopped 30 years previously. Apart from osteoarthritis of her left hip and a BMI of 40, she appeared well with no other symptoms. The orthopaedic consultant organised a CT scan of thorax and has referred her to you for advice about the nodule. The CT scan shows a 6 mm nodule in the left upper lobe of the lung with no lymphadenopathy. The nodule is described as smooth with no calcification by the consultant radiologist. How would you manage this patient?

A Reassure and discharge the patient
B Organise a CT guided biopsy
C Organise a bronchoscopy for bronchoalveolar lavage
D Organise a CT-PET scan
E Arrange for an interval CT scan of thorax in 6 months

Answer: E

All SPNs in the lung may be malignant, especially in someone over the age of 40 years and who has a smoking history. This nodule is only 6 mm and smooth and was found incidentally. It will not be easy to biopsy, especially in someone with a BMI of 40. It may also be too small for CT-PET resolution. As she is asymptomatic and stopped smoking some time ago, she is in the low risk group. The Fleischner Society guidelines recommends an interval CT scan in 12 months to see if it changes.

FURTHER READING

American College of Chest Physicians (ed.) (2013). Diagnosis and Management of Lung Cancer, 3rd ed: American College of Chest Physicians Evidence-Based Clinical Practice Guidelines. *Chest* 143 (5): 1S–50S.

Cancer Research UKs (2016) [online]. https://www.cancerresearchuk.org (accessed 13 March 2017).

Doll, R. and Hill, A.B. (1954). The mortality of doctors in relation to their smoking habits. *British Medical Journal* 1 (4877): 1451–1455.

Gould, M.K., Fletcher, J., Iannettoni, M.D. et al. (2007). Evaluation of patients with pulmonary nodules: when is it lung cancer?: ACCP evidence-based clinical practice guidelines (2nd edition). *Chest* 132 (3): 108S–130S.

MacMahon, H., Austin, J.H., Gamsu, G. et al. (2005). Guidelines for management of small pulmonary nodules detected on CT scans: a statement from the Fleischner Society. *Radiology* 237 (2): 395–400.

Macmillan Cancer Support (n.d.) Home – Macmillan Cancer Support, 2016 [online]. Available at: www.macmillan.org.uk (accessed 11 March 2017).

National Institute for Health and Care Excellence (2011). Lung cancer: diagnosis and management. NICE Guideline (CG121), Clinical Guideline, (April), [online]. Available at: http://nice.org.uk/guidance/cg121.

Ost, D., Fein, A.M., and Feinsilver, S.H. (2003). The solitary pulmonary nodule. *New England Journal of Medicine* 348 (25): 2535–2542.

Rami-Porta, R. and Crowley, J.G.P. (2009). The revised TNM staging system for lung cancer. *Annals of Thoracic and Cardiovascular Surgery* 15 (1): 4–9.

Rivera, M., Mehta, A., and American College of Chest Physicians (2007). Initial diagnosis of lung cancer: ACCP Evidence-Based Clinical Practice Guidelines (2nd edition). *Chest* 132 (3 Supplement): 131S–148S.

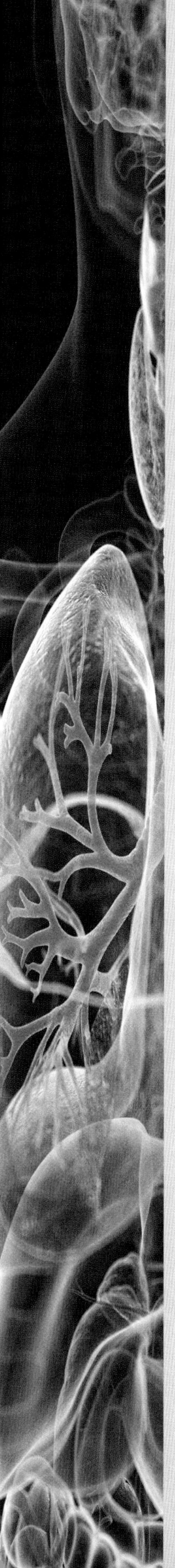

CHAPTER 10
Pleural disease

Learning objectives

- To understand the composition and formation of pleural fluid
- To know the mechanisms of injury to the pleura
- To understand the aetiology, diagnosis, and management of primary and secondary pneumothoraces
- To recognise the diagnosis and management of a tension pneumothorax
- To learn the aetiology, diagnosis, and management of a pleural effusion
- To understand the management of a malignant pleural effusion
- To understand the management of pleural infection, including empyema
- To appreciate asbestos-related pleural disease
- To understand the aetiology, diagnosis, and management of malignant mesothelioma

Essential Respiratory Medicine, First Edition. Shanthi Paramothayan.

Companion website: www.wiley.com/go/paramothayan/essential_respiratory_medicine

Abbreviations

ARDS	adult respiratory distress syndrome
BTS	British Thoracic Society
CAP	community acquired pneumonia
CCF	congestive cardiac failure
CPR	cardiopulmonary resuscitation
CRP	C-reactive protein
CT	computed tomography
DNA	deoxyribonucleic acid
EPP	extra pleural pneumonectomy
FDG	^{18F}-Fluorodeoxy glucose
HIV	human immunodeficiency virus
HRCT	high-resolution computed tomography
ICU	intensive care unit
IGRA	interferon gamma release assay
ILD	interstitial lung disease
IMRT	intensity modulated radiotherapy
LAM	lymphangioleiomyomatosis
LDH	lactate dehydrogenase
LMWH	low molecular weight heparin
MRI	magnetic resonance imaging
MRSA	methicillin-resistant *Staphylococcus aureus*
NIV	non-invasive ventilation
NPSA	National Patient Safety Agency
PCR	polymerase chain reaction
PET-CT	positron emission tomography with computed tomography
PLCH	Pulmonary Langerhans cell histiocytosis
PleurX	tunnelled pleural catheter
PSP	primary spontaneous pneumothorax
RCT	randomised controlled trial
SMRP	soluble mesothelin-related protein
SP	secondary pneumothorax
SPN	solitary pulmonary nodule
SVCO	superior vena cava obstruction
TB	*Mycobacterium tuberculosis*
TED	thromboembolic disease
VATS	video-assisted thoracoscopic surgery

Normal pleura and pleural fluid

The pleura is a thin, serous membrane comprising of the visceral pleura, which covers the lungs and the mediastinum, and the parietal pleura which lines the inside of the thoracic cage and diaphragm. Chapter 2 has more details on the anatomy and physiology of the lung.

Pleural fluid is filtered from blood in the capillaries supplying the parietal pleura down a pressure gradient into the pleural space. Pleural fluid drains out of the pleural space through stomata in the parietal lymphatics which lie between the parietal mesothelial cells. These stomata merge into small lymphatic channels which form larger vessels which connect areas of the parietal, mediastinal and diaphragmatic pleura, ultimately draining into the mediastinal lymph nodes. In health, there is a thin layer of pleural fluid in the pleural space, approximately 1–5 ml and 10 μm thick, which acts as a lubricant, allowing expansion of the lungs without friction. There is a turnover of 1–2 L of pleural fluid each day. More pleural fluid is secreted at the apices of the lungs and more fluid is resorbed at the bases as there are a greater number of parietal lymphatics in the diaphragm and mediastinum.

In health, pleural fluid contains the same amount of protein and glucose as interstitial fluid, but a lower amount of sodium and a greater amount of lactate dehydrogenase (LDH). Pleural fluid also contains mesothelial cells, macrophages, and lymphocytes. The pH of healthy pleural fluid is 7.6. Water and small molecules move passively between the layers while larger particles are transported across by cytoplasmic transport mechanisms.

Pleural effusion

Definition

A pleural effusion is fluid in the pleural cavity. A pleural effusion occurs if more fluid is produced than is resorbed. A pleural effusion can be unilateral or bilateral.

Aetiology of pleural effusion

Analysis of pleural fluid and applying Light's criteria can differentiate between an exudate and a transudate. Box 10.4 summarises what constitutes an exudate and a transudate. There are many different causes for an exudative and transudative pleural effusion.

Clinical assessment of a patient presenting with a pleural effusion

The main symptom associated with a pleural effusion is breathlessness. The patient may also complain of chest pain and other symptoms depending on the cause of the effusion. It is important to elicit the following information from the history: (Boxes 10.1 and 10.2).

Diagnostic pathway for management of a unilateral pleural effusion

Figure 10.1 shows the BTS diagnostic algorithm for investigation of a unilateral pleural effusion. There are several clinical signs that indicate a pleural effusion (Box 10.3).

Box 10.1 Symptoms of Pleural Effusion.

- Smoking history (pack years)
- History of asbestos exposure: a full and comprehensive occupational history is required
- Symptoms suggestive of infection
- Symptoms suggestive of malignancy
- Drug history

Box 10.2 Clinical Examination of patient with a pleural effusion.

- Clubbing of fingernails
- Clinical signs of pleural effusion can be detected when there is more than 300 ml of fluid
- Clinical signs of cardiac failure

Investigations for a pleural effusion

Chest X-ray (CXR): A pleural effusion with more than 300 ml fluid can be seen on a postero-anterior (PA) CXR as an area of whiteness. The fluid accumulates at the lung base because of gravitational forces, so the costophrenic angle is usually obliterated first. If the effusion is extensive, the CXR can show as a complete 'white-out' of the hemithorax. A small effusion, with only 50 ml of fluid, may be detected on a lateral decubitus CXR (Figure 10.2). A pleural effusion may be difficult to detect on a CXR taken when the patient is supine, for example, on the intensive care unit (ICU), as the fluid lies posteriorly. An ultrasound may be better at detecting fluid under these circumstances.

In a patient with congestive cardiac failure (CCF), bilateral pleural effusions can occur and there may be other radiological evidence of heart failure, such as an enlarged heart, Kerley B lines and fluid in the horizontal fissure.

Thoracic ultrasound is an essential investigation in the management of a pleural effusion as it is more sensitive than a CXR at identifying small effusions, including sub-pulmonic effusions (Figure 10.3). Thoracic ultrasound is also better at differentiating between pleural fluid and pleural thickening. Features such as septation seen on thoracic ultrasound may help distinguish between an exudate and a transudate and between a malignant and a benign pleural effusion with greater sensitivity than a contrast CT scan. Thoracic ultrasound is also essential for successful and safe thoracocentesis.

CT thorax with contrast should be conducted if the fluid is an exudate and if there are other abnormalities on the chest X-ray, such as a mass (Figure 10.4). Ideally, the CT scan should be done before the pleural fluid is completely drained. Septation, due to fibrin deposition, appears as suspended air bubbles. Contrast CT can reliably distinguish between an empyema and a lung abscess, as the former appears as a lenticular opacity with pleural enhancement around it. Contrast enhancement of the pleura can distinguish between benign and malignant pleural thickening, with malignant pleura showing areas of pleural nodularity. Mediastinal, parietal, and circumferential pleural thickening of >1 cm suggests a malignant process. Pleural enhancement can also occur when there is inflammation of the pleura secondary to infection. A CT thorax with contrast is essential if a surgical pleural biopsy is required and in the management of complicated pleural infections, including empyema.

An **MRI** is not routinely required in the management of a pleural effusion but can distinguish between a malignant and a benign pleural effusion when CT with contrast is contraindicated. An MRI can also give anatomical information about chest wall and diaphragmatic involvement when the effusion is secondary to malignancy, especially if surgery is being contemplated.

A **PET-CT** is not routinely used in the management of a pleural effusion as there are many false positives but, as with MRI, can be occasionally used for staging when there is a malignant pleural effusion.

Pleural Aspiration (Thoracocentesis)

This is an essential investigation in the diagnosis of a pleural effusion and should be conducted using direct ultrasound guidance as this increases the chance of successful aspiration, reduces the need for repeated aspiration, and reduces the risk of pneumothorax and injury to the heart, liver, and spleen. A 21G fine bore needle attached to a 50 ml syringe should be used. Appendix 10.A describes the methodology of pleural fluid collection. Table 10.1 describes the analysis of pleural fluid.

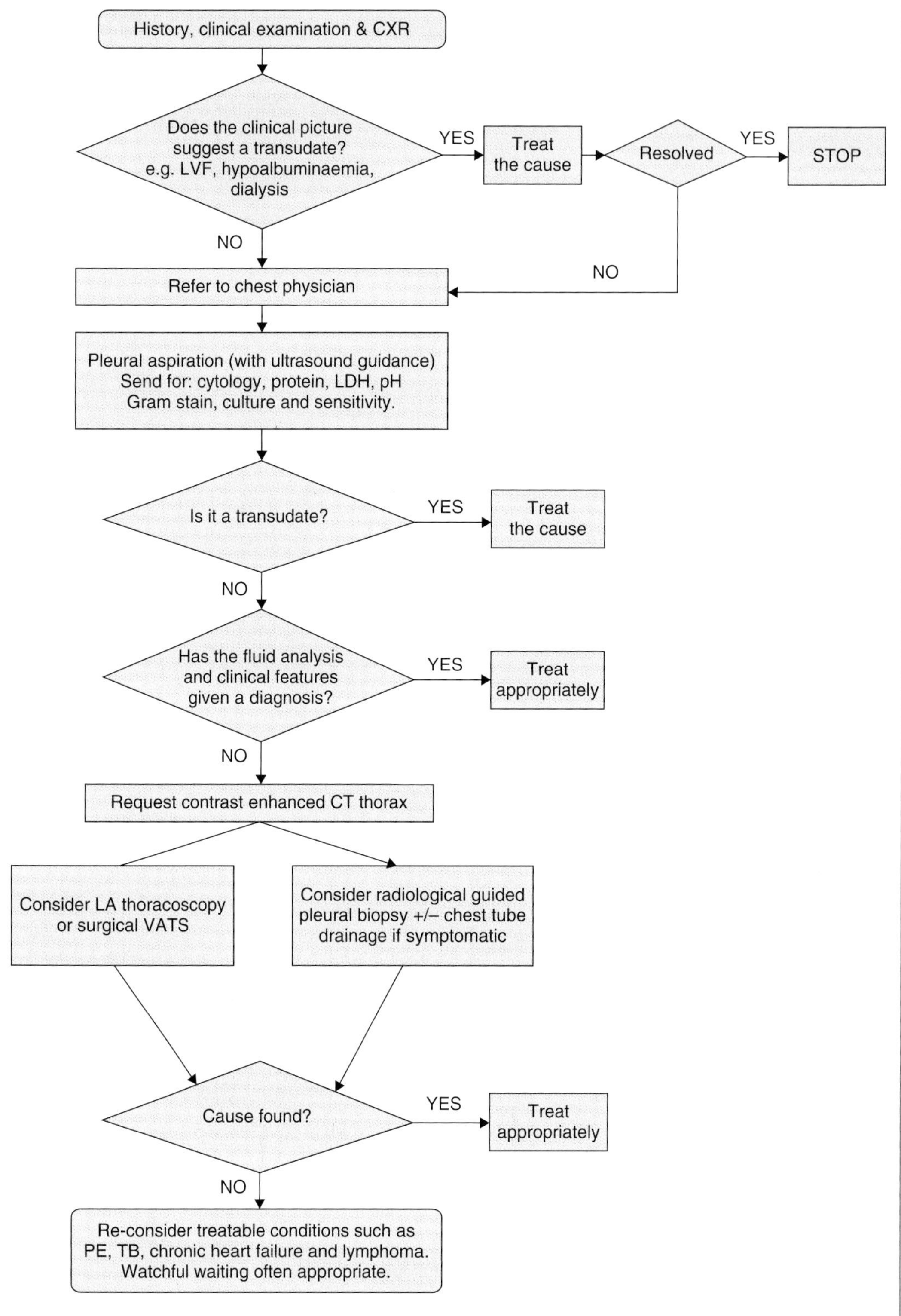

Figure 10.1 BTS diagnostic algorithm for investigation of a unilateral pleural effusion.

Box 10.3 Clinical signs of a pleural effusion.

- Reduced chest wall movement on the side of the effusion
- Reduced air entry on the side of the effusion
- Dullness on percussion on the side of the effusion: this is the most reliable clinical finding
- Decreased tactile vocal fremitus and vocal resonance on the side of the effusion
- Bronchial breathing above the effusion
- Tracheal deviation away from side of a large effusion

Classification of the fluid into either an exudate or a transudate is essential for diagnosis and further management. This can be done by applying Light's criteria (Box 10.4).

Pleural biopsy

Histological and microbiological analysis of pleura is essential in the management of an exudate as this can usually distinguish between malignancy, infection, and benign pleural fibrosis. Pleural biopsy can be obtained through an Abram's needle, with a CT-guided biopsy or a VATS biopsy.

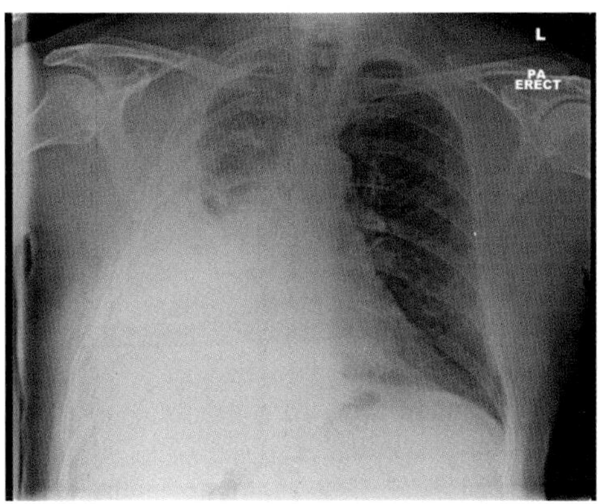

Figure 10.2 CXR showing a unilateral (right-sided) pleural effusion.

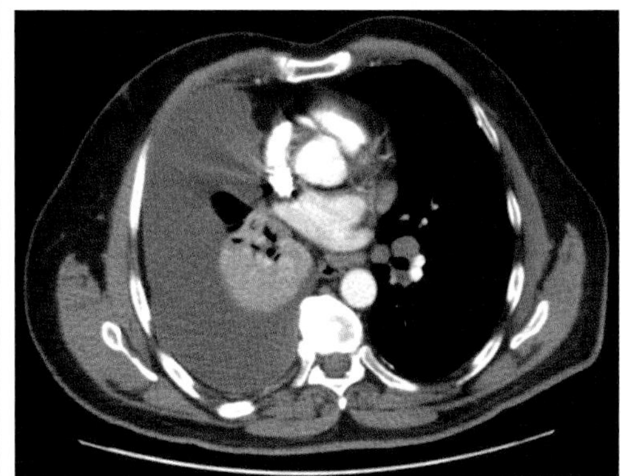

Figure 10.4 CT thorax showing a unilateral (right-sided) pleural effusion.

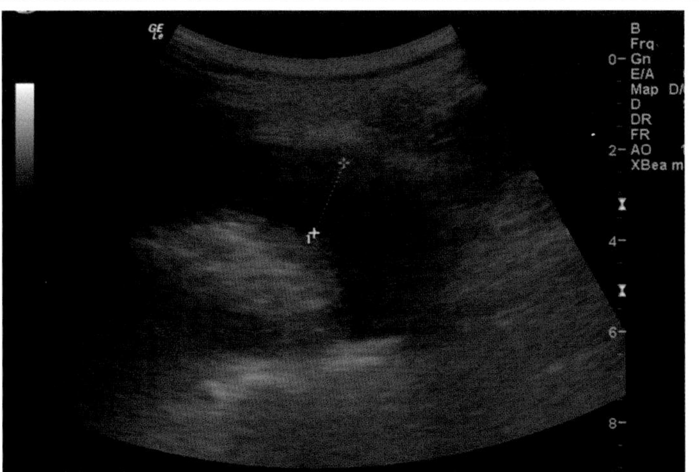

Figure 10.3 Thoracic ultrasound scan showing a pleural effusion with underlying lung atelectasis.

Table 10.1 Analysis of pleural fluid from thoracocentesis.

Measurement	Result of pleural fluid analysis
Appearance	Serous (clear)
	Turbid suggests infection or empyema
	Pus suggests empyema
	Milky suggests chylothorax or pseudo chylothorax
	Blood-stained suggests malignancy, mesothelioma, pulmonary embolus with infarction, trauma, or post-cardiac surgery
	Bloody: if the pleural fluid haematocrit is >50% of the blood haematocrit, then it is classified as a haemothorax.
Odour	Malodour suggests anaerobic infection
Biochemistry	Pleural fluid protein and pleural fluid protein /serum protein ratio
	Pleural fluid lactate dehydrogenase (LDH) and pleural fluid LDH/serum LDH ratio
	Pleural fluid glucose will be low (<3.3 mmol/L) in a chronic effusion with a pleural fluid/serum glucose ratio < 0.5.
	Common causes of a low fluid glucose include empyema, malignancy, or mycobacterium tuberculosis infection.
	Rheumatoid arthritis is associated with a very low fluid glucose level < 1.6 mmol/L
Cytology	Malignant cells may be detected in 60% of malignant effusions
	Differential cell count may be helpful, but is very non-specific and not diagnostic
	Neutrophilia (>50%) suggests an acute process. This includes parapneumonic effusions secondary to a bacterial infection, pulmonary embolus, acute mycobacterium tuberculosis infection or benign asbestos pleural effusion
	Lymphocytosis (>50%) suggests a chronic effusion secondary to mycobacterium tuberculosis infection or malignancy. Significant lymphocytosis (>80%) suggests mycobacterium tuberculosis infection, lymphoma, sarcoidosis, chronic rheumatoid pleurisy, or post-cardiac bypass surgery.
	Eosinophilia (>10%) is usually due to air or blood in the pleural space but could indicate parapneumonic effusions, eosinophilic granulomatosis with polyangiitis, lymphoma, drugs, parasitic infestation, pulmonary infarction, or benign asbestos pleural effusion
	Mesothelial cells predominate in transudates
Microbiology	Gram stain
	Ziehl-Neelsen stain
	Microscopy, culture, and sensitivity, including TB culture
pH	Normal pleural fluid pH is 7.6
	pH can vary significantly between locules in a complicated effusion pH < 7.3 in chronic malignant effusions, rheumatoid arthritis, mycobacterium tuberculosis infection and oesophageal rupture pH < 7.2 is the best indicator of an empyema and the need for a chest drain
	pH > 7.6 when there is infection with proteus spp. which produces ammonia

Table 10.1 (*Continued*)

Measurement	Result of pleural fluid analysis
Other tests as indicated	Adenosine deaminase if TB suspected (>45 IU l^{-1})
	Polymerase chain reaction (PCR) for *Mycobacterium tuberculosis*
	Interferon-gamma assay for *Mycobacterium tuberculosis*
	Pancreatic amylase if pancreatitis is suspected or salivary amylase for oesophageal rupture
	Chylomicrons will be seen with a chylothorax (milky effusion)
	Pleural fluid triglyceride level will be >110 mg dl^{-1} in a chylothorax
	Pleural fluid cholesterol will be elevated in a pseudo chylothorax

Box 10.4 Light's criteria.

The fluid is an exudate if one or more of the following criteria are met:

- Pleural fluid protein/serum protein >0.5
- Pleural fluid LDH/serum LDH > 0.6
- Pleural fluid LDH > two-thirds of upper limit of normal serum LDH

Light's criteria, used most often to differentiate between an exudate and a transudate, has a sensitivity of 98% and a specificity of 80%. It can falsely categorise a transudate as an exudate in 20% of cases, especially in patients with partially treated heart failure or those on diuretics as this increases the concentration of protein and LDH.

Measurement of N-terminal pro-brain natriuretic peptide in pleural fluid or serum can be helpful in borderline cases as this is raised in systolic and diastolic cardiac failure. Comparison of albumin and cholesterol in the pleural fluid to serum levels may also be helpful in differentiating between an exudate and a transudate.

An Abrams needle biopsy with a local anaesthetic is only recommended if mycobacterium tuberculosis is strongly suspected, if there is diffuse pleural enhancement on a contrast CT scan, and alternative methods of obtaining tissue are not feasible. Generally, this method of obtaining pleural tissue has a low yield and a high complication rate and is done much less now than it was a few years ago.

A CT-guided percutaneous pleural biopsy, which is less invasive than a surgical biopsy, can be performed if there is obvious pleural disease on imaging and if the patient is not fit for surgery. This has a better yield than an Abram's blind biopsy and is much safer. A CXR is required after any invasive procedure to ensure that there is no iatrogenic pneumothorax.

A thoracoscopic pleural biopsy has the best yield and is a safe procedure. A therapeutic pleurodesis can be carried out at the same time if indicated, for example, for a malignant pleural effusion, avoiding two separate procedures. A medical thoracoscopic pleural biopsy with local anaesthetic and sedation can be carried out by a trained respiratory physician and is a safer procedure than a blind pleural biopsy, with a reasonable yield of 92% in experienced hands. The main complications are infection and haemorrhage.

A VATS pleural biopsy, carried out by a thoracic surgeon, is the investigation of choice for a patient with an exudate, so long as they can tolerate a general anaesthetic. The pleura can be directly visualised, and this gives the best yield of 95%, with a low complication rate. If there is a trapped lung, this can be freed, and a talc pleurodesis can be conducted at the same time as the biopsy.

Bronchoscopy is indicated if the patient with an exudative pleural effusion presents with haemoptysis, if aspiration pneumonia or inhalation of a foreign body is suspected, or if there are radiological changes suggestive of an endobronchial lesion.

Differential diagnosis of a transudate

A transudate occurs either due to an increase in the hydrostatic pressure in the parietal pleura or due to reduced oncotic pressure of the fluid, usually from hypoalbuminaemia. Table 10.2 lists the differential diagnosis of a transudate.

Table 10.2 Differential diagnosis of a transudate.

• Left ventricular failure: unilateral or bilateral pleural effusions
• Liver failure: right pleural effusion commoner then left. Ascites may be present
• Nephrotic syndrome
• Post cardiac surgery
• Hypothyroidism
• Constrictive pericarditis
• Meig's syndrome: right>left, often associated with ascites, occurs with ovarian tumours
• Peritoneal dialysis
• Urinothorax

Management of a transudate

Management of a transudate is that of the underlying condition. Bilateral pleural effusions are usually transudates, most commonly secondary to CCF. The BTS guidelines do not recommend pleural aspiration in this situation unless there are atypical features, or the effusion does not respond to diuretics. CT thorax and pleural biopsy are not required in most cases of a transudate.

Differential diagnosis of an exudate

An exudate occurs when there is increased permeability of the capillaries, usually due to inflammation, with reduced fluid resorption. Table 10.3 lists the differential diagnosis of an exudate.

Table 10.3 Differential diagnosis of an exudate.

• Malignancy: commonest cause in patients over 60 years
• Parapneumonic effusion: occurs in 50% of bacterial pneumonias and the commonest cause in patients <40 years
• Mesothelioma: often blood-stained fluid
• Pulmonary embolus
• *Mycobacterium tuberculosis*: lymphocytic effusion, acid-fast bacilli positive in 10% of cases and culture positive in 25% of cases. Pleural biopsy and culture often diagnostic
• Rheumatoid arthritis: low pleural fluid glucose <1.6 mmol/L
• Systemic lupus erythematosus
• Other connective tissue disorders
• Sarcoidosis: an effusion is very rare but when present will be lymphocytic
• Acute pancreatitis or pancreatic pseudocyst: increase in pancreatic amylase in the fluid
• Oesophageal rupture (Boerhaave's syndrome): pH < 7.2 and an increase in salivary amylase
• Sub-phrenic abscess
• Eosinophilic granulomatosis with polyangiitis: increased eosinophils in pleural fluid
• Dressler's syndrome: occurs post cardiac surgery, blood-stained fluid
• Post-myocardial infarction
• Chylothorax: chylomicrons in fluid with elevated triglyceride levels
• Cryptogenic organising pneumonia
• Yellow nail syndrome
• Familial Mediterranean fever
• Drug-induced: amiodarone, bromocriptine, methotrexate, phenytoin, nitrofurantoin

Management of malignant pleural effusion

Malignant cells reach the visceral pleura either haematogenously or through the lymphatic network and spread to the parietal pleural through pleural adhesions. Malignant cells, cytokines, and vascular endothelial growth factor (VEGF) increase endothelial permeability, disrupt the lymphatic network, and promote angiogenesis, thereby causing accumulation of fluid, which is often blood-stained. Involvement of the regional lymph nodes is usually associated with the presence of a pleural effusion.

The presence of malignant cells in the pleura or pleural fluid suggests advanced metastatic disease with a median survival of 3–12 months, depending on the cancer. The commonest cause of a malignant pleural effusion in men is lung cancer (40%) and in women is breast cancer (17%). Other causes of a malignant pleural effusion include lymphoma, tumours of the gastrointestinal system, and tumours of the genitourinary system. In 10% of cases of a malignant pleural effusion, no primary malignancy is identified.

A large pleural effusion is most likely to be malignant, but in 25% of cases of a malignant pleural effusion, the patient is asymptomatic. Overall, 60% of malignant effusions can be diagnosed by pleural fluid cytology, with a greater diagnostic rate for adenocarcinoma of the lung than for mesothelioma or other types of lung cancers. Measurement of tumour markers in pleural fluid is not routinely done for lung cancer. Mesothelin levels may be elevated in epithelioid mesothelioma. A pH < 7.3 in a malignant pleural effusion confers a worse prognosis and a lower chance of successful pleurodesis.

Malignant pleural effusions recur within weeks after drainage and repeated aspirations are not ideal in most cases. There are several therapeutic options which will depend on the fitness of the patient and their overall prognosis. Patients who are relatively asymptomatic from their effusion can be observed.

In symptomatic patients who have a poor performance status and life expectancy of only a few weeks, repeated pleural aspirations can be carried out as a palliative procedure to remove some fluid to improve breathlessness. Patients who are not surgical candidates should have a small bore intercostal chest drain inserted to remove 500 ml to 1.5 L of fluid in a controlled way to avoid re-expansion pulmonary oedema. A low-pressure, high-volume suction device and regular flushing may be helpful. Chemical pleurodesis using talc, bleomycin or tetracycline should be considered as this will reduce the chance of recurrence, even if the effusion cannot be completely drained because of a trapped lung.

Patients who have a reasonable performance status and life expectancy of at least several months should have a VATS pleurodesis, as any trapped lung can be freed and the outcome is better, with fewer complications. A systematic review of 46 randomised controlled trials (RCTs) with 2053 patients concluded that talc pleurodesis was associated with fewer recurrences than bleomycin or tetracycline and that a thoracoscopic pleurodesis was better than a pleurodesis done via an intercostal chest drain.

Patients with a recurrent malignant pleural effusion who cannot have a medical or surgical pleurodesis because of poor performance status or a trapped lung, should have a tunnelled pleural catheter (PleurX) inserted. This will improve symptoms and allow the patient to go home. Rarely, when pleurodesis fails, a pleuroperitoneal shunt can be considered.

Pleural infection and empyema

Definitions

Pleural infection is an infection in the pleural space. Empyema is frank pus in the pleural space.

The annual incidence of pleural infection in the UK and the USA is 80 000 cases. Pleural infections are commoner in the very young, the elderly, and commoner in men compared to women. The morbidity and mortality of pleural infection are high, especially for empyema, which has a mortality of 20%. Prompt diagnosis and management by an expert reduce the morbidity and mortality. Box 10.5 lists the risk factors for developing pleural infections and empyema.

Aetiology of pleural infection

Most pleural infections result from sub-optimally treated pneumonia, with progression of a parapneumonic effusion to frank empyema. Over 50% of patients with community acquired pneumonia (CAP) develop a parapneumonic effusion which usually resolves over a few weeks with prompt antibiotic treatment. If there is a delay in treatment or if there are underlying risk factors, some parapneumonic effusions can progress to pleural infection and empyema.

Box 10.5 Risk factors for developing pleural infection and empyema.

- Diabetes mellitus
- Immunosuppression
- Alcohol abuse
- Gastro-oesophageal reflux
- Intravenous drug use
- Aspiration pneumonia
- Poor oral hygiene

Iatrogenic causes of pleural infection include any pleural intervention, especially repeated aspirations, thoracic surgery, oesophageal surgery, and oesophageal perforation.

Pathophysiology of pleural infection

Although the majority of parapneumonic effusions resolve with antibiotic treatment, some can progress through a fibrinopurulent stage to an empyema. Pro-inflammatory cytokines increase capillary vascular permeability resulting in fluid entering the pleural cavity. If the patient does not receive prompt antibiotics at this stage, then bacteria invade the pleural cavity, followed by neutrophils. There is activation of the coagulation cascade with deposition of fibrin, causing septation. The increased metabolic activity in the pleural space results in an increase in LDH, a decrease in the glucose content of the fluid, a lactic acidosis, and a decrease in the fluid pH. There is gradual organisation of the fluid with fibroblast proliferation and the formation of a pleural peel, which can encase the lung and reduce lung expansion.

Hypoalbuminaemia ($<30\,g\,l^{-1}$), thrombocytosis (platelet count $>400 \times 10\ 9\,l^{-1}$) and hyponatraemia (sodium <130 mmol/L) predispose to the development of an empyema.

Pleural infection should be suspected in any patient with a pneumonia who fails to improve after 3 days of antibiotic treatment, with continuing fever and high CRP. Table 10.4 describes the process whereby a simple parapneumonic effusion becomes an empyema.

Appendix 10.A describes how pleural fluid should be collected for analysis.

Management of pleural infection

Pleural infections can be complicated, have a high morbidity and mortality, and should be managed by a respiratory physician and a thoracic surgeon. Poor prognostic factors include older age, co-morbid disease, poor nutrition, and a serum albumin of less than $30\,g\,l^{-1}$.

Management

- Antibiotics
- Nutrition
- Thromboprophylaxis
- Intercostal chest drainage
- Surgical drainage

Antibiotics for pleural infection

Pleural fluid should be sent in a blood culture bottle as this increases the diagnostic yield of anaerobic infections. Samples will be culture positive in 60% of cases and this guides antibiotic treatment. When pleural fluid cultures are negative, blood cultures may be helpful in 15% of cases. Pleural fluid samples should always be stained for acid-fast bacilli (Ziehl-Neelsen stain) and sent for *Mycobacterium tuberculosis* culture.

Community acquired pleural infections are usually secondary to community acquired pneumonia. The commonest infections are Gram positive organisms, such as *Streptococcus milleri* and *Staphylococcus aureus*, which account for 65% of cases. Co-infection with anaerobic infections occurs in up to 76% of cases, often associated with aspiration pneumonia or poor dental hygiene and can have a more insidious onset. Gram-negative organisms, such as Enterobacteriaceae, *Escherichia coli* and *Haemophilus influenza*, can occur in patients with co-morbidities.

Hospital acquired pleural infections are often associated with pleural or other interventions. *Staphylococcus aureus* and methicillin-resistant *Staphylococcus aureus* (MRSA) infections account for two-thirds of these cases. Gram-negative infections, such as *Escherichia coli*, Enterobacter Spp and Pseudomonas Spp occur in older, immunocompromised patients and have a high morbidity and mortality. Fungal empyema, which is usually due to candida, is uncommon (<1%) and occurs in the immunocompromised.

Prompt antibiotics should be prescribed for empyema after discussion with the microbiologist, taking note of local prescribing guidelines and resistance patterns. Penicillin antibiotics with beta lactamase inhibitors, metronidazole and cephalosporins, which have good penetration into the pleural space, are usually the first choice. Patients with a penicillin allergy should be prescribed clindamycin. Macrolides are not usually required and aminoglycosides do not penetrate the pleural space well. Intravenous antibiotics should be given for at least 48 hours followed by oral antibiotics for up to 6 weeks, until there is complete resolution of symptoms, normalisation of inflammatory markers and radiological improvement. Intra-pleural antibiotics are not recommended.

Table 10.4 Pathophysiology of pleural infection.

Diagnostic tests	Simple parapneumonic effusion	Fibrinopurulent effusion	Empyema
Appearance of fluid	Clear	Turbid	Pus
Appearance on ultrasound	Fluid	Echogenic with septation and loculation	Fibrous pleural peel, multi-loculated with numerous septation
Appearance on CT scan	No pleural thickening	Pleural thickening in 56%	Pleural thickening in 86–100% Split pleura sign with enhancement of visceral and parietal pleura
Protein	$>30\,g\,l^{-1}$	$>30\,g\,l^{-1}$	$>30\,g\,l^{-1}$
LDH	50% of serum LDH	Raised	Markedly raised
Glucose	Normal	<2.2 mmol/L	<2.2 mmol/L
pH	7.6	<7.2	Unable to analyse
Differential cell count	Normal	Predominantly neutrophils	Predominantly neutrophils. If lymphocytes predominate, suspect mycobacterium tuberculosis infection
Organisms	None	Positive in 60%	Positive in 60%
Management	Antibiotics	Antibiotics and chest drain	Antibiotics and chest drain. Surgery for debridement and pleurodesis may be required

Indications for chest drain insertion in pleural infection

A chest drain should be considered in all patients who show no clinical improvement after 3 days of treatment with antibiotics, with continuing fever, high respiratory rate, and high CRP (Figure 10.5). Indications for a chest drain include pleural fluid pH < 7.2, frank pus in the pleural cavity, pleural fluid glucose of <2.2 mmol/L, and features of a complicated effusion on thoracic ultrasound, such as septation and loculation.

The BTS and the National Patient Safety Agency (NPSA) recommend that a small bore (10–14F) chest drain is inserted using thoracic ultrasound guidance (Figure 10.6). Regular flushing with 20–30 ml of normal saline every 6 hours, together with suction of −20 cm H_2O, is recommended.

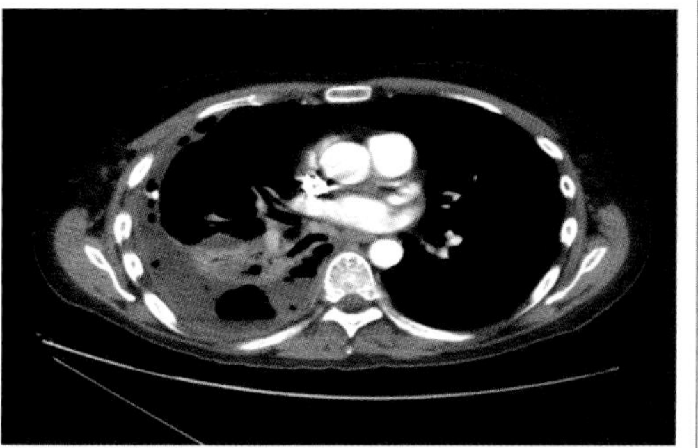

Figure 10.5 CT thorax showing right-sided empyema with inserted drain.

Indications for surgery for pleural infection

There are no clear, evidence-based guidelines as to when a patient with an infective pleural effusion should be referred for surgery, although there is some evidence that surgery may have better long-term outcome than more conservative approaches.

Patients who have clinical evidence of persistent sepsis and radiological evidence of infection despite antibiotics and a chest drain for more than 4 or 5 days should be discussed with a thoracic surgeon. A patient who is compromised because of a fibrinous peel causing compression of the lung may also warrant surgical decortication. The thoracic surgeon will need to decide between a VATS procedure and a thoracotomy with decortication depending on the fitness of the patient, their co-morbidities, and the extent of the pleural disease.

Intrapleural fibrinolytic drugs

The use of intrapleural fibrinolytic drugs in the management of pleural infection is controversial. A large British RCT did not find any long term benefit with intrapleural streptokinase, with no reduction in the need for surgical intervention, length of stay or mortality, but with significant side

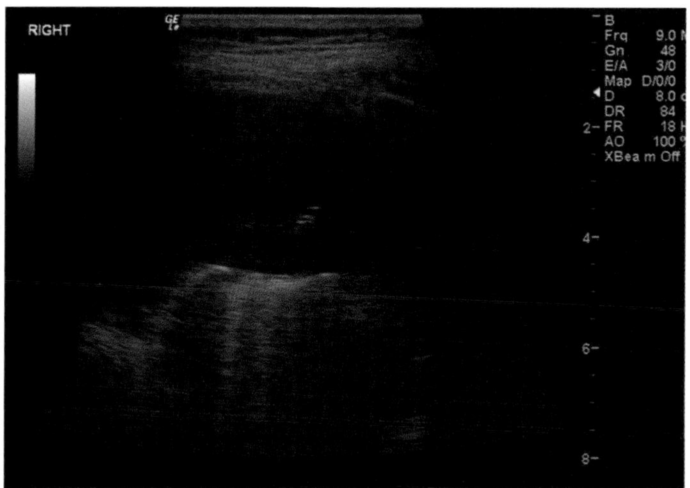

Figure 10.6 Thoracic ultrasound scan of empyema with air-bubbles post aspiration.

effects of fever and malaise. Some argue that this was because a heterogeneous group of patients, at various stages of organisation of the pleural fluid, were included. Several smaller RCTs using streptokinase and urokinase have reported benefits, with increased volume of fluid drained and reduced need for surgical decortication compared to placebo. A Cochrane meta-analysis with a small number of trials also concluded that intrapleural fibrinolytic drugs reduced the hospital stay, and resulted in radiological and symptomatic improvement.

The BTS recommendation is that intrapleural fibrinolytic drugs should not be given routinely to patients with pleural infection. However, fibrinolytic drugs could be used by experienced physicians in selected patients, for example, in elderly patients who have a complex, loculated effusion who are unfit for surgery.

Long term sequelae of pleural effusion secondary to pleural infection

Some 13% of patients with a pleural infection and empyema develop pleural thickening which can, over time, become calcified. In rare cases, a bronchopleural fistula can develop. An extensive fibrothorax can cause breathlessness and a restriction in breathing. If severe, patients may require surgical decortication.

Empyema necessitans results from a disruption of the parietal pleura, with spontaneous discharge of the pleural contents into the subcutaneous tissue of the chest wall. The commonest cause is *Mycobacterium tuberculosis*. Actinomycosis and aspergillus can also be the causative organisms. A CXR will show a soft tissue density. Management is surgical drainage and a prolonged course of antibiotics.

Mycobacterium tuberculosis *pleural effusion (tuberculous effusion)*

An exudative pleural effusion with a high lymphocyte count and low glucose is a common presentation of mycobacterium tuberculosis infection. The number of organisms in the fluid is very low, and acid-fast bacilli will be detected in less than 5% of cases. The pleural fluid culture has a slightly better yield of 10–20%.

If a tuberculous effusion is suspected, it is essential to obtain pleural biopsies for microbiological staining and culture. This will be positive in 70% of cases and will give information about drug sensitivities and resistance, thus dictating therapy. If TB is suspected, the pleural fluid should be sent for adenosine deaminase testing, an enzyme present in lymphocytes, which is elevated (>45 U l^{-1}) and has a sensitivity of 92% and specificity of 90%. This test may be a particularly useful in those with HIV or those who are immunosuppressed. Pleural fluid should also be sent for unstimulated interferon-gamma levels and PCR. Interferon-gamma release assays (IGRA) are more expensive and have not been validated for the diagnosis of pleural TB. TB is discussed in more detail in Chapter 8.

Rheumatoid arthritis pleural effusion

Although rheumatoid arthritis is commoner in women compared to men, pleural effusion associated with rheumatoid arthritis is commoner in men. Acute rheumatoid pleurisy can occur in 50% of cases and the exudate will have a very low glucose of <1.6 mmol/L, a high lymphocyte count, and low C4 complement levels. A chronic rheumatoid effusion may present as a pseudochylous effusion with a high cholesterol level and the presence of cholesterol crystals.

Pulmonary emboli and pleural effusion

A third of patients with a pulmonary embolus will develop either a unilateral, or bilateral small exudates. Pulmonary emboli should be suspected in patients whose symptoms of breathlessness are out of proportion to the size of the effusion. Thromboembolic disease is discussed in Chapter 11.

Chylothorax

Chylothorax is the accumulation of chyle, which is lymphatic fluid of intestinal origin, in the pleural cavity. It appears as a milky pleural fluid which remains milky after centrifuging. It occurs as the result of damage to the thoracic duct, often after thoracic surgery (particularly oesophageal), malignancy or disorders of the lymphatic system. The diagnosis is confirmed by the presence of chylomicrons in the pleural fluid or elevated triglyceride levels of >1.24 mmol/L. Lymphangiography and a CT scan are essential to identify where the lymph is coming from. Management depends on the cause and includes conservative management, drainage of chyle with pleurodesis, a period of fasting, a high protein-low fat diet supplemented by medium chain triglycerides, octreotide analogues, such as somatostatin, and surgical repair of the thoracic duct.

Pseudo chylothorax can occur in rheumatoid arthritis and with mycobacterium tuberculosis infection. The fluid appears milky, as with a chylothorax, but there are cholesterol crystals in the fluid.

Benign asbestos pleural effusion

This condition, unlike the other asbestos-related pleural diseases, has a much shorter latency period, occurring 10–20 years after asbestos exposure. It is also dose-related, so more likely to occur with a greater exposure to asbestos. The patient is usually asymptomatic and presents with a small, unilateral, bloody, effusion, which resolves within 6–12 months, leaving diffuse pleural thickening. As the differential diagnosis for this presentation includes mesothelioma, patients will require surgical pleural biopsies, perhaps several, and long term follow-up before mesothelioma can be excluded.

Idiopathic pleural effusion

In about 8% of cases no obvious cause for the effusion is identified. Most of these will resolve spontaneously.

Pneumothorax

Definition

A pneumothorax is air in the pleural space, either from air leaking through a hole in the lung or from a penetrating chest injury. The sudden entry of air into the pleural space causes collapse of the underlying lung.

Primary spontaneous pneumothorax (PSP)

The incidence of primary spontaneous pneumothorax is 10/100 000/year, with a male to female ratio of 5 : 1. PSP occurs in patients with apparently normal lungs, although high resolution CT scan shows apical sub-pleural blebs and bullae in 90% of cases (Box 10.6). The aetiology of these blebs is unclear.

PSP is commonest in tall, thin men between the ages of 20–40 years because there is more negative intrapleural pressure at the apex of the lung causing the blebs to burst.

Box 10.6 Risk factors for primary spontaneous pneumothorax.

- Tall and thin
- Asthma
- Smoking
- Collagen vascular disease, for example, Marfan's disease
- Trauma
- Occupational, for example, deep sea diving

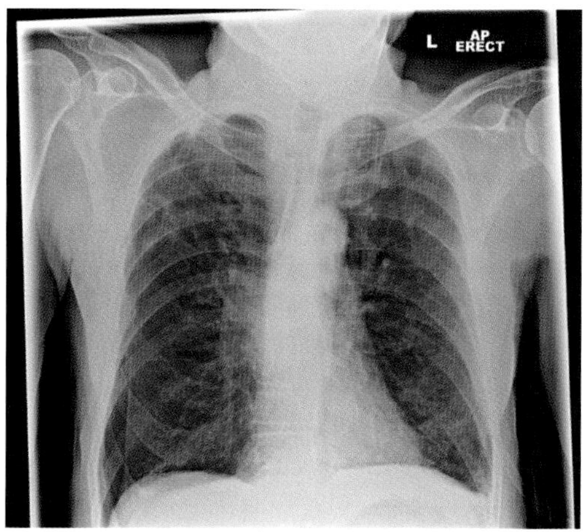

Figure 10.7 CXR of a small, unilateral (right-sided) pneumothorax.

Those over 1.9 m in height have a greater incidence. Smoking increases the risk of a pneumothorax significantly, probably by the development of small bullae and secondary to obstruction of small airways (Figure 10.7, Figure 10.8). There is no association with physical exertion.

Secondary pneumothorax (SP)

SP occurs in individuals with underlying chronic lung disease. The incidence of SP is 17/100 000 in males and 6/100 000 in females. Patients with SP are considerably older than those with PSP, with more significant co-morbidities. They have little respiratory reserve, so are often unable to tolerate even a small pneumothorax. The morbidity and mortality of a secondary pneumothorax are, therefore, much greater, with patients developing respiratory failure. Box 10.7 lists those conditions

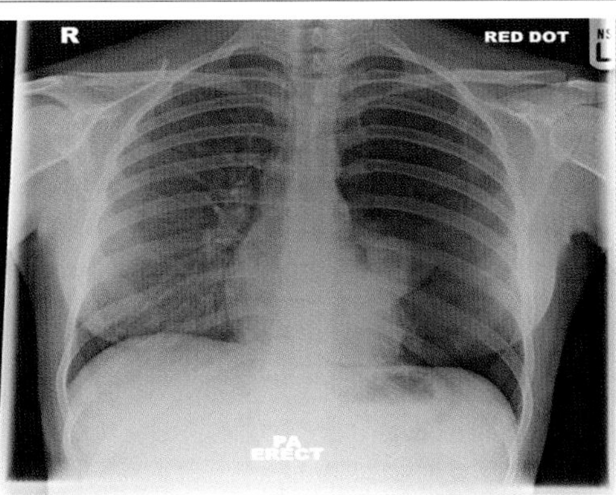

Figure 10.8 CXR showing a large, left-sided pneumothorax with complete collapse of the left lung.

Box 10.7 Lung conditions predisposing to the development of a pneumothorax.

- Chronic obstructive pulmonary disease (COPD)
- Chronic asthma
- Interstitial lung disease (ILD)
- Lymphangioleiomyomatosis (LAM)
- Pulmonary Langerhans cell histiocytosis (PLCH)
- Cystic fibrosis
- *Mycobacterium tuberculosis*
- HIV, particularly with pneumocystis jiroveci infection
- Catamenial pneumothorax

that predispose to developing pneumothorax. Interventional procedures can also result in pneumothorax. Box 10.8 lists these.

Clinical presentation of pneumothorax

Box 10.9 details some important points in the history of pneumothorax.

Patients with a tension pneumothorax will present with collapse and cardiac arrest. This is a clinical diagnosis requiring immediate insertion of a needle. The emergency management of a tension pneumothorax is discussed later in the chapter.

The clinical history is not a reliable indicator of the size of the pneumothorax (Box 10.10). Patients with PSP may not be excessively breathless and 40–50% of patients wait for more than two days before they seek medical attention. These patients may be at risk of re-expansion pulmonary oedema when the lung is re-inflated. Patients with even a small secondary pneumothorax may be very breathless because of their underlying lung disease

Box 10.8 Iatrogenic causes of pneumothorax.

- Percutaneous needle biopsy of lung
- Transbronchial biopsy
- Pleural aspiration
- Pleural biopsy
- Subclavian line insertion
- Central line insertion
- Percutaneous liver biopsy
- Mechanical ventilation on ICU
- Tension pneumothorax can occur after CPR, NIV or hyperbaric oxygen treatment

Box 10.9 Important points in the history.

- Pleuritic chest pain, sudden in onset and unilateral
- Breathlessness
- Associated symptoms, such as cough
- Smoking history
- Underlying lung disease
- Occupational history, such as diving
- Trauma
- Previous pneumothorax

Box 10.10 Clinical signs of pneumothorax.

- Tachypnoea
- Tachycardia
- Decreased air entry on side of pneumothorax
- Hyper-resonance on side of pneumothorax
- Hamman's sign, a click heard on auscultation due to movement of pleural surfaces with a left-sided pneumothorax
- Severe signs of respiratory distress with tracheal deviation, mediastinal shift, distended neck veins, cyanosis, and hypotension heralding cardiac arrest in a tension pneumothorax

and older age. As the management depends on whether it is a primary or secondary pneumothorax, this distinction needs to be made at the beginning of treatment.

Investigations for a pneumothorax

- Chest X-ray: postero-anterior (PA), lateral or lateral decubitus
- Oxygen saturation on air
- Arterial blood gas on air
- High-resolution computed tomography (HRCT).

A PA CXR usually confirms the diagnosis of a pneumothorax. There will be an area of hypolucency, with a pleural line running parallel to the chest wall and no lung markings. There may also be blunting of the costophrenic angle due to bleeding into the pleural space. If there is doubt and the clinical suspicion is high, then a lateral or lateral decubitus CXR may be helpful. An expiratory CXR is not recommended. When there is underlying chronic lung disease, it may be difficult to distinguish between a small pneumothorax and a bulla. In these cases, it is essential to organise an urgent high-resolution CT thorax (HRCT) prior to any intervention.

The PaO_2 is <10.9 kPa in 75% of patients with a pneumothorax and 16% of patients with secondary pneumothorax will develop type 2 respiratory failure, with PaO_2 < 7.5 kPa and $PaCO_2$ > 6.9 kPa.

Classification of pneumothorax

- Small: if the rim of air is <2 cm between the edge of the lung and the chest wall at the level of the hilum.
- Large: if the rim of air is >2 cm between the edge of the lung and the chest wall at the level of the hilum.

As the volume of the pneumothorax approximates to the ratio of the cube of the lung diameter to the diameter of the hemithorax, the appearance on the CXR underestimates the volume of lung involved. A 1 cm pneumothorax occupies 27% of the hemithorax volume and a 2 cm pneumothorax occupies 49% of the hemithorax volume (Figure 10.9).

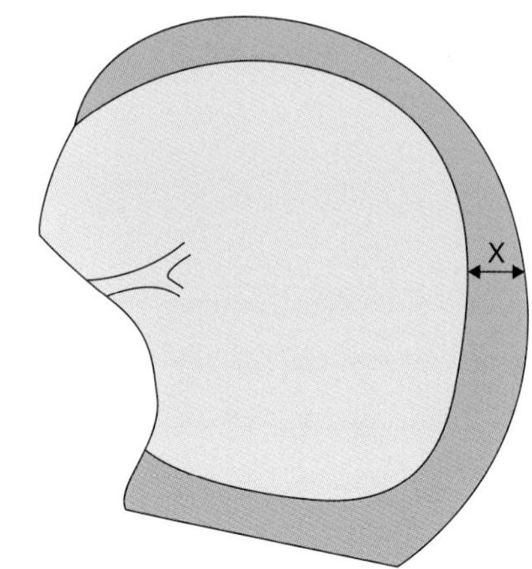

X = Interpleural distance at the level of the hilum

Figure 10.9 Measurement of the size of a pneumothorax from BTS Guidelines.

Management of pneumothorax

The management of a pneumothorax will depend on

- Whether it is a primary or secondary pneumothorax
- Whether the patient is symptomatic or not
- The age of patient
- Associated co-morbidities
- The size of the pneumothorax, although this is less important than the amount of clinical compromise

Management of primary spontaneous pneumothorax (PSP)

Most young patients with a PSP have minimal symptoms and tolerate a pneumothorax well. Young patients (<50 years) with a small pneumothorax (<2 cm), who are not breathless, could be discharged from hospital with clear written advice about returning if they should become symptomatic (Box 10.11). These patients should be reviewed in the respiratory clinic with a repeat CXR to ensure that the pneumothorax has resolved and to identify any underlying lung abnormalities. An HRCT may be necessary to identify early, minor abnormalities. Patients should also be carefully assessed to identify any risk factors, including features of Marfan's disease or other collagen vascular disease. Patients with asthma should have lung function testing and asthma treatment optimised. Smokers should be encouraged and supported to stop smoking, prescribed appropriate pharmacological support, and referred to a smoking cessation clinic.

Box 10.11 Written advice to patients on discharge after pneumothorax.

- Advise the patient to return immediately to the emergency department if the symptoms recur
- Advise the patient to stop smoking
- Advise the patient to avoid flying for at least one week after complete resolution of pneumothorax on CXR or two weeks for a traumatic pneumothorax
- Advise the patient to avoid deep sea diving unless they have had a definite bilateral surgical procedure and have satisfactory lung function test and CT scan at follow-up
- Patients with a SP may be at risk of a recurrent pneumothorax for one year. Patients who have had a definitive surgical procedure have a lower risk. Patients with lymphangioleiomyomatosis (LAM) are at increased risk

A small pneumothorax spontaneously resolves at a rate of 1–2% each day, with a median of 8 days for complete resolution. A large pneumothorax can take several weeks to resolve completely. The risk of recurrence is 40% in the first two years and is greater in those who smoke. The risk of recurrence increases with each subsequent pneumothorax, and up to 60% after a third pneumothorax.

Older patients with a small pneumothorax who are not breathless can be observed in hospital with high flow oxygen and have a repeat CXR to ensure that the pneumothorax has not enlarged.

Patients who are breathless should be admitted, given high flow oxygen ($10\,L\,min^{-1}$), given analgesia for the chest pain, and should undergo a simple aspiration with a 16F cannula inserted into the second intercostal space in the mid-clavicular line which is connected to a three-way tap. The cannula can also be inserted in the 8th, 9th or 10th intercostal space in the mid-axillary line. Aspiration should be continued until there is resistance to aspiration or until >2.5 L of air is aspirated as this suggests a persistent air leak from a bronchopleural fistula. Aspiration should also be stopped if the patient coughs or complains of worsening chest pain. A CXR should always be performed after an aspiration to ensure that there has been resolution of the pneumothorax. Inhalation of oxygen reduces the partial pressure of nitrogen in the blood and increases the absorption of air from the pleural cavity, thus expediting resolution.

Success rates for aspiration in PSP are between 50% and 69%. If the first aspiration is not successful, then a repeat aspiration is not recommended according to BTS Guidelines unless there was a technical reason for the failure. However, it is worth noting that a second aspiration is successful in a third of patients with a PSP. Aspiration is not recommended for very small pneumothorax of <1 cm as there is a risk of injury to the lung and the development of a larger pneumothorax.

Intercostal chest drain insertion for pneumothorax

If the aspiration fails, a small (8–14F) intercostal chest drain should be inserted in the triangle of safety using a Seldinger technique. There is no evidence that a large drain (20–24F) is any better than a small drain (8–14F). The drain should be attached to an underwater sealed unit. Swinging of the drain indicates that it is in the pleural space, and bubbling on inspiration and coughing will confirm the drainage of air. A CXR is necessary to ensure that the drain is in an optimal position.

Management of secondary pneumothorax (SP)

Most patients with SP will be symptomatic because of their underlying lung disease and poor respiratory reserve. The commonest cause of a SP is COPD. In these patients it can sometimes be difficult to differentiate between a small pneumothorax and a bulla and it would be catastrophic to put a chest drain into a bulla (Figure 10.10, Figure 10.11). These patients should have an urgent HRCT to confirm the presence of a pneumothorax and should be discussed with a respiratory physician prior to any intervention.

A small SP (<2 cm) could be managed with simple aspiration. However, the majority are likely to require an intercostal chest drain (as above for PSP). If there is a large and persistent air leak, a larger drain may be necessary, especially in a ventilated patient on ICU.

Rates of pneumothorax recurrence correlate with age and are particularly high in patients with severe emphysema, cystic fibrosis, LAM, and PLCH.

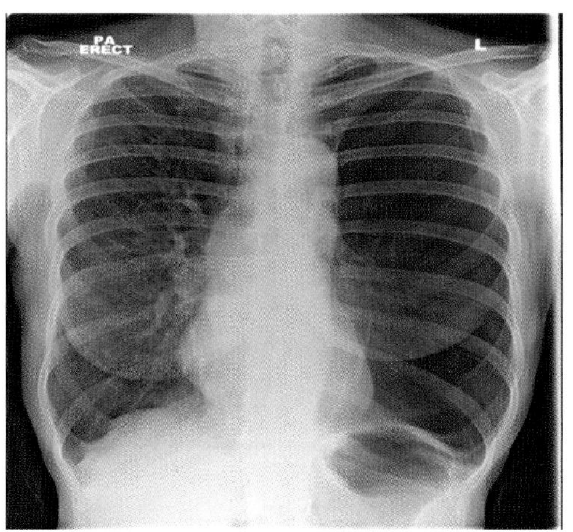

Figure 10.10 CXR showing a large, left-sided emphysematous bulla.

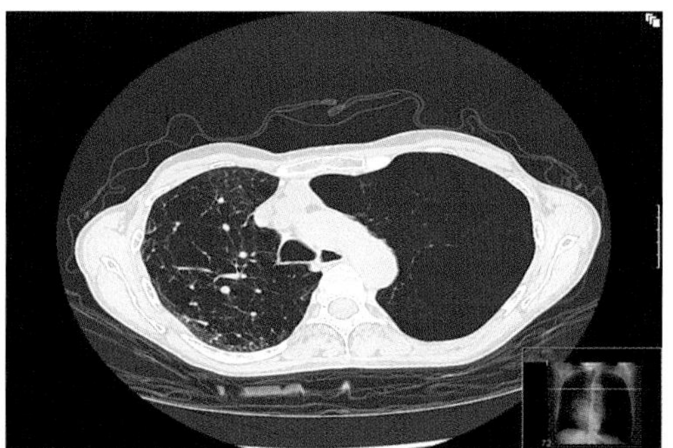

Figure 10.11 CT thorax showing a large, left-sided emphysematous bulla.

Management of patients with a chest drain for pneumothorax

Patients should be observed carefully on a specialist ward with nurses who are trained to manage chest drains. High flow oxygen should be prescribed if not contra-indicated by the development of type 2 respiratory failure. Analgesia should always be prescribed as chest drain insertion is painful. As the air in the pleural space comes out through the drain into the sealed bottle with sterile water, there will be bubbling of air. The chest drain should never be clamped because of the risk of creating a tension pneumothorax. Patients should be clinically reviewed daily to see whether their breathing is back to normal and whether their chest drain has stopped bubbling. A CXR will be necessary to see if the lung has come up. If the chest drain is not swinging or bubbling but the CXR shows a persistent pneumothorax, then the drain should be checked to ensure that it is not kinked or that it has not been displaced.

Suction using a high volume, low pressure system (–10 to –20 cm H_2O) is recommended if there is continued air leak (bubbling) 48 hours after chest drain insertion. This removes air from the pleural cavity and helps the parietal and visceral pleural surfaces to come together. Suctioning before 48 hours is not recommended as this may precipitate the development of re-expansion pulmonary oedema which can occasionally affect the contralateral lung. This serious, and occasionally fatal, complication is commonest in young patients who present late with a large pneumothorax and therefore have had the collapsed lung for several days. This can occur in up to 14% of cases and presents with cough and breathlessness. It usually resolves without treatment in most cases. Once the pneumothorax has resolved, the chest drain can be removed, sutures inserted if necessary, and a sterile dressing placed.

Complications of chest drain for pneumothorax

Complications of chest drain for pneumothorax include surgical emphysema, with air tracking subcutaneously due to pressure from the pleural space. This is more likely if there is an air leak, if the chest drain is displaced, or if there is significant underlying lung disease. A crackling sensation can be felt on palpating the chest wall and neck, and a crunch can be heard on auscultation. High flow oxygen and re-positioning of the chest drain will result in resolution in most cases. Severe surgical emphysema can cause upper airway obstruction and respiratory distress and may require skin incision decompression (Figure 10.12).

In a significant number of patients, particularly with a secondary pneumothorax, the pneumothorax will not resolve. These patients should be referred to a respiratory physician. A thoracic surgical opinion should be sought in patients who have a persistent air leak for more than 4 days.

Surgery for persistent pneumothorax

The aim of surgery is to repair the damaged pleura and obliterate the pleural space in patients with a persistent air leak or when the lung fails to

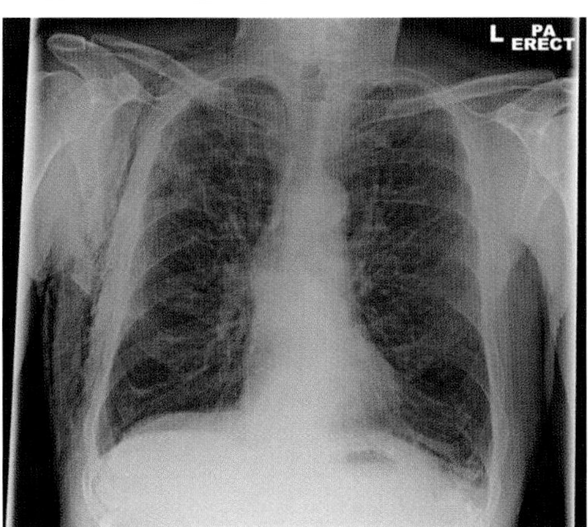

Figure 10.12 CXR showing surgical emphysema.

re-expand several days after drain insertion. Surgical intervention may also be indicated in patients who have had more than two pneumothoraces on the same side, in those who develop bilateral pneumothoraces, or who have an underlying lung disease that predisposes to the development of a pneumothorax.

Open thoracotomy with resection of apical blebs, pleural abrasion, or apico-lateral pleurectomy has a recurrence rate of only 1% without compromising lung function. However, it is a major procedure with a hospital stay of a few days. VATS pleural abrasion with pleurectomy is better tolerated with a shorter hospital stay, but has a recurrence rate of 4%. Surgical pleurodesis with talc can also be considered although it is less effective than pleural abrasion and there is a risk of ARDS and emphysema. These procedures do not compromise future lung transplantation in patients with cystic fibrosis, LAM, or PLCH.

Patients who have a persistent air leak but are unfit for surgery could have a bedside chemical pleurodesis, although this has a failure rate of 10–20%. An alternative would be to have a Heimlich flutter valve which will allow the patient to mobilise and to go home.

Traumatic pneumothorax

A traumatic pneumothorax, usually the result of rib fractures, may be complicated by haemothorax and other injuries. Such patients should be looked after by the Trauma Team. Traumatic pneumothorax may also be complicated by pneumomediastinum and/or pneumopericardium. Figure 10.13 shows the BTS algorithm for the management of a primary and a secondary pneumothorax.

Tension pneumothorax

A tension pneumothorax occurs when air leaks into the pleural space during inspiration but is not able to re-enter the lung on expiration because the hole in the lung behaves like a valve. This results in accumulation of air in the pleural cavity which gradually compresses the lungs and the mediastinal structures, causing tracheal and mediastinal shift away from the side of the pneumothorax. Eventually the pressure on the heart impedes venous return with a reduction in cardiac output, resulting in a cardiac arrest, usually of the pulseless electrical activity type.

A tension pneumothorax is a medical emergency. The patient will present with severe dyspnoea, tachycardia, and will collapse. Clinical examination will reveal reduced air entry on the side of the pneumothorax with hyper-resonance on percussion and signs of mediastinal shift away from the side of the pneumothorax, such as deviated trachea and displaced apex beat.

Management of tension pneumothorax

As with all respiratory emergencies, the airways, breathing, and circulation should be assessed. If the clinical diagnosis is one of a tension pneumothorax, a 16G cannula attached to a 20 ml syringe containing 5 ml saline should be inserted into the second intercostal space in the mid-clavicular line on the side of the pneumothorax without delay. The plunger should be removed from the syringe and a hissing sound will indicate that it is in the correct position and that air is leaking out.

Intravenous access should be gained, the patient given high flow oxygen and arterial blood gas measurement obtained. A CXR should be performed to confirm the size of the pneumothorax once the patient is stable. An intercostal chest drain, using the Seldinger technique, should be inserted as soon as possible.

Recurrent pneumothorax

More than one pneumothorax, either on the same side or on the contralateral side, will warrant referral to the thoracic surgeon for consideration of

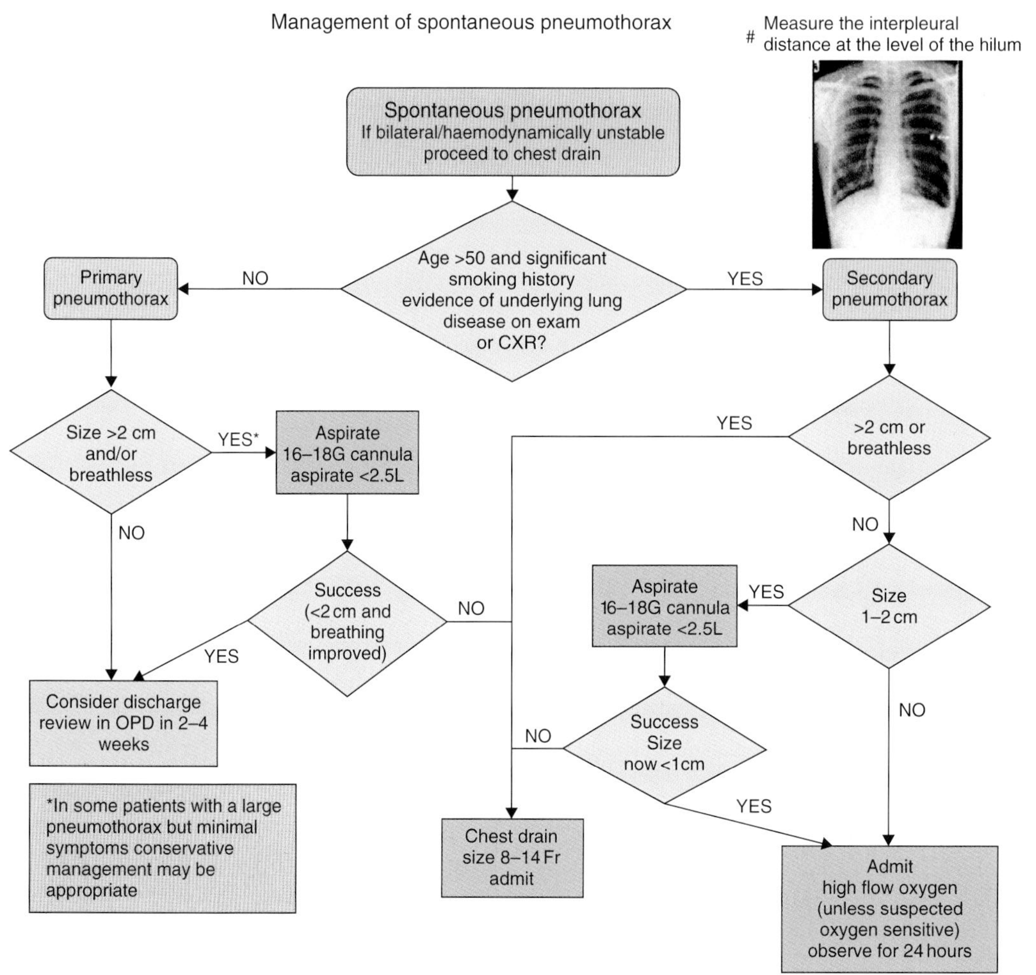

Figure 10.13 BTS algorithm for management of primary and secondary pneumothorax.

VATS pleural abrasion, talc pleurodesis, pleurectomy, or bullectomy. The risk of recurrence of a primary pneumothorax is 54% within the first 4 years and increases up to 60% after the third pneumothorax.

Catamenial pneumothorax occurs during menstruation and may be due to pleural endometriosis. This should be considered in young women with recurrent pneumothoraces. Surgical intervention, together with hormonal management, may be required.

There is an increased risk of pneumothorax in pregnancy. The woman should be looked after by both the respiratory physician, and the obstetrician. Management should be conservative, if possible, or with simple aspiration. Patients should have a caesarean section with regional anaesthesia as near term as possible.

Asbestos-related pleural disease

Asbestos is a common cause of a variety of pleural diseases, benign and malignant. Patients should always be questioned in detail about their possible exposure to asbestos.

Benign pleural plaque

Benign pleural plaques, caused by thickening of the parietal pleura, are the commonest manifestation of asbestos exposure. The pleural plaques can occur all over the parietal pleural surface but are commonest on the postero-lateral chest wall, over the mediastinal pleura, and on the dome of the diaphragm. These occur in 50% of those exposed to asbestos and develop 20–30 years after exposure to asbestos, but not in a dose-dependent way. They can calcify heavily (Figure 10.14). Pleural plaques are usually asymptomatic and identified incidentally on a chest X-ray. Rarely, if the pleural plaques are extensive and calcified, they can result in restriction of the thoracic cavity and breathlessness (Figure 10.15). There is no evidence that pleural plaques predispose to the development of mesothelioma. Patients with benign pleural plaques are not eligible for compensation.

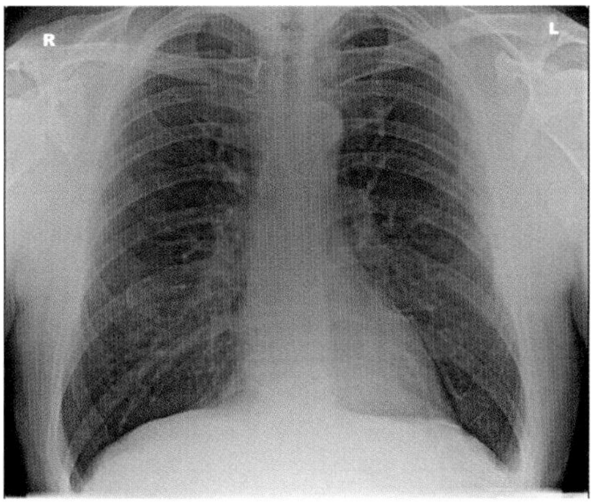

Figure 10.14 CXR showing benign, calcified, pleural plaques.

The differential diagnosis for unilateral calcified pleural plaque includes previous tuberculous effusion or secondary to a haemothorax.

Diffuse pleural thickening

Asbestos exposure can result in adhesion of the visceral and parietal pleura, with obliteration of the pleural space and fibrosis. This process can be extensive and involve much of the pleural surface, including the costophrenic angles, the apices, and the inter-lobar fissures. This occurs in a dose-dependent way and may follow recurrent asbestos pleurisy.

Patients with diffuse pleural thickening may present with breathlessness and pleuritic chest pain. A chest X-ray and a contrast CT scan will show smooth pleural thickening with no enhancement (Figure 10.16).

Pulmonary function testing may show a restrictive process. As the differential diagnosis for pleural thickening includes mesothelioma, these patients will need a pleural biopsy and careful monitoring. Management is symptomatic as there is no definite treatment that will reverse this process. Patients with diffuse pleural thickening are eligible for compensation (see Appendix 10.B).

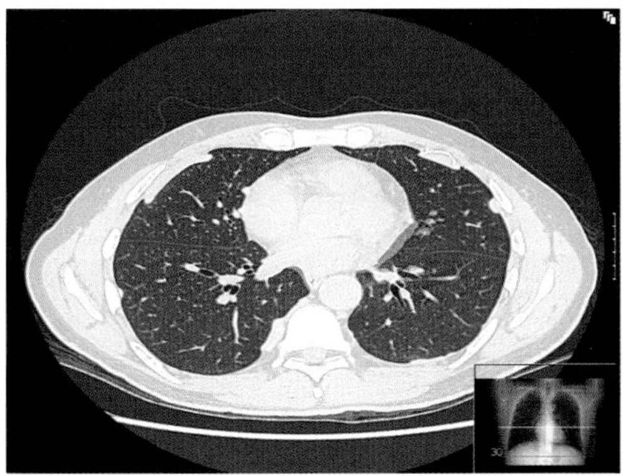

Figure 10.15 CT thorax showing benign, calcified pleural plaques.

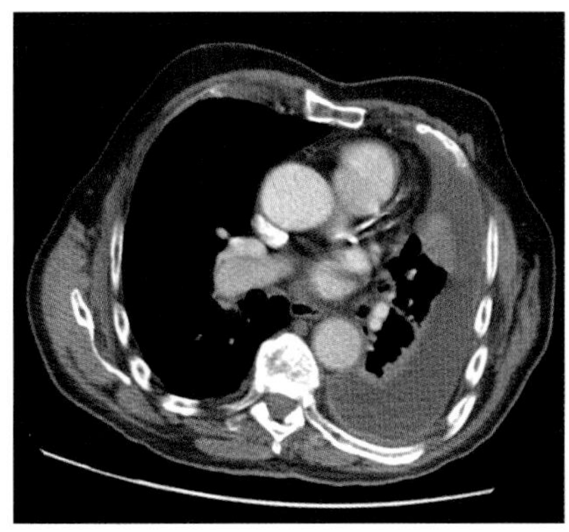

Figure 10.16 CT thorax showing left-sided pleural thickening.

Benign asbestos-related pleural effusion

Rounded atelectasis (folded lung/ Blesovsky syndrome)

Rounded atelectasis can develop secondary to any cause of pleural fibrosis, including asbestos. Contraction of fibrotic areas of the visceral pleura can entrap a segment of lung and twist it into a distinctive, rounded, pleural-based mass of 2.5–5 cm in diameter, which can appear like a solitary pulmonary nodule (SPN) (Figure 10.17, Figure 10.18). Patients are usually asymptomatic. A contrast CT scan shows a characteristic "comet-tail" appearance of vessels and bronchi converging towards lesion and adjacent thickened pleura (Figure 10.19). There may be volume loss in the affected lobe.

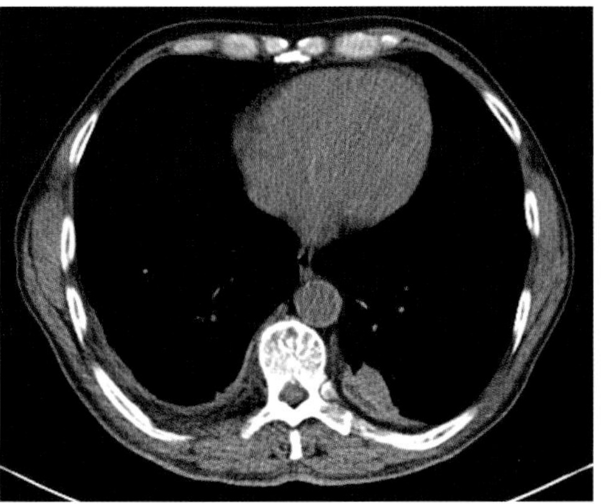

Figure 10.17 CT thorax showing round atelectasis with adjacent left-sided pleural thickening (mediastinal window).

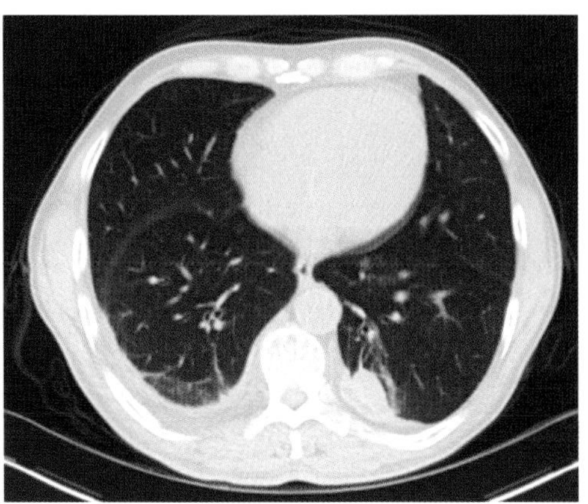

Figure 10.18 CT thorax showing round atelectasis with adjacent left-sided pleural thickening (parenchymal window).

Asbestosis, pulmonary fibrosis caused by inhalation of asbestos fibres, is discussed in Chapter 15.

Mesothelioma

Mesothelioma is a malignant tumour of the pleura with a poor prognosis and median survival of 8–14 months from diagnosis. In rare cases, the tumour can arise in the peritoneum, pericardium, or tunica vaginalis. Peritoneal mesothelioma, which occurs after prolonged asbestos exposure, presents with abdominal pain, ascites, and weight loss. It has a median survival of 7 months.

- **Incidence and prevalence:** The Mesothelioma Register was established in the 1960s. The number of cases of malignant mesothelioma continues to increase, with approximately 2000 deaths per year in the UK. It is estimated that the number of new cases will peak around 2020, after which time numbers are likely to decrease in the UK, reflecting the ban on asbestos use in the 1970s. The prevalence of mesothelioma is likely to be much greater in developing countries where asbestos is still widely used.
- **Age:** mesothelioma commonly presents in people aged between 50 and 70 years. It has been known to occur very rarely in children.
- **Male: Female:** mesothelioma is commoner in men as it is due to occupational exposure to asbestos in 90% of cases. It accounts for 0.7% of all deaths in men born in the late 1930s and early1940s.

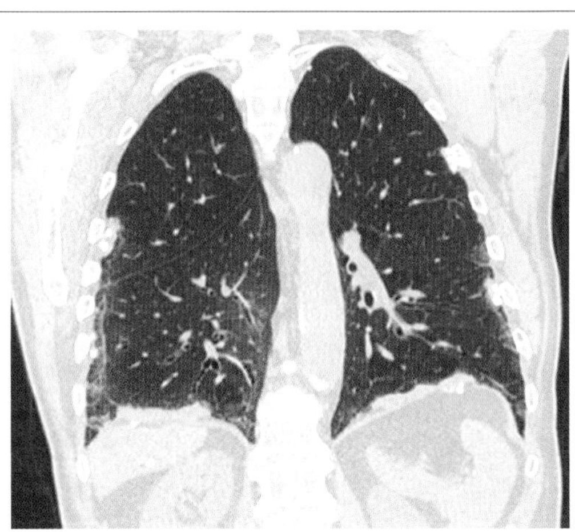

Figure 10.19 Coronal reconstruction of CT thorax showing sub-pleural reticulation and multiple, bilateral, calcified pleural plaques.

Women exposed to asbestos while washing their husbands' work clothes have also been known to develop mesothelioma. Ambient asbestos levels in the environment are low, but many old buildings, including schools, have asbestos.

- **Geographical variation:** the incidence of mesothelioma is higher in areas of shipbuilding, railway construction, asbestos manufacture and building construction.
- The **responsibility of employers** towards their employees in these industries is laid out in the Control of Asbestos Regulations 2006 (Statutory Instrument 2006 No. 2739).

Aetiology of mesothelioma

Asbestos, a naturally occurring material formed of crystalline hydrated silicates in fibrous form, was used extensively because it was cheap and resistant to acid, alkali, and heat. Box 10.10 lists the occupations associated with asbestos exposure. Inhalation of asbestos fibres can be attributed to be the cause of mesothelioma in up to 90% of cases. The latency period from first exposure to developing mesothelioma ranges from 15 to 67 years, with a median of 32 years, although the development is not dose-related.

Chrysotile, white asbestos with a serpentine structure, was the most commonly used asbestos type in construction. It clears rapidly from the lungs, so has a low risk of malignancy. Crocidolite, blue asbestos with an amphibole structure, takes longer to be degraded from the lungs and has a higher risk of malignancy, even with lower exposure. Erionite, a non-asbestos fibre found in rock in some areas of Turkey, appears to cause mesothelioma in up to 25% of residents in that region.

Pathophysiology of mesothelioma

It is postulated that asbestos fibres are inhaled, reach the terminal bronchioles, irritate the pleura, and damage the DNA, resulting in genetic changes. Mesothelioma arises from sub-mesothelial cells which proliferate and grow as a rind around the chest wall. The tumour invades locally into the mediastinum, pericardium, chest wall, and diaphragm. At an advanced stage, the tumour can spread haematogenously to distant sites.

A full occupational history, detailing all the jobs the patient has ever done, should be obtained. The patient should be questioned specifically about professions associated with asbestos exposure (Box 10.12). The chest pain may be referred to the shoulder or abdomen, may be pleuritic in nature, or have a neuropathic component if intercostal, thoracic, or brachial plexus nerves are involved. Box 10.13 lists the symptoms of mesothelioma and Box 10.14 lists the clinical signs of mesothelioma.

Box 10.12 Occupations associated with asbestos exposure.

- Construction: insulation, fireproofing, electrical, lagging, plumbing, welding, carpentry
- Shipbuilding
- Brake lining
- Mining
- Milling asbestos fibres

Investigations in the diagnosis of malignant mesothelioma

A **CXR** will show a unilateral pleural effusion in 90% of cases. The differential diagnosis includes benign asbestos pleural effusion and lung cancer (adenocarcinoma) with pleural metastases. The CXR may also show pleural thickening, a lobulated pleural mass, volume loss, and a contracted hemithorax. Bilateral pleural involvement is rare.

Box 10.13 Symptoms of mesothelioma.

- Dull, persistent, and progressively worsening chest pain
- Worsening breathlessness
- Weight loss
- Lethargy
- Excessive sweating
- Fever
- Cough
- Hoarseness
- Dysphagia

Box 10.14 Clinical signs in mesothelioma.

- Clubbing of fingers (<1%)
- Signs consistent with a unilateral pleural effusion
- Volume loss on the side of the effusion
- Cachexia
- Pericardial involvement resulting in cardiac tamponade
- Superior vena cava obstruction

A **contrast CT scan** usually shows a unilateral pleural effusion with enhancing, nodular, circumferential pleural thickening of >1 cm which may involve the mediastinal pleura, the pericardium, and the diaphragm. This can result in volume loss and contraction of the hemithorax. Mesothelioma can also appear as a lobulated pleural mass with lymphadenopathy (Figure 10.20, Figure 10.21). The CT scan is poor at distinguishing mediastinal nodal metastases from adjacent mediastinal pleural involvement. A mediastinoscopy will be required for accurate staging if surgery is being contemplated. Local invasion of chest wall can also be seen on a CT scan. In 20% of patients with mesothelioma, there will other radiological signs of asbestos exposure, such as pleural plaques or interstitial fibrosis.

An **MRI** may provide additional anatomical information when there is chest wall invasion. There will be enhancement with gadolinium-based contrast material. This may useful if surgery is being contemplated.

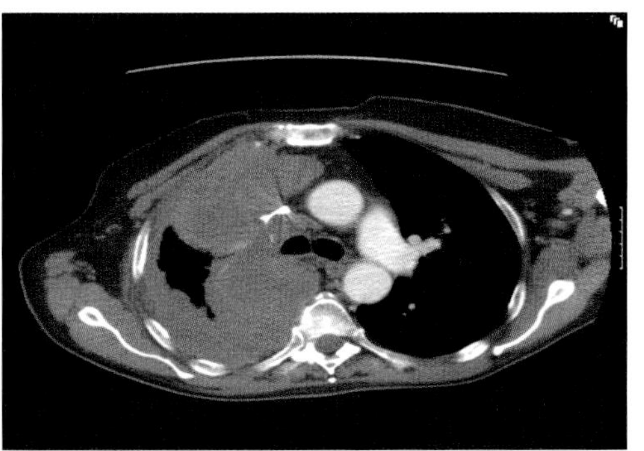

Figure 10.20 CT thorax showing right-sided malignant mesothelioma associated with external compression of the superior vena cava.

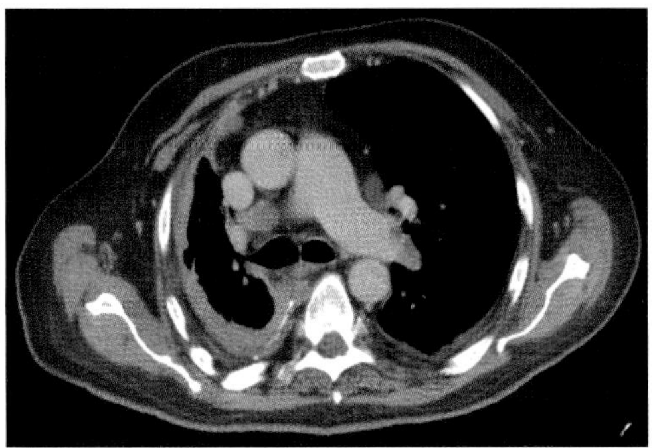

Figure 10.21 CT thorax showing right-sided malignant mesothelioma.

A **PET-CT** can be helpful when pleural biopsies have been negative as areas of FDG uptake may guide the surgeon to where to take further biopsies. A PET-CT is also important for accurate staging when surgery is being considered. However, false positive FDG uptake can occur with parapneumonic effusions and false negative results can occur with sarcomatoid mesothelioma.

Ultrasound guided pleural aspiration will reveal an exudate which is often blood-stained. Pleural cytology is positive in 50% of cases but it can be difficult to differentiate between reactive mesothelial cells, malignant mesothelial cells, and adenocarcinoma of the lung. Immunocytochemistry, using a panel of antibodies applied to cell blocks obtained from pleural fluid, may differentiate between mesothelioma cells and metastatic adenocarcinoma cells. Positive staining for calretinin, epithelial membrane antigen (EMA) and CK5/6 suggests epithelioid mesothelioma, whereas adenocarcinoma is CEA and TTF 1 positive.

Mesothelin levels may be elevated in the pleural fluid and blood of patients with malignant mesothelioma, although the sensitivity is only 48–84% and the specificity is 70–100%. False negative results occur in sarcomatoid mesothelioma and false positive results in adenocarcinoma, pancreatic carcinoma, lymphoma, and ovarian cancer. Soluble mesothelin-related protein (SMRP) levels are increased in mesothelioma with a sensitivity of 84%, but this is only used in clinical trials currently.

Pleural biopsy

A pleural biopsy is necessary in most cases to establish a firm histological diagnosis of mesothelioma. This will determine the course of treatment, the prognosis, and is helpful when seeking compensation. A VATS pleural biopsy is usually definitive and has the best yield as the tumour appears as white nodules on the parietal pleura on direct visualisation. The VATS procedure also has the advantage that a pleurodesis can be carried out at the same time, reducing the risk of recurrence of the effusion.

If the patient is not fit for surgery, then a medical thoracoscopy with a local anaesthetic and sedation can be attempted. If this is not available, then a CT-guided pleural biopsy should be considered. A blind Abram's biopsy is not recommended. The number of attempts at pleural aspiration should be limited as seeding of tumour in the subcutaneous tissue can occur, causing pain.

It is common to have negative pleural biopsies with mesothelioma, and repeat pleural biopsies may be required over a period of months to confirm the diagnosis if there is clinical suspicion. A mediastinoscopy may be required to sample mediastinal nodes as part of staging if surgery is being considered as CT and PET-CT are not good at detecting tumour involvement of mediastinal nodes.

Pathological types of malignant mesothelioma

- Epithelioid (50–70%)
- Sarcomatoid (10–15%)
- Mixed (biphasic) (20–40%)

Within each of these histological types there are several subtypes, but these do not have any prognostic significance. Sarcomatoid mesothelioma has a particularly aggressive course and a poor prognosis, with median time from diagnosis to death of only 6 months. Poor prognostic features include trans-diaphragmatic spread, involvement of mediastinal lymph nodes, male gender, poor performance status, and sarcomatoid histology.

Management of malignant mesothelioma

Currently there is no curative treatment available, and limited evidence of benefit with surgery, chemotherapy, or radiotherapy. Once the diagnosis of mesothelioma is confirmed, the patient should be discussed at the lung multidisciplinary meeting and referred to a specialist centre with expertise in managing mesothelioma.

The patient and their relatives should be given verbal and written information about the diagnosis and prognosis, as well as information about compensation. The patient should be referred to the palliative care team for symptom control and be followed up by the lung cancer or mesothelioma nurse specialist. Patients with mesothelioma will benefit from counselling, rehabilitation, complementary therapies, referral to social services, and to Macmillan Cancer Support. After death, all patients should be referred for a Coroner's post mortem.

See Appendix 10.B for details on obtaining compensation. See Chapter 9 for details on the lung MDT.

Palliative care

Pain should be managed with opioids, non-steroidal anti-inflammatory drugs (with proton pump cover) and steroids. Neuropathic pain can be managed with carbamazepine, amitriptyline, or gabapentin. When there is persistent pain due to chest wall invasion, the patient should be referred to a specialist pain service for consideration of nerve blocks (intercostal, paravertebral, or brachial plexus), intrapleural, epidural or intrathecal analgesic infusions or percutaneous cervical cordotomy. Transcutaneous electrical nerve stimulation (TENS) machines may help. Palliative radiotherapy has been shown to improve pain in 60–90% of patients.

Dyspnoea can be difficult to manage and does not respond to palliative radiotherapy. Opioids, steroids, and oxygen may be required. Drainage of the pleural effusion with talc pleurodesis, undertaken at the same time as the pleural biopsy, can improve breathlessness. If the patient is frail, pleurodesis can be done via a small bore (16–18F) intercostal drain. Sometimes, a chronic pleural effusion can result in a trapped lung which fails to expand. An indwelling pleural catheter, which can be managed at home, can be used although there is a risk of pleural infection. Pleuroperitoneal shunts are occasionally used when there is a trapped lung or when pleurodesis has failed, but are associated with a risk of shunt occlusion and infection.

Radical radiotherapy may improve local control of disease in 60–90% of patients. As the volume of disease in mesothelioma is considerable, irradiation to the pleura is limited by toxicity to the underlying lung and the mediastinal structures. This could be improved by using intensity modulated radiotherapy (IMRT). **Prophylactic radiotherapy** used to be offered to patients within 4 weeks of pleural aspiration or biopsy in order to reduce the risk of tumour seeding in the scar tissue. Recent trials do not support this practice.

Palliative radiotherapy improves pain in 50% of patients but does not improve symptoms of breathlessness.

Chemotherapy

All patients with histologically-verified malignant mesothelioma and a good performance status of 0–2 should be referred to an oncologist for consideration of chemotherapy. A combination of pemetrexed and cisplatin results in tumour regression and improvement in symptoms in 40% of cases and prolongs survival by 3 months. A combination of gemcitabine and cisplatin has also shown good response in recent trials.

Surgery

The role of surgery in malignant mesothelioma is controversial. Radical extra-pleural pneumonectomy (EPP) involves removal of all macroscopic disease, a pneumonectomy with resection of all parietal and visceral pleura, the diaphragm, and pericardium. The operative mortality is 4–9% and more than 60% have serious complications. The recent Mesothelioma and Radical Surgery (MARS) randomised feasibility study found no benefit with EPP versus no EPP as part of tri-modal therapy. Although only 50 patients participated in this study between 2005 and 2008, EPP was associated with a higher morbidity and mortality compared to the group not having surgery.

Debulking/cytoreductive surgery can be done by open thoracotomy or by a VATS procedure and involves removal of as much of the tumour as possible. This decortication may allow the re-expansion of the trapped lung and may reduce the re-accumulation of fluid.

The MesoVATS multicentre, randomised controlled trial compared VATS partial pleurectomy against talc pleurodesis. The results showed no difference in survival between the two groups. Partial pleurectomy was more expensive, and the patients had more complications with a longer hospital stay, but some improvement in symptoms at 6 months. Partial pleurectomy may be a more effective treatment for trapped lung.

Compensation

Patients with mesothelioma and some other asbestos-related lung diseases are eligible for compensation. See Appendix 10.B for details on compensation.

SUMMARY OF LEARNING POINTS

- Investigation of a unilateral pleural effusion includes contrast CT thorax, pleural aspiration, and pleural biopsy.
- Pleural fluid analysis and applying Light's criteria is the critical first step in management of a unilateral pleural effusion.
- The commonest cause of an exudate in patients over 60 years is malignancy and in younger patients is infection.
- The commonest cause of a transudate is CCF.
- Parapneumonic effusions are common and occur in 50% of patients with CAP.
- If a parapneumonic effusion is not treated optimally with antibiotics, or if the patient has risk factors, then this can progress to an empyema.
- An empyema can be diagnosed if there is pus in the pleural cavity or if the pleural fluid pH < 7.2.
- Empyema should be managed aggressively with intravenous antibiotics and intercostal chest drain insertion.
- Patients with pleural infection who do not improve with antibiotics and chest drain will require surgery.
- The management of a spontaneous pneumothorax will depend on whether it is primary or secondary, whether the patient is symptomatic or not, the age of the patient, the co-morbidities of the patient, and the size of the pneumothorax.
- Primary spontaneous pneumothorax occurs in young patients with no obvious underlying lung disease and is commoner in tall thin men.
- Primary spontaneous pneumothorax can be managed conservatively if the patient is not symptomatic, but will require intervention if the patient is breathless, regardless of the size of the pneumothorax.
- Secondary pneumothorax has a higher morbidity and mortality and is more difficult to manage.
- Most patients with a secondary pneumothorax will require intercostal chest drain insertion.
- Patients with a chest drain should be managed on a specialist respiratory ward by a respiratory physician and specialist nurses.
- If the pneumothorax does not resolve within 3–5 days, the patient should be referred to a thoracic surgeon for pleural abrasion, pleurectomy, pleurodesis, or bullectomy.
- Patients who have recurrent pneumothoraces should be referred to the thoracic

surgeon for pleural abrasion, pleurectomy, pleurodesis, or bullectomy.
- Mesothelioma, a malignant tumour of the pleura, is associated with asbestos exposure and has a terrible prognosis.
- Mesothelioma should be suspected in any patient presenting with chest pain and a unilateral pleural effusion, and/or pleural thickening.

MULTIPLE CHOICE QUESTIONS

10.1 Compared to interstitial fluid, pleural fluid has?

A Higher concentration of lactate dehydrogenase
B Higher concentration of neutrophils
C Higher concentration of sodium
D Lower concentration of glucose
E Lower concentration of protein

Answer: A

Pleural fluid has the same concentration of protein and glucose as interstitial fluid but a slightly lower concentration of sodium and a higher lactate dehydrogenase level. An increased neutrophil count in pleural fluid indicates an acute effusion secondary to bacterial infection.

10.2 A bilateral pleural effusion is most likely to be due to what cause?

A Congestive cardiac failure
B Meig's syndrome
C Mesothelioma
D Pulmonary embolus
E Rheumatoid arthritis

Answer: A

The commonest cause of a bilateral pleural effusion is congestive cardiac failure and it will be a transudate. Pleural aspiration is not necessary unless there are atypical features, or the effusion does not respond to diuretics. Meig's syndrome can present with bilateral pleural effusions but is a rare condition. Bilateral effusions are rare in mesothelioma.

10.3 What is the ideal management of a simple parapneumonic effusion?

A Give intravenous antibiotics and insert a Seldinger intercostal chest drain
B Give intravenous antibiotics and refer to a thoracic surgeon for VATS debridement
C Give intravenous antibiotics and monitor closely
D Give intra-pleural antibiotics through a Seldinger intercostal chest drain
E Give intra-pleural fibrinolytic drug through a Seldinger intercostal chest drain

Answer: C

The majority of parapneumonic effusions are secondary to bacterial pneumonia and will resolve with intravenous antibiotics without the need for an intercostal chest drain or surgery. Intra-pleural antibiotics have no proven benefit and intra-pleural fibrinolytic drugs are not indicated for most pleural infections.

10.4 Which of the following statements about an empyema is true?

A The commonest cause of an empyema is from a pleural intervention
B Empyema should always be managed by a thoracic surgeon with a VATS debridement
C A pH of <7.2 suggests that the pleural fluid is an empyema
D The mortality associated with an empyema is 1%
E Intra-pleural fibrinolytic drugs are always recommended as they break down the septation

Answer: C

Most empyemas arise from parapneumonic effusions that have not been optimally treated. A pH < 7.2 is an indication for drainage in the first instance and patients should be referred to a thoracic surgeon only if there is no improvement after several days. The use of an intrapleural fibrinolytic drug is controversial with insufficient evidence of long term benefit. Empyema has a significant mortality of up to 20% in immunocompromised patients.

10.5 According to the BTS pneumothorax guidelines, what should you do with a young patient with a primary spontaneous pneumothorax who is breathless?

A He can be discharged home if the pneumothorax is small, with follow-up in two weeks
B He should have an intercostal chest drain inserted without delay
C He should have an intercostal chest drain inserted and attached to suction to speed up recovery
D He should be observed on the ward and given high flow oxygen
E He should have simple aspiration in the first instance

Answer: E

The clinical state of the patient is more important than the size of the pneumothorax. Breathless patients should never be discharged home and will require an intervention. The first intervention is simple aspiration and an intercostal chest drain is indicated only if that fails. Suction is not recommended in the first 48 hours as it may precipitate re-expansion pulmonary oedema.

10.6 In a patient presenting with a unilateral pleural effusion, which of the following is most important?

A A bronchoscopy is always indicated.
B The differential cell count can be diagnostic
C Several samples of fluid should be sent for cytology
D The fluid protein and LDH to serum protein and LDH ratio should be measured
E Pleural fluid amylase level can be diagnostic

Answer: D

The essential investigation is pleural fluid analysis for the protein and LDH ratio compared to serum levels (Light's criteria) as this distinguishes an exudate from a transudate and guides management. A bronchoscopy is only indicated if the patient has symptoms such as haemoptysis, or if there is a mass on the CXR. The differential cell count can narrow the differential diagnosis but will not be diagnostic. There is no benefit in sending more than two samples of fluid for cytology, and amylase levels are not routinely sent.

10.7 A 55-year-old man with emphysema presents to hospital with breathlessness and is found to have a 2 cm pneumothorax on the right side. How would you manage this patient?

A Simple aspiration as many times as necessary as chest drain insertion is dangerous when there are bullae
B Prescribe high flow oxygen and observe the patient carefully on the ward
C Insert a Seldinger intercostal chest drain, ensuring that it is a pneumothorax
D Insert a large bore chest drain as there is likely to be a significant leak
E Refer the patient to the thoracic surgeon for a VATS pleurodesis

Answer: C

Patients with a secondary pneumothorax who are symptomatic require intervention. Although one simple aspiration could be attempted, most patients with a secondary pneumothorax are likely to require a Seldinger chest drain. There is no evidence that a large drain is better and, in fact, may cause more complications. Thoracic surgical intervention should be considered if the pneumothorax does not resolve 3–5 days after insertion of the chest drain.

10.8 When managing a chest drain inserted for a secondary pneumothorax, what is the procedure?

A Swinging indicates that the drain is not working properly

B Persistent bubbling after 48 hours suggests a bronchopleural fistula
C The development of surgical emphysema is a life-threatening complication
D The drain should be clamped when the patient mobilises to avoid too much air leaking out
E The chest drain should be connected to a high pressure low volume suction device

Answer: B

Swinging of the drain indicates that it is correctly positioned in the pleural space. Surgical emphysema is usually a minor complication and resolves once the drain has been re-positioned. A bubbling chest drain should never be clamped as this might create a tension pneumothorax. A low pressure high volume suction device could be used, but only after 48 hours to prevent re-expansion pulmonary oedema. Persistent bubbling after 48 hours suggests the development of a bronchopleural fistula and thoracic surgery may be indicated.

10.9 In making a histological diagnosis of mesothelioma, what should you do?
A Pleural fluid cytology is diagnostic in most cases
B Repeat CT guided pleural biopsies are advised to ensure that the diagnosis is correct
C An MRI scan can be helpful in obtaining adequate samples
D A PET-CT is essential prior to obtaining biopsies as it has a high sensitivity and specificity
E A VATS pleural biopsy has the best yield and is the preferred investigation

Answer: E

A VATS pleural biopsy, done under direct visualisation, is the investigation of choice. Pleural fluid cytology is positive in only 50% of patients with mesothelioma and repeated biopsies can result in tumour seeding so should be avoided. MRI scan and PET-CT do not have a role in the histological diagnosis of mesothelioma.

10.10 What should a patient discharged home after a primary spontaneous pneumothorax be told?
A They must not participate in any physical activity for 4 weeks
B They should be able to fly on a commercial flight after 1 week if the chest X-ray is normal
C They must not fly in a helicopter for 6 weeks
D They can go scuba diving after 1 year
E Their risk of a recurrent pneumothorax is 10%

Answer: B

Patients with no chronic lung disease, and whose CXR confirms that the pneumothorax has resolved, are considered safe to fly after 1 week. There is no evidence that the development of a pneumothorax is related to physical exertion. Flying in a helicopter is safe as they do not fly at high altitude. Patients should not participate in any diving activity unless they have had a definitive surgical procedure, such as a pleural abrasion, pleurectomy or pleurodesis.

Appendix 10.A Analysis of pleural fluid

Biochemistry

- 2–5 ml of pleural fluid should be sent in a plain container for measurement of protein and lactate dehydrogenase (LDH). A blood sample should also be sent for total protein and LDH so that the fluid: serum ratio can be calculated (Light's criteria).
- 1–2 ml of pleural fluid should be sent in a fluoride oxalate tube for glucose measurement. A serum glucose sample should be sent at the same time.

Microbiology

- 5 ml of pleural fluid should be sent in a plain container and 5 ml in anaerobic and aerobic blood culture bottles to the microbiology department for microscopy, culture, and sensitivity, including Ziehl-Neelsen stain and culture for tuberculosis if indicated.

Cytology

- 20–40 ml of pleural fluid (or more if available) should be sent in a plain universal container without delay. Samples taken out of hours should be refrigerated. Yield for malignancy increases if cell blocks formed by centrifuging and extracting the solid cellular portion are examined. Smears are also prepared from pleural fluid samples.
- 5 ml pleural fluid in an anti-coagulated tube for differential cell count.

pH

- pH should be measured in non-purulent samples only as pus can damage the blood gas analyser. 0.5–1 ml of fluid should be drawn up into a heparinised blood gas syringe. Contamination with local anaesthetic must be avoided. Exposure to air must be minimised by keeping the syringe capped.

Haematocrit

- 1–2 ml of pleural fluid should be sent in an EDTA container to the Hematology department if a haemothorax is suspected.

Appendix 10.B Compensation for asbestos-related disease

Compensation is available for the following conditions:

- Malignant mesothelioma.
- Diffuse pleural thickening.
- Asbestos-related pulmonary fibrosis (asbestosis).

Pathological diagnosis is not mandatory but helpful. The patient must identify occupational exposure or another source of asbestos to satisfy the 'balance of probabilities' test. The individual must also show that the employer was negligent in not maintaining appropriate standards required by common law and in breach of safety regulations.

The following compensation is available

1. Industrial Injuries Disablement Benefit (IIDB) is payable to individuals with asbestos-related illnesses, including mesothelioma, if they have been exposed to asbestos at work. It is not applicable if the patient was self-employed. This payment is made weekly, monthly, or quarterly by the Department of Work and Pensions.
2. The Pneumoconiosis etc. (Worker's Compensation) Act 1979 entitles the patient to a lump sum if they have been awarded Industrial Injuries Disablement Benefit and their employer is no longer in business or if the compensation claim has not been settled.
3. Diffuse Mesothelioma Scheme 2008 is for patients who cannot claim benefits under either of the above two schemes because their exposure to asbestos was not occupational but through contact with relatives who were exposed to asbestos (for example, wives washing their husbands' work clothes) or individuals who were self-employed. The claim must be made within 12 months of the diagnosis of mesothelioma.
4. War Pensions Scheme is applicable if the individual was exposed to asbestos while working in the armed forces.
5. Common Law Claim is compensation from a previous employer or their insurers, usually through a specialist solicitor. Individuals will need accurate dates regarding their period of employment that resulted in exposure to asbestos. The individual will need to log a claim within three years of the time they first became aware of their illness.

As well as these compensation schemes, individuals may be entitled to statutory sick pay, incapacity and disability benefits, and employment and support allowance – called the Universal Credit from October 2013.

The next of kin of an individual who has died from mesothelioma can claim compensation for their relative's pain and suffering and for financial losses within 6 months of death of the individual.

FURTHER READING

American Thoracic Society, Guidotti, T.L., Miller, A. et al. (2004). Diagnosis and initial management of nonmalignant diseases related to asbestos. *American Journal of Respiratory and Critical Care Medicine* 170 (6): 691–715.

Bouros, D., Antoniou, K., and Light, R.W. (2006). Intrapleural streptokinase for pleural infection. *BMJ (Clinical Research ed.)* 332 (7534): 133–134.

British Thoracic Society (2007). BTS statement on malignant mesothelioma in the UK, 2007. *Thorax* 62 (Suppl 2): ii1–ii19.

British Thoracic Society, MacDuff, A., Arnold, A., and Harvey, J. (2010a). Management of spontaneous pneumothorax: British Thoracic Society pleural disease guideline 2010. *Thorax* 65 (Suppl 2): ii18–ii31.

British Thoracic Society, Roberts, M.E., Neville, E. et al. (2010b). Management of a malignant pleural effusion: British Thoracic Society pleural disease guideline 2010. *Thorax* 65 (Suppl_2): ii32–ii40.

British Thoracic Society Standards of Care Committee, Ahmedzai, S. et al. (2011). Respiratory diease: managing passengers with stable respiratory disease planning air travel: British Thoracic Society recommendations. *Thorax* 66 (Suppl 1): i1–i30.

Davies, H.E., Davies, R.J.O., Davies, C.W.H., and on behalf of the BTS Group (2010). Management of pleural infection in adults: British Thoracic Society pleural disease guideline 2010. *Thorax* 65 (Suppl 2): ii41–ii53.

Health and Safety Executive and Local Authorities Enforcement Liaison Committee (HELA) (2012) Control of Asbestos Regulations 2012: General enforcement guidance and advice, pp. 1–23, [online]. Available at: www.hse.gov.uk/foi/internalops/ocs/200-299/oc265-50.pdf.

Hooper, C., Lee, Y.C.G., and Maskell, N. (2010). Investigation of a unilateral pleural effusion in adults: British Thoracic Society pleural disease guideline 2010. *Thorax* 65 (Suppl 2): ii4–ii17.

Light, R.W. (2002). Pleural effusion. *New England Journal of Medicine* 346 (25): 1971–1977.

Maskell, N.A., Davies, C.W., Nunn, A.J. et al. (2005). U.K. controlled trial of Intrapleural streptokinase for pleural infection. *The New England Journal of Medicine* 352 (9): 865–874.

Porcel, J.M. and Light, R.W. (2006). Diagnostic approach to pleural effusion in adults. *American Family Physician* 73 (7): 1211–1220.

Tan, C., Sedrakyan, A., Browne, J. et al. (2006). The evidence on the effectiveness of management for malignant pleural effusion: a systematic review. *European Journal of Cardio-thoracic Surgery* 29 (5): 829–838.

Zocchi, L. (2002). Physiology and pathophysiology of pleural fluid turnover. *European Respiratory Journal* 20 (6): 1545–1558.

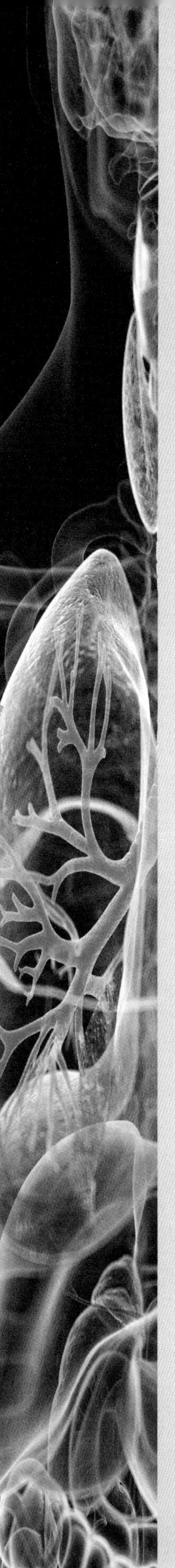

CHAPTER 11
Pulmonary embolus, pulmonary hypertension, and vasculitides

Learning objectives

- To understand the risk factors for thromboembolic disease and how to calculate the probability score
- To understand the clinical presentation of an acute pulmonary embolus
- To understand the investigations for diagnosing acute pulmonary embolus
- To understand the management of acute pulmonary embolus
- To recognise the clinical presentation, investigations and management of chronic pulmonary emboli
- To understand the aetiology and clinical presentation of pulmonary hypertension
- To appreciate the investigations and diagnosis of pulmonary hypertension
- To understand the management of pulmonary hypertension
- To appreciate the differential diagnoses of pulmonary haemorrhagic syndromes
- To appreciate the clinical presentation, diagnosis and management of granulomatosis with polyangiitis
- To recognise the clinical presentation, diagnosis and management of eosinophilic granulomatosis with polyangiitis
- To understand the clinical presentation, diagnosis and management of anti-glomerular basement membrane antibody disease
- To understand the clinical presentation, diagnosis and management of hereditary haemorrhagic telangiectasia

Essential Respiratory Medicine, First Edition. Shanthi Paramothayan.

Companion website: www.wiley.com/go/paramothayan/essential_respiratory_medicine

Abbreviations

ABG	arterial blood gas
ABPA	allergic bronchopulmonary aspergillosis
ANCA	anti-neutrophil cytoplasmic antibodies
APTT	activated partial thromboplastin time
AVM	arterio-venous malformation
BMPR2	bone morphogenetic protein receptor 2
CO	carbon monoxide
COPD	chronic obstructive pulmonary disease
CPFE	combined pulmonary fibrosis and emphysema
CTEPH	chronic thromboembolic pulmonary hypertension
CTPA	computed tomography pulmonary angiogram
CUS	compressive lower extremity ultrasound
CXR	chest X-ray
DVT	deep vein thrombosis
ECG	electrocardiogram
ECHO	echocardiogram
eGFR	estimated glomerular filtration rate
EGPA	eosinophilic granulomatosis with polyangiitis
ELISA	enzyme linked immunosorbent assay
GPA	granulomatosis with polyangiitis
Hb	haemoglobin
HDU	high dependency unit
HHT	hereditary haemorrhagic telangiectasia
HIT	heparin induced thrombocytopaenia
HIV	human immunodeficiency virus
HRCT	high-resolution computed tomography
ICU	intensive care unit
ILD	interstitial lung disease
INR	International Normalised Ratio
IVC	inferior vena cava
JVP	jugular venous pressure
IVUFH	intravenous unfractionated heparin
KCO	transfer coefficient
kPA	kilopascals
LMWH	low molecular weight heparin
LTOT	long term oxygen therapy
MPA	microscopic polyangiitis
MPO	myeloperoxidase
MRPA	magnetic resonance pulmonary angiogram
NICE	National Institute for Health and Care Excellence
NYHA	New York Heart Association
OSA	obstructive sleep apnoea
PAH	pulmonary arterial hypertension
PAP	pulmonary artery pressure
PDGF	platelet derived growth factor
PE	pulmonary embolus
PESI	Pulmonary Embolism Severity Index
PGI_2	prostaglandin
PHT	pulmonary hypertension
PPH	primary pulmonary hypertension
PPV	positive predictive value
PR3	proteinase 3
PVOD	pulmonary veno-occlusive disease
SCUFH	subcutaneous unfractionated heparin
SLE	systemic lupus erythematosus
SSRI	selective serotonin reuptake inhibitors
TED	thromboembolic disease
TGF	transforming growth factor
TLCO	carbon monoxide transfer factor (diffusing capacity)
TTE	transthoracic echocardiogram
UFH	unfractionated heparin
UK	United Kingdom
VEGF	vascular endothelial growth factor
VQ	ventilation perfusion
VTE	venous thromboembolism
WHO	World Health Organisation

Introduction

Diseases of the pulmonary vasculature can present with symptoms of breathlessness, chest pain and haemoptysis. In some cases, these disorders can be life-threatening. Some conditions, such as pulmonary emboli, are relatively common. Pulmonary vasculitides, which can present with pulmonary haemorrhage and life-threatening haemoptysis, can involve other organs and are much rarer. Pulmonary embolism, pulmonary hypertension and some of the commoner pulmonary vasculitic conditions are discussed in this chapter.

Pulmonary embolism

A pulmonary embolus (PE) is caused by the obstruction of one, or both, of the pulmonary arteries or one of its branches by thrombus. Pulmonary arteries can also be blocked by air, fat or tumour cells, but these will not be discussed in this chapter.

Thromboembolic disease is a term used for the development of deep vein thrombosis (DVT) in the deep veins of the legs and pelvis which then break off and travel to the lungs, causing obstruction of

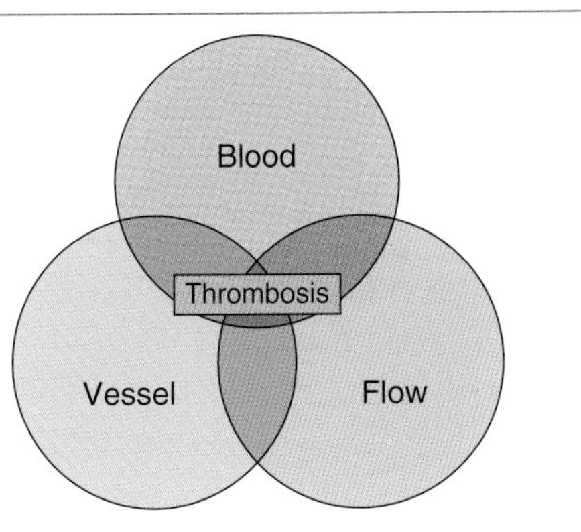

Figure 11.1 Virchow's triad.

the pulmonary vasculature. DVT and PE develop when there is venous stasis, endothelial damage, and hypercoagulability, described as Virchow's Triad (Figure 11.1). Table 11.1 lists the risk factors for developing DVT and PE.

It is estimated that there are 120 cases of PE/100 000 population with the incidence increasing to 500/100 000 in those aged over 75 years. PE is estimated to be responsible for 0.5% of all deaths in Europe, the majority of which occur in hospitals. It is estimated that 1% of patients admitted to hospital develop an acute pulmonary embolus (PE), which is responsible for 5% of all deaths in hospital. There is a higher incidence of PE in African Americans and the incidence is less common in Asians.

All patients admitted to hospital should have a careful assessment and documentation of their risk of developing thromboembolic disease. Patients who have had surgery and who are immobile are at a particularly high risk of developing venous thromboembolism (VTE) because of venous stasis. Pregnant women also have an increased risk because of their hypercoagulable state and the occlusion of the pelvic veins caused by the enlarging uterus. Acute pulmonary embolus is the leading cause of maternal deaths in the UK. Patients with inherited thrombotic disorders, such as Factor V Leiden and prothrombin gene mutations, who may have a family history of thromboembolic disease, are also at an increased risk of developing PE, as are those with malignancy.

Prophylaxis with a low dose of low molecular weight heparin (LMWH) is recommended for those who are at risk, unless they have a risk of bleeding. Most patients who are going to have elective surgery and those who are immobile should be prescribed LMWH. It should be continued for a period after discharge from hospital. Patients who are ambulant with no specific risk factors may not require LMWH prophylaxis. Thromboembolic disease (TED) stockings are also used to prevent the development of DVT. If LMWH is contraindicated, for example because of an increased risk of bleeding or renal failure, then intravenous unfractionated heparin (UFH) infusion, which has a shorter half-life and can be reversed more quickly, can be considered. Patients who have had a stroke should be offered graded elastic compression stockings (TED stockings) and mechanical calf pumps. All patients should be encouraged to mobilise as early as possible.

Thromboprophylaxis is not required for most patients who are undertaking long journeys, including long-haul flights. Travellers should be reminded to keep hydrated, mobilise frequently, and do calf exercises to prevent venous stasis. High risk patients may require LMWH prior to a flight that is more than 12 hours long.

Table 11.1 Risk factors for developing thromboembolic disease.

Hypercoagulability	Stasis	Endothelial damage
Malignancy	Immobility	Previous DVT
Thrombophilia	Obesity	Thrombophlebitis
Pregnancy	Pregnancy	Lower limb trauma
Oral contraceptive pill	Long haul flight	
Sepsis	Low cardiac output	

Acute pulmonary embolus

An acute PE is a common, and sometimes fatal, form of venous thromboembolism which should be considered in anyone presenting with dyspnoea, pleuritic chest pain, haemoptysis, hypotension, or cardiac arrest. The severity of symptoms will depend on how much the pulmonary circulation is occluded and where the emboli are. The clinical presentation can be highly variable and often non-specific.

Symptoms of a PE can occur acutely (within seconds or minutes), sub-acutely (over days or weeks), or occur slowly over many months, resulting in chronic thromboembolic pulmonary hypertension (CTEPH), which is discussed later in this chapter.

Prompt diagnosis and treatment of PE will reduce morbidity and mortality. A comprehensive history should include ascertaining the risk factors for developing thromboembolic disease and the calculation of a probability score.

Box 11.1 lists the commonest symptoms of a pulmonary embolus as determined in the Prospective Investigation of Pulmonary Embolism Diagnosis 11 (PIOPED 11) Study.

Patients usually develop sudden onset of breathlessness within minutes, especially if the thrombus blocks the main or lobar pulmonary vessels. However, patients may experience very mild symptoms or be asymptomatic, even with a large PE, and present after a delay of days or weeks. In a systematic review of studies, one-third of patients with DVT were found to have an asymptomatic PE.

Pleuritic chest pain is more likely to develop with smaller, more peripheral emboli, which result in inflammation of the visceral pleural membrane. This can lead to pulmonary infarction in 10% of cases, resulting in haemoptysis.

Box 11.1 Common symptoms of pulmonary embolus.

- Dyspnoea at rest or exertion (73%)
- Pleuritic chest pain (44%)
- Calf or thigh pain and swelling (44%)
- Dry cough (37%)
- Orthopnoea (28%)
- Wheezing (21%)
- Haemoptysis (13%)

Box 11.2 Common clinical signs on examination in PE.

- Tachypnoea (54%)
- Calf/thigh swelling (47%)
- Tachycardia (24%)
- Crackles (18%)
- Loud P_2 (15%)
- Raised JVP (14%)
- Cardiovascular collapse (8%)
- Fever (3%)

The differential diagnoses for anyone presenting with pleuritic chest pain and dyspnoea includes a variety of common respiratory conditions, such as acute asthma, pneumothorax, exacerbation of COPD, community acquired pneumonia, and heart failure.

The clinical signs of pulmonary embolus are relatively non-specific and include tachypnoea and a pleural rub if the patient presents late and has developed pulmonary infarction. Oxygen saturation measurement at rest may appear normal if the embolus is small, but a desaturation of more than 4% on exertion should alert the clinician to the possibility of a PE. PE should be suspected when there is hypotension and the JVP is elevated. If pulmonary embolus is suspected, then the lower limbs should be examined for evidence of a DVT which presents with leg swelling and pain on palpation. Box 11.2 lists the frequency of the common presenting signs on clinical examination.

A large saddle embolus, which lodges at the bifurcation of the main pulmonary artery and extends into the right and left main pulmonary arteries, occurs in 3–6% of cases and carries a mortality of 5%. These emboli can move distally and lodge in the segmental or sub-segmental branches.

Diagnosis of pulmonary embolus

It is recommended by NICE that a pre-test clinical probability score should be calculated in all patients with a suspected PE. In combination with simple investigations, this score can be used to decide whether further investigations are required. This is important as this avoids unnecessary investigations, such as a computed tomography pulmonary angiogram (CTPA), which exposes the patient to a high dose of radiation. However, it is important

Table 11.2 Modified Wells score.

Clinical feature	Points
Clinical symptoms of DVT	3
Other diagnosis less likely than PE	3
Heart rate > 100 bpm	1.5
Immobilisation or surgery within last 4 weeks	1.5
Previous DVT or PE	1.5
Haemoptysis	1
Malignancy	1

Score 2 or less: Low risk of PE.
Score 2–4: Intermediate risk of PE.
Score > 6: High risk of PE.

that a patient with risk factors for PE has appropriate investigations so that a PE is not missed.

The NICE guidelines recommend the use of a two-level modified **Wells score** (Table 11.2) to assess the probability of an individual patient having a PE. A score greater than 4 indicates that a PE is likely and a score less than 4 suggests that a PE is unlikely. The Geneva score is an alternative score that is sometimes used.

Investigations in the diagnosis of pulmonary embolus

Most of the routine investigations that a patient will have when presenting to hospital are non-specific and therefore not useful on their own in making or excluding a diagnosis of PE.

The ECG is often normal. The commonest ECG abnormality is sinus tachycardia. Other ECG changes, which occur in 70% of patients with a PE, include right heart strain, right axis deviation, depression of the ST segment, and T wave inversion in leads V1–V3. The S1Q3T3 pattern occurs in less than 10% of patients (Figure 11.2). Patients who develop bradycardia, atrial arrhythmias, new right bundle branch block, inferior Q-waves, and anterior ST-segment changes have a worse prognosis.

The chest X-ray (CXR) is normal in approximately 20%, and is an essential investigation to exclude pneumothorax, consolidation, and cardiac failure. A small pleural effusion is found in 47% of patients with a PE; this is often blood-stained if aspirated. Other radiological changes include atelectasis, pruning of the pulmonary vasculature with distal hypoperfusion, and a wedge-shaped opacity in the lung periphery (Figure 11.3).

Arterial blood gas (ABG) analysis is not a sensitive or specific test in the diagnosis of PE, but 74% of patients will be hypoxic. Approximately 41%

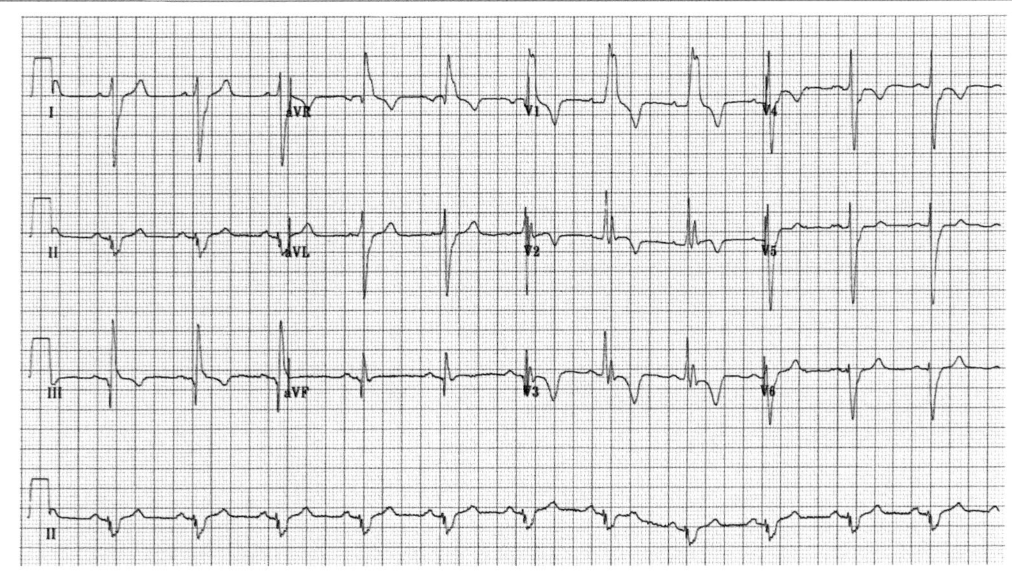

Figure 11.2 ECG changes seen in pulmonary embolus.

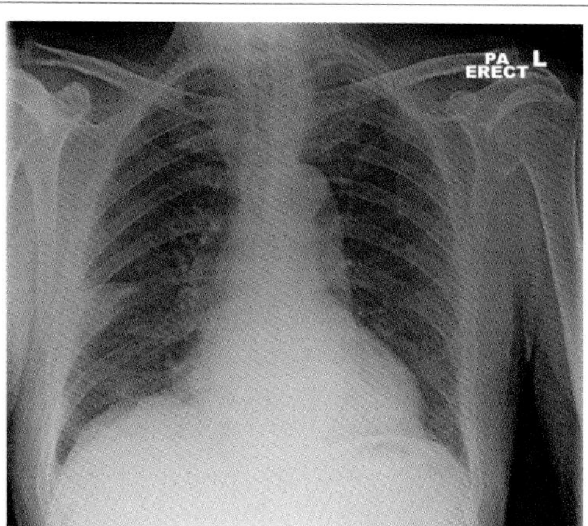

Figure 11.3 CXR showing right lower lobe infarction after a pulmonary embolism.

will have hypocapnia and a respiratory alkalosis. PE should be considered in anyone who has a normal CXR and unexplained hypoxaemia. Ventilation perfusion mismatch will result in widening of the Alveolar-arterial (A-a)gradient in the majority. The calculation of the A-a gradient is described in Chapter 13. Although not helpful on its own to make a diagnosis, the ABG at presentation may be of prognostic value. As patients with an initial oxygen saturation of less than 95% have an increased risk of respiratory failure and death, it is recommended that such patients are admitted to hospital for careful monitoring while undergoing investigations and treatment.

D-dimer is a breakdown product of cross-linked fibrin and levels will be elevated in patients with thromboembolism. Sensitive D-dimer testing using ELISA (enzyme-linked immunosorbent assay) is recommended. Although it is a sensitive test, with a greater increase in those with larger PEs, it lacks specificity. D-dimer levels will be elevated in those with any acute illness and in pregnant women. D-dimer levels will be falsely positive in patients with chronic renal failure with an estimated glomerular filtration rate (eGFR) $<60\,\text{ml}\,\text{min}^{-1}/1.73\,\text{m}^2$. The D-dimer level also increases gradually in patients over the age of 50 years. Age-adjusted D-dimer values may increase the specificity of the test, but this is not routinely done in the UK.

The D-dimer level is only useful in excluding a PE and should not be used to make a diagnosis of PE. According to the NICE guidelines, the D-dimer should be used in conjunction with the modified Wells score to determine the need for further investigations. If the modified Wells score is greater than or equal to 4, then the patient should go on to have further investigations to confirm the diagnosis of PE, regardless of the D-dimer level. In those with a high clinical suspicion of PE and a normal D-dimer level, the prevalence of PE is 20–28%.

If the probability of PE is considered unlikely (modified Wells score of less than 4), then a D-dimer level should be obtained. If this is negative, then no further testing is required. In those in whom the D-dimer level is elevated, a CTPA is required.

Although not sensitive or specific, serum Troponin I and T levels may indicate right ventricular dysfunction. Raised levels may be elevated in 30–50% of patients with a large PE and may be of prognostic value. The levels are rarely as high as would be after a myocardial infarction and return to normal within 2 days.

Imaging to confirm a diagnosis of PE

Computed tomography pulmonary angiogram (CTPA)

CTPA with intravenous contrast is a rapid test that is available in all hospitals in the UK. CTPA is the imaging of choice in a non-pregnant patient with normal renal function who is haemodynamically stable and not allergic to contrast. CTPA may not be the optimal investigation in the morbidly obese patient and in women under the age of 40 because of the high dose of radiation to the breasts, which may increase the risk of breast cancer.

An algorithmic approach which combines CTPA with clinical assessment and D-dimer levels increases the sensitivity and specificity of the test. CTPA has a sensitivity of over 90% for the diagnosis of PE, which increases to 96% when combined with a clinical probability assessment. The specificity of CTPA is 95%. When the modified Wells score is <2, the positive predictive value (PPV) of CTPA is 58%. If the Wells score is 2–6, then the PPV is 92% and for a Wells score >6, the PPV rises to 96%.

A PE will appear as a filling defect in a branch of the pulmonary artery which is otherwise filled with contrast (Figure 11.4). CTPA is most accurate

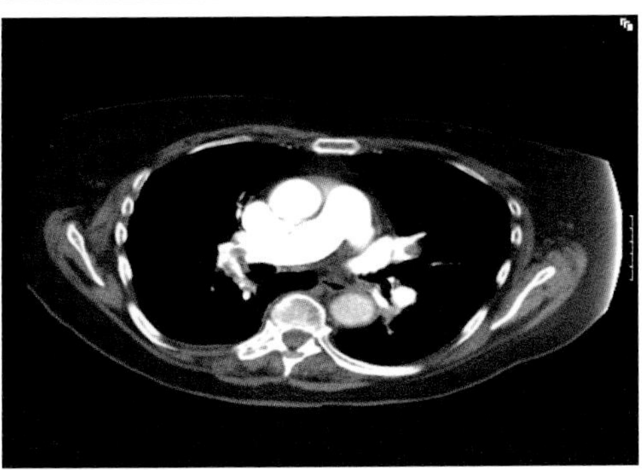

Figure 11.4 CTPA showing bilateral filling defects seen with multiple pulmonary emboli.

for the detection of a large PE blocking the main, lobar, and segmental pulmonary arteries. It is less accurate for detecting smaller, peripheral, sub-segmental PEs. The modern multi-detector scanners can detect smaller, more peripheral emboli. The CTPA also has the advantage of finding other abnormalities which may be responsible for the clinical symptoms and signs.

A positive CTPA will confirm a diagnosis of PE and a negative CTPA means that a PE is unlikely. When the clinical suspicion is high but the CTPA is negative, 5% will have a PE. Therefore, patients with a high Wells score and a negative CTPA may require further investigations, which may include a VQ scan or a contrast-enhanced pulmonary angiogram.

Ventilation perfusion scan (VQ scan)

A VQ scan should be considered in any patient in whom a CTPA is contraindicated as discussed above. It should also be considered in women under the age of 40. A normal CXR is necessary when interpreting the VQ images and is, therefore, not a suitable investigation in a patient with chronic lung disease. A VQ scan may occasionally be indicated if the clinical suspicion of a PE is high but the CTPA is negative. A VQ scan is a nuclear medicine scan that is not available in all centres and not available out of hours because radioactive isotopes are required.

The PIOPED 11 study is the largest study to date which looked at the sensitivity and specificity of VQ scanning. A VQ scan has a moderately high sensitivity but a poor specificity, with a high number of false positive test results. As with CTPA, diagnostic accuracy was greater when the results of the VQ scan was combined with a clinical probability score.

A VQ scan is reported according to whether there are areas which have normal ventilation but abnormal perfusion (VQ mismatch). Patients with underlying lung disease, for example, COPD, will have matched ventilation and perfusion defects. A VQ scan can be reported as normal, low-probability of PE, intermediate probability of PE, or high-probability of PE.

A normal VQ scan means that a PE is unlikely, and no further investigations are required. A patient with a Wells score<2 and a normal or low-probability VQ scan will have <4% chance of having a PE. If this is combined with a normal D-dimer level, then the chance of a PE is <3%. A high probability VQ scan in a patient with a high clinical probability score means that there is a 96% chance of a PE (Figure 11.5). Patients with a low probability or inconclusive VQ scan will need further investigations (Figure 11.6).

Patients with a high clinical suspicion of PE in whom a CTPA is either negative or contra-indicated and in whom the VQ scan is inconclusive will require further imaging.

A **contrast-enhanced pulmonary angiogram** is historically the definitive test for diagnosing PE and has a good sensitivity and specificity. Although it is an invasive test and is associated with a small risk of harm, it is safe and well tolerated in haemodynamically stable patients with <2% mortality. Complications include catheter-related events, contrast-related complications, and cardiac complications. One advantage of this test is that if a clot is directly visualised, it can be lysed by embolectomy and/or thrombolysis if anticoagulation is contra-indicated.

A **magnetic resonance pulmonary angiogram (MRPA)** is less sensitive and specific and is rarely used. **Proximal vein compressive lower-extremity ultrasound (CUS)** can detect a DVT so can indirectly make a diagnosis of PE. It is not recommended in routine practice for diagnosing PE as only 9–12% of patients with PE are found to have a DVT by this method. However, in those in whom other investigations are contra-indicated, serial CUS done weekly for several weeks could be useful to detect DVT if the clinical suspicion is high. It is a valuable test in pregnant women as there is no exposure to radiation.

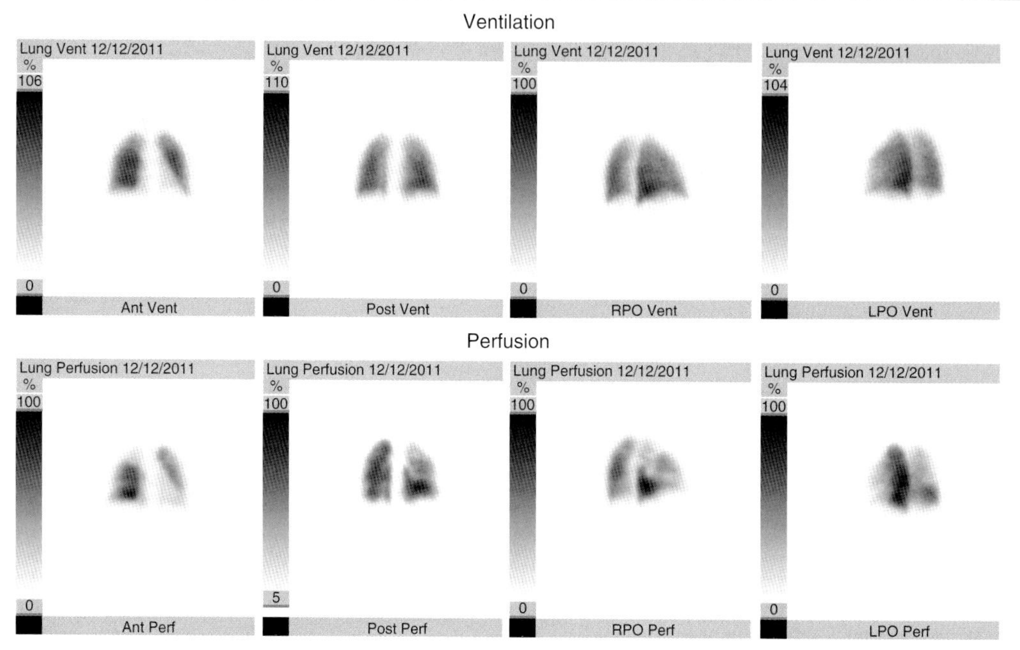

Figure 11.5 : Ventilation perfusion scan showing perfusion defects in pulmonary emboli.

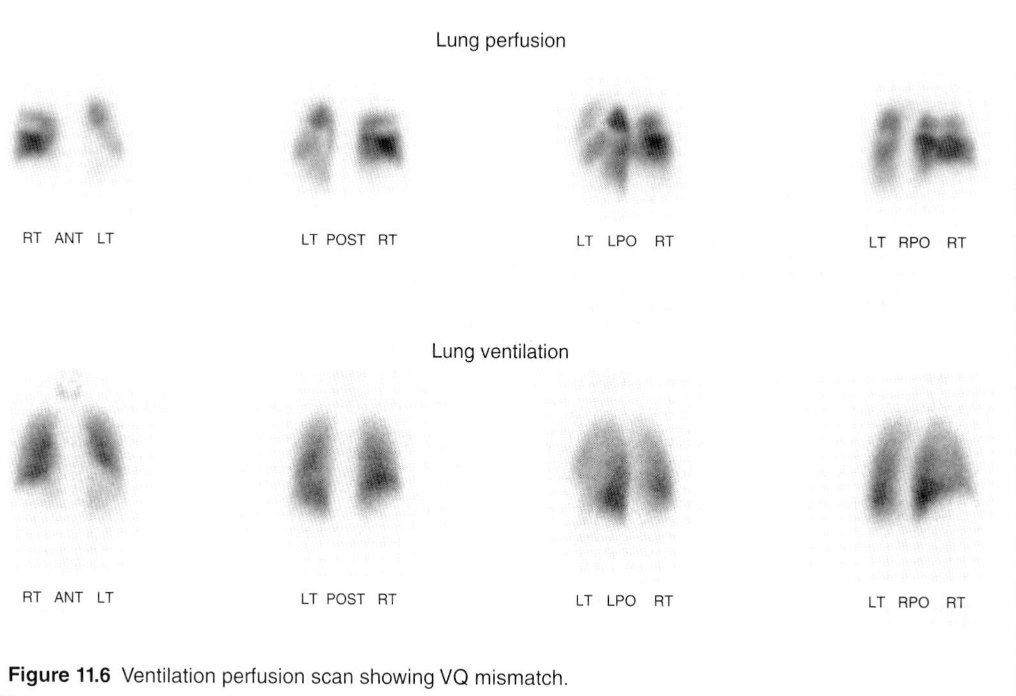

Figure 11.6 Ventilation perfusion scan showing VQ mismatch.

A transthoracic echocardiogram cannot make a diagnosis of PE, but in 30–40% of patients with a PE there will be changes consistent with right ventricular strain, which includes regional wall motion abnormalities that spare the right ventricular apex. In severe PE, there may be evidence of elevated right ventricular pressures, an increase in right ventricular size, tricuspid regurgitation, and pulmonary hypertension. In 4% of cases, a thrombus may be seen in the right ventricle, which confers a poor prognosis. The echo changes may be of prognostic value and resolution of changes can be used to monitor improvement with anticoagulation and, sometimes, to guide the length of anticoagulation. An echocardiogram can also diagnose other causes of hypotension and cardiovascular collapse, including aortic dissection and pericardial tamponade.

PE is a leading cause of mortality during pregnancy and in the 6 weeks post-partum, accounting for 20–30% of maternal deaths. It is difficult for the clinician to calculate the clinical probability of a pregnant woman having a PE as there are no validated scores in this group of patients. The imaging to use in a pregnant woman often causes much concern for the doctor and the patient. All pregnant women who present with possible PE should have a CXR (with lead protection for the foetus) which may suggest an alternative diagnosis. Both CTPA and VQ scan will expose the foetus to some radiation. CTPA exposes the mother's breasts to a significant dose of radiation at a time when they are particularly metabolic, thus increasing the future risk of breast malignancy. It is recommended that a CUS of legs and pelvis is a useful initial investigation in a pregnant woman if PE is suspected. If this is normal but the presentation is suggestive of a PE, then a half-dose perfusion scan is recommended. CTPA is reserved for pregnant women who are clinically unwell and in whom other investigations are indeterminate.

Management of acute pulmonary embolus

Patients with suspected PE should receive oxygen and analgesia as required. Those with a high probability of PE (Wells score > 6) should receive LMWH while they are having investigations. Those with a moderate clinical probability (Wells score of 2–6) should be anticoagulated if the diagnosis is going to take more than 4 hours. It is recommended that all the diagnostic tests should be done within 4 hours. Patients with a low risk of PE should undergo investigations within 24 hours and do not require anticoagulation while waiting for the results.

Anticoagulation

Anticoagulation is the main treatment for PE. The risk of PE recurrence is 25% in patients with a high probability score and anticoagulation has been shown to reduce this. The main complication of anticoagulation is bleeding, and intracranial bleeding may be life-threatening. The risk of bleeding is estimated to be 1.6% in the first 3 months in those with no risk factors for bleeding and will be up to 3% in those with risk factors. Minor haemoptysis, epistaxis, and menstruation are not contraindications to anticoagulation. Anticoagulation has also been shown to reduce mortality, the benefits outweighing the risk of major bleeding.

The aim of anticoagulation is to reach a therapeutic level within 24 hours of treatment using either LMWH, subcutaneous fondaparinux, intravenous unfractionated heparin (IVUFH), or subcutaneous unfractionated heparin (SCUFH). A patient diagnosed with PE with a high risk of haemorrhage should be discussed with an expert prior to anticoagulation.

LMWH is recommended in haemodynamically stable patients with normal renal function. It is not indicated in patients who are morbidly obese as there is decreased absorption of medication given subcutaneously. Advantages of LMWH over IVUFH include lower mortality, fewer recurrent thromboembolic events, fewer major bleeding episodes, and a lower incidence of heparin induced thrombocytopaenia (HIT). LMWH has more predictable pharmacokinetics than UFH, requires twice daily administration of a fixed dose, and monitoring of anti-Xa levels is not required. The choice of which LMWH to use will be dictated by the cost and clinical experience. The dose is calculated according to the patient's weight and given subcutaneously by injection.

LMWH is also recommended for the treatment of PE in a pregnant woman and more careful monitoring is recommended. Anticoagulation should be continued for 3 months after birth if pregnancy is the only risk factor for developing the PE. Those with other risk factors may need a longer period of anticoagulation. Warfarin is teratogenic so is contraindicated in pregnancy, particularly in the first trimester. Warfarin is, however, considered to be safe in breastfeeding mothers.

IVUFH is recommended in patients with massive PE and hypotension as they may require thrombolysis and the effects of the UFH can be reversed with protamine sulphate more rapidly than when patients receive LMWH or fondaparinux. IVUFH is also indicated in those in whom there is an increased risk of bleeding, those with renal failure (creatinine clearance less than 30 ml min^{-1}) and in the morbidly obese. Patients on UFH will require monitoring of their activated partial thromboplastin time (APTT).

Oral anticoagulation

Warfarin, a vitamin K antagonist, which blocks the production of the vitamin-K dependent clotting factors (11, V11, 1X and X), is the drug most commonly used for the long term treatment of PE. It is effective in preventing recurrent PEs and DVTs. Warfarin can be started as soon as the diagnosis of PE is confirmed while the patient is on the treatment dose of LMWH but should not be started without prior treatment with LMWH as there is evidence that this may increase the incidence of PE and/or DVT. It is recommended that LMWH treatment should continue for at least 5 days after starting treatment and until the International Normalised Ratio (INR) has been therapeutic (between 2 and 3) for at least 24 hours. This is because it takes at least 5 days for the intrinsic clotting pathway activity to be suppressed. It is recommended that the starting dose of warfarin should be 5 mg for 2 days and then the dose calculated according to the INR. The effects of warfarin can be reversed by giving vitamin K. Fresh frozen plasma can also be given if necessary.

Warfarin is a cheap drug but has a narrow therapeutic range and requires monitoring. Warfarin is a drug that has interactions with other commonly used drugs which are metabolised through the cytochrome P450 system. Doctors should be aware of these interactions. Certain food items, particularly those containing vitamin K, can also alter warfarin levels, so patients should be given information booklets with details of foods to avoid.

Increasingly, Factor Xa inhibitors, such as rivoroxaban, apixaban, and edoxaban are being used. Dabigatran, a direct thrombin inhibitor, is also being used in certain circumstances. These are fixed dose agents that do not require monitoring. However, the effects cannot be easily reversed. It is not within the scope of this book to discuss these newer anticoagulants in detail.

Patients with PE who are haemodynamically stable, not hypoxaemic, not in respiratory distress, who do not have significant co-morbidities, no increased risk of bleeding, and who do not live alone can be safely anticoagulated at home.

Duration of anticoagulation

The length of time that anticoagulation should be continued depends on the underlying cause of the PE. Rates of clot resolution with anticoagulant therapy are variable. It is estimated that there is resolution of the PE in 40% of patients within 1 week, in 50% within 2 weeks and in 73% within 4 weeks. Thrombi can also move during anticoagulation.

If the DVT and/or PE is due to an identifiable risk factor, such as immobility or surgery, the guidelines recommend 3 months of anticoagulation, so long as the INR is therapeutic during this period. The patient should be reviewed after this period to ensure that the symptoms have resolved and that there is no evidence of pulmonary hypertension.

Patients who have an ongoing risk of thromboembolism, such as an inherited clotting disorder, will require lifelong anticoagulation. Patients with an unprovoked PE, with no obvious risk factors, should have a thorough clinical assessment and appropriate investigations to exclude malignancy. They may require life-long anticoagulation as the risk of recurrence is 25% at 5 years without anticoagulation. The risk of bleeding is estimated to be 1.2% at 5 years. The risk of PE recurrence if anticoagulation is stopped, together with the risk of bleeding with continuing anticoagulation, should be discussed.

Patients with malignancy have an increased risk of PE. LMWH is recommended for patients with malignancy who develop PE. These patients also have an increased risk of bleeding, so the decision as to which anticoagulation to use, and for how long, must be made after weighing up the pros and cons for each patient.

Inferior vena cava filter

An IVC filter should be considered in anyone with a diagnosis of PE who has a significant risk of haemorrhage if commenced on anticoagulation. This includes those who are more than 65 years old, those with recent surgery, known haematological risk factors, liver failure, and malignancy. Patients who have extensive DVT and pelvic malignancy may also have recurrent episodes of PE as the clot breaks off and travels to the lungs. Retrievable filters are recommended, and the majority are placed infra-renally to prevent further emboli from reaching the lungs. This is usually a temporary solution and the filter will need to be removed once anticoagulation has been optimised.

Management of massive life-threatening pulmonary embolus

Approximately 8% of patients with a PE present with shock and collapse. Patients who have a systolic blood pressure of less than 90 mmHg may not be well enough for a CTPA to confirm the diagnosis but must rely on a bedside transthoracic echocardiogram which will show signs of right heart strain. Patients who present with a suspected massive pulmonary embolus with haemodynamic compromise, signs of right heart strain on transthoracic echocardiogram and or bilateral or saddle embolus on CTPA should be thrombolysed.

Patients should have immediate, but careful, intravenous fluid resuscitation, oxygen therapy to maintain the oxygen saturation between 94% and 98% and vasopressor support. If the intravenous fluid is given too aggressively, there is a risk of right ventricular failure. While waiting for confirmation of a PE, the patient should be commenced on IVUFH. Patients should receive 50 mg of alteplase as a bolus via a peripheral vein followed by intravenous heparin infusion. The activated partial thromboplastin time (APTT) should be maintained at between 1.5–2.5 times normal. Analgesia will be required for pain. Oral anticoagulation, usually with warfarin, should be started with a loading dose of 10 mg, with an aim to maintain the INR between 2 and 3.

Thrombolysis can increase the risk of cerebral and pulmonary haemorrhage. The decision to thrombolyse should be made by a senior respiratory physician after consultation with a radiologist and intensivists. Such patients should be managed in a high dependency unit (HDU) or intensive care unit (ICU).

If thrombolysis is contra-indicated, for example, in a pregnant patient, or it fails, then catheter-directed embolectomy or surgical embolectomy should be considered. These procedures are only available in tertiary centres and are associated with a high mortality.

Prognosis after acute PE

The overall mortality without treatment is 30% but reduces to 2–11% with anticoagulation. The risk of death is highest in the first week due to cardiogenic shock. The risk of recurrent PE is also greatest in the first 2 weeks. In the longer term, mortality is due to the underlying condition that caused the PE, such a malignancy.

The Pulmonary Embolism Severity Index (PESI) can be used to calculate the risk of death. Poor prognostic factors include age more than 65 years, co-morbid conditions, shock, right ventricular failure, hypoxaemia, thrombus in the right ventricle, elevated brain natriuretic peptide and N-terminal pro-brain natriuretic peptide, and elevated troponin I and T levels.

Recurrent pulmonary emboli

Patients with recurrent, acute PE may require life-long anticoagulation. Compliance with treatment should be checked, ensuring that the INR is therapeutic. Some patients, especially those with malignancy or pelvic DVTs, may have recurrent pulmonary emboli despite anticoagulation. In some patients it can be difficult to maintain the INR in the therapeutic range. In these patients, and those in whom anticoagulation is contra-indicated, an inferior vena cava filter should be considered. If a patient with a known diagnosis of PE, who is already being anticoagulated, presents with symptoms and signs of a PE, the same diagnostic approach should be taken. Images should be carefully reviewed by the radiologist as interpretation may be difficult.

Chronic pulmonary emboli

Patients with chronic pulmonary emboli will present with progressively worsening breathlessness and clinical features of pulmonary hypertension, which includes raised JVP, peripheral oedema, and parasternal heave. The ECG may show right ventricular hypertrophy and right axis deviation. The CXR will show prominent pulmonary arteries. A VQ scan will demonstrate unmatched defects. These patients are at risk of developing chronic thromboembolic pulmonary hypertension (CTEPH), which will be discussed in the next section.

Pulmonary hypertension

Pulmonary vascular tone is dependent on the balance of vasoconstrictors and vasodilators. Oxygen is a potent vasodilator, therefore hypoxia results in vasoconstriction.

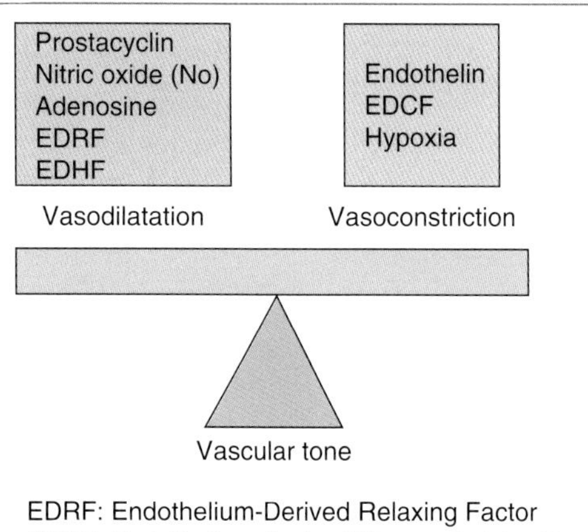

Figure 11.7 Regulation of pulmonary vascular tone.

Pulmonary hypertension presents with insidious onset of breathlessness, fatigue, and pre-syncope (Figure 11.7). When severe, patients can also experience atypical chest pains, peripheral oedema, palpitations, and syncope. Pulmonary hypertension can be due to a variety of different aetiologies as described in the WHO classification in Table 11.3. The NYHA Functional Classification (Box 11.3) is used to describe the severity of the dyspnoea.

Pulmonary hypertension can affect patients of all ages and ethnicities but occurs more commonly in African-Americans. The prevalence of pulmonary hypertension is estimated to be around 5–7/100 000 of population. Pulmonary hypertension has a poor prognosis if not diagnosed and treated promptly.

Normal pressure in the pulmonary artery system is 20/8 mmHg. The mean pulmonary artery pressure is 12–15 mmHg. Pulmonary hypertension is defined as a mean pulmonary artery pressure (PAP) of greater than 3.3 kPa (25 mmHg) at rest or greater than 4.0 kPa (30 mmHg) on exercise. Pulmonary hypertension can occur due to pulmonary

Table 11.3 WHO classification of pulmonary hypertension.

Type	Aetiology	Management
Group 1: Pulmonary arterial hypertension	Familial Appetite suppressants	Prostacyclin Endothelin receptor antagonist Phosphodiesterase-5 inhibitor
Group 2: Left heart disease: elevated left atrial pressure and pulmonary venous hypertension	Congenital cardiomyopathies Valvular heart disease Outflow tract obstruction Left ventricular systolic dysfunction Left ventricular diastolic dysfunction	Management of underlying condition Anticoagulation LTOT
Group 3: Severe lung disease	All causes of hypoxaemia, including COPD, ILD, sleep disordered breathing, alveolar hypotension	Management of underlying condition Anticoagulation LTOT
Group 4: Thromboembolic disease (CTEPH)	Develops secondary to chronic occlusion of proximal or distal pulmonary vessels	Thromboendarterectomy
Group 5: Multifactorial	Sickle cell disease β-thalassaemia Spherocytosis Myeloproliferative disorders Sarcoidosis Glycogen storage disease Chronic kidney disease	Management of underlying condition Anticoagulation LTOT

Box 11.3 NYHA functional classification.

Class	Functional capacity	Objective assessment
I	No symptoms with normal physical activity	No objective evidence of cardiovascular disease
II	Minimal symptoms on physical exertion	Some evidence of cardiovascular disease
III	Moderately severe symptoms on physical exertion	Evidence of moderately severe cardiovascular disease
IV	Severe symptoms on exertion, symptoms present at rest	Evidence of severe cardiovascular disease

arterial hypertension alone or occur due to pulmonary venous hypertension.

In patients presenting with symptoms suggestive of pulmonary hypertension a detailed history should include that of underlying lung disease (COPD, ILD, OSA), heart disease (including congenital heart disease), chronic thromboembolic disease, connective tissue disorders, and human immunodeficiency virus infection.

Clinical examination will reveal tachypnoea, tachycardia, and a loud second heart sound (P_2, the pulmonary component). In severe pulmonary hypertension there will be signs of right heart failure, which includes a parasternal heave, raised JVP, peripheral oedema, tricuspid regurgitation, and hepatomegaly. When pulmonary hypertension is due to an underlying condition, such as a connective tissue disorder, signs of that disease may be present.

Several investigations are required to make a diagnosis of pulmonary hypertension and to elucidate the cause of the pulmonary hypertension. The CXR in pulmonary hypertension will show large pulmonary arteries with pruning of the pulmonary vessels in the lung fields (Figure 11.8). The ECG will show tall p wave in leads 11, 1 V, AVF (p pulmonale) with a tall R wave in V1, ST segment depression with T wave inversion in V1–V3 (Figure 11.9).

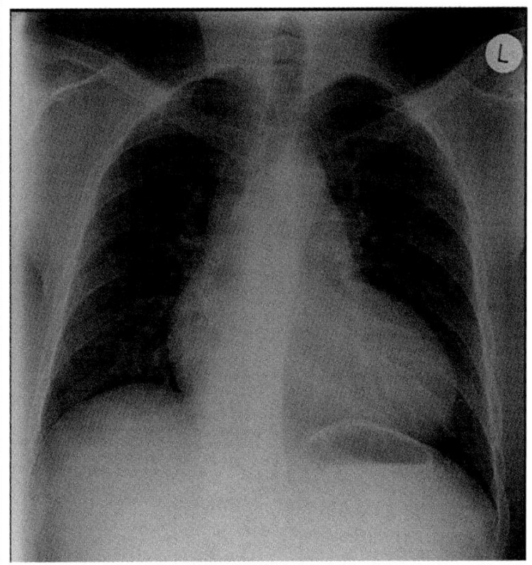

Figure 11.8 CXR showing right ventricular hypertrophy in a patient with severe pulmonary hypertension.

A transthoracic echocardiogram (TTE) is an essential investigation in a patient suspected of having pulmonary hypertension. It will show an enlarged right ventricle with right ventricular hypertrophy. The PA pressure can be estimated from the velocity of the tricuspid regurgitant jet. Right heart catheterisation is required to measure the mean pulmonary artery pressure, the pulmonary vascular resistance, to see if there are any thrombotic lesions and to assess the response to vasodilators. This is a specialist investigation that is conducted in a pulmonary hypertension centre.

An HRCT may be required to confirm the diagnosis of an ILD. A CTPA can confirm an acute pulmonary embolus and a VQ scan will be required to diagnose chronic pulmonary emboli.

Classification of pulmonary hypertension

Table 11.3 describes the WHO classification of Pulmonary Hypertension.

Group 1: Pulmonary Arterial Hypertension

Pulmonary hypertension due to **pulmonary arterial hypertension** (PAH) can occur due to a variety of different aetiologies that affect the small, muscular pulmonary arterioles. Box 11.4 lists these causes. This group was previously called Primary

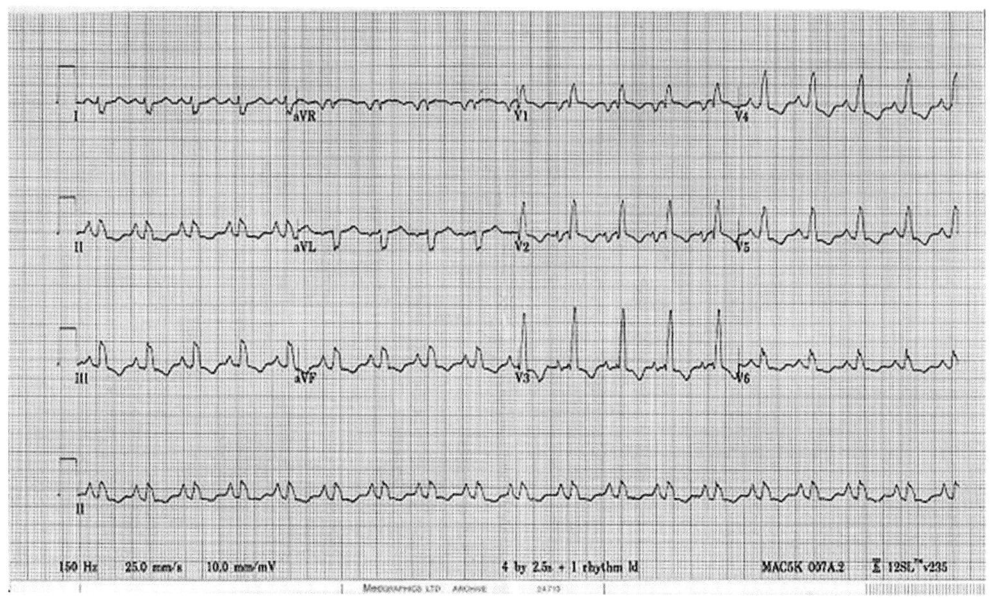

Figure 11.9 ECG changes seen in pulmonary hypertension.

Box 11.4 Aetiology of pulmonary arterial hypertension.

- Idiopathic (sporadic)
- Familial (hereditary)
- Drugs and toxins
- Connective tissue diseases
- Human immunodeficiency virus infection
- Portal hypertension
- Congenital heart disease
- Schistosomiasis

Pulmonary Hypertension. The incidence of PAH is 1–2/million of population, with a prevalence of 8/million of population. The peak incidence is in the 3rd and 4th decades of life with a female:male ratio of 2.4 : 1. There appears to be an increased incidence in Afro-Caribbean women. Patients with PAH should be managed in a centre with expertise in the management of this condition.

In genetically predisposed individuals, endothelial injury results in the release of a variety of cytokines, including endothelin and thromboxane, which are potent vasoconstrictors, and a reduction in the release of nitric oxide and prostaglandin I_2, which are potent vasodilators. These vasoconstrictors cause smooth muscle hyperplasia, medial hypertrophy, intimal thickening, and plexiform lesions of the muscular pulmonary arterioles (Figure 11.10, Figure 11.11). With time, there is vascular remodelling and increase in pulmonary vascular resistance. In addition, there is increased production of platelet-derived growth factor (PDGF), vascular endothelial growth factor (VEGF) and transforming growth factor (TGF) which results in a hypercoagulable state with in situ thrombosis, which causes further damage to the vessels.

The idiopathic and familial types cannot be clinically separated. Of these, 90% of cases are sporadic and 10% of cases are familial. The majority (80%) of the familial group occur due to a mutation of the bone morphogenetic protein receptor 2 (BMPR2) which is inherited as an autosomal dominant trait with incomplete penetrance of 10–20%. The remaining 20% of the familial group is due to other genetic defects.

Some 25% of the sporadic cases also have a genetic mutation in BMPR2 gene. Most individuals with the mutation never acquire the disease but may transmit the mutation to their progeny. The estimated risk of acquiring the disease is 10%.

Some cases of pulmonary arterial hypertension have been associated with the use of appetite suppressant drugs, including aminorex, fenfluramines, dexfenfluramine, toxic rapeseed oil, diethylproprion,

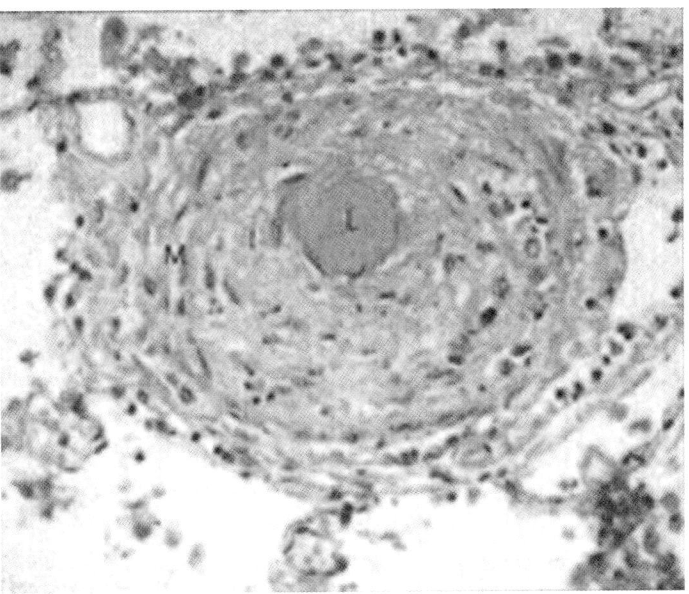

Figure 11.10 Histology showing intimal proliferation in pulmonary hypertension.

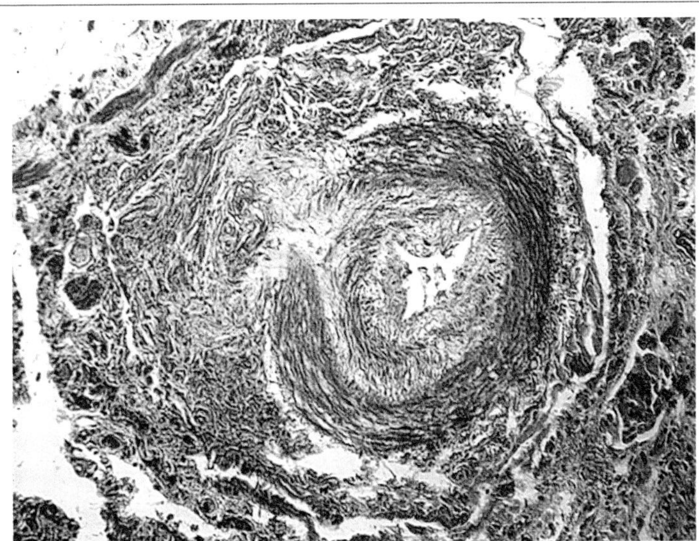

Figure 11.11 Histology showing changes of pulmonary arterial hypertrophy.

and benfluonex. Other drugs which have been implicated include L-tryptophan, amphetamines, methamphetamines, cocaine, and St. John's Wort. When a pregnant woman takes selective serotonin reuptake inhibitors (SSRIs), this may result in persistent pulmonary hypertension of the newborn child. SSRIs can also worsen existing pulmonary arterial hypertension in adults.

Several connective tissue disorders, for example, rheumatoid arthritis and systemic lupus erythematosus, can result in pulmonary hypertension secondary to interstitial lung disease. This is more likely in females and more likely in those with Raynaud's phenomenon. It is estimated that approximately 10–15% of patients with systemic sclerosis (scleroderma) develop pulmonary arterial hypertension caused by fibrous destruction of the alveolar capillaries, small arterioles, and arteries. The prognosis is very poor.

Approximately 0.5% of patients with HIV develop PAH through an unknown mechanism as do 1–6% of patients with portal hypertension secondary to chronic liver disease: this improves with liver transplantation. Congenital heart disease secondary to defects in the vascular system results in PAH due to an increase in pulmonary blood flow and pressure overload. Approximately 10% of children born with heart defects leading to left-to-right intracardiac shunts, for example, Eisenmenger's syndrome, will develop PAH, even if the defect is repaired.

Schistosomiasis is the commonest cause of PAH worldwide, mainly affecting those with hepato-splenic involvement. The schistosome ova embolize to the lungs and cause a granulomatous reaction in the pulmonary arterioles.

A rare cause of PAH is pulmonary veno-occlusive disease (PVOD) resulting from the occlusion of the pulmonary veins and tortuous dilatation of the pulmonary capillaries.

Patients with Group 1 PAH have a worse prognosis than those in the other groups if no treatment is given, with a median survival of 3 years.

Group 2: Pulmonary hypertension secondary to left heart disease

In this group, pulmonary hypertension develops due to elevation of the left atrial pressure and pulmonary venous pressure. This can develop secondary to left ventricular systolic or diastolic dysfunction, valvular heart diseases (particularly severe mitral regurgitation), inflow or outflow tract obstruction, and congenital and restrictive cardiomyopathies. Rarer causes include left atrial myxoma, constrictive pericarditis, and morbid obesity which can cause pulmonary hypertension by causing severe diastolic dysfunction. It is important to measure the pulmonary capillary wedge pressure and the left ventricular end-diastolic pressure accurately.

Group 3: Pulmonary hypertension secondary to lung disease

Common causes of pulmonary hypertension in this group include COPD, ILD combined pulmonary fibrosis and emphysema (CPFE), obstructive sleep apnoea (OSA) and disorders of alveolar hypoventilation. Hypoxaemia is a powerful stimulus for pulmonary vasoconstriction, which can result in pulmonary hypertension.

Mild pulmonary hypertension is prevalent in patients with COPD and confers a worse outcome. Patients with severe pulmonary hypertension, with a mean pulmonary artery pressure (PAP) of more than 45 mmHg, have less than 10% 5-year survival. Patients with ILD can develop pulmonary hypertension secondary to hypoxaemia or develop PAH directly due to the involvement of the pulmonary vascular bed as discussed earlier. Patients with CPFE have a particularly high risk of developing pulmonary hypertension which carries a poor prognosis. It is estimated that up to 20% of patients with severe OSA develop PH.

Group 4: Pulmonary hypertension secondary to chronic thromboembolic disease (CTEPH)

Approximately 1–5% of patients who survive an acute pulmonary embolus will develop chronic thromboembolic pulmonary hypertension (CTEPH) due to occlusion of the proximal or distal pulmonary vasculature. It is hypothesised that abnormally elevated Factor VIII levels or the presence of antiphospholipid antibodies may predispose to the development of CTEPH.

Patients who develop CTEPH will present with progressively worsening dyspnoea, initially on exertion, but eventually at rest and develop symptoms and signs of right heart failure. A history of possible previous PE should be sought. As the differential diagnosis for this presentation is huge, the patient will usually undergo many investigations to exclude primary cardiac problems, obstructive airways disease, and restrictive airways disease. A ventilation perfusion (VQ) scan is the imaging modality of choice and will show several mismatched defects. Patients will require right heart catheterisation to measure the pulmonary artery pressure and to determine whether the thrombotic lesions can be surgically removed.

Group 5: Multifactorial pulmonary hypertension

Pulmonary hypertension can develop due to a variety of other aetiologies. Haematological causes include chronic haemolytic anaemia, sickle cell disease, β-thalassaemia, spherocytosis, and myeloproliferative diseases. Other causes include sarcoidosis and glycogen storage diseases.

Management of pulmonary hypertension

Medical management of pulmonary hypertension includes optimal management of the underlying condition that caused the pulmonary hypertension to limit progression. Specific management of right heart failure and pulmonary hypertension includes anticoagulation, diuretics, and long term oxygen therapy (LTOT).

Advanced therapy is recommended for patients with Group 1 PAH. These treatments are generally not recommended for those with other types of pulmonary hypertension. Patients must be assessed in a specialised unit and have a diagnostic right heart catheter and vasoreactivity testing to determine which medications are likely to be beneficial.

Calcium channel antagonists, which cause vasodilation, may be beneficial and will demonstrate vasodilatation during right heart catheterisation. Diltiazem is the most commonly used agent.

Prostacyclin (PGI_2), an endogenous substance derived from arachidonic acid and produced by vascular endothelial cells, is reduced in pulmonary hypertension. PGI_2 has a variety of effects, including vascular smooth muscle relaxation resulting in vasodilatation, inhibition of smooth muscle proliferation and inhibition of platelet activity. Prostacyclin has a very short half-life *in vivo*.

Prostacylin (epoprostenol) is most effective when given intravenously through an in-dwelling catheter. Epoprostenol improves cardiopulmonary haemodynamics by causing vasodilation, and reduces pulmonary vascular resistance, thereby improving breathlessness and exercise capacity. Epoprostenol also improves life expectancy. This treatment is reserved for patients who are symptomatic with a NYHA stage of III or IV. Catheter-related sepsis, haemodynamic instability, and thrombosis are common complications. Iloprost, the inhaled form of prostacyclin and treprostanil, given subcutaneously, also improve exercise capacity and cardiopulmonary haemodynamics, with fewer systemic side effects. The oral form (Beraprost) is less effective. The oral and inhaled prostacyclins are usually given to patients who are WHO functional class II or III.

Oral endothelin receptor antagonists, such as bosenten, ambrisentan, or macitentan, reduce vascular tone, intimal proliferation, pulmonary artery pressure and pulmonary vascular resistance. Selective oral phosphodiesterase-5 inhibitors, such as sildenafil and tadalafil, also decrease pulmonary artery pressure and can be taken orally. Oral guanylate cyclase inhibitor, riociguat, is also available.

Surgical treatment of pulmonary hypertension

Endarterectomy is indicated for patients with CTEPH. Atrial septostomy has also shown benefits in patients with severe pulmonary hypertension, especially as a bridge to lung transplantation. Heart or heart lung transplantation may be an option for young patients with severe pulmonary hypertension.

Pulmonary haemorrhagic syndromes

There are several pulmonary haemorrhagic syndromes which can present with life-threatening haemoptysis. Pulmonary vasculitic diseases usually occur as part of a generalised systemic vasculitis which may involve the kidneys and other organs. Systemic lupus erythematosus (SLE) can cause pulmonary haemorrhage while rheumatoid arthritis rarely causes pulmonary haemorrhage.

Most patients with a vasculitis will have antineutrophil cytoplasmic antibodies (ANCA), which are immunoglobulin G antibodies against antigens in the cytoplasm of the neutrophil granulocyte. Antibodies to the perinuclear antigens, including myeloperoxidase (MPO), results in a p-ANCA vasculitis, and antibodies to proteinase 3 (PR3) results in a c-ANCA vasculitis.

Severe pulmonary haemorrhage results in blood in the alveolar spaces which compromises oxygenation, resulting in hypoxaemia and respiratory failure. Diffusing capacity (TLCO) and transfer coefficient (KCO) will be increased and blood-stained fluid will be seen when bronchoalveolar lavage is performed.

Management of pulmonary haemorrhage secondary to a vasculitis is with immunosuppressive treatment and plasmapheresis to remove circulating antibodies. Supportive treatment includes oxygen, bronchodilators, reversal of any coagulopathy, blood transfusion, and mechanical ventilation in severe cases. Management of life threatening haemoptysis is discussed in Chapter 5.

Granulomatosis with polyangiitis (GPA)

Granulomatosis with polyangiitis, previously known as Wegener's Granulomatosis, is a necrotising vasculitis affecting the upper airways, lungs, and kidneys. GPA presents with symptoms of rhinitis, sinusitis, blood-stained nasal discharge, epistaxis, and haemoptysis, which can result in extensive and life-threatening pulmonary haemorrhage.

The CXR and CT thorax often show cavitating nodules, the differential diagnosis for which includes malignancy, especially squamous cell carcinoma (see Chapter 9), infections such as *Staphylococcus aureus, Mycobacterium tuberculosis* and aspergillus fumigatus (see Chapter 8), and occupational lung diseases (see Chapter 15). A CT-PET will generally show increased FDG uptake and a CT-guided biopsy of the pulmonary nodule will show fibrinoid necrosis (Figure 11.12).

GPA also results in focal, necrotising glomerulonephritis, progressing rapidly to end-stage renal failure without treatment. Urea and electrolytes will be consistent with renal failure. Some 90% of patients with GPA will be c-ANCA positive and less than 10% will be p-ANCA positive. Renal biopsy will show fibrinoid necrosis.

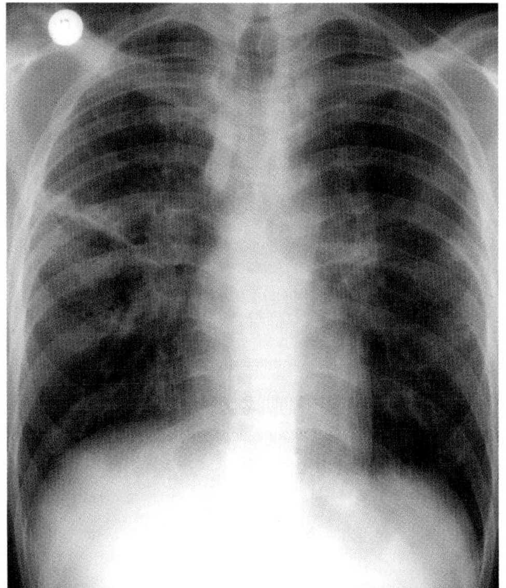

Figure 11.12 CXR of a patient with granulomatosis with polyangiitis.

Management of GPA is with immediate immunosuppression with high doses of intravenous cyclophosphamide in combination with methylprednisolone. Most patients (70–90%) will achieve remission, and immunosuppression can be maintained with less toxic drugs, such as azathioprine, rituximab, or methotrexate. Relapses are common, especially in patients with involvement of the upper airways and lungs and those with *Staphylococcus aureus* in their nasal passages.

Other vasculitides

Polyarteritis nodosa is a vasculitis affecting medium and small arteries resulting in aneurysm formation, glomerulonephritis, and vasculitic lesions in various organs. Pulmonary involvement is unusual but may result in haemoptysis, pulmonary haemorrhage, fibrosis, and pleurisy. **Microscopic polyangiitis** (MPA) is a systemic, ANCA-positive vasculitis resembling GPA.

Anti-glomerular basement membrane antibody (Goodpasture's) syndrome

Anti-glomerular basement membrane disease presents with rapidly progressive crescentic glomerulonephritis and alveolar haemorrhage due to circulating anti-basement membrane antibodies that bind to lung and renal tissue. Patients who are not diagnosed and treated promptly will progress to end-stage renal failure. There is clinical correlation between the initial plasma creatinine concentration and the severity of the renal disease.

Pulmonary involvement is more common in smokers, resulting in severe pulmonary haemorrhage and life-threatening haemoptysis. The CXR typically shows parenchymal infiltrates secondary to alveolar haemorrhage. Patients may become anaemic and require a blood transfusion. Type 1 respiratory failure can develop rapidly. A lung function test will show increased diffusing capacity (TLCO) because of the binding of inhaled CO to haemoglobin in the alveoli, and the transfer coefficient (KCO) will be increased. Bronchoalveolar lavage will reveal blood-stained fluid.

Management is with plasmapheresis to remove the circulating anti-basement membrane antibodies and complement. Immunosuppression with high dose methylprednisolone, followed by 1 mg kg^{-1} of oral prednisolone and oral cyclophosphamide will reduce the production of new antibodies. Smoking cessation is essential.

Anti-GBM levels should be monitored periodically until they are negative on two occasions. Approximately half of patients treated with plasmapheresis and immunosuppression will recover, but may be left with renal failure and abnormal lung function.

Patients receiving high dose immunosuppression for any of these conditions are at risk of developing pneumocystis jiroveci infection, so prophylaxis with co-trimoxazole is required. Intravenous fluids can reduce the risk of bladder toxicity, which can occur with intravenous cyclophosphamide.

Eosinophilic granulomatosis with polyangiitis (Churg-Strauss syndrome)

Eosinophilic granulomatosis with polyangiitis (EGPA), or allergic granulomatosis, was previously called Churg-Strauss syndrome. It is a multisystem, autoimmune condition causing inflammation of small and medium-sized blood vessels and usually develops in an individual with a history of atopy. The majority (>90%) have a history of asthma which precedes the development of the vasculitis by approximately 9 years.

In the initial prodromal stage, the majority of patients develop allergic rhinitis presenting with rhinorrhoea, nasal obstruction, nasal polyps, sinusitis, and worsening asthma. Patients may also develop fever and dyspnoea.

This initial stage is followed by marked peripheral blood eosinophilia, with more than 1500 cells ml^{-1}, or greater than 10% eosinophils on a differential white cell count. This may be masked if the patient is on corticosteroids for asthma.

This stage is followed by an eosinophilic vasculitis, which occurs due to eosinophilic infiltration of organs, causing damage. Eosinophilic infiltration of the lungs results in flitting pulmonary infiltrates on the CXR (see Figure 11.9). An HRCT thorax will show ground-glass changes and patchy areas of consolidation. Symptoms of dyspnoea, wheeze, cough, night sweats, fever, malaise, and weight loss occur.

Infiltration of other organs can result in severe vasculitic complications and infarction of organs. Some 75% of patients develop mononeuritis multiplex, and two-thirds of patients will develop skin involvement, with subcutaneous nodules, granuloma formation, and palpable purpura. Cardiac involvement, which may be asymptomatic, results in myocarditis, cardiomyopathy, and pericardial tamponade, and is fatal in 50% of cases. Myositis, eosinophilic infiltration of the gastrointestinal tract, neuritis, glomerulonephritis, and central nervous system involvement can all occur. Patients with EGPA will have symptoms related to the organs involved as well as systemic symptoms of fever, night sweats, malaise, and weight loss.

Five-year mortality is 12%. Renal involvement, proteinuria, involvement of the central nervous system and gastrointestinal system confer a worse prognosis, with a 5-year mortality rising to 50% if more than two organs are involved.

Diagnosis is made by recognising the clinical presentation, noting the marked peripheral eosinophilia, and demonstrating organ eosinophilia by biopsy of an organ. The lung and skin are most usually biopsied as these are often involved. P-ANCA levels, suggesting antibodies against myeloperoxidase, may be elevated in 40–60% of cases. Box 11.5 lists the American College of Rheumatology criteria for diagnosing EGPA. The presence of at least four of these has a sensitivity of 85% and a specificity of 99.7%.

The main differential diagnosis of EGPA includes allergic asthma, ABPA, granulomatosis with polyangiitis, microscopic polyangiitis and eosinophilic pneumonias. The differential diagnosis of eosinophilic pulmonary disorders is discussed in Chapter 7.

Box 11.5 Diagnosis of EGPA.

- Asthma
- Peripheral eosinophilia >10%
- Mononeuropathy or polyneuropathy
- Flitting pulmonary infiltrates
- Paranasal sinus abnormalities
- Extravascular eosinophils

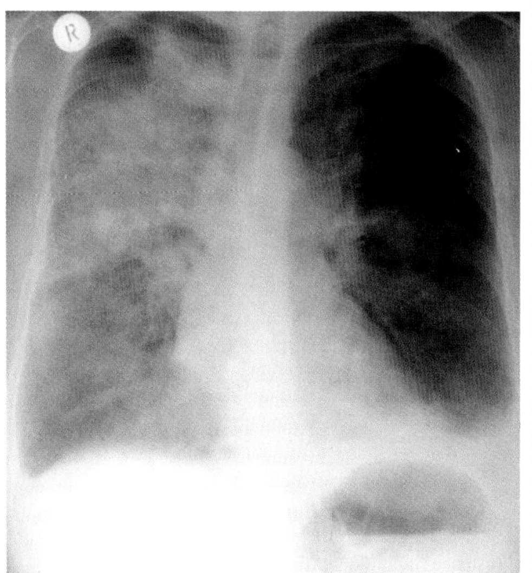

Figure 11.13 CXR showing acute haemorrhage in right lung in a patient with HHT.

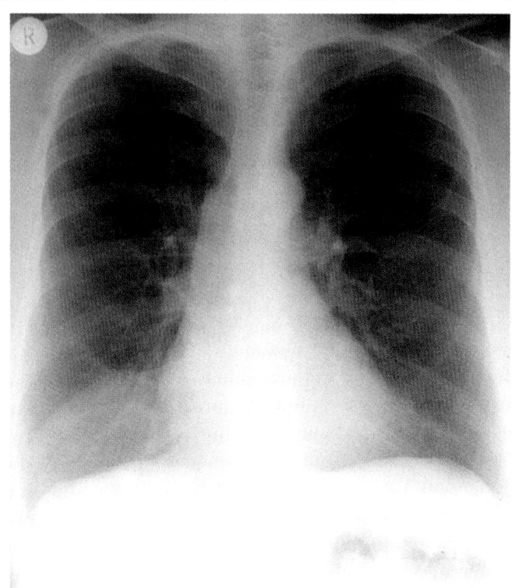

Figure 11.14 CXR showing changes of chronic pulmonary haemorrhage.

EGPA responds well to immunosuppression with intravenous corticosteroids, intravenous azathioprine and or cyclophosphamide, although relapse is common. Most patients suffer with chronic disease, with relapses and remissions throughout their lifetime.

Hereditary haemorrhagic telangiectasia (HHT)

Hereditary haemorrhagic telangiectasia (HHT), also called Osler-Weber-Rendau Syndrome, is a vasculitis which presents with multiple pulmonary arteriovenous malformations (AVMs). The exact prevalence is unknown but is estimated to be approximately 1 : 5000 to 1 : 8000.

HHT is an autosomal dominant disorder with mutations of the endoglin, ALK-1 and SMAD4 genes. For a diagnosis to be made, the International Consensus diagnostic criteria require the individual to have a first degree relative with HHT, suffer with spontaneous, recurrent epistaxis, have several mucocutaneous telangiectasias, and have arterio-venous malformations affecting the lungs, brain, liver, or the gastrointestinal tract. Most patients with HHT are asymptomatic in childhood but develop spontaneous and recurrent epistaxis during adolescence. Pulmonary AVMs are abnormal, thin-walled, saccular vessels that connect the pulmonary and systemic circulations. Many individuals with pulmonary AVMs are asymptomatic, but a third can develop clinically relevant right-to-left shunts with hypoxaemia which can progress to heart failure and secondary polycythaemia. These patients will develop clubbing and cyanosis. Pulmonary AVMs can also bleed into the lungs in 1.4%, resulting in haemoptysis and haemothorax, especially in pregnancy. AVMs increase in size during pregnancy, increasing the risk of haemorrhage, with a 1% risk of death (Figure 11.13, Figure 11.14).

The biggest risk is the development of embolic strokes and cerebral abscess secondary to paradoxical embolism. Management of pulmonary AVMs is with embolisation of the vessels to reduce the risk of cerebrovascular accidents. Chapter 5 describes the management of massive haemoptysis.

Individuals with HHT may present with iron deficiency anaemia secondary to gastrointestinal bleeding and with cerebral haemorrhage. It is important to screen family members to identify those at risk. There is some evidence that hormones and antifibrinolytic agents reduce the risk of gastrointestinal and nasal haemorrhage. Patients who suffer recurrent epistaxis, haemoptysis and haemothorax are advised not to embark on air travel.

SUMMARY OF LEARNING POINTS

- Thromboembolic disease is common in patients admitted to hospital, with 1% developing deep vein thrombosis and/or pulmonary emboli.
- Patients who are admitted to hospital should be assessed for their risk of developing VTE and offered prophylactic LMWH as appropriate.
- Acute pulmonary embolus should always be in the differential diagnosis of any patient presenting with acute breathlessness, pleuritic chest pain, unexplained hypoxia, hypotension, or collapse.
- The modified Wells score should be used to determine the probability of the patient having VTE.
- A CTPA is usually used to confirm the diagnosis of pulmonary embolus.
- Patients who present with acute pulmonary embolus should receive anticoagulation with low molecular weight heparin and warfarin or a NOAC.
- Patients who develop massive, life-threatening pulmonary embolus and who are haemodynamically unstable may require thrombolysis.
- Patients who develop pulmonary embolus without an obvious risk factor should receive anticoagulation indefinitely.
- Chronic thromboembolic disease should be considered in anyone presenting with insidious dyspnoea.
- A VQ scan is the investigation of choice for patients suspected of having chronic pulmonary emboli.
- Patients with acute or chronic pulmonary emboli can develop pulmonary arterial hypertension.
- Pulmonary hypertension is defined as a mean pulmonary artery pressure of greater than 25 mmHg.
- There are many different causes of pulmonary hypertension.
- Pulmonary arterial hypertension has a bad prognosis with a mean life expectancy of 3 years without treatment.
- A definitive diagnosis of pulmonary hypertension is made with a right heart catheter which directly measures the PAP and the response to vasodilators.
- Management of PH is with treatment of the underlying cause, anticoagulation, calcium antagonists (in some cases), and LTOT.
- Patients with pulmonary arterial hypertension and WHO functional class III or IV must be assessed in a specialist centre and receive advanced treatments.
- Pulmonary haemorrhagic syndromes can affect many organs and may present with life-threatening haemoptysis.
- Most of these conditions are ANCA-positive and respond well to immunosuppression and plasmapheresis.
- Hereditary haemorrhagic telangiectasia is an inherited condition with the development of AVMs which can present with haemorrhage into the lungs, brain, and gastrointestinal system.

MULTIPLE CHOICE QUESTIONS

11.1 Which of the following statements about acute pulmonary emboli is true?

A A CXR is a sensitive test in making a diagnosis of PE

B ECG changes can be used to make a diagnosis of PE

C Patients with a PE always present with symptoms of breathlessness

D Symptoms of PE always occur within minutes of occlusion of the pulmonary artery

E About 70% of patients with a PE will be hypoxaemic

Answer: E

PE often presents with non-specific symptoms which can occur within minutes, although many patients present after days, weeks or months. Only 73% of patients with a PE present with symptoms of breathlessness. Neither a CXR or ECG changes are specific for PE and can be confidently used to make a diagnosis of a PE on their own.

11.2 Which of the following statements about the diagnosis of PE is true?

A A positive D-dimer level is helpful in making a diagnosis of PE
B A normal troponin level means that a PE can be ruled out
C A modified Wells score, used together with imaging and D-dimer level, increases the sensitivity of the test
D VQ scan is the imaging modality of choice in most patients
E Patients with a high Wells score and negative D-dimer will not require any further investigations

Answer key: C

The D-dimer level may be high for many reasons so cannot be used to make a diagnosis of PE. A negative D-dimer in a patient with a low Wells score rules out PE. Troponin may be elevated in patients with a large PE, but cannot be used to exclude PE. CTPA is the main imaging modality for PE, with a higher sensitivity and specificity than VQ scan and because it is available in most centres. Patients with a high clinical probability of PE will require further investigations (CTPA) regardless of the D-dimer result.

11.3 Which of the following statements about acute PE is true?

A All patients presenting with an acute PE should be hospitalised
B Patients with an acute PE should be started on warfarin as the first anticoagulant
C LMWH is the initial treatment of choice for most haemodynamically stable patients with PE
D Patients who are hypotensive should be commenced on LMWH
E Rivaroxaban is the treatment of choice for patients with severe PE

Answer: C

Patients who are haemodynamically stable and not hypoxaemic can be anticoagulated safely at home. The guidelines recommend that patients with acute PE are started on LMWH first, which should be continued for at least 48 hours after the INR level is therapeutic. Patients with severe PE and hypotension should be given IVUFH as they may require thrombolysis, and UFH has a shorter half-life and the effects can be reversed more quickly. Rivoroxaban, a Factor Xa inhibitor, is contra-indicated as the effects cannot be easily reversed.

11.4 Which of the following statements is true?

A All patients with acute PE should be anticoagulated for 12 months
B Patients who develop PE after surgery should be anticoagulated for 6 months
C Patients with recurrent PEs should be anticoagulated for life
D The risk of PE recurrence is 5% in the first 5 years
E Most patients who have a PE are found to have a DVT

Answer: C

The recommendations are that patients with a known specific cause for the PE, such as surgery, should receive 3 months of anticoagulation. If the cause is unknown, then they should receive 6 months and then be reviewed. The risk of recurrence is up to 20% over the first 5 years, so patients with unprovoked or recurrent PEs may need lifelong anticoagulation. Only 10% of patients with PE are found to have a DVT.

11.5 Which of the following statements about chronic thromboembolic disease (CTED) is true?

A Patients with CTED should receive intravenous prostacyclin
B Thrombolysis is the treatment of choice for those with CTEPH
C Some 50% of patients with acute PE develop CTED
D A diagnosis of CTED can be made with an echocardiogram
E Embolectomy should be considered in a patient with CTEPH

Answer: E

Only 1–5% of patients with acute PE go on to develop CTED, but the majority of these will have evidence of pulmonary hypertension which requires a right heart catheter for a definitive diagnosis. Embolectomy is often successful in these patients where neither prostacyclin or thrombolysis is indicted.

11.6 Which of the following statements about pulmonary hypertension is true?

A Hereditary pulmonary hypertension is the commonest aetiology
B Median survival of Group 1 PAH is 10 years without treatment
C Group 1 PAH has a worse prognosis than the other types of PH
D Some 50% of those who survive an acute pulmonary embolus develop PH
E The diagnosis of pulmonary hypertension can be made rapidly in the clinic

Answer: C

Hereditary (familial) pulmonary hypertension accounts for a minority of all cases of pulmonary hypertension. Group 1 PAH has the worst prognosis, with a median survival of 3 years without treatment. Some 1–5% of patients who survive an acute pulmonary embolus develop pulmonary hypertension. The diagnosis of pulmonary hypertension can be difficult as the symptoms are often vague and insidious. There is evidence that it can take more than 2 years before a definitive diagnosis is made.

11.7 Which of the following is consistent with a diagnosis of pulmonary hypertension?

A Mean PAP > 15 mmHg at right heart catheter
B Increased pulmonary vasculature on CXR
C ECG showing ST elevation in the anterior leads
D Pan-systolic murmur throughout the praecordium
E Enlarged right ventricle on transthoracic echocardiogram

Answer: E

Patients with pulmonary hypertension will have pruning of the pulmonary vessels on CXR, ECG will show tall p wave in leads II, IV, AVF (p pulmonale) with a tall R wave in V1, ST segment depression with T wave inversion in V1–V3. The mean PAP will be greater than 25 mmHg at rest or greater than 30 mmHg on exertion. A pan-systolic murmur is not associated specifically with pulmonary hypertension.

11.8 Which of the following is NOT indicated as management of established Group 1 pulmonary arterial hypertension?

A Endothelin inhibitor
B Fibrinolytic agent
C Heart lung transplantation
D Phosphodiesterase-5 inhibitor
E Prostacyclin analogues

Answer: B

Fibrinolytic agents are not indicated in the management of PAH. All the others are indicated.

11.9 Which of the following statements about granulomatosis with polyangiitis (GPA) is true?

A Relapse is commoner in those with upper airway and lung involvement
B GPA commonly presents with nephritic syndrome
C A history of atopy is uncommon in patients with GPA
D Nasal involvement is rare with GPA
E Majority of patients with GPA will be p-ANCA positive

Answer: A.

Most patients with GPA are c-ANCA positive and present with necrotising glomerulonephritis. Nasal involvement is common, and relapse is commoner in those with upper airway and lung involvement. History of atopy is common in those with Eosinophilic granulomatosis with polyangiitis and not in GPA.

11.10 Which of the following statements about hereditary haemorrhagic telangiectasia (HHT) is NOT true?

A HHT is an autosomal recessive disorder
B HHT increases the risk of cerebrovascular accidents secondary to paradoxical embolism

C HHT increases the risk of haemoptysis and haemothorax in pregnancy
D Most patients with HHT are asymptomatic in childhood
E Iron deficiency anaemia can occur secondary to gastrointestinal bleeding

Answer: A

HHT is an autosomal dominant disorder. Arteriovenous malformations (AVMs) develop in many organs, including the lungs, the brain, and the gastrointestinal tract which can bleed, resulting in haemoptysis cerebrovascular accidents and gastrointestinal bleeding. HHT can present with iron-deficiency anaemia. The risk of bleeding is increased in pregnancy. Children are relatively asymptomatic, and symptoms develop progressively after puberty.

FURTHER READING

Ageno, W., Gallus, A.S., Wittkowsky, A. et al. (2012). Oral anticoagulant therapy—antithrombotic therapy and prevention of thrombosis, 9th ed: American College of Chest Physicians evidence-based clinical practice guidelines. *Chest* 141 (2 SUPPL): e44S–e88S.

Allen, J.N. and Davis, W.B. (1994). Eosinophilic lung diseases. *American Journal of Respiratory and Critical Care Medicine* 150 (5): 1423–1438.

Badesch, D.B., Champion, H.C., Sanchez, M.A.G. et al. (2009). Diagnosis and assessment of pulmonary arterial hypertension. *Journal of the American College of Cardiology* 54 (1 Suppl): S55–S66.

British Thoracic Society Standards of Care Committee Pulmonary Embolism Guideline Development Group (2003). British Thoracic Society guidelines for the management of suspected acute pulmonary embolism. *Thorax* 58 (6): 470–483.

Churg, J. and Strauss, L. (1951). Allergic granulomatosis, allergic angiitis, and periarteritis nodosa. *The American Journal of Pathology* 27 (2): 277–301.

Dartevelle, P., Fadel, E., Mussot, S. et al. (2004). Chronic thromboembolic pulmonary hypertension. *European Respiratory Journal* 23 (4): 637–648.

Federman, D. and Kirsner, R. (2001). An update on hypercoagulable disorders. *Archives of Internal Medicine* 161 (8): 1051–1056.

Galiè, N., Corris, P.A., Frost, A. et al. (2013). Updated treatment algorithm of pulmonary arterial hypertension. *Journal of the American College of Cardiology* 62 (25 Suppl): D60–D72.

Garcia, D.A., Baglin, T.P., Weitz, J.I., and Samama, M.M. (2012). Parenteral anticoagulants-antithrombotic therapy and prevention of thrombosis, 9th ed: American College of Chest Physicians evidence-based clinical practice guidelines. *Chest* 141 (2 SUPPL): e24S–e43S.

Guérin, L., Couturaud, F., Parent, F. et al. (2014). Prevalence of chronic thromboembolic pulmonary hypertension after acute pulmonary embolism. Prevalence of CTEPH after pulmonary embolism. *Thrombosis and Haemostasis* 112 (3): 598–605.

Jiménez, D., Kopecna, D., Tapson, V. et al. (2014). Derivation and validation of multimarker prognostication for normotensive patients with acute symptomatic pulmonary embolism. *American Journal of Respiratory and Critical Care Medicine* 189 (6): 718–726.

Kearon, C., Akl, E.A., Comerota, A.J. et al. (2012). Antithrombotic therapy for VTE disease: antithrombotic therapy and prevention of thrombosis, 9th ed: American College of Chest Physicians evidence-based clinical practice guidelines. *Chest* 141 (2 SUPPL): 419–494.

Kemmeren, J., Algra, A., and Grobbee, D. (2001). Third generation oral contraceptives and risk of venous thrombosis: meta-analysis. *British Medical Journal* 323 (7305): 131–139.

Kucher, N. and Goldhaber, S.Z. (2005). Management of massive pulmonary embolism. *Circulation* 112 (2): e28–e32.

Kyrle, P.A., Rosendaal, F.R., and Eichinger, S. (2010). Risk assessment for recurrent venous thrombosis. *Lancet* 376 (9757): 2032–2039.

Lang, I.M., Pesavento, R., Bonderman, D., and Yuan, J.X.-J.J. (2013). Risk factors and basic mechanisms of chronic thromboembolic pulmonary hypertension: a current understanding. *European Respiratory Journal* 41 (2): 462–468.

Liu, C., Chen, J., Gao, Y. et al. (2013). Endothelin receptor antagonists for pulmonary arterial hypertension. *The Cochrane Database of Systematic Reviews* (2): CD004434. http://www.ncbi.nlm.nih.gov/pubmed/23450552.

Masi, A.T., Hunder, G.G., Lie, J.T. et al. (1990). The American College of Rheumatology 1990 criteria for the classification of Churg-Strauss syndrome (allergic granulomatosis and angiitis). *Arthritis & Rheumatism* 33 (8): 1094–1100.

Paramothayan, N.S., Lasserson, T.J., Wells, A.U., and Walters, E.H. (2003). Prostacyclin for pulmonary hypertension. The Cochrane Database of Systematic Reviews CD002994.

Quinlan, D.J., McQuillan, A., and Eikelboom, J.W. (2004). Low-molecular-weight heparin compared with intravenous unfractionated heparin for treatment of pulmonary embolism: a meta-analysis of randomized, controlled trials. *Annals of Internal Medicine* 140 (3): 175–183.

Rubin, L.J., Badesch, D.B., Fleming, T.R. et al. (2011). Long-term treatment with sildenafil citrate in pulmonary arterial hypertension: the SUPER-2 study. *Chest* 140 (5): 1274–1283.

Sanchez, O., Trinquart, L., Planquette, B. et al. (2013). Echocardiography and Pulmonary Embolism Severity Index have independent prognostic roles in pulmonary embolism. *The European Respiratory Journal* 42 (3): 681–688.

Sekhri, V., Mehta, N., Rawat, N. et al. (2012). Management of massive and nonmassive pulmonary embolism. *Archives of Medical Science* 8 (6): 957–969.

Stein, P.D., Beemath, A., Matta, F. et al. (2007). Clinical characteristics of patients with acute pulmonary embolism: data from PIOPED II. *The American Journal of Medicine* 120 (10): 871–879.

Taichman, D.B., Ornelas, J., Chung, L. et al. (2014). Pharmacologic therapy for pulmonary arterial hypertension in adults: CHEST guideline and expert panel report. *Chest* 146 (2): 449–475.

Wells, P.S., Anderson, D.R. et al. (2000). Derivation of a simple clinical model to categorize patients probability of pulmonary embolism: increasing the models utility with the SimpliRED D-dimer. *Thrombosis and Haemostasis* 83 (3): 416–420.

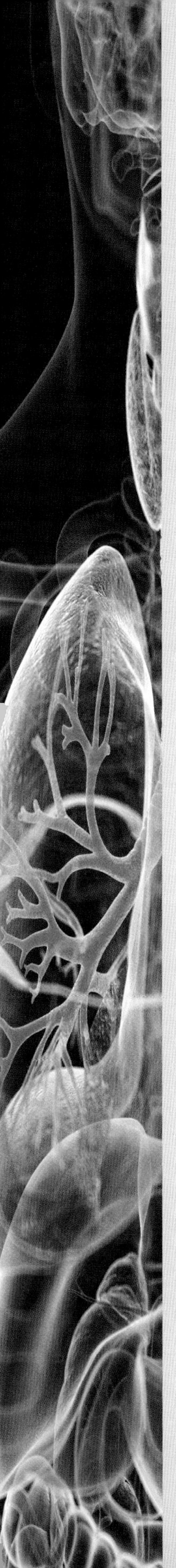

CHAPTER 12

Suppurative lung disease

Learning objectives

- To understand the aetiology and predisposing factors for suppurative lung diseases
- To understand the structure and function of cilia and the consequences of abnormally functioning cilia
- To recognise the aetiology, diagnosis, and management of bronchiectasis
- To understand the inheritance, diagnosis, and management of cystic fibrosis
- To understand the inheritance, diagnosis, and management of primary ciliary dyskinesia
- To understand the aetiology, diagnosis, and management of lung abscess

Essential Respiratory Medicine, First Edition. Shanthi Paramothayan.

Companion website: www.wiley.com/go/paramothayan/essential_respiratory_medicine

Abbreviations

A1AT	alpha 1 antitrypsin
ABC	ATP binding cassette
ABPA	allergic bronchopulmonary aspergillosis
ATP	adenosine triphosphate
BiPAP	bi-level positive airway pressure
cAMP	cyclic adenosine monophosphate
CAP	community acquired pneumonia
CF	cystic fibrosis
CFTR	cystic fibrosis transmembrane conductance regulator
COPD	chronic obstructive pulmonary disease
CRP	C-reactive protein
CT	computed tomography
CVID	common variable immunodeficiency
CXCR1	chemokine receptor
CXR	chest X-ray
DNA	deoxyribonucleic acid
FEV_1	forced expiratory volume in one second
FVC	forced vital capacity
HIV	human immunodeficiency virus
HRCT	high-resolution computed tomography
LTOT	long term oxygen therapy
MAC	*Mycobacterium avium complex*
MCE	mucociliary escalator
MDCT	multi detector computed tomography
NMCC	nasal mucociliary clearance test
NO	nitric oxide
NTM	non-tuberculous mycobacteria
PCD	primary ciliary dyskinesia
SGRQ	St. George's Respiratory Questionnaire
SLE	systemic lupus erythematosus
UK	United Kingdom

Introduction

Suppurative lung diseases are a group of disorders which result in chronic lung infection, with pus in the lungs. Individuals with suppurative lung diseases present with chronic purulent sputum and recurrent respiratory tract infections. The aetiology of these conditions is variable. Bronchiectasis is a relatively common condition whereas primary ciliary dyskinesia (PCD) is rare. Cystic fibrosis is a relatively common inherited condition which results in severe bronchiectasis. Empyema is pus in the pleural cavity. This is discussed in Chapter 10. Box 12.1 lists some suppurative lung diseases.

Box 12.1 Suppurative lung diseases.

- Bronchiectasis
- Cystic fibrosis
- Primary ciliary dyskinesia
- Lung abscess
- Empyema

Bronchiectasis

Bronchiectasis is a chronic lung disease which occurs after destruction and dilatation of bronchi due to a cycle of recurrent infection and inflammation (Figure 12.1).

The healthy bronchial epithelium is lined with fine, hair-like structures called cilia. The cilium has a structure identical to that of a flagellum and is composed of nine pairs of microtubular doublets, each with an A and B sub-unit attached as a semi-circle. A central sheath contains a pair of microtubules which attach to the outer doublet by radial spokes with the outer doublets interconnected by nexin links. The A subunit is attached to two dynein arms (inner and outer) that contain adenosine triphosphate (ATP) which are responsible for ciliary motion. The central sheath, radial spokes, and nexin links maintain the structural integrity of the cilium. The cilium is anchored at its base by cytoplasmic microtubules and a basal body comprised of a basal foot and rootlet. The orientation of the basal foot indicates the direction of effective cilial stroke (Figure 12.2).

Cilia line the entire respiratory system: the nasal mucosa, paranasal sinuses, middle ear, the Eustachian tube, pharynx, trachea, and bronchi down to the respiratory bronchioles. Each ciliated cell has 200 cilia, 5–6 μm long. Cilia line the Fallopian tubes and important in the movement of the fertilised ovum. The structure of the spermatozoan tail is identical to that of the cilium.

Ciliary motion is responsible for the rotation of organs in embryogenesis so that the organs end up in their usual positions, with the heart on the left side of the thoracic cavity and the liver on the right side of the abdomen.

Healthy lungs have fully functioning cilia that beat synchronously in a two-part ciliary beat cycle: the power stroke and then the recovery stroke. This ciliary action propels the overlying mucus up the bronchial tree, up the trachea until it reaches the

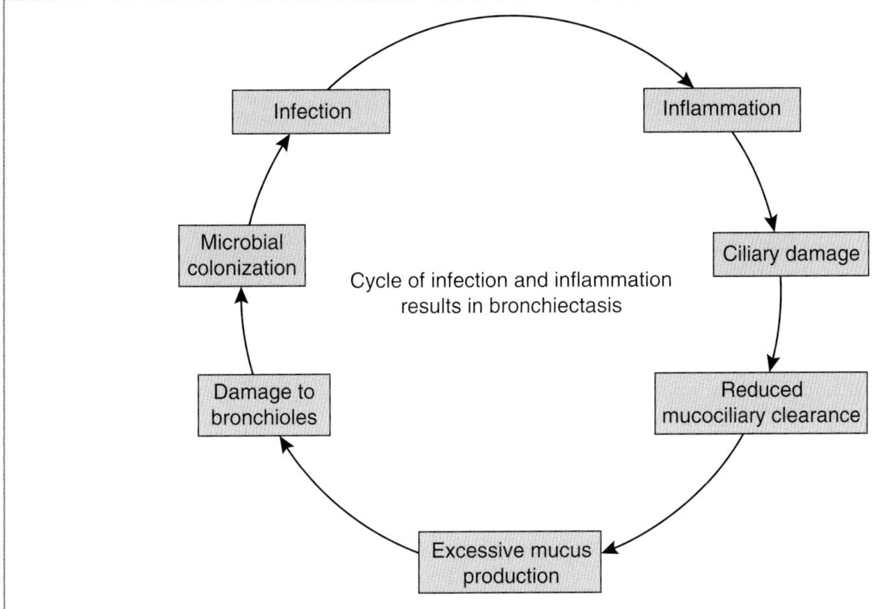

Figure 12.1 Progression of bronchiectasis with cycle of infection and inflammation.

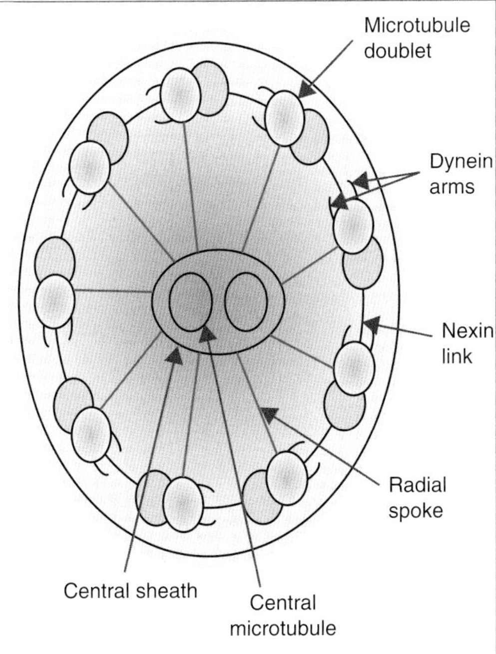

Figure 12.2 Electron microscopy image of cilium (diagram).

pharynx and is swallowed. The amount of mucus produced by normal lungs is relatively small. This constant movement and clearance of mucus forms the mucociliary escalator (MCE), which is an essential part of the lungs' clearance and defence mechanisms. Bacteria, viruses, pollen, dust, and other particulate matter become trapped in the mucus layer and are cleared. The lungs' defence mechanism is discussed more fully in Chapter 2.

Pathogenesis of bronchiectasis

Ciliary function is impaired by cigarette smoke, bacterial toxins, and viral antigens that cause the shedding of ciliated respiratory cells and disruption to the MCE. Damage to the epithelial cells can take several weeks to repair, even after the common cold. Impaired ciliary function results in a build-up of mucus within the dilated bronchi. Bacteria and viruses get trapped in the mucus, multiply rapidly and colonise the lung, causing persistent infection and chronic mucus production. Bacteria prevent the healing of the damaged respiratory epithelium by binding to, and disrupting, the functioning of certain epithelial receptors: fibronectin, which is important in cell migration, and integrin, which is necessary for the adhesion of cells.

Bronchiectasis results in inflammation of the airways and airflow obstruction. Bacterial infection results in the outpouring of inflammatory cytokines, including interleukin 8 and interleukin 6, which recruit neutrophils through interaction with the chemokine receptor CXCR1. Proteases from bacterial pathogens, for example, Pseudomonas aeruginosa, cleave and disable CXCR1, resulting in a reduction in neutrophil recruitment, ineffective neutrophil function, and failure of bacterial killing. Neutrophils release proteases and reactive oxygen intermediates, such as hydrogen peroxide, as well as several inflammatory cytokines. High levels of human neutrophil peptides, called alpha defensins, are found in the sputum of patients with bronchiectasis. These impair neutrophil phagocytosis and reduce antimicrobial activity. Anti-proteases, such as alpha -1 antitrypsin, restore CXCR1 and enhance bacterial killing. Increased neutrophil elastase activity results in mucus which is more viscous and harder to clear. Collagen deposition in the bronchial wall causes permanent distortion and dilatation of major bronchi.

Aetiology of bronchiectasis

Bronchiectasis that results from infection and inflammation is referred to as non-cystic fibrosis bronchiectasis, thus differentiating it from the severe bronchiectasis that occurs in cystic fibrosis. The prevalence of bronchiectasis is unknown as it can arise from several different causes. The prevalence of bronchiectasis has declined in the developed world but is a common cause of morbidity and mortality in developing countries. Bronchiectasis is commoner in females compared to males, perhaps because of the higher prevalence of rheumatoid arthritis and related conditions in the female population. Bronchiectasis can occur after damage to the bronchial mucosa, due to immunodeficiency states which predispose to recurrent infections, abnormal ciliary function or abnormal viscosity of the respiratory secretions. Table 12.1 lists these conditions.

Bronchiectasis may be localised to a small area of the lung or be more diffuse due to generalised infection and inflammation. Localised bronchiectasis can occur after inhalation of a foreign body, such as a peanut, which traps purulent material within that segment, causing bronchial wall damage. An enlarged lymph node can compress a bronchus, resulting in bronchiectasis more distally.

Several international studies which looked at how often a specific aetiology for the bronchiectasis could be identified found a specific cause in 60–93% of patients after comprehensive tests. Severe and recurrent respiratory tract infections are the commonest cause of ciliary and bronchial wall damage, accounting for 20% of bronchiectasis. Bronchiectasis secondary to childhood infections, particularly measles and pertussis (whooping cough), was common prior to immunisation in the UK and still is a common cause of bronchiectasis in developing countries. In adults, bronchiectasis can develop after community acquired pneumonia, especially after infections with *Staphylococcus aureus* and *Klebsiella pneumonia*, although severe bronchiectasis is much less common now with prompt antibiotic treatment. Tuberculosis is still a common cause of bronchiectasis, especially in developing countries.

A heterozygous mutation in the cystic fibrosis transmembrane conductance regulator (CFTR) gene may contribute to the development of diffuse bronchiectasis through dysfunction of the airway sodium and chloride channels.

Vitamin D deficiency may predispose to increased colonisation with bacteria, including Pseudomonas, and increase the frequency of exacerbations. Increased markers of neutrophilic inflammation were found in the sputum of those with bronchiectasis and vitamin D deficiency.

Recurrent aspiration pneumonia is a common cause of bronchiectasis in the elderly. The risk of aspiration pneumonia is increased in patients with reduced consciousness, for example, after a stroke, after a seizure, or when intoxicated with alcohol or other drugs. Neurological and neuromuscular conditions, such as Parkinson's disease, multiple sclerosis, and motor neurone disease, result in impaired swallowing and aspiration, as do oesophageal diseases, such as reflux and achalasia.

Foreign body aspiration is more likely to occur in small children and the elderly. Common items aspirated include small toys, nut and seeds in children, and bones and a bolus of food in the elderly. There is usually a history of choking and coughing preceding the development of chronic symptoms, often weeks earlier. The foreign body is more likely to enter the right lung and lodge in the middle lobe. Clinical examination may reveal a monophonic wheeze. The CXR and CT thorax will be abnormal, showing signs of collapse or atelectasis. Flexible bronchoscopy may be required to remove the foreign body. In some cases, if the foreign body

Table 12.1 Aetiology of bronchiectasis.

Underlying cause	**Diagnosis**	**Management**
Infection	Childhood infections (pertussis, measles)	Childhood vaccination
Infection	Recurrent respiratory infections	Treatment of underlying cause Prompt antibiotics, mucolytics, bronchodilators and chest physiotherapy Prophylactic antibiotics
Infection	ABPA	Corticosteroids and antifungals
Allergic reaction	*Mycobacterium tuberculosis*	BCG vaccination in high risk groups Anti-tuberculous treatment
Infection	Non-tuberculous mycobacterial infection (NTM)	Anti-tuberculous treatment for 24 months
Infection	Aspiration pneumonia	Prevention by identifying groups at risk Prompt antibiotic treatment and chest physiotherapy
Bronchial obstruction	Foreign body inhalation Carcinoid tumour Enlarged lymph node	Bronchoscopy Surgical resection
Systemic disease	Rheumatoid arthritis Sjögren's disease Crohn's disease HIV	Treatment of underlying condition (immunosuppression) Anti-retroviral treatment
Abnormal cartilage	Tracheobronchomalacia Bronchomalacia Tracheobronchomegaly	Tracheal or bronchial stent Tracheobronchoplasty
Abnormal immune system	Congenital hypogammaglobulinaemia Combined variable immune deficiency (CVID) Selective immunoglobulin deficiencies Lymphoma Myeloma Post-transplant	Intravenous immunoglobulins Prophylactic antibiotics Prompt treatment of infections
Ciliary dysfunction	Primary Ciliary Dyskinesia Young syndrome	Treatment of bronchiectasis
Abnormal respiratory secretions	Cystic fibrosis	Treatment of severe bronchiectasis Lung transplantation

is lodged very far down the bronchial tree, rigid bronchoscopy under general anaesthetic, or surgery may be indicated. Post-obstructive pneumonia can progress to bronchiectasis or to a lung abscess.

While non-tuberculous mycobacteria (NTM) infection can result in bronchiectasis with the characteristic *tree in bud* appearance, bronchiectasis from a different aetiology can predispose to NTM infection, particularly with *Mycobacterium avium complex* (MAC). These patients are more likely to develop ABPA and aspergilloma.

Tracheobronchomalacia (Williams-Campbell syndrome) and tracheobronchomegaly (Mounier-Kuhn syndrome) are diffuse or segmental weaknesses of the trachea or main stem bronchi due to anatomic defects of the airways arising from a deficiency of cartilage in the fourth to sixth order bronchi. Deficient cartilage support results in airway collapse during forced exhalation. This results in inefficient clearance of respiratory secretions and predisposes to the development of bronchiectasis. The CXR will show dilated trachea and bronchi. The diameter of the trachea (measured 2 cm above the main carina) will be greater than 3 cm, the right main bronchus greater than 2.5 cm and the left main bronchus greater than 2 cm. CT thorax with expiratory views will demonstrate airway collapse and narrowing. Placement of a tracheal stent will improve symptoms by reducing airway collapse. Tracheobronchoplasty could be considered in some patients.

Connective tissue disorders, particularly rheumatoid arthritis and Sjögren's syndrome, predispose to the development of bronchiectasis, although the exact mechanism is unknown. Symptoms of bronchiectasis occur years after the diagnosis of the underlying condition is made. In one study, the frequency of an abnormal CFTR allele was increased in patients with bronchiectasis and rheumatoid arthritis relative to patients with rheumatoid arthritis but without bronchiectasis and normal controls. Bronchiectasis is a rare complication of other connective tissue disorders, especially systemic lupus erythematosus (SLE) and Marfan's syndrome. Bronchiectasis is also associated with Crohn's disease, ulcerative colitis, and yellow nail syndrome. It is assumed that optimal treatment of the underlying systemic disease will prevent the deterioration of bronchiectasis, although there are no studies supporting this assumption.

Alpha 1 antitrypsin (A1AT) deficiency is associated with bronchiectasis. A1AT deficiency is discussed in Chapter 6. Adult polycystic kidney disease (APKD), which is an autosomal dominant disease, occurs because of defective cilia and ciliary protein expression of polycystin-1 and polycystin-2, with the formation of renal cysts. Patients with APKD are more likely to develop bronchiectasis.

Congenital hypogammaglobulinaemia and selective immunoglobulin deficiencies present with recurrent upper and lower respiratory tract infections in childhood and, if undetected, will result in bronchiectasis. Hypogammaglobulinaemia may be associated with thymoma. Common variable immunodeficiency (CVID) results in small airway changes and bronchiectasis. It is not clear whether an isolated IgG subclass deficiency, for example, IgG_2 deficiency, can result in bronchiectasis as the levels of these vary greatly in normal adults. Investigation for bronchiectasis includes measurement of IgG, IgA, and IgM with serum electrophoresis and other specialist immunology assessments as indicated. Immunoglobulin deficiencies can be managed with intravenous or subcutaneous immunoglobulin replacement therapy, vaccination as well as prompt treatment of infections.

To evaluate the patient's response to infection, baseline specific antibody levels to tetanus toxoid and the capsular polysaccharides of *Streptococcus pneumonia* and *Haemophilus influenza* type b should be measured. If baseline levels are low, the adequacy of the humoral response should be assessed by immunisation with the appropriate vaccines and re-measurement of antibody levels after four weeks.

Immunoglobulin deficiency can occur because of haematological malignancies, such as lymphoma and myeloma. Human immunodeficiency virus (HIV) also predisposes to recurrent bacterial infections and bronchiectasis.

Primary ciliary dyskinesia (PCD) is a rare, inherited abnormality of the cilium which will be discussed later in this chapter.

Abnormally viscid mucus, as occurs in cystic fibrosis (CF), is a cause of severe bronchiectasis and will be discussed later in this chapter.

Diagnosis of bronchiectasis

A careful history of presenting complaints, childhood infections, past medical history and family history should be taken. A meticulous clinical examination is essential. Box 12.2 lists the common symptoms and signs of bronchiectasis.

Box 12.2 Symptoms and signs of bronchiectasis.

- Cough (98%)
- Copious sputum production (78%)
- Wheezing (22%)
- Dyspnoea (62%)
- Rhinosinusitis (73%)
- Haemoptysis (27%)
- Fatigue (43%)
- Coarse crackles (75%)
- Digital clubbing (2%)
- Recurrent pleurisy (20%)
- Anosmia

Patients usually present with chronic, productive cough, recurrent chest infections, and minor haemoptysis. Information about hearing loss, sinusitis, gastrointestinal symptoms, and infertility should be ascertained. Only 2% of patients with bronchiectasis will have finger clubbing, although the majority will have coarse crackles on auscultation.

Table 12.2 lists the investigations that are routinely carried out to make a diagnosis of bronchiectasis and the investigations that should be done if PCD, immunodeficiency or CF is suspected.

The diagnosis of bronchiectasis is made on clinical history and radiological appearance. In early, mild, disease the CXR may appear normal. If the clinical presentation suggests bronchiectasis, then a high resolution computed tomography (HRCT) or multi-detector computed tomography (MDCT) scan of the thorax should be done which will be more sensitive at detecting changes. Expiratory scans best demonstrate air trapping and mosaic attenuation.

Box 12.3 lists the characteristic radiological finding in bronchiectasis, the abnormalities typically affecting the lower lobes (Figure 12.3, Figure 12.4, Figure 12.5). Airway dilatation results in the appearance of parallel lines, referred to as tram lines, and ring shadows when the airway is seen in cross-section. When the diameter of the airway is more than 1.5 times greater than the diameter of the adjacent blood vessel, this is termed **cylindrical bronchiectasis**. With severe bronchiectasis there is the formation of cysts, and this is termed **cystic bronchiectasis**.

Bronchiectasis predominantly affecting the upper lobes of the lungs suggests post-tuberculous bronchiectasis or CF, whereas a middle lobe distribution is consistent with PCD (Box 12.3). A tree in bud appearance is often seen with non-tuberculous mycobacterial infection. This is discussed in Chapter 8.

Nitric oxide (NO) levels can be measured quite simply by blowing into a NO monitor. Levels of NO are increased in patients with bronchiectasis because of airway inflammation, although raised exhaled NO is not diagnostic. Very low levels <77 nl min^{-1} in a patient with bronchiectasis is consistent with PCD and should prompt the doctor to do ciliary studies.

Lung function tests will show obstruction, with a reduced forced expiratory volume in one second (FEV_1) and a reduced FEV_1/FVC ratio. The severity of clinical disease correlated well with HRCT changes and poor lung function in several studies. Individuals with severe bronchiectasis may develop type 1 respiratory failure, with hypoxia and normocapnia on arterial blood gas measurement.

The result of the shuttle walking test correlates well with the severity of bronchiectasis and may be of prognostic value. Shuttle walking test can be used to monitor the response to treatment and is used as an end-point in many trials. A validated respiratory questionnaire, for example, the St. George's Respiratory Questionnaire (SGRQ), can be used to monitor the patient's response to treatment. The details of these investigations are discussed in Chapter 4.

Differential diagnoses of bronchiectasis

The differential diagnosis of bronchiectasis includes other conditions which cause bronchial wall dilatation. Chronic obstructive pulmonary disease (COPD) can have a similar presentation to bronchiectasis, with chronic sputum production and frequent exacerbations but with a history of cigarette smoking. A quarter of patients with alpha 1 antitrypsin deficiency (A1AT) present with daily, chronic sputum production, and the majority have radiological evidence of bronchiectasis. It is therefore recommended that testing for A1AT deficiency is carried out in patients presenting with bronchiectasis with no obvious underlying cause.

Allergic bronchopulmonary aspergillosis (ABPA), which results in proximal bronchiectasis, with dilatation of central airways, develops in patients with asthma and is caused by an allergic

Table 12.2 Investigations for the diagnosis of bronchiectasis.

Diagnosis	Bloods	Radiology	Other
Diffuse bronchiectasis	Full blood count Differential cell count C-reactive protein Immunoglobulins G, M, A, and E Protein electrophoresis Antibody titres to pneumococcal vaccine Aspergillus precipitins (IgE and IgG antibodies) Total serum IgE IgG subclasses Rheumatoid factor Alpha-1 antitrypsin level	CXR: ring shadows, tram lines, mucus plugging HRCT: airway dilatation with bronchial wall thickening, mucus plugging, tree in bud and cysts CT sinus: opacification and mucosal oedema	Sputum for microscopy, culture, sensitivity, and differential cell count Lung function tests Nitric Oxide (NO) Bronchial lavage
Localised bronchiectasis		CXR CT thorax	Bronchoscopy
Immunodeficiency	Full blood count C-reactive protein Immunoglobulins Protein electrophoresis Immune function tests Specialist immune tests	CXR HRCT	Refer to Immunologist Refer to Haematologist
PCD	Full blood count C-reactive protein Immunoglobulins Protein electrophoresis Immune function test	CXR HRCT CT sinus	Nitric Oxide (NO) Ciliary studies: saccharin test, ultrastructure of cilia, microscopic photometry of ciliary function
CF	Full blood count C-reactive protein Immunoglobulins Protein electrophoresis Immune function tests Aspergillus precipitins	CXR HRCT	Sweat chloride test Sweat sodium test Nitric Oxide (NO) DNA analysis

reaction to the fungus *Aspergillus fumigatus*. COPD, A1AT deficiency, and ABPA are discussed in more detail in Chapter 6. Traction bronchiectasis describes stretching and distortion of bronchi due to pulmonary fibrosis, and is discussed in Chapter 7.

Management of bronchiectasis

The management of bronchiectasis depends on the underlying cause. For example, bronchiectasis that occurs due to immunodeficiency will respond to intravenous or subcutaneous immunoglobulin therapy. However, there are several evidence-based treatments that improve symptoms, reduce the frequency of infections, thus preventing further bronchial wall damage. The management is summarised in Box 12.4.

The aim of the management of bronchiectasis is to improve the symptoms of breathlessness and productive cough, and to prevent recurrent chest infections. Long-acting bronchodilators, in combination with inhaled corticosteroids, should be

Box 12.3 Characteristic HRCT findings in bronchiectasis.

- Bronchial wall thickening
- Dilatation of bronchi
- Lack of airway tapering
- Tree in bud appearance
- Mucus plugging
- Post-operative air trapping
- Mosaic attenuation
- Cystic changes

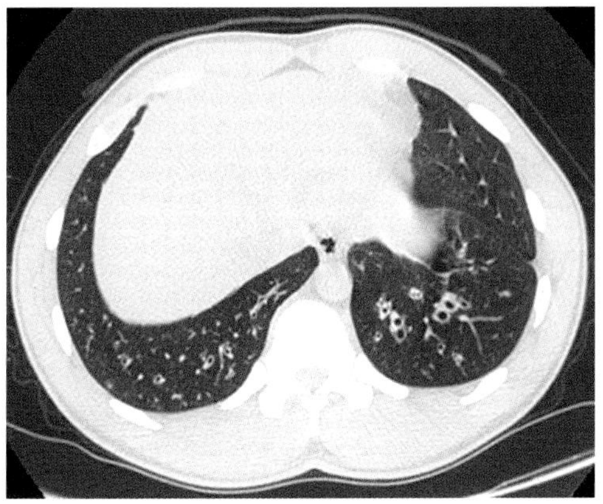

Figure 12.3 CT showing dilated bronchi in bronchiectasis.

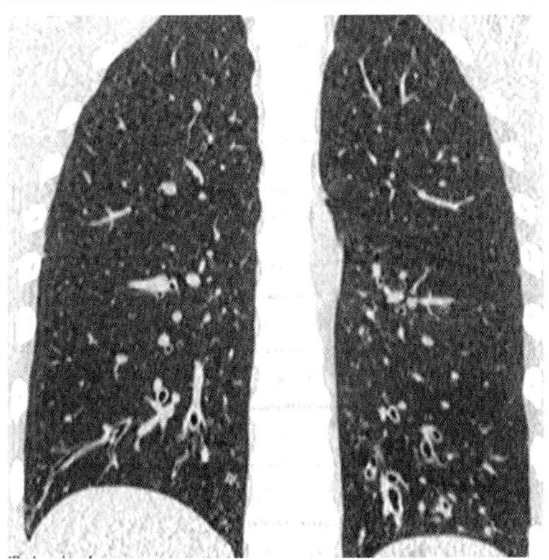

Figure 12.4 Coronal CT thorax showing bronchiectasis.

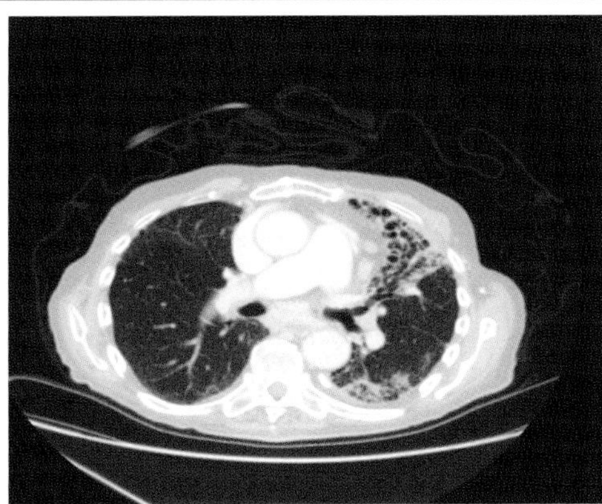

Figure 12.5 CT thorax showing cylindrical bronchiectasis.

Box 12.4 Management of bronchiectasis.

- Short-acting inhaled bronchodilators (β_2-agonists)
- Long-acting β_2-agonists
- Inhaled corticosteroids
- Long-acting anticholinergic medication
- Mucolytic drugs
- Sputum culture and sensitivity for exacerbations
- Prompt antibiotics, often longer course (rescue pack)
- Prophylactic antibiotics
- Chest physiotherapy
- Surgery for localised bronchiectasis

prescribed to those with airway obstruction. Short-acting bronchodilators will improve the symptoms of breathlessness and wheeze. There is no evidence for the routine use of oral corticosteroids in the management of chronic bronchiectasis.

Annual influenza vaccination is recommended for all chronic respiratory diseases. Pneumococcal vaccination should be offered.

Pulmonary rehabilitation is effective in bronchiectasis, as it is in all chronic respiratory diseases, and will result in improvement in exercise tolerance and quality of life measures. Pulmonary rehabilitation has been shown to improve endurance capacity, breathlessness, the distance walked in the shuttle walk test, and the six-minute walk test.

However, a regular exercise regime is required to sustain any improvement.

Nutritional supplementation with a high protein diet may benefit those with bronchiectasis which is often associated with a poor appetite and weight loss. The recurrent infection and raised inflammation drive a catabolic process, therefore extra calories are required. Supplementation with hydroxyl-beta-methylbutyrate, which has anti-inflammatory and anti-catabolic effects, may help.

If the bronchiectasis is confined to one lobe of the lung, wedge resection or lobectomy can be very effective and potentially curative. Recurrent, massive haemoptysis could be one indication for surgery. Single or double lung transplantation could be considered in those with severe diffuse bronchiectasis.

Infective exacerbations of bronchiectasis

An infective exacerbation should be suspected when the patient reports an increase in the volume of sputum, a change in the colour of sputum to yellow or green, sputum that is purulent, worsening breathlessness, chest pain, haemoptysis, and systemic symptoms, such as fever and decreased appetite.

Bacterial pathogens, including opportunistic organisms, are the main cause of exacerbations, although viruses, such as coronavirus, rhinovirus, and influenza can also cause infections. Bacteria often associated with exacerbations in bronchiectasis include *Haemophilus influenza, Staphylococcus aureus, Moraxella catarrhalis*, and the mucoid type of *Pseudomonas aeruginosa*. Many of these organisms will be resistant to the usual oral antibiotics; therefore, it is important to culture sputum to determine antibiotic sensitivities.

Infective exacerbations should be treated with prompt antibiotics for 10–14 days. The exact length of the treatment and the route of antibiotic therapy will depend on the clinical condition of the patient and the antibiotic sensitivities. Patients who become clinically unwell with hypotension, tachypnoea, and respiratory failure will need to be admitted for intravenous antibiotics, intravenous fluids, oxygen therapy, and chest physiotherapy to clear retained secretions, thus improving oxygenation. Blood cultures should be taken in patients who are febrile or show other signs of sepsis.

If information is available about the antibiotic sensitivities of the bacterial pathogen colonising the lungs of the patient, this should guide the choice of antibiotics given. If no sputum culture result is available, then a fluoroquinolone, amoxicillin, or a macrolide would be a suitable initial choice. The initial antibiotic therapy may need to be modified when sputum culture results become available. If there is a beta-lactamase-positive organism, then a second or third generation cephalosporin or macrolide should be used.

Pseudomonas aeruginosa colonises the lungs of patients with bronchiectasis and its presence in the sputum of a patient with bronchiectasis signifies a worse prognosis. Pseudomonas can overcome the lungs' defence mechanisms by interacting with the CFTR, thus altering the milieu of the lungs. Patients colonised with Pseudomonas aeruginosa have decreased quality of life, severe bronchiectasis on HRCT, worse lung function tests, increased number of exacerbations and hospitalisations, and increased mortality compared to patients with bronchiectasis colonised with other organisms.

The usual choice of antibiotics for Pseudomonas is oral ciprofloxacin, 500 or 750 mg twice a day for 14 days. Resistance to ciprofloxacin can develop rapidly, so further sputum samples should be sent if there is no clinical improvement. Pseudomonas can be treated with nebulised colomycin.

The choice of intravenous antibiotic therapy will depend on the patient's previous history of antibiotic resistance and the results of sputum culture and sensitivities. An anti-pseudomonal penicillin, such as ceftazidime, together with an aminoglycoside or fluoroquinolone, is the usual combination given. Aminoglycosides should not be given alone, and the level should be monitored carefully to avoid renal toxicity and ototoxicity.

If the sputum grows Aspergillus fumigatus, then a course of Itraconazole or Voriconazole should be given, with careful monitoring of liver function tests.

Other treatments during an exacerbation include nebulised bronchodilators, controlled oxygen therapy, regular chest physiotherapy, intravenous fluids, and systemic corticosteroids in some cases. Corticosteroids must be used with care as they are immunosuppressive drugs and therefore can worsen infection.

Prevention of exacerbations

There is evidence that meticulous attention to sputum clearance techniques will reduce the bacterial load in the lungs and reduce the frequency of exacerbations. Regular sputum clearance improves symptoms, improves lung function, and reduces infective exacerbations.

There are various mucolytic drugs that have been shown in *in vitro* studies to aid the clearance of mucus from the lungs, although trial evidence is limited. Carbocysteine, a commonly used mucolytic drug, reduces the viscosity of mucus and the number of exacerbations. *In vitro* studies have shown that nebulised hypertonic saline (6–7%) improves the flow of mucus, increases ciliary motility, and improves hydration of the secretions, thereby potentially improving expectoration. Although clinical trials have not shown a benefit, once-daily nebulised mannitol, which is a hyperosmolar agent, hydrates airway secretions and aids sputum clearance. Care must be taken not to use mannitol in patients with co-existing asthma as this can result in mast cell mediator release and bronchoconstriction. N-Acetylcysteine, a mucolytic agent that cleaves disulphide bonds in glycoproteins, has not demonstrated benefit in patients with CF and there are no studies using this in non-CF bronchiectasis. Aerosolised recombinant deoxyribonuclease (DNase), which breaks down DNA, improves lung function and decreases hospitalisation in patients with CF, and is not effective in non-CF bronchiectasis.

Chest physiotherapy, an essential part of the management of bronchiectasis, involves techniques of chest percussion, active cycle of breathing, and the use of various devices which break up the mucus into smaller particles, making it easier to expectorate. Standard physiotherapy applied by trained experts is time-consuming and not possible for patients who are at home. Devices which aid sputum clearance include positive expiratory pressure devices, high frequency chest wall oscillation devices, oral high frequency oscillation devices, intrapulmonary percussive ventilation, incentive spirometry, the flutter valve, the Acapella device, and the cornet. These devices are less time-consuming, easier for the patient to use after training, and a good alternative to standard chest physiotherapy. These devices can be used by children, for example, those with cystic fibrosis, under the supervision of their parents. It is not within the scope of this book to discuss these devices in detail. The physiotherapist will recommend the most appropriate device for the individual.

There is trial evidence that patients who have more than two infective exacerbations every year benefit from low-dose prophylactic Azithromycin, 250 mg two or three times a week. Low-dose azithromycin appears to work by a mechanism other than the antimicrobial one, although the exact way it works is unclear. Three small randomised trials using prophylactic macrolide antibiotics, two of them using Azithromycin (EMBRACE and BAT) and one using erythromycin (BLESS) have shown a reduction in the number of exacerbations, reduction in the volume of sputum, improved symptoms using the SGRQ, and an improved dyspnoea index.

Side effects of macrolides include gastrointestinal discomfort, hepatotoxicity, ototoxicity, and bacterial resistance. Patients should be informed of the potential side effects and asked to report any adverse effects, such as change in hearing. It is recommended that liver function tests are monitored and the drug discontinued if there is any evidence of hepatotoxicity. Macrolide antibiotics are associated with a risk of prolongation of QT interval and *torsades de pointes* and should not be given to those with hypokalaemia, hypomagnesaemia, bradycardia, and heart failure. The length of treatment should be for 3–6 months with careful assessment of the patient at the end of this period. It is important to give a break after this period to reduce the risk of developing resistance to macrolide antibiotics.

If macrolide prophylaxis is contraindicated, amoxicillin 500 mg twice a day or doxycycline 100 mg twice a day should be considered.

The role of inhaled antibiotics in patients with non-CF bronchiectasis who are colonised with Pseudomonas aeruginosa is unclear. Inhaled tobramycin, ciprofloxacin and colistin have been shown to reduce the volume of sputum and reduce the bacterial load but are associated with bronchoconstriction. In patients with three or more exacerbations a year with Pseudomonas aeruginosa, a therapeutic trial of inhaled antibiotics could be considered. Spirometry 15 and 30 minutes after administration of the drug should be carried out and the drug stopped if there is evidence of significant bronchoconstriction with a reduction in FEV_1 by more than 15% or >200 mL. Administering inhaled β_2-agonist prior to giving the inhaled antibiotic will reduce the risk of bronchoconstriction. There is less evidence for the use of inhaled Aztreonam and inhaled gentamicin, so their use in this way is not recommended.

As gastro-oesophageal reflux may be a factor in the development of bronchiectasis, treatment with a proton pump inhibitor is recommended to reduce the risk of aspiration of gastric contents. In one small, single-centre, pilot study, atorvastatin 80 mg daily for six months resulted in improvement in cough compared to the placebo group but there were significant side effects. A larger, randomised, double-blind controlled study is required before the routine use of a statin is recommended in bronchiectasis.

It is essential to reiterate the importance of compliance with all these treatments to the patient. Annual influenza vaccination and regular pneumonia vaccination should be offered to the patient.

Cystic fibrosis

Cystic fibrosis (CF) is the commonest inherited genetic disorder in the United Kingdom's Caucasian population, occurring at a frequency of 1 in 2500 live births. It is inherited as an autosomal recessive disorder, which means that the individual has inherited a defective gene from each parent. One in 25 of the Caucasian population is an asymptomatic carrier of the defective gene. There are approximately 9000 individuals with CF in the UK.

CF occurs due to a mutation in a gene on the long arm of chromosome 7 resulting in a defect in the cystic fibrosis transmembrane conductance regulator (CFTR), which is a protein comprising of 1480 amino acids. This CFTR protein is a member of the ATP Binding Cassette (ABC) family, and is an essential regulator of membrane physiology. CTFR sits in the membrane of epithelial cells and regulates the transport of chloride ions through activation of cyclic adenosine monophosphate (cAMP) and through calcium-activated chloride channels (Figure 12.6). CTFR also inhibits the transport of sodium through the sodium channels in the epithelial cell membrane and regulates the movement of bicarbonate anions.

Approximately 1800 different mutations of the gene have been identified which are classified into five groups based on their effect on CFTR function. The severity of the disease and the clinical presentation depend on the nature of the mutation. The most common mutation is a deletion of phenylalanine at position 508 of the protein, described as Delta F508, which is a Class 1 defect.

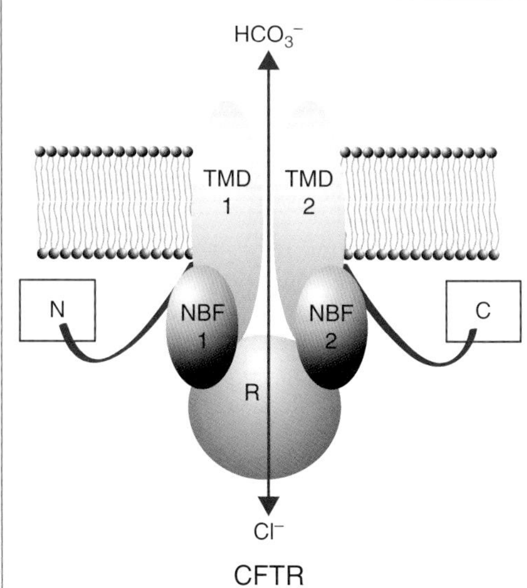

Figure 12.6 The structure of the cystic fibrosis transmembrane conductance regulator.

This results in the degradation of the CFTR protein in the endoplasmic reticulum of the cell so that no protein reaches the cell membrane.

Other mutations result in defective protein processing (Class 2), defective protein activation (Class 3), impaired chloride conductance (Class 4), and reduced amount of CFTR protein (Class 5). Defects belonging to Classes 4 and 5 will result in some active protein being produced so that the patient presents with less severe clinical disease than mutations in Classes 1, 2, and 3.

Epithelial cells line the bronchial mucosa, the gastrointestinal tract, the pancreas, the hepatobiliary system, the reproductive tract, and the sweat glands in the skin. Therefore, a defect in the CFTR gene will affect all these systems.

Abnormal CFTR protein results in decreased chloride reabsorption and increased sodium reabsorption, resulting in secretions that have a very high viscosity and reduced water content. This impedes mucociliary clearance in the bronchi so that respiratory secretions are stagnant. The high salt content of the secretions also disrupts the functioning of antimicrobial peptides which are part of the defence system of the respiratory tract. Therefore, the individual with CF is at a high risk of developing frequent respiratory infections, which will inevitably progress to severe bronchiectasis within a few years. Individuals with CF are particularly prone to developing infections with Gram-negative organisms, such as Pseudomonas aeruginosa and Burkholderia cepacia. There is a risk of this infection progressing to life-threatening necrotising pneumonia (Cepacia syndrome).

Defective CFTR also results in abnormal chloride transport in the pancreas leading to destruction of the pancreas, pancreatic exocrine insufficiency, reduction of lipase activity, and decreased absorption of fat in the small intestine, resulting in steatorrhoea. This, together with decreased water content in the intestines, results in thick faecal material which can cause intestinal obstruction, called the 'meconium ileus equivalent' in adults as it mimics meconium ileus in neonates. Lack of fat absorption will lead to nutritional deficiencies, especially of the fat-soluble vitamins, and failure to thrive. Over time, there is failure of endocrine pancreatic function, resulting in diabetes.

Clinical presentation of CF

The presentation of CF will depend on the severity of the genetic defect. The delta F508 mutation will present with symptoms and clinical signs in the neonate or young child. In 7% of cases, the mutation results in less severe disease so that the diagnosis may not be made until adolescence or even adulthood. Table 12.3 lists some of the features of CF in the different age groups.

Diagnosis of CF

A diagnosis of CF is made based on clinical features consistent with CF, an abnormal CXR, a positive sweat test, an abnormal potential difference across the nasal epithelium and DNA analysis. The commonest symptoms are sinusitis and bronchiectasis (Figure 12.7, Figure 12.8) which predominantly affects the upper lobes. Sputum samples usually grow *Staphylococcus aureus* in children and *Pseudomonas aeruginosa* in adolescents and adults. A sweat test involves instilling pilocarpine on the skin and stimulating the sweat glands by a small electric current which increases the production of sweat. A chloride content more than 60 mmol/L is abnormal, and two such readings confirms a diagnosis of CF. A chloride level of between 40 and 60 mmol/L may indicate one of the less severe forms of CF.

Genotyping can be done for the common mutations but would not be possible for all the known different types. Prenatal diagnosis can be offered when DNA analysis is conducted on a sample of the chorionic villus. Neonatal screening is done by measuring serum immunoreactive trypsin activity on a Guthrie card. This will be elevated in those with CF.

Management of CF

The care of patients with CF should be undertaken in a specialist centre with a multidisciplinary team of doctors, specialist nurses, physiotherapists, occupational therapists, dieticians, and psychologists. Patients with CF should be seen in the clinic at regular intervals and have assessments, which includes chest imaging, sputum culture, spirometry, oximetry, weight, height, body mass index measurement, and blood glucose. Compliance with the management plan can be ascertained and its importance reinforced.

The aim with CF is to reduce the number of respiratory exacerbations, thus preventing the progression of bronchiectasis, to give nutritional support, and give emotional and psychological support to the individual and their family.

Patients are taught techniques of sputum clearance which is the most important aspect of managing the bronchiectasis and will reduce the risk of infection. This includes chest percussion, postural drainage, active cycle of breathing technique, and the use of oscillating positive expiratory pressure devices (flutter valve or Acapella device). The use of mucolytic drugs will aid sputum clearance. Nebulised recombinant human DNase has been shown in clinical trials to reduce sputum viscosity, reduce exacerbations, and improve lung function. The DNase works by degrading the high concentrations of DNA in the sputum from dying cells. Nebulised bronchodilators and inhaled corticosteroids improve symptoms.

Infective exacerbations must be managed rapidly and effectively with intravenous antibiotics. Macrolide antibiotics, such as Azithromycin, can be effective in preventing exacerbations in the early stages of the disease in the same way as for those with non-CF bronchiectasis. Patients with frequent exacerbations may require permanent intravenous access so that antibiotics and fluids can be administered without delay and for long periods.

Individuals who have become colonised with the Gram-negative organisms (Pseudomonas aeruginosa and Burkholderia cepacia), are treated with

Table 12.3 Clinical presentation of cystic fibrosis.

Age of patient	Respiratory system	Upper airways	Gastrointestinal system	Endocrine/Metabolic	Fertility
Neonate	Respiratory infection with *Staphylococcus aureus, Haemophilus influenzae* and *Streptococcus pneumonia*		Meconium ileus (10%) Rectal prolapse		
Child	Recurrent respiratory infection with *Staphylococcus aureus*, *Haemophilus influenzae* and *Streptococcus pneumonia*, chronic productive cough, severe airway obstruction	Sinusitis	Intestinal obstruction Abdominal distension Malabsorption Failure to thrive	Short stature Heat prostration in hot weather due to excessive loss of salt in sweat	
Adolescent	Development of severe bronchiectasis, colonisation with *Pseudomonas aeruginosa, Burkholderia cepacia* and *Aspergillus fumigatus*	Sinusitis Nasal polyps	Abdominal distension Malabsorption Failure to thrive	Diabetes mellitus Delayed puberty Short stature Heat prostration in hot weather due to excessive loss of salt in sweat	
Adult	Clubbing Severe bronchiectasis Colonisation with *Pseudomonas aeruginosa, Burkholderia cepacia, Aspergillus fumigatus* and *Mycobacterium abscessus* Recurrent pneumothorax (5–10%) Massive haemoptysis Type 1 and type 2 respiratory failure Cor pulmonale	Nasal polyps (20%) Sinusitis (25%)	Pancreatic insufficiency (85%) Malabsorption Underweight Distal intestinal obstruction (meconium ileus equivalent) Gall stones (10–30%) Multinodular cirrhosis (5%) Hepatosplenomegaly, portal hypertension, oesophageal varices	Diabetes mellitus Short stature Osteoporosis Hypertrophic osteoarthropathy (15%) Amyloidosis	Infertility in males: absent vas deferens and epididymis (98%) Cervical mucus abnormalities in females

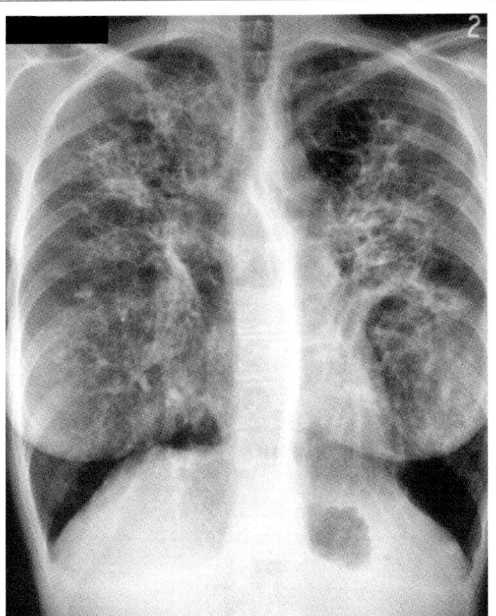

Figure 12.7 CXR of patient with CF showing extensive bronchiectasis.

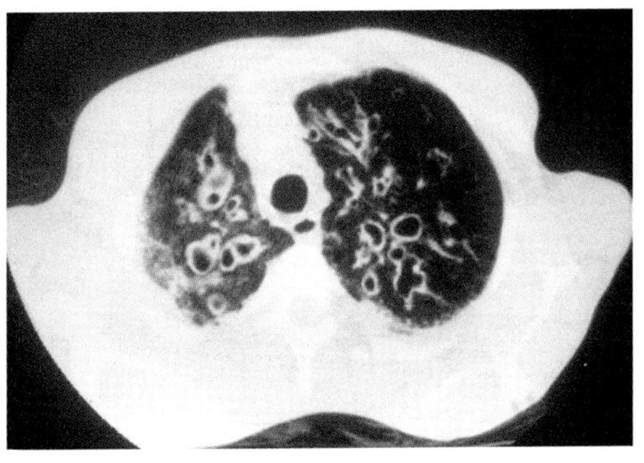

Figure 12.8 CT of patient with CF.

long term nebulised colistin and nebulised tobramycin but will require intravenous antibiotics during exacerbations. They are usually treated with third generation cephalosporins, piperacillin, and aminoglycoside, but development of resistance is a major concern.

As these severe infections can be transmitted from one patient to another, patients who are known to be colonised with a particular organism are segregated in different clinics and on different wards to prevent cross-transmission. Babies with CF should receive all their immunisation and all patients should have their annual influenza vaccination.

As the bronchiectasis gets progressively worse, there is a risk of recurrent pneumothoraces. Pleurodesis could be considered, although this may make lung transplantation difficult in the future. Massive haemoptysis due to hypertrophy of the bronchial arteries can be life-threatening and difficult to manage. Bronchial artery embolisation is the most effective treatment for this complication.

Patients who develop type 1 respiratory failure will require long term oxygen therapy (LTOT). Many patients develop type 2 respiratory failure requiring bi-level positive pressure ventilation (BiPAP).

Single lung, double lung or heart and lung transplantation is the only real hope for patients with respiratory failure and cor pulmonale secondary to CF. Patients should be referred for transplant assessment and, if suitable, put on to the transplant register.

Pancreatic insufficiency is treated with pancreatic supplements, for example, Creon, Pancrease or Nutrizym, which is taken with every meal. These supplements contain lipases which will help digest and absorb fat. Patients should receive advice and support from the dietician and take other dietary supplements, including vitamins A, D and E. Patients with severe malnutrition will require enteral feeding.

Patients may require specific treatment for intestinal obstruction with intravenous rehydration and intestinal lavage with Gastrograffin and N-acetylcysteine. Diabetes is managed with insulin and the complications of diabetes are actively treated.

CF is a serious and life-threatening condition and therefore a diagnosis in a baby or child can be extremely harrowing for the parents. Individuals and families will need a lot of emotional support from trained therapists. The Cystic Fibrosis Trust offers support and advice to these families.

All attempts should be made to ensure that children, adolescents, and adults live their lives as normal as possible, attend school, participate in physical activity, take up employment, and get married. It is not uncommon for women with CF to have a normal pregnancy, although there are associated risks, and they will need careful medical attention.

Despite all available treatments, most patients with the commonest forms of CF will deteriorate and die. Those approaching end of life should be referred to the palliative care team.

Prognosis of CF

Most individuals with CF die of progressive respiratory failure. The 2-year survival of those with severe airway obstruction is less than 50%. The prognosis has improved significantly in the past few decades, largely due to early diagnosis, prompt treatment of infections with antibiotics, chest physiotherapy, nutritional support, a multidisciplinary approach, and management in specialist centres with considerable expertise. The median survival in 2015 was approaching 40 years.

Future therapy for CF

A lot of research is being conducted into gene therapy, whereby a normal copy of the gene is placed into the lungs through liposomal or viral carriers. There is some optimism that this technique will significantly improve the prognosis of those with CF in the future.

Primary ciliary dyskinesia

Primary ciliary dyskinesia (PCD) is also called the immotile cilia syndrome. PCD is an autosomal recessive disorder with a prevalence of 1 in 16000 live births. The commonest genetic defect is a deficiency of the dynein arm which results in immotile cilia or cilia which move in an abnormal way. This condition will affect all the organs that rely on normal ciliary motion.

Failure of normal ciliary function results in recurrent otitis media leading to deafness, recurrent sinusitis, anosmia, and bronchiectasis. Most men with PCD will be infertile and women will be sub-fertile. As cilia are responsible for the rotation of the internal organs during embryogenesis, there is a random rotation of organs in PCD. So, 50% of those with PCD will have dextrocardia and situs inversus (Figure 12.9). The triad of bronchiectasis, dextrocardia, and sinusitis is called Kartagener's syndrome.

There are at least eight categories of cilia in the human body. Defects in the ependymal cilia will result in hydrocephalus whereas defective cilia in the retinal photoreceptor cells will result in retinitis pigmentosa. Abnormal ciliary protein is also important in the development of APKD

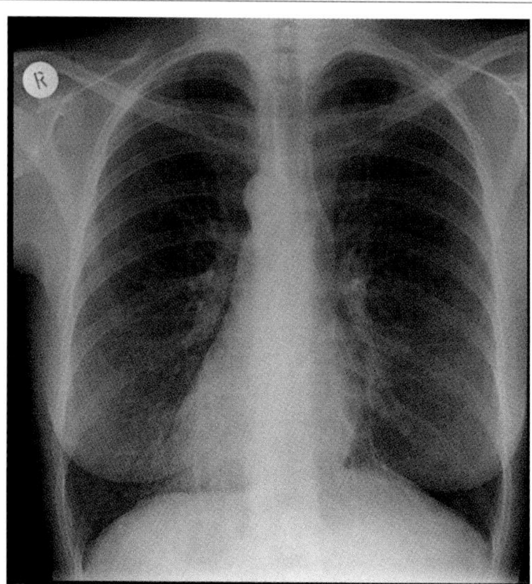

Figure 12.9 CXR of patient with PCD showing dextrocardia.

Diagnosis of PCD

Patients with PCD are usually diagnosed in adolescence or early adulthood when they present with bronchiectasis, sinusitis, otitis media, and infertility. These patients should have the same investigations as for bronchiectasis, but should in addition have nasal mucociliary clearance test (NMCC), also called the saccharin test. A 0.5 mm particle of saccharin is placed on the lateral nasal wall, 1 cm behind the anterior end of the inferior turbinate. In a normal individual, the mucociliary mechanism will transport the saccharin to the nasopharynx and pharynx where it can be tasted within 30 min. In PCD there will be a considerable delay, or the saccharin may never reach the pharynx.

Using nasal or turbinate brush biopsies, the ultrastructure of the cilium can be looked at through electron microscopy, and phase contrast microscopy can be used to determine cilial beat frequency. Exhaled nitric oxide levels will be low ($< 77\,nL\,min^{-1}$) in patients with PCD. CF is always in the differential diagnosis of this presentation and should be excluded.

Early diagnosis and prompt treatment of bronchiectasis will minimise symptoms and morbidity. Life expectancy is normal. Genetic counselling is available.

Young syndrome may be a variant of PCD or may have been caused by exposure to mercury in childhood. It results in bronchiectasis, sinusitis, and obstructive azoospermia, and is now rare.

Lung abscess

Lung abscess is a chronic lung condition due to a localised collection of pus within a cavity in the lung parenchyma. Patients will present with symptoms of productive cough, fever, malaise, cachexia, chest pain, haemoptysis, and weight loss. The patient will appear unwell and may be clubbed. If untreated, it can result in significant morbidity and mortality. Box 12.5 lists the aetiology of lung abscess.

The commonest cause of lung abscess is that secondary to community acquired pneumonia, which is discussed in Chapter 8. CAP due to *Staphylococcus aureus* and *Klebsiella pneumonia* especially predispose to the formation of a lung abscess. Aspiration of anaerobic organisms, which includes Fusobacteria and Prevotella, also predisposes to the formation of a lung abscess. Septic emboli can travel to the lungs from any source of bacteraemia. Individuals who use infected needles for intravenous drug use are at a high risk of developing abscesses.

Transdiaphragmatic spread of infection may occur from a subphrenic abscess, for example, after biliary surgery. Amoebic hepatic abscess also has the potential to spread to the lungs if untreated.

Box 12.5 Aetiology of lung abscess.

- Aspiration pneumonia
- Community acquired pneumonia (CAP)
- Intravenous drug use
- Secondary to bronchial obstruction
- Secondary to sepsis
- Dental infection
- Chronic sinus infection
- Subphrenic abscess
- Hepatic abscess
- Infected bulla
- Lung infarction
- Penetrating trauma to chest
- Bronchopulmonary sequestration

Bronchial obstruction secondary to tumour or foreign body can result in chronic infection distal to the obstruction which causes lung infarction and cavitation, resulting in formation of a lung abscess. Pulmonary embolus can also result in lung infarction and the development of an abscess. Pulmonary embolus is discussed in Chapter 11.

Diagnosis of lung abscess is made based on the clinical presentation, a history suggestive of chronic sepsis, and a CXR showing a thick-walled cavity. Such a cavity can be seen more clearly on a CT scan (Figure 12.10, Figure 12.11, Figure 12.12).

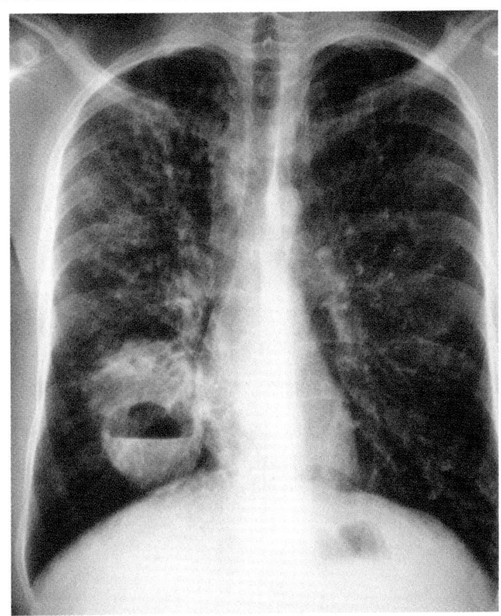

Figure 12.10 CXR of right-sided lung abscess.

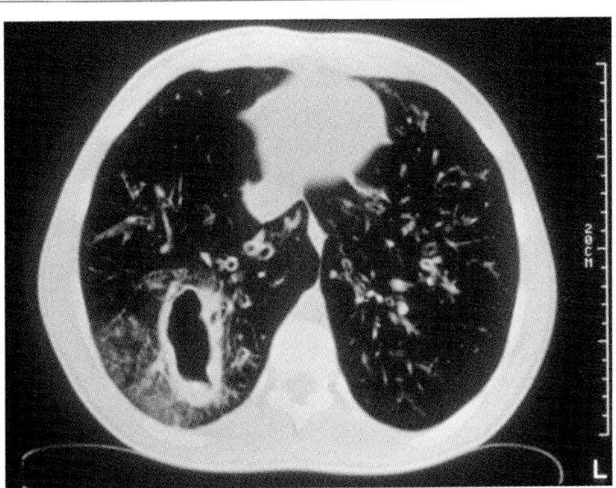

Figure 12.11 CT of right-sided lung abscess.

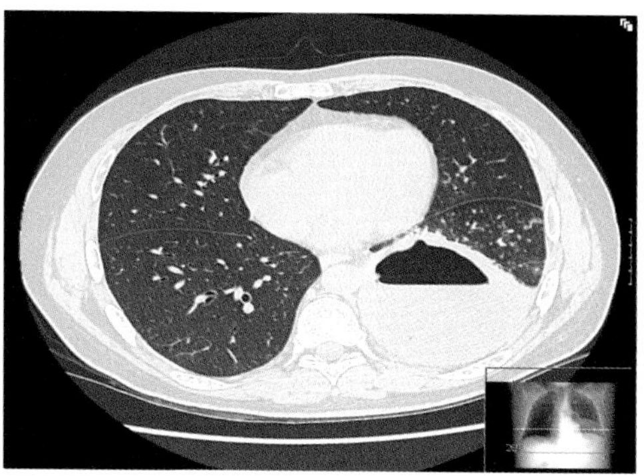

Figure 12.12 CT of left lung abscess.

Causative organisms in lung abscess

A variety of organisms result in the formation of a lung abscess; anaerobic organisms, *Staphylococcus aureus*, *Klebsiella pneumonia* and Gram-negative bacteria. Actinomyces and Nocardia are rarer causes of lung abscess.

Bronchopulmonary sequestration is a congenital anomaly when an area of the lung is not connected to the bronchial tree and has an anomalous blood supply, usually from the aorta. Infection of the sequestered area predisposes to abscess formation as there is inadequate drainage. Bronchial arteriography will identify the anomalous blood supply. Surgery will be required to remove the infected area of lung.

Box 12.6 Differential diagnosis of lung abscess.

- Cavitating lung cancer
- Pulmonary tuberculosis
- Pulmonary infarct
- Infected bullae
- Hiatus hernia
- Granulomatosis with polyangiitis (previously called Wegener's Granulomatosis)

There are several conditions that can resemble a lung abscess, both clinically and radiologically. These are listed in Box 12.6.

Management of lung abscess

A prolonged course of appropriate antibiotics is indicated. A combination of high dose penicillin and metronidazole is usually recommended for at least six weeks, with careful monitoring of clinical and radiological improvement. The CRP level is often used as a marker of improvement. Percutaneous drainage of the abscess under radiological guidance should be undertaken whenever possible. Surgery to remove the abscess should also be considered.

Lung abscess has a significant morbidity and mortality, especially in the immunocompromised and malnourished individual. The abscess can rupture into the lungs causing severe infection.

SUMMARY OF LEARNING POINTS

- Suppurative lung diseases are those with chronic purulent material in the lungs.
- Suppurative lung diseases present with chronic sputum production, recurrent chest infections, and systemic symptoms of anorexia and weight loss.
- Cilia are fine, hair-like structures that line the epithelial cells in the upper and lower respiratory tract, the tail of the spermatozoa, and Fallopian tubes and are responsible for the rotation of organs in embryogenesis.
- A cilium, which resembles a flagellum, is comprised of nine pairs of microtubules arranged in a circle with a central pair of microtubules all linked together.
- The commonest suppurative lung disease is bronchiectasis.
- There are many different causes of bronchiectasis; careful history, clinical examination and investigations are required to make the diagnosis.
- Recurrent respiratory infections, community acquired pneumonia, and aspiration pneumonia are common causes of bronchiectasis in the UK.
- *Mycobacterium tuberculosis* is a common cause of bronchiectasis worldwide.
- Typical HRCT appearance of bronchiectasis includes bronchial wall thickening, dilatation of bronchi, lack of airway tapering, and mucus plugging.
- The management of bronchiectasis includes chest physiotherapy, bronchodilators, mucolytic agents, prompt treatment of infection after sputum microbiology, and prophylactic antibiotics.
- Cystic fibrosis is a common autosomal recessive condition that affects 1:2500 live births in the UK.
- CF is caused by a defect in the CFTR protein resulting in a high concentration of chloride in the secretions from epithelial cells.
- Prenatal diagnosis of CF is possible, as is genetic counselling.
- There are over 1800 genotypes of CF and the clinical presentation will depend on the actual defect.
- The diagnosis of CF is made with an abnormal sweat test and DNA analysis.
- The commonest genetic abnormality in CF, the F508 mutation, presents with recurrent respiratory infections leading to severe bronchiectasis in early adulthood, colonisation with mucoid Pseudomonas aeruginosa, and development of respiratory failure.
- Patients with CF also develop pancreatic exocrine deficiency requiring pancreatic supplements, fat soluble vitamins, and nutritional supplements.
- Patients with CF develop diabetes mellitus requiring insulin therapy.
- Patients with CF develop other complications, including liver cirrhosis, gallstones, intestinal obstruction, and infertility.
- The management of CF is optimising the management of bronchiectasis with antibiotics, chest physiotherapy, mucolytic agents, including DNase, management of recurrent pneumothorax, management of haemoptysis, and lung transplantation.
- PCD is a rare, autosomal recessive condition which occurs because of an abnormality in the dynein arm of the cilium.
- PCD presents with bronchiectasis, sinusitis, otitis media, infertility, and in 50% dextrocardia and situs inversus.
- The diagnosis of PCD is made when there is a very low exhaled NO, abnormal mucociliary clearance test, and abnormal ciliary structure and function.
- PCD is managed by early diagnosis and management of bronchiectasis, sinusitis, and otitis media.
- Lung abscess is an infected cavity within the lung parenchyma.
- Lung abscess occurs as a complication of CAP, secondary to aspiration pneumonia, secondary to sepsis, and after dental infections.
- A diagnosis of lung abscess is made on clinical presentation, and a CT thorax showing a fluid-filled cavity.
- The management of lung abscess is with drainage, surgical resection, and prolonged course of antibiotics.

MULTIPLE CHOICE QUESTIONS

12.1 Which of the following is NOT a clinical feature of bronchiectasis?

A Clubbing
B Coarse crackles
C Chronic productive cough
D Haemoptysis
E Steatorrhoea

Answer: E

Bronchiectasis is due to the destruction and dilatation of the bronchi. Patients have retained secretions which get infected. Symptoms of bronchiectasis include chronic productive cough and haemoptysis. Clinical signs include clubbing in a small percentage and coarse crackles. Steatorrhoea is not seen with bronchiectasis but is a feature of cystic fibrosis due to pancreatic insufficiency, which results in an inability to absorb fat.

12.2 Which of the following statements about Primary Ciliary Dyskinesia is true?

A It is an autosomal dominant condition
B Individuals with PCD will require pancreatic supplements
C Life expectancy is reduced
D Individuals with PCD can present with deafness
E 100% of those affected will have dextrocardia

Answer: D

PCD is a rare, autosomal recessive condition which results in abnormal cilia which cannot beat synchronously. As a result, all the parts of the body which have ciliated epithelium are affected. PCD can result in repeated otitis media which can result in deafness. Cilia are also responsible for rotation of the organs during embryogenesis and therefore 50% of individuals with PCD will have dextrocardia and situs inversus. If detected early and the bronchiectasis treated adequately, individuals with PCD will have a normal life expectancy.

12.3 Which one of the following statements about cilia is NOT true?

A Cilia are responsible for the rotation of organs in embryogenesis
B A cilium is composed of five pairs of microtubules linked together
C Ciliary motion is essential for the normal functioning of the mucociliary escalator
D Cilia are structured in the same way as flagella
E Defective ciliary protein expression results in adult polycystic kidney disease

Answer: B

A cilium is composed of nine pairs of microtubules (sub-units A and B) in a circle with a central pair of microtubules, all linked by dynein arms. A defect in these proteins will result in abnormal cilia. The structure of the cilium is identical to that of a flagellum. Abnormalities result in a non-functioning mucociliary escalator, random rotation of organs during embryogenesis, and adult polycystic kidney disease.

12.4 Which of the following statements about cystic fibrosis is true?

A It is inherited as an autosomal recessive condition
B Carriers of the condition have some clinical symptoms
C CF results in decreased chloride concentration in respiratory secretions
D Patients with CF have abnormal cilia
E Patients with CF are always infertile

Answer: A

CF is inherited as an autosomal recessive condition, so carriers have no symptoms. Abnormality of the CFTR protein results in an increased amount of chloride in the respiratory secretions. The cilia are normal in structure and function in CF. A significant number of male patients with CF are infertile, but not all, and only a small proportion of female patients are infertile.

12.5 Which of the following statements about the management of bronchiectasis is true?

A There is no evidence for the use of prophylactic antibiotics
B Chest physiotherapy is a key part of managing this condition

C Long term oral corticosteroids prevent recurrent infections
D Inhaled long-acting bronchodilators are contra-indicated
E Surgery is never an option

Answer: B

The key in preventing recurrent infections is chest physiotherapy and sputum clearance. Inhaled bronchodilators and inhaled corticosteroids may by indicated in those with airway obstruction, co-existing asthma, and reversibility. Prophylactic macrolide antibiotics, given twice or three times a week, has been shown to reduce the number of exacerbations. Surgery in the form of wedge resection or lobectomy is a option in those with localised bronchiectasis.

12.6 Which one of the following investigations confirms the diagnosis of primary ciliary dyskinesia?
A High-resolution computed tomography.
B Nitric oxide breath test
C Nasal mucociliary clearance test
D Microscopy of ciliary structure and function
E Sweat test

Answer: D

HRCT will show features of bronchiectasis but will not determine the reason for the bronchiectasis. NO and the nasal mucociliary clearance test will be abnormal in PCD, but it is the ultrastructure of the cilium through an electron microscope and the movement of cilia with scanning electron microscopy that will diagnose that it is PCD.

12.7 Which of the following statements about CF is true?
A *Staphylococcus aureus* is the commonest pathogen to colonise the lungs of adults
B Prenatal diagnosis of CF is still not possible
C Meconium ileus occurs in 90% of neonates with CF
D Individuals with CF thrive in hot weather
E 20% with CF develop nasal polyps

Answer: E

Staphylococcus aureus occurs in children with CF but in adolescent and adult CF patients, *Pseudomonas aeruginosa* is the commonest pathogen to colonise the lungs. DNA analysis of chorionic villus sample is possible to make a prenatal diagnosis. Meconium ileus occurs in 10% of neonates. CF results in a loss of salt in sweat with a risk of heat prostration and severe dehydration. Some 20% of those with CF develop nasal polyps and 20% develop sinusitis.

12.8 Which of the following statements about bronchiectasis is true?
A Rheumatoid arthritis predisposes to the development of bronchiectasis
B Haemophilus influenza is the commonest pathogen in sputum
C NO levels can be diagnostic
D The aetiology of bronchiectasis is rarely found
E Traction bronchiectasis suggests an infection with non-tuberculous mycobacteria

Answer: A

The aetiology of bronchiectasis can be determined in most patients if the appropriate investigations are carried out. Connective tissue disorders, including rheumatoid arthritis, predispose to the development of bronchiectasis. Common pathogens include *Staphylococcus aureus* and *Klebsiella pneumonia*. NO level is high in bronchiectasis but is not diagnostic. Traction bronchiectasis is a term used to describe the distortion of the bronchi in pulmonary fibrosis. Non-tuberculous mycobacterial infections cause a 'tree-in-bud' appearance.

12.9 Which of the following statements about lung abscess is true?
A Surgery is the only treatment
B It can be treated with a long course of oral antibiotics
C It presents most commonly in young children
D It is a collection of pus in the pleural cavity
E It can be associated with abnormal cilia

Answer: B

Lung abscess is commoner in the elderly. It is an infected cavity within the lung parenchyma. Pus in the pleural space is called an empyema. Although surgery should be considered, it is not the only option. If the patient is not fit for surgery, then drainage through a chest drain and a long course of oral antibiotics are indicated. A lung abscess is not caused by abnormal cilia.

12.10 Which one of the statements about lung abscess is NOT true?

A It can occur due to inhaled foreign body
B It can occur after aspiration pneumonia
C It is a common complication of community acquired pneumonia
D Diagnosis is made at bronchoscopy
E CT thorax is the diagnostic test of choice

Answer: D

Lung abscess can occur as a complication of CAP, aspiration pneumonia and inhaled foreign body. The diagnosis is made on the history, CXR and CT thorax. Bronchial washings taken at bronchoscopy may be helpful in identifying the organism but will not make the diagnosis of an abscess.

FURTHER READING

Altenburg, J., de Graaff, C.S., Stienstra, Y. et al. (2013). Effect of azithromycin maintenance treatment on infectious exacerbations among patients with non-cystic fibrosis bronchiectasis: the BAT randomized controlled trial. *JAMA* 309 (12): 1251–1259.

Anwar, G.A., Bourke, S.C., Afolabi, G. et al. (2008). Effects of long-term low-dose azithromycin in patients with non-CF bronchiectasis. *Respiratory Medicine* 102 (10): 1494–1496.

Barbato, A., Frischer, T., Kuehni, C.E. et al. (2009). Primary ciliary dyskinesia: a consensus statement on diagnostic and treatment approaches in children. *European Respiratory Journal* 34 (6): 1264–1276.

Barker, A. (2002). Bronchiectasis. *New England Journal of Medicine* 346 (18): 1383–1393.

Bienvenu, T., Sermet-Gaudelus, I., Burgel, P.-R. et al. (2010). Cystic fibrosis transmembrane conductance regulator channel dysfunction in non-cystic fibrosis bronchiectasis. *American Journal of Respiratory and Critical Care Medicine* 181 (10): 1078–1084.

Chalmers, J.D., Goeminne, P., Aliberti, S. et al. (2014). The bronchiectasis severity index an international derivation and validation study. *American Journal of Respiratory and Critical Care Medicine* 189 (5): 576–585.

Chalmers, J.D., McHugh, B.J., Docherty, C. et al. (2013). Vitamin-D deficiency is associated with chronic bacterial colonisation and disease severity in bronchiectasis. *Thorax* 68 (1): 39–47.

Chalmers, J.D., Smith, M.P., McHugh, B.J. et al. (2012). Short- and long-term antibiotic treatment reduces airway and systemic inflammation in non-cystic fibrosis bronchiectasis. *American Journal of Respiratory and Critical Care Medicine* 186 (7): 657–665.

Cohen, M. and Sahn, S.A. (1999). Bronchiectasis in systemic diseases. *Chest* 116 (4): 1063–1074.

Davies, G. and Wilson, R. (2004). Prophylactic antibiotic treatment of bronchiectasis with azithromycin. *Thorax* 59 (6): 540–541.

Driscoll, J.A., Bhalla, S., Liapis, H. et al. (2008). Autosomal dominant polycystic kidney disease is associated with an increased prevalence of radiographic bronchiectasis. *Chest* 133 (5): 1181–1188.

Elphick, H.E. and Tan, A. (2005). Single versus combination intravenous antibiotic therapy for people with cystic fibrosis. *The Cochrane Database of Systematic Reviews* (2): CD002007. http://www.ncbi.nlm.nih.gov/pubmed/15846627.

Flude, L.J., Agent, P., and Bilton, D. (2012). Chest physiotherapy techniques in bronchiectasis. *Clinics in Chest Medicine* 33 (2): 351–361.

Gonska, T., Choi, P., Stephenson, A. et al. (2012). Role of cystic fibrosis transmembrane conductance regulator in patients with chronic sinopulmonary disease. *Chest* 142 (4): 996–1004.

King, P.T., Holdsworth, S.R., Freezer, N.J. et al. (2006). Characterisation of the onset and presenting clinical features of adult bronchiectasis. *Respiratory Medicine* 100 (12): 2183–2189.

Knowles, M.R., Daniels, L.A., Davis, S.D. et al. (2013). Primary ciliary dyskinesia: recent advances in diagnostics, genetics, and characterization of clinical disease. *American Journal of Respiratory and Critical Care Medicine* 188 (8): 913–922.

Leigh, M.W., Hazucha, M.J., Chawla, K.K. et al. (2013). Standardizing nasal nitric oxide measurement as a test for primary ciliary dyskinesia. *Annals of the American Thoracic Society* 10 (6): 574–581.

Loebinger, M.R., Wells, A.U., Hansell, D.M. et al. (2009). Mortality in bronchiectasis: a long-term study assessing the factors influencing survival. *European Respiratory Journal* 34 (4): 843–849.

Lonni, S., Chalmers, J.D., Goeminne, P.C. et al. (2015). Etiology of non-cystic fibrosis bronchiectasis in adults and its correlation to disease severity. *Annals of the American Thoracic Society* 12 (12): 1764–1770.

Martínez-García, M.Á., Soler-Cataluña, J.J., Donat Sanz, Y. et al. (2011). Factors associated with bronchiectasis in patients with COPD. *Chest* 140 (5): 1130–1137.

Murray, M.P., Pentland, J.L., and Hill, A.T. (2009a). A randomised crossover trial of chest physiotherapy in non-cystic fibrosis bronchiectasis. *European Respiratory Journal* 34 (5): 1086–1092.

Murray, M.P., Turnbull, K., MacQuarrie, S., and Hill, A.T. (2009b). Assessing response to treatment of exacerbations of bronchiectasis in adults. *European Respiratory Journal* 33 (2): 312–317.

Parr, D.G., Guest, P.G., Reynolds, J.H. et al. (2007). Prevalence and impact of bronchiectasis in α1-antitrypsin deficiency. *American Journal of Respiratory and Critical Care Medicine* 176 (12): 1215–1221.

Pasteur, M.C., Bilton, D., Hill, A.T., and British Thoracic Society Bronchiectasis non-CF Guideline Group (2010). British Thoracic Society guideline for non-CF bronchiectasis. *Thorax* 65 (Suppl 1): i1–i58.

Primary Ciliary Dyskinesia Family Support Group (2017) Primary Ciliary Dyskinesia, [online] Available at: http://pcdsupport.org.uk.

Shoemark, A., Ozerovitch, L., and Wilson, R. (2007). Aetiology in adult patients with bronchiectasis. *Respiratory Medicine* 101 (6): 1163–1170.

Vallilo, C.C., Terra, R.M., de Albuquerque, A.L.P. et al. (2014). Lung resection improves the quality of life of patients with symptomatic bronchiectasis. *The Annals of Thoracic Surgery* 98 (3): 1034–1041.

Wilczynska, M.M., Condliffe, A.M., and McKeon, D.J. (2013). Coexistence of bronchiectasis and rheumatoid arthritis: revisited. *Respiratory Care* 58 (4): 694–701.

Wilkinson, M., Sugumar, K., Sj, M. et al. (2014). Mucolytics for bronchiectasis (review). *Cochrane Database of Systematic Reviews* (5): CD001289. doi: 10.1002/14651858.CD001289.pub 2.

Wong, C., Jayaram, L., Karalus, N. et al. (2012). Azithromycin for prevention of exacerbations in non-cystic fibrosis bronchiectasis (EMBRACE): a randomised, double-blind, placebo-controlled trial. *Lancet* 380 (9842): 660–667.

Wu, Q., Shen, W., Cheng, H., and Zhou, X. (2014). Long-term macrolides for non-cystic fibrosis bronchiectasis: a systematic review and meta-analysis. Respirology 19 (3): 321–329.

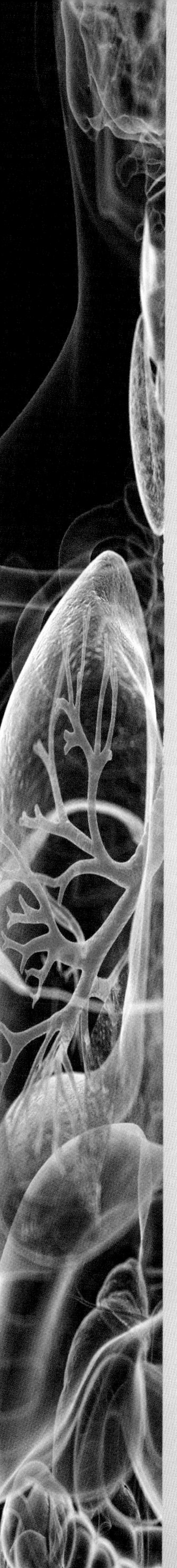

CHAPTER 13
Respiratory failure

Learning objectives

- To understand the definition of respiratory failure
- To understand the physiology of respiratory failure
- To be able to interpret arterial blood gas results
- To be able to calculate the alveolar-arterial oxygen gradient
- To understand the difference between type 1 and type 2 respiratory failure
- To understand the causes, diagnosis, and management of acute type 1 respiratory failure
- To understand the causes, diagnosis, and management of acute type 2 respiratory failure
- To appreciate the management of chronic type 2 respiratory failure
- To understand how oxygen should be safely prescribed, delivered, and monitored
- To understand the indications and contraindications for non-invasive ventilation
- To appreciate the ethical dilemmas in the management of patients with type 2 respiratory failure

Essential Respiratory Medicine, First Edition. Shanthi Paramothayan.

Companion website: www.wiley.com/go/paramothayan/essential_respiratory_medicine

Abbreviations

ABG	arterial blood gas
APACHE	acute physiology and chronic health evaluation
ARDS	adult respiratory distress syndrome
BiPAP	Bi-level positive airway pressure
BPM	breaths per minute
BTS	British Thoracic Society
CO_2	carbon dioxide
COPD	chronic obstructive pulmonary disease
CTPA	computed tomography pulmonary angiogram
ECG	electrocardiogram
EPAP	expiratory positive airway pressure
FEV_1	forced expiratory volume in one second
FiO_2	fractional inspired oxygen concentration
GCS	Glasgow Coma Scale
H^+	hydrogen ions
H_2O	water
HDU	high dependency unit
HRCT	high-resolution computed tomography
ICU	intensive care unit
IPAP	inspiratory positive airway pressure
kPa	kilo pascals
LTOT	long term oxygen therapy
mm Hg	millimetres of mercury
NICE	National Institute for Health and Care Excellence
NIPPV	non-invasive positive pressure ventilation
NIV	non-invasive ventilation
NPSA	National Patient Safety Agency
O_2	oxygen
PCO_2	partial pressure of carbon dioxide
PO_2	partial pressure of oxygen
RCT	randomised controlled trial
SaO_2	oxygen saturation
UK	United Kingdom
V-Q	ventilation-perfusion

Respiratory failure

Respiratory failure occurs due to inadequate gas exchange resulting in an abnormally low oxygen (O_2) level in blood. It is a potentially life-threatening condition that can lead to respiratory arrest and death if untreated. It can be categorised into type 1 respiratory failure or type 2 respiratory failure which can be acute or chronic at presentation. The diagnosis of type 1 and type 2 respiratory failure can be made by arterial blood gas (ABG) measurement. The mechanisms for developing these two types of respiratory failure are different (Box 13.1).

Table 13.1 depicts the results of a normal ABG measurement and ABG in patients with type 1 and type 2 respiratory failure.

Box 13.1 Key definitions.

- **Hypoxaemia** is an arterial oxygen level that is below normal and which can result in hypoxia.
- **Hypoxia** is a reduction in the oxygen delivery to tissues despite adequate perfusion.
- **Hypocapnoea** is a reduced level of carbon dioxide (CO_2) in blood.
- **Hypercapnoea** is an elevated level of CO_2 in blood.
- **Respiratory failure** is defined as hypoxaemia, with a partial pressure of oxygen (PaO_2) of <60 mmHg or 8.0 kPa.
- **Type 1 respiratory failure** is hypoxaemia (PaO_2 < 60 mmHg or 8.0 kPa) with a normal or reduced CO_2 level. It arises from a disturbance of the ventilation and perfusion of the lungs and can be the result of any acute respiratory illness, such as pulmonary embolus, acute asthma, heart failure or pneumonia.
- **Type 2 respiratory failure** is defined as hypoxaemia (PaO_2 < 60 mmHg or 8.0 kPa) with hypercapnoea, with a $PaCO_2$ of >48 mmHg or 6.5 kPa. A patient who has type 2 respiratory failure is at risk of developing respiratory acidosis (pH < 7.35) which can be life-threatening. Type 2 respiratory failure can occur from any cause of alveolar hypoventilation as a result of ventilatory failure.

The regulation of breathing

The physiology and control of breathing are discussed in Chapter 2. The respiratory centre consists of neurones in the medulla and in the floor of the fourth ventricle which initiate automated breathing activity under the regulation of chemical and physical reflexes. These can be overridden by voluntary cortical control, for example when sighing or breath-holding.

Table 13.1 Arterial blood gas measurements.

	Normal	Type 1 respiratory failure	Acute type II respiratory failure
PaO_2 mmHg (kPa)	80–100 (10.5–13.3)	<60 (8.0)	< 60 (8.0)
$PaCO_2$ mmHg (kPa)	35–45(4.5–6.0)	35–45 (4.5–6.0)	>48 (6.5)
pH	7.35–7.45	7.35–7.45	<7.35
HCO_3^- mmol/L	24	22–26	22–26

During inspiration, the inspiratory muscles contract, resulting in an increase in the volume of the thoracic cavity. This generates negative pressure in the alveoli and flow of air into the lungs. During expiration, the intra-alveolar pressure becomes slightly higher than atmospheric pressure and air flows out of the lungs.

The relationship between the partial pressure of oxygen in blood (PO_2) and the oxygen saturation measured by pulse oximetry (SaO_2) is described as the oxyhaemoglobin dissociation curve. Oxygen saturation is closely related to the partial pressure of oxygen in blood only over a short range of about 3–7 kPa. Above this level the dissociation curve begins to plateau and there is only a small increase in oxygen saturation as PO_2 rises. See Chapter 2 for details of the oxyhaemoglobin dissociation curve.

CO_2 is carried in blood dissolved in plasma and is in equilibrium with the bicarbonate anion (HCO_3^-), which is an important buffer, ensuring acid–base homeostasis. The Henderson-Hasselbalch equation shows this:

$$CO_2 + H_2O \leftrightarrow H_2CO_3 \leftrightarrow H^+ + HCO_3^-$$

In 1868, Pfluger was the first to show that the CO_2 content of arterial blood directly affected breathing in animals. In 1905, Haldane and Priestley established that the respiratory centre was extremely sensitive to small changes in alveolar CO_2 concentrations. CO_2 readily crosses the blood-brain barrier, rapidly increasing the concentration of H^+ in the cerebrospinal fluid. The chemoreceptors on the antero-lateral surfaces of the medulla are extremely sensitive to hydrogen ions (H^+). A small rise in PCO_2, therefore, results in an increase in the concentration of H^+ in the cerebrospinal fluid and an increase in ventilation.

The peripheral chemoreceptors in the carotid and aortic bodies are also sensitive to CO_2 and H^+ but are activated only when there is a significant fall in the O_2 level of arterial blood (< 60 mmHg or 8.0 kPa). These chemoreceptors do not play an important role in the regulation of breathing under normal physiological conditions.

Patients with type 2 respiratory failure have chronically elevated CO_2 levels in their blood and in the extracellular fluid surrounding the central chemoreceptors in the respiratory centre. These chemoreceptors, therefore, become relatively insensitive to the raised levels of CO_2. Under these circumstances the response to hypoxia by the peripheral chemoreceptors becomes the key stimulant to breathing. Correcting the hypoxia by giving uncontrolled oxygen can prevent the response to hypoxia and worsen the hypoventilation, eventually resulting in respiratory arrest (see Chapter 2).

Mechanisms of respiratory failure

Respiratory failure can occur because of a disturbance of gas exchange at the alveolar level (type 1) or due to failure of the ventilatory muscle pump that enables air to enter and leave the lungs (type 2).

Type 1 respiratory failure

Type 1 respiratory failure occurs due to ventilation-perfusion (V-Q) mismatch in the lungs, resulting in a reduction in gas exchange (Box 13.2). It is necessary to have an adequate surface area and sufficient blood flow through the pulmonary capillaries to maintain oxygenation. Any condition that results in a reduction in blood flow in the pulmonary arteries (such as pulmonary emboli) or a reduction in the surface area for gas exchange (such as emphysema) will result in type 1 respiratory failure.

Box 13.2 Causes of type 1 respiratory failure.

- Obstructive airways disease: severe asthma, COPD, bronchiectasis
- Parenchymal disease: pulmonary fibrosis of any cause, ARDS, pulmonary oedema, pneumonia
- Vascular disease: pulmonary hypertension, pulmonary emboli
- Other: pneumothorax, right-to-left shunt

Box 13.3 Calculating the Alveolar-arterial oxygen gradient.

$$PAO_2 - PaO_2 = \frac{[FiO_2 - PaCO_2]}{0.8} - PaO_2$$

FiO_2 = fractional inspired oxygen concentration, which is 21% when breathing room air at atmospheric pressure

PAO_2 = partial pressure of oxygen in the alveolus

PaO_2 = partial pressure of arterial oxygen (obtained from ABG)

$PaCO_2$ = partial pressure of arterial carbon dioxide (obtained from ABG)

R is the Respiratory Quotient and is 0.8 in an individual on a normal diet

Clinical presentation of type 1 respiratory failure

Patients with type 1 respiratory failure will usually present with breathlessness, increased respiratory rate and symptoms and signs of the underlying cause. This may include wheeze in asthma and crackles in patients with pulmonary oedema or pulmonary fibrosis. If the hypoxia is severe, the patient may appear cyanosed.

Investigations in type 1 respiratory failure

Initial investigations should include a full history, a thorough examination, pulse oximetry, ABG on air, chest X-ray, full blood count, urea and electrolytes, and blood glucose.

Further investigations can be carried out as indicated by the initial findings and may include a high-resolution CT scan (HRCT) if underlying fibrotic lung disease is suspected, ventilation-perfusion (VQ) scan or CTPA if a pulmonary embolus is suspected, or echocardiogram if left ventricular failure or pulmonary hypertension is suspected.

Alveolar-arterial oxygen gradient

The alveolar (A)-arterial (a) oxygen gradient is the difference between the alveolar concentration of oxygen (A) and the arterial concentration of oxygen (a). It is a more sensitive indicator of disturbance of gas exchange (VQ mismatch) than arterial blood gas measurement alone and can be particularly helpful in patients who appear breathless and are hypoxic without having respiratory failure ($PaO_2 > 8\,kPa$). Calculation of the A-a gradient in a patient with acute type 2 respiratory failure may also be helpful in determining the underlying cause of the lung disease.

In a young, healthy individual the A-a gradient will be around 2 or 3, increasing up to 4 with age. A high A-a gradient suggests a diffusion defect, a VQ mismatch or a right-to-left shunt. In routine clinical practice it is not unusual for the extent of the VQ mismatch to be underestimated because too much reliance is placed on simple oximetry and ABG measurement alone. A slightly reduced PaO_2, for example between 10 and 12 kPa, is often ignored. Box 13.3 explains how to calculate the A-a gradient.

It is assumed that the $PaCO_2$ is equal to the $PACO_2$ because carbon dioxide crosses rapidly from the pulmonary vasculature to the alveoli. This equation can be simplified for ease of calculation as follows:

$$\mathbf{A - a\ gradient = FiO_2 - PaCO_2 \times 1.2 - PaO_2}$$

Appendix 13.A gives some examples of how to calculate the A-a gradient.

Management of type 1 respiratory failure

Type 1 respiratory failure can present as an emergency, requiring prompt assessment and treatment. Management of type 1 respiratory failure consists of immediately correcting the hypoxaemia and treating the underlying cause. The aim in type 1 respiratory failure is to maintain the oxygen saturation in the range of 94–98% using a suitable device. These patients are usually not at risk of developing hypercapnoea, so the concentration of oxygen that is required can be safely given, so long as the ABG is monitored regularly.

Oxygen therapy and monitoring in type 1 respiratory failure

Hypoxaemia (PaO_2 < 60 mmHg or 8.0 kPa) must always be corrected to avoid the consequences, which includes respiratory arrest. Oxygen is a drug and must be prescribed, just like any other drug. Oxygen is indicated for all patients with hypoxaemia but is not a panacea for breathlessness in the absence of hypoxaemia except in the palliative care setting. The British Thoracic Society (BTS) Oxygen Guidelines, with agreement from 21 other societies, including the British Association for Emergency Medicine, the British Cardiovascular Society and the Royal College of Anaesthetists, has been disseminated nationally and these should be followed. The BTS oxygen audit is available at http://www.brit-thoracic.org.uk.

It is the responsibility of the doctor to ensure that oxygen has been prescribed, specifying the appropriate target saturation range and the device through which oxygen is to be delivered.

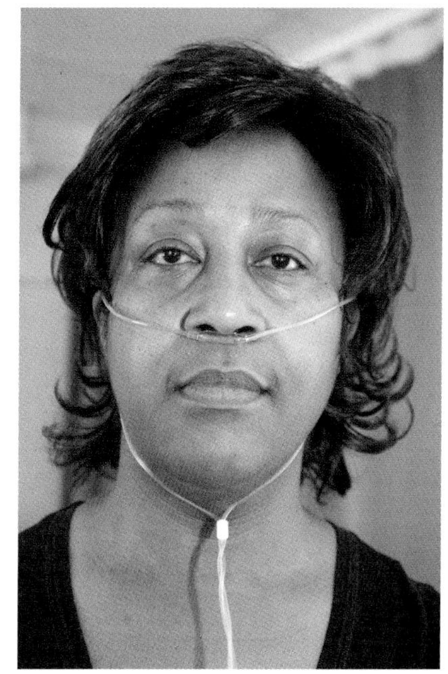

Figure 13.1 Patient using a nasal cannulae.

Devices for giving oxygen

Patients who are hypoxic can be given oxygen through a variety of devices. **Nasal cannulae** are suitable for most patients with type 1 respiratory failure (Figure 13.1).

A flow rate of 2–6 L min^{-1} of oxygen can be delivered, giving a fractional inspired oxygen concentration (FiO_2) of between 24 and 50%. The exact FiO_2 will depend on the patient's minute volume, inspiratory flow, and pattern of breathing. Nasal cannulae are cheap, comfortable to wear and well-tolerated. A **simple face mask** can also be used for patients with type 1 respiratory failure (Figure 13.2).The flow rate must be set at between 5 and 10 L min^{-1} to deliver an oxygen concentration of between 35 and 60%. A lower flow rate may result in CO_2 build up. A **reservoir** or **re-breathe mask** (Figure 13.3) is used to deliver a higher concentration of oxygen of between 60% and 80% in patients with severe hypoxaemia who are not at risk of retaining CO_2. It is often used in patients who are critically ill. Patients who are extremely hypoxic and require very high concentrations of inspired oxygen may benefit from continuous positive airways pressure (CPAP) device which can deliver over 90% of oxygen, often on the high dependency unit (HDU) (Figure 13.4). If oxygenation is inadequate through any of these devices, intubation and ventilation on

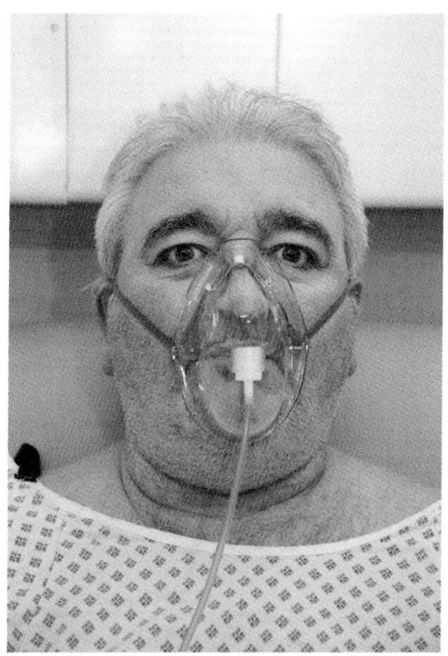

Figure 13.2 Patient using a simple face mask.

the intensive care unit (ICU) should be considered. Patients who are at risk of type 2 respiratory failure should be given controlled oxygen via a venturi mask (see section on management of Type 2 respiratory failure).

Nursing staff are responsible for monitoring and documenting the oxygen saturation on the observation chart. In addition, the prescription chart should be signed at each drug round. This is to ensure that the oxygen prescription is being carefully followed and that the amount of oxygen given is adjusted according to the oxygen saturation measurement.

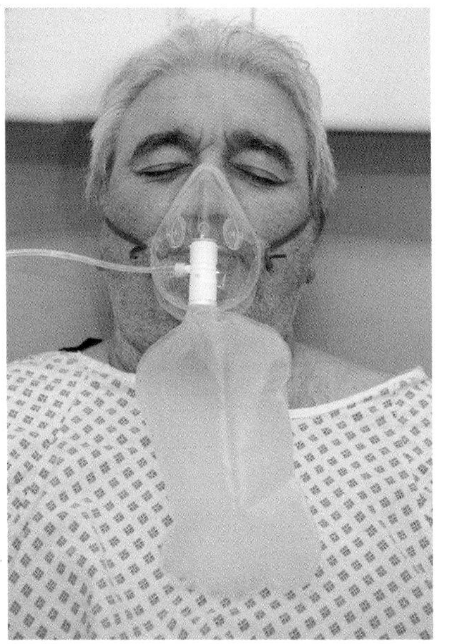

Figure 13.3 Patient using a reservoir (re-breathe) mask.

It must be remembered that high concentrations of oxygen given over a prolonged period may be harmful, resulting in coronary vasoconstriction, reduced cardiac index, and re-perfusion injury after a myocardial infarction. It may also have adverse effects in patients who have suffered a stroke.

Chronic type 1 respiratory failure

Patients with severe lung disease may be chronically hypoxic and are at risk of developing complications, such as cor pulmonale. They will require long term oxygen therapy (LTOT) at home. These patients should have a formal LTOT assessment, which is usually carried out by a respiratory nurse or physiotherapist. These patients are prescribed the amount of oxygen required (usually 1–4 L min^{-1}) via a concentrator which is installed in their home to use for a specified number of hours. Chapter 3 discusses oxygen as a drug, how it is prescribed and delivered.

Type 2 respiratory failure

Type 2 respiratory failure occurs because of failure of ventilation resulting in alveolar hypoventilation. It can be acute or chronic, or present with an acute component overlying the chronic condition.

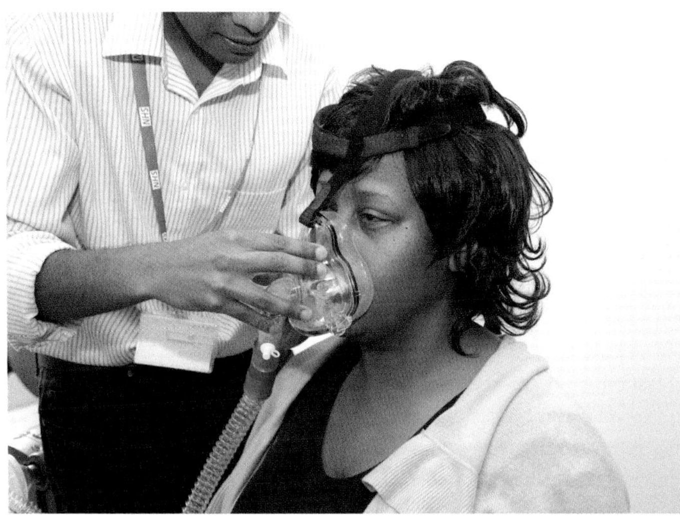

Figure 13.4 Patient being fitted with a CPAP device.

Patients who present with acute type 2 respiratory failure will be symptomatic and unwell.

Exacerbation of COPD is the commonest cause of acute type 2 respiratory failure in hospitals in the UK and is associated with significant morbidity and mortality. These patients may develop type 2 respiratory failure in transit to hospital or in the emergency department because they are given uncontrolled oxygen. The uncontrolled oxygen stops the hypoxic drive that the patient is reliant on, resulting in hypoventilation, hypercapnoea, and eventually respiratory arrest. It is therefore essential to be aware of the risk factors for developing type 2 respiratory failure. Box 13.4 lists the common causes of type 2 respiratory failure.

Acute type 2 respiratory failure can develop within minutes to hours. There is insufficient time for the renal buffering system to compensate, so the bicarbonate level remains in the normal range and the pH drops. **Chronic type 2 respiratory failure** develops over several days to weeks, during which period the kidneys excrete carbonic acid and reabsorb bicarbonate ions so that the pH is only slightly reduced and the bicarbonate level is elevated. Table 13.2 gives a quick and simple guide to working out ABG results in acute and chronic respiratory acidosis and in metabolic acidosis.

Box 13.4 Causes of type 2 respiratory failure.

- Chronic lung disease: COPD, severe chronic asthma, bronchiectasis, cystic fibrosis
- Chest wall deformity: kyphoscoliosis, thoracoplasty, extensive pleural calcification, chest wall trauma, obesity
- Neuromuscular and peripheral nerve disorders: myopathies, muscular dystrophy, motor neurone disease, spinal cord injury, poliomyelitis, Guillain-Barré syndrome, phrenic nerve injury, damage to diaphragm
- Disorders of the neuromuscular junction: myasthenia gravis, botulism
- Disorders of the respiratory centre: anaesthetics, respiratory depressants and sedatives, head injury, central sleep apnoea, cerebrovascular accident, multiple sclerosis

Clinical presentation of acute type 2 respiratory failure

Patients presenting with type 2 respiratory failure are hypoventilating rather than hyperventilating, so may not appear dyspnoeic. Patients who initially present with type 1 respiratory failure and tachypnoea may become tired and thus begin to retain CO_2, as occurs in life-threatening asthma discussed in Chapter 6. Patients may have symptoms and signs of the underlying cause of respiratory failure, for example, neuromuscular weakness, an abnormal chest wall or paradoxical abdominal movement suggesting diaphragmatic weakness. Patients with type 2 respiratory failure may display symptoms and signs of CO_2 retention, which includes drowsiness, confusion, irritability, a CO_2 retention flap, and a bounding pulse caused by vasodilatation. If untreated, the patient will become comatose when the $PaCO_2$ rises above 10 kPa and will ultimately die.

Investigations for acute type 2 respiratory failure

Immediate investigations include a chest X-ray, measurement of oxygen saturation (pulse oximetry) and baseline ABG taken while breathing room air.

Table 13.2 Comparison of arterial blood gases in acute and compensated respiratory and metabolic acidosis.

	PaO_2	$PaCO_2$	pH	HCO_3^-
Acute Respiratory Acidosis	↓	↑↑	↓↓	Normal
Compensated (Chronic) Respiratory Acidosis	↓	↑	Normal but <7.40	↑
Metabolic Acidosis	Normal	Normal	↓	↓
Compensated Metabolic Acidosis	Normal	Normal or↓	Normal but<7.40	↓

The initial ABG measurement will act as a guide to how much oxygen should be prescribed. Further, regular ABG measurements are compulsory once the patient has been commenced on oxygen. If the cause of the respiratory failure is not clear, then further investigations, such as a CT scan of the thorax or thoracic ultrasound may be indicated when the patient is stable.

Immediate management of acute type 2 respiratory failure

Once it has been established from an ABG measurement that the patient has acute type 2 respiratory failure, it is essential to treat it without delay. The key point in the management of type 2 respiratory failure is the use of **controlled oxygen** and treating the underlying cause, for example, with bronchodilators, antibiotics, corticosteroids, theophyllines, diuretics, and anticoagulants.

Controlled oxygen therapy and monitoring in type 2 respiratory failure

The challenge is to maintain the oxygen saturation between 88% and 92% without a significant increase in the level of CO_2 and the development of respiratory acidosis. Controlled oxygen should be given by the use of a venturi (fixed performance) mask, which gives controlled inspired oxygen of 24%, 28%, 35% or 40%. These venturi masks are colour-coded to make it easier to identify which one to use (Figure 13.5, Figure 13.6).

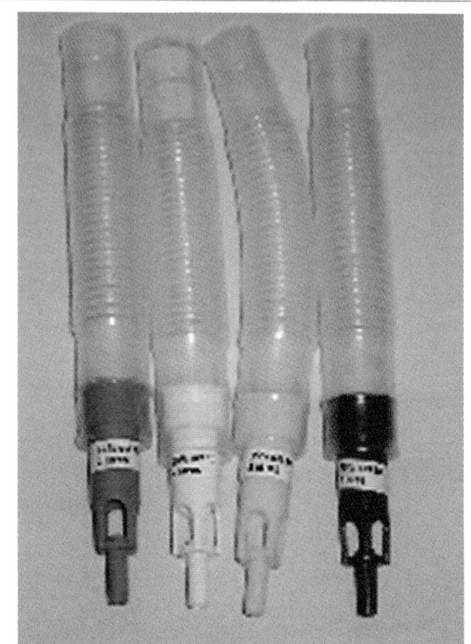

Figure 13.5 A range of venturi valves. *Source: ABC of COPD*, 3rd Edition. Figure 11.4.

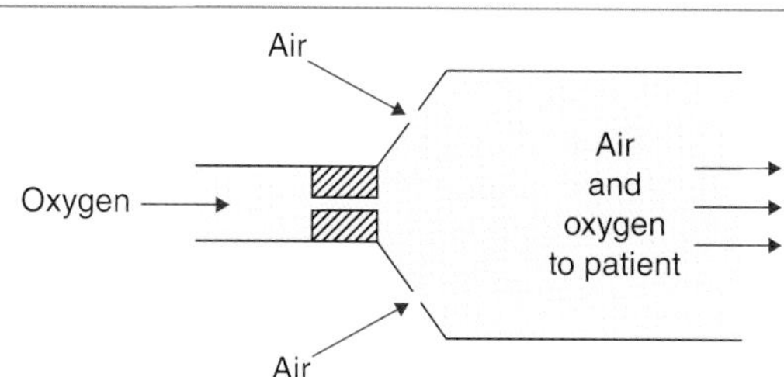

Figure 13.6 The venturi principle. *Source: ABC of COPD*, 3rd Edition, Figure 11.5.

If the patient is tachypnoeic with a respiratory rate of >30 breaths per minute, the oxygen supply should be increased by 50%. This does not increase the amount of inspired oxygen. If the patient is unable to tolerate a venturi mask, then a small concentration of inspired oxygen (0.5–1 L) can be given by nasal cannulae with careful monitoring. Once the patient has been commenced on oxygen therapy, the ABG should be measured every 20–30 minutes and the oxygen prescription adjusted until the patient is stable.

The risk of developing acute type 2 respiratory failure can be reduced by educating all healthcare professionals about those patients at risk, by always prescribing oxygen in the correct oxygen saturation range, and by carefully monitoring oxygen saturation to ensure that it is in the range prescribed. The British Thoracic Society (BTS) audit in 2008 highlighted concerns regarding the inappropriate prescription and monitoring of oxygen therapy in most UK hospitals. The BTS Guidelines (2008) have been disseminated to all Trusts with a recommendation to complete regular audits to ensure compliance. The National Patient Safety Agency (NPSA) has also emphasised the risk of oxygen therapy which can result in the development of type 2 respiratory failure.

Type 2 respiratory failure: to treat or not to treat?

As many patients who develop type 2 respiratory failure have severe chronic lung disease, some will deteriorate despite optimal management of the underlying condition and careful oxygen therapy. Their CO_2 level will go up and they will develop respiratory acidosis. A decision has to be made by a senior doctor regarding the ceiling of treatment; whether to commence non-invasive ventilation (NIV), refer for intubation and ventilation, or whether palliative care is indicated. This decision should be based on the patient's pre-morbid state (including their quality of life), the severity of their underlying disease, any co-morbid disease (particularly cardiac and neurological), any reversible component to their acute illness, any relative contra-indications to NIV, and their wishes.

Unless there are contraindications, non-invasive ventilation is the treatment of choice. Many patients with type 2 respiratory failure secondary to severe, chronic disease are not considered suitable for ventilation on the ICU as they can develop severe nosocomial infections and weaning them off the ventilator can be very difficult. Prior to the introduction of NIV, most of these patients would have died without any form of ventilation.

If it is clear that it is an 'end-of-life' situation, then palliative care should be the priority, with the aim of symptom control, especially relieving distressing breathlessness with medication such as opiates. Clear, careful, and sympathetic communication with the family and the patient is crucial. The palliative care team should be involved.

There should be clear documentation in the notes of the treatment decision and management plan. If NIV is to be initiated, there should be a clear plan regarding how long to continue with NIV, what to do if it fails and whether referral to the ICU for intubation and ventilation should be considered. A decision about the patient's resuscitation status should be made and documented. Ideally, the decision regarding the ceiling of treatment in patients with end-stage lung disease should be made prior to an acute admission after a detailed discussion with the patient and their family, and should be clearly documented in the notes.

Non-invasive ventilation (NIV)

The term non-invasive positive pressure ventilation (NIPPV) is synonymous with non-invasive ventilation (NIV). A variety of ventilator units are available (Figure 13.7), but the commonest in UK hospitals is the bi-level positive airways pressure (BiPAP) unit. Negative-pressure tank-type ventilators were first developed by Dalziel in 1832 and Drinker-Shaw used the iron lung for patients with respiratory failure secondary to poliomyelitis in 1928. The tank ventilator was further developed by Emerson in 1931.

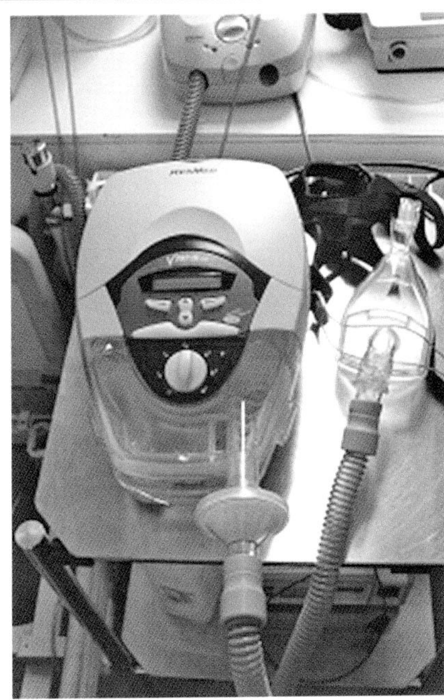

Figure 13.7 A non-invasive ventilator. *Source: ABC of COPD*, 3rd Edition, Figure 13.1.

NIV has revolutionised the management of type 2 respiratory failure and is the treatment of choice for patients with acute type 2 respiratory failure and decompensated respiratory acidosis, with a $pH < 7.35$ and a $PaCO_2$ of > 6.5 kPa, who have not responded to optimal medical treatment and careful oxygen therapy. NIV improves clinical parameters within a few hours of being commenced, with a reduction in respiratory rate, reduction in the work of breathing, an increase in tidal volume, improvement in oxygenation, a reduction in the CO_2 level and improvement in acidosis. NIV has been shown in randomised controlled trials (RCTs) to reduce the need for intubation, reduce the length of stay in hospital, and reduce mortality in patients with type 2 respiratory failure secondary to a variety of causes, but particularly COPD. NICE recommends that NIV is available in all hospitals treating patients with acute type 2 respiratory failure. Box 13.5 lists the inclusion and exclusion criteria for NIV.

Box 13.5 Inclusion and exclusion criteria for NIV.

Inclusion criteria	Exclusion criteria
pH < 7.35 and $PaCO_2$ > 6 kPa	Metabolic acidosis
Conscious	Unconscious
Not requiring immediate intubation and ventilation	Requires immediate intubation and ventilation
Co-operative	Not co-operative
Relatively calm	Severe agitation
Not cognitively impaired	Severe cognitive impairment
Little or no confusion	Severe confusion
Patient and/or their relatives wish to have NIV	Patient and/or their relatives do not wish to have NIV
Able to protect airways	Unable to protect airways
Reasonable quality of life	Poor quality of life
	Facial surgery
	Pneumothorax
	Vomiting
	Haemodynamically unstable

Some of these are relative contraindications and the benefit versus the risks of NIV should be considered carefully by a senior doctor after full discussion with the patient and/or their relatives. NIV is not indicated for patients with metabolic acidosis.

Table 13.2 describes the differences in ABG measurements between respiratory and metabolic acidosis. It is beyond the scope of this book to discuss the causes and management of metabolic acidosis.

It is important to be realistic about the use of BiPAP in patients with severe type 2 respiratory failure and patient selection is essential. Factors predicting a successful outcome include a co-operative patient with normal neurological function, a moderately high APACHE II score (acute physiology and chronic health evaluation) and a pH > 7.10. If the patient deteriorates despite NIV, there should be a clear decision regarding the ceiling of treatment made by a senior physician after discussion with the patient and their family. If it is felt that the patient is a candidate for invasive ventilation, then referral to ICU should be made without delay.

There is evidence that the prognosis is better if the patient is commenced on NIV within 60 minutes of presentation. There is also evidence that patients who are managed on a high dependency unit (HDU) by experienced doctors and nurses have a better outcome. NIV may also be indicated for patients who are slow to wean from ventilation as it reduces the total length of time on a ventilator and reduces mortality.

BiPAP

The usual device used is a bi-level positive airways pressure device (BiPAP) which can be set to deliver different pressures during inspiration and expiration. BiPAP should be readily available in the emergency department, acute medical unit, and respiratory ward in all hospitals and should be initiated by an experienced doctor or other healthcare professional. The patient should be in a sitting or semi-recumbent position and should have a full face mask fitted in the first instance which can be changed to a nasal mask after 24 hours if the patient prefers it.

It is recommended that the inspiratory positive airways pressure (IPAP), which blows off the CO_2, is commenced at 10 cm water (H_2O), and then increased incrementally, by 2 cm, up to a maximum of 24 cm H_2O if there is persistent hypercapnia. The expiratory positive airways pressure (EPAP) should be set at 4 cm H_2O to begin with and then increased up to 10 cm H_2O (Figure 13.8). The number of breaths per minute (BPM) is set between 12 and 18 in the patient flow-triggered/time-triggered (S/T) mode and the synchrony of ventilation should be checked. The limiting factor is often patient tolerance. As patient comfort will improve compliance and the success of this treatment, it is important to begin with the low settings to allow

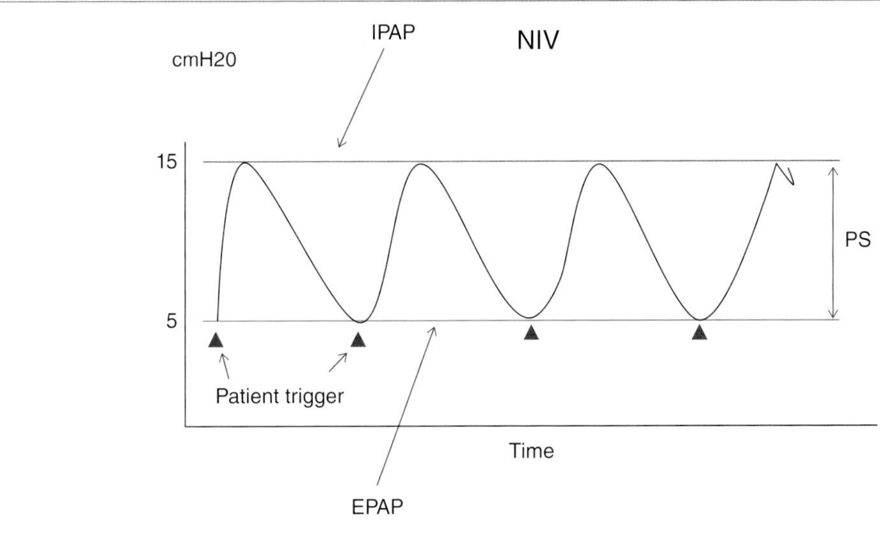

Figure 13.8 NIV pressures.

the patient time to get used to the feeling of the mask and the ventilator as this can be quite frightening and uncomfortable. The exact settings of the BiPAP will depend on the individual patient and includes factors such as the size of the patient and the severity of bullous disease.

A variety of full face and nasal masks in small, medium and large sizes are available. Measurement of the facial dimension should be taken to ensure that the mask fits properly. A mask that fits firmly but comfortably will improve compliance and prevent the leakage of air which will compromise the close circuit functioning of the system. A well-fitting mask will reduce pressure sores and skin lacerations from developing in areas of close fitting, such as the bridge of the nose. Other types of patient-ventilator interfaces, such as mouthpieces, nasal pillows, total face masks, and helmet devices are also available.

Patients who feel claustrophobic should be given reassurance, encouragement, and frequent (but short) breaks to allow them to get used to the mask and the device. This can be time-consuming for the doctor or nurse who initiates the BiPAP. Patients on BiPAP can become dry, so will need intravenous fluids, humidification, and nasal saline. Gastric insufflation, aspiration, and pneumothorax are rare complications of NIV.

Most patients in type 2 respiratory failure will require supplemental oxygen while on BiPAP in order to correct their hypoxaemia without worsening the hypercapnoea and acidosis. This is given through a port on the BiPAP mask until oxygen saturation in the range of 88–92% is achieved.

Monitoring on NIV

NIV should be prescribed on a chart with documentation of the initial IPAP and EPAP settings, the flow rate of supplemental oxygen given, the baseline ABG measurement, respiratory rate, heart rate and GCS. It must be emphasised that a patient commenced on BiPAP must have ABG measurement done 30–60 minutes later, and after every change in setting. Acutely unwell patients may require more frequent ABG measurements and may benefit from an arterial line. It is recommended that these patients are monitored on the HDU by experienced nurses. There should be documentation of any change in the settings and a record of the hours of use and time taken for breaks. Clinical progress can be gauged by observing the patient's respiratory rate, heart rate and use of accessory muscles. Patients on BiPAP should have continuous oxygen pulse oximetry and cardiac monitoring.

OXYGEN ALERT CARD

Name: ____

I have a chronic respiratory condition and I am at risk of having a raised carbon dioxide level in my blood during flare-ups of my condition (exacerbations)

Please use my _____% Venturi mask to achieve an oxygen saturation of

_____% to _____ % during exacerbations of my condition

Use compressed air to drive nebulisers (with nasal oxygen a 2 l/min)
If compressed air is not available, limit oxygen-driven nebulisers to 6 minutes

Figure 13.9 Oxygen Alert Card. *Source: ABC of COPD*, 3rd Edition, Figure 11.3.

Weaning off NIV

Patients should be continued on BiPAP until there is clinical improvement and their acidosis resolves. On average, this takes 48–72 hours. Patients are usually weaned off BiPAP gradually, with extended periods off BiPAP, initially during the day and then at night, until they no longer require it. Some patients improve very quickly and may only require NIV for a few hours. Some patients with severe lung disease may remain in type 2 respiratory failure and may require **domiciliary ventilatory support.**

Respiratory stimulants

Doxapram stimulates the respiratory centre in the medulla to increase the tidal volume and respiratory rate. Although not used as first line treatment, doxapram can be used in patients with type 2 respiratory failure who are unable to tolerate BiPAP or when there is a contra-indication to BiPAP. Doxapram should be initiated after consultation with a senior doctor who has experience in using the drug. Doxapram is given intravenously at 1–3 mg min^{-1} and usually for a short period of time. Careful monitoring of the patient will be required.

Prognosis and outcome

In many cases, patients with acute type 2 respiratory failure will improve over a few days if their respiration is supported over the critical period. However, their prognosis depends on their underlying disease and they may be at risk of developing respiratory failure again. They should be made aware of this, given written information about their condition and the dangers of uncontrolled oxygen therapy. Before discharge from hospital, they should be given an oxygen alert card (Figure 13.9) specifying how much oxygen they can have and a venturi mask to use at home if they are on long term oxygen or if they become acutely unwell and require oxygen, for example, while being transferred to hospital via an ambulance.

Management of chronic type 2 respiratory failure

Patients with musculoskeletal abnormalities, neuromuscular problems and obesity can develop type 2 respiratory failure gradually over a period of time. These patients hypoventilate at night when they are supine. Patients with chronic type 2 respiratory failure may not appear particularly breathless or very unwell despite high CO_2 levels because of the compensatory mechanisms which correct the acidosis (Table 13.2 describes the ABG in a patient with a compensated respiratory acidosis). These patients often report symptoms of tiredness, lethargy, and morning headaches from the high CO_2 levels overnight. An overnight full sleep study, which includes pulse oximetry and nocturnal CO_2 monitoring, will be required to make the diagnosis.

If they become unwell, for example, with an infection, they can present with an acute respiratory failure and acidosis on top of their chronic respiratory failure. Once the acute element has been treated with antibiotics, diuretics, and NIV, the patient will return to their baseline but will continue to have elevated CO_2 levels. Patients with chronic type 2 respiratory failure are managed with domiciliary NIV with regular follow up in a dedicated centre.

SUMMARY OF LEARNING POINTS

- Respiratory failure can be defined as a PaO_2 of less than 8.0 kPA.
- Type 1 respiratory failure is hypoxia with normal CO_2 levels and is caused by a diffusion defect, VQ mismatch or a right-to-left shunt.
- Type 2 respiratory failure is hypoxia with hypercapnoea ($PaCO_2$ level above 6.5 kPA) and is due to failure of ventilation.
- Type 2 respiratory failure can occur if a patient is given uncontrolled oxygen which can stop their hypoxic drive.
- Interpretation of the ABG measurement is critical in deciding what the diagnosis is and in prescribing the correct concentration of oxygen.
- The widened alveolar-arterial (A-a) oxygen gradient is more sensitive than ABG measurement at detecting a VQ mismatch, a diffusion defect or a right-to-left shunt in a breathless patient who is hypoxic.
- Patients with type 1 respiratory failure should be prescribed oxygen to maintain their oxygen saturation in the range of 94–98%.
- Oxygen is not indicated for breathlessness alone except in the palliative context.
- When prescribing oxygen, it is important to use the correct device.
- Patients at risk of developing type 2 respiratory failure should be identified and prescribed oxygen to maintain their oxygen saturation in the range of 88–92%.
- It is possible to work out from the ABG measurement whether the patient has an acute or chronic type 2 respiratory failure.
- Patients with type 2 respiratory failure have a high morbidity and mortality and should be managed by specialists on the HDU.
- Controlled oxygen should be prescribed for type 2 respiratory failure using a venturi mask. Serial ABG measurements should be made and oxygen concentration titrated accordingly.
- Patients with type 2 respiratory failure should be commenced on NIV if pH<7.35, so long as there are no absolute contraindications.
- Supplemental oxygen can be given via nasal cannulae in a patient on BiPAP.
- It is essential to choose the right mask to ensure a firm and comfortable fit and to get the settings right in order to ensure compliance. This can take time.
- Type 2 respiratory failure can be prevented by educating doctors, nurses, and patients about the risks, issuing alert cards and by giving the patient a venturi mask to take home.
- Patients with type 1 or type 2 respiratory failure who do not respond to any treatment should be discussed with the intensivists for consideration of intubation and ventilation.
- In patients with type 2 respiratory failure and severe lung disease, a decision will have to be made by a senior doctor regarding the ceiling of treatment.

MULTIPLE CHOICE QUESTIONS

13.1 In a healthy individual the chemoreceptors in the medulla oblongata are most sensitive to changes in the concentration of what in the blood?

A Bicarbonate
B Carbon dioxide
C Carbonic acid
D Hydrogen ion
E Oxygen

Answer: B

The chemoreceptors in the medulla are sensitive to hydrogen ions, CO_2 and O_2. However, CO_2 crosses the blood-brain barrier more quickly than hydrogen ions and therefore changes in CO_2 level in the blood result in the most rapid change in ventilation.

13.2 Which of the following statements about the alveolar-arterial gradient is true?

A The A-a gradient decreases with age
B The A-a gradient increases in Type 2 respiratory failure

C The A-a gradient decreases in Type 1 respiratory failure
D The A-a gradient can be calculated using the Henderson-Hasselbalch equation
E The A-a gradient is a more sensitive measure of VQ mismatch than arterial blood gas measurement

Answer: E

The A-a gradient increases with age, from two up to four in those with normal lungs. It increases in any condition that causes a diffusion defect, a VQ mismatch or a right-to-left shunt, all of which present with type 1 respiratory failure. It can be calculated using the PaO_2, $PaCO_2$, and the FiO_2. It is a more sensitive measure of VQ mismatch than ABG measurement.

13.3 A 65-year-old woman with kyphoscoliosis is admitted to hospital and has ABG measurement while breathing 2 l oxygen via nasal cannulae. The results show a pH of 7.38 kPa, PaO_2 of 8.6 kPa, $PaCO_2$ of 10.0 kPa and a HCO3- (bicarbonate) of 41.2 mmol/L. What does this indicate?

A Respiratory acidosis
B Compensated respiratory acidosis
C Respiratory alkalosis
D Compensated respiratory alkalosis
E Metabolic acidosis

Answer: B

The ABG indicates that although the CO_2 is high, the pH is within normal limits and the bicarbonate is high. This is consistent with a compensated respiratory acidosis.

13.4 A 50-year-old man with severe COPD exacerbation is rushed into the emergency department and is given 10 l oxygen via a re-breathe mask. His ABG is as follows: pH 7.25, PaO_2 of 10.82 kPa, $PaCO_2$ of 8.50 kPa and HCO3- of 31.2 mmol/L. How would you manage this patient?

A Commence BiPAP
B Commence CPAP
C Give oxygen via a venturi mask and redo ABG
D Give intravenous bicarbonate
E Call ICU

Answer: C

This patient with COPD has developed type 2 respiratory failure because he has been given uncontrolled oxygen. He is over-oxygenated as his PaO_2 is well above 8 kPa. Although he is acidotic, the oxygen should be reduced in the first instance using a venturi device and the ABG should be rechecked. Only if the patient and the ABGs do not improve should BiPAP be commenced. If that does not work, then intubation and ventilation should be considered.

13.5 A 68-year-old man with moderately severe COPD is admitted with an infective exacerbation. His respiratory rate is 22 and his GCS is 15. His ABG on air is as follows: pH 7.38, $PaCO_2$ 6.92 kPa, PaO_2 6.50 kPa, HCO3–24.2 mmol/L. What would you do?

A Commence BiPAP alone
B Commence BiPAP and 2 l of oxygen via nasal cannulae
C Give controlled oxygen via nasal cannulae
D Give controlled oxygen via face mask
E Give controlled oxygen via a venturi device

Answer: E

This man is in type 2 respiratory failure and therefore needs controlled oxygen. This can only be delivered safely through a venturi device. It is not possible to know the exact concentration of oxygen delivered through the face mask or nasal cannulae. He is not acidotic enough to need BiPAP.

13.6 Which of the following statements about type 1 respiratory failure is true?

A It can occur in patients with COPD
B One should aim for a target oxygen saturation range of 88–92%
C Any patient with a PaO_2 of <10 kPa should receive oxygen
D It can be alleviated by BiPAP and oxygen
E It should always be managed by giving high concentration of oxygen through a re-breathe mask

Answer: A

Type 1 respiratory failure can occur in any respiratory disease, including COPD, although these patients are at risk of developing type 2 respiratory failure so should be monitored closely with regular ABG measurements. The target oxygen saturation to aim for is 94–98% in those who do not retain Co_2. The definition of respiratory failure is a $PaO_2 < 8.0$ kPA so a patient with a PaO_2 of 10 kPa does not require oxygen. BiPAP is not indicated in type 1 respiratory failure.

13.7 Which of the following statements about type 2 respiratory failure is true?

A It is possible to predict who will develop type 2 respiratory failure from the initial ABG measurement
B It can be managed with CPAP and controlled oxygen on the HDU
C A $PaCO_2$ of >6.5 kPA is an indication for immediate BiPAP
D A bicarbonate level of >35 in the ABG suggests a chronic type 2 respiratory failure
E Chronic type 2 respiratory failure responds well to respiratory stimulants, such as doxapram

Answer: D

It is not possible to predict whether someone will retain CO_2 from the first ABG measurement which is why serial readings are required. CPAP is not a treatment for type 2 respiratory failure. Slight hypercapnoea in the absence of acidosis is not an indication for BiPAP. A high bicarbonate level is indicative of a chronic process as there has been time for the kidneys to retain bicarbonate. Respiratory stimulants will not have a significant effect on chronic type 2 respiratory failure.

13.8 Which of the following statements about NIV is true?

A It is recommended for all patients with type 2 respiratory failure
B It should be used with sedation in an agitated and non-compliant patient
C It has significantly improved the mortality of patients with type 2 respiratory failure
D It is contra-indicated if the patient is very hypoxic with a $PaO_2 < 5$ kPa
E It is commonly complicated by a pneumothorax

Answer: C

NIV has improved the management of type 2 respiratory failure and reduced the need for intubation. It is only recommended for patients who are acidotic with a pH < 7.35 and who can tolerate it. Sedation is contra-indicated in any patient with respiratory failure and no patient should be forced to have NIV. Patients who are very hypoxic and in type 2 respiratory failure can have NIV and supplemental oxygen as required. Pneumothorax can occur, especially in patients with bullous disease, but is not a common complication.

13.9 Which of the following factors best predicts a successful outcome with NIV for a patient presenting with type 2 respiratory failure?

A The APACHE 11 score
B The initial PaO_2 on air
C The age of the patient
D The length of time they have had their lung disease
E Their baseline FEV_1

Answer: A

A moderately high APACHE 11 score best predicts a successful outcome. The other factors may also indicate severity of disease and influence prognosis.

13.10 Which of the following statements about metabolic acidosis is true?

A It can never occur together with respiratory acidosis
B The bicarbonate in the ABG is usually low
C The $PaCO_2$ in ABG is usually high though the compensatory mechanism
D It can be successfully managed with NIV.
E It can improve slightly with respiratory stimulants

Answer: B

Metabolic acidosis can occur together with respiratory acidosis and results in a low bicarbonate. The $PaCO_2$ is usually normal or slightly low from the increased respiratory rate. Neither NIV nor respiratory stimulants are indicated for metabolic acidosis.

Appendix 13.A Calculation of the alveolar-arterial oxygen gradient

The equation for calculating the A-a gradient

Example 13.1:

Normal individual breathing room air.

$FiO_2 = 21$

$PaCO_2 = 4\,kPa$

$PaO_2 = 13\,kPa$

A-a gradient = 21 - (5 × 1.2) - 13 = 2

Example 13.2:

Young woman with a small pulmonary embolus making her breathless, breathing room air. Her PaO2 appears to be almost normal.

$FiO_2 = 21$

$PaCO_2 = 3\,kPa$

$PaO_2 = 12\,kPa$

A-a gradient = 21 – (3 × 1.2) – 12 = 5.4

Example 13.3:

A young man with a right-to-left shunt breathing room air.

$FiO_2 = 21$

$PaCO_2 = 4\,kPa$

$PaO_2 = 9\,kPa$

A-a gradient = 21 – (4 × 1.2) – 9 = 7.2

FURTHER READING

Albert, R., Spiro, S., and Jett, J. (2001). *Comprehensive Respiratory Medicine*. St. Louis, MO: Mosby Chapter 12.

Bott, J., Carroll, M.P., Conway, J.H. et al. (1993). Randomised controlled trial of nasal ventilation in acute ventilator failure due to chronic obstructive airways disease. *Lancet* 341: 1555–1557.

Brochard, L., Mancebo, J., Wysocki, M. et al. (1995). Noninvasive ventilation for acute exacerbations of chronic obstructive pulmonary disease. *New England Journal of Medicine* 333: 817–822.

Flenley, D.C. (1978). Interpretation of blood-gas and acid–base data. *British Journal of Hospital Medicine* 20: 384–394.

Kramer, N., Meyer, T.J., Meharg, J. et al. (1995). Randomised, prospective trial of noninvasive positive pressure ventilation in acute respiratory failure. *American Journal of Respiratory and Critical Care Medicine* 151 (6): 1799–1806.

Lumb, A.B. (2000). *Nunn's Applied Respiratory Physiology*, 5the. Oxford: Butterworth-Heinemann Chapter 5.

Martin, T.J., Hovis, J.D., Constantino, J.P. et al. (2000). A randomised, prospective evaluation of noninvasive ventilation for acute respiratory failure. *American Journal of Respiratory and Critical Care Medicine* 161 (3): 807–813.

National Institute for Health and Care Excellence (2010). Guideline on Chronic Obstructive Pulmonary Disease, June 2010, clinical guideline 12.

Nava, S., Bruschi, C., Orlando, A. et al. (1998). Noninvasive mechanical ventilation (NINMV) facilitates the weaning of patients with respiratory failure due to chronic obstructive pulmonary disease. *Annals of Internal Medicine* 128: 721–728.

O'Driscoll, B.R., Howard, L.S., and Davison, A.G. (2008). BTS guidelines for emergency oxygen use in adult patients. *Thorax* 68: vi1–vi 68.

Pingleton, S.K. (1988). Complications of acute respiratory failure. *American Review of Respiratory Diseases* 137: 1463–1493.

Royal College of Physicians (2008). *Non-invasive ventilation in chronic obstructive pulmonary disease: management of acute type 2 respiratory failure, National Guidelines*, Concise Guidance to Good Practice, vol. 11. London: Royal College of Physicians.

Soo Hoo, G.W., Santiago, S., and Williams, J. (1994). Nasal mechanical ventilation for hypercapnic respiratory failure in chronic obstructive pulmonary disease: determinants of success and failure. *Critical Care Medicine* 27: 417–434.

Woollam, C.H.M. (1976). The development of apparatus for intermittent negative pressure respiration. *Anaesthesia* 3: 666–668.

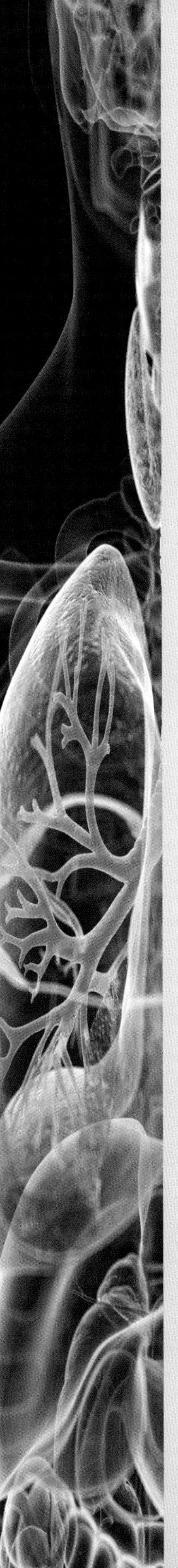

CHAPTER 14
Sleep-related disorders

Learning objectives

- To gain an understanding of normal sleep physiology and its impact on breathing
- To understand the causes of, and investigations for, excessive daytime sleepiness
- To understand the causes of and investigations for snoring
- To differentiate between upper airways resistance syndrome and obstructive sleep apnoea/hypopnoea syndrome (OSAHS)
- To understand the pathophysiology, diagnosis, and management of obstructive sleep apnoea/hypopnoea syndrome (OSAHS)
- To gain some understanding of other causes of excessive daytime sleepiness
- To differentiate between central sleep apnoea and obstructive sleep apnoea

Essential Respiratory Medicine, First Edition. Shanthi Paramothayan.

Companion website: www.wiley.com/go/paramothayan/essential_respiratory_medicine

Abbreviations

AHI	apnoea/hypopnoea index
BiPAP	bilevel positive airways pressure
BMI	body mass index
CPAP	continuous positive airways pressure
CSA	central sleep apnoea
DVLA	Driver and Vehicle Licensing Agency
ECG	electrocardiogram
EDS	excessive daytime sleepiness
EEG	electroencephalogram
EMG	electromyelogram
ENT	Ear, Nose, and Throat
EOG	electro-oculogram
ESS	Epworth Sleepiness Scale
HDU	high dependency unit
ICU	intensive care unit
IH	idiopathic hypersomnia
IOD	intra-oral device
LAUP	laser-assisted uvulopalatopharyngoplasty
MAD	mandibular advancement device
MSLT	multiple sleep latency test
MWT	maintenance of wakefulness test
OSA	obstructive sleep apnoea
OSAHS	obstructive sleep apnoea hypopnoea syndrome
PO_2	partial pressure of oxygen
PCO_2	partial pressure of carbon dioxide
PLMD	periodic limb movement disorder
PSG	polysomnography
RBD	REM behaviour disorder
RDI	respiratory disturbance index
REM	rapid eye movement
RLS	restless leg syndrome
UARS	upper airways resistance syndrome
UPP	uvulopalatopharyngoplasty

Introduction

In this chapter, there will be a description of normal sleep physiology and the autonomic changes that occur during sleep. The symptoms and conditions that can affect people when they sleep will be discussed. Upper airways resistance syndrome (UARS) and obstructive sleep apnoea/hypopnoea syndrome (OSAHS) are common conditions that present with snoring and excessive daytime sleepiness (EDS). OSAHS can lead to systemic hypertension and can severely impair the individual's quality of life. Treatment with continuous positive airways pressure (CPAP) can be effective in severe cases, while milder cases may benefit from an intra-oral device and lifestyle modifications. Rarer causes of hypersomnia include narcolepsy, periodic limb movement disorder, and idiopathic hypersomnia. Central sleep apnoea (CSA), which is much rarer than OSAHS, can be differentiated from OSAHS by the absence of ventilatory drive. These conditions are all classified according to the International Classification of Sleep Disorders.

Sleep physiology

Sleep is essential, but the physiology of sleep and the reasons why it is necessary are poorly understood. Sleep architecture varies with age, hormonal factors, and with external factors, such as sedatives and alcohol, so it can be difficult to define what is normal.

During sleep, consciousness is partly or totally suspended and muscle tone, including that of the respiratory muscles, is reduced. The respiratory centre in the medulla becomes less responsive to cortical, chemical, and mechanical stimuli, resulting in a fall in minute ventilation, a reduction in respiratory rate, a slight reduction in pO_2 and a small increase in pCO_2. These changes occur predominantly during rapid eye movement (REM) sleep. Individuals with respiratory disease which compromises their breathing when awake can become decompensated during sleep, with nocturnal hypoxaemia and hypercapnia, resulting in ventilatory failure.

The stages of sleep can be divided into non-rapid eye movement (non-REM) and rapid eye movement (REM) sleep. An understanding of these stages of sleep has been gained by monitoring brain wave activity during sleep using an electroencephalogram (EEG). An electro-oculogram (EOG) can accurately differentiate between REM and non-REM sleep.

Non-REM sleep

Non-REM sleep is subdivided into four stages during which the individual goes from a relaxed, but awake, state to being deeply asleep and less able to be roused (Figure 14.1). There is a progressive loss of alpha wave activity, with a slowing in the frequency of, and an increase in the amplitude of the waves measured on EEG. During Stage 2, the individual is completely asleep, and the EEG shows a further decrease in frequency of the waves, with spindles and k-complexes. During this period there is a decrease in muscle tone, pulse rate, respiratory rate, and temperature. Stages 3 and 4 are characterised by the presence of lower frequency delta waves. Nightmares, parasomnias, sleep walking, and nocturnal enuresis can occur during this stage. Each stage of non-REM sleep lasts between 5 and 15 minutes.

It generally takes about 70 minutes to drift from wakefulness through the stages of non-REM sleep before entering REM sleep. The individual spends 30 minutes in REM sleep before entering non-REM sleep again.

REM sleep

REM sleep is characterised by rapid eye movements as demonstrated by EOG monitoring and vivid dreams. EEG demonstrates high frequency, low amplitude waves (Figure 14.1). There are several autonomic changes during REM sleep, including a decrease in ventilatory drive, decrease in body temperature, reduction in muscle tone, and an increase in pulse rate and blood pressure. Apnoeic episodes lasting for up to 20 seconds occur, which can compromise breathing. Each period of REM sleep lasts about 30 minutes after which the individual awakes briefly before returning to Stage 1 of non-REM sleep. There are four to five cycles of REM sleep during a typical night which occupies 20–25% of total sleep time, predominantly during the second half of the night. REM sleep occupies 80% of sleep in infants and it is postulated that it may be important in learning and memory. Table 14.1 lists the causes of excessive sleepiness during the day (hypersomnia).

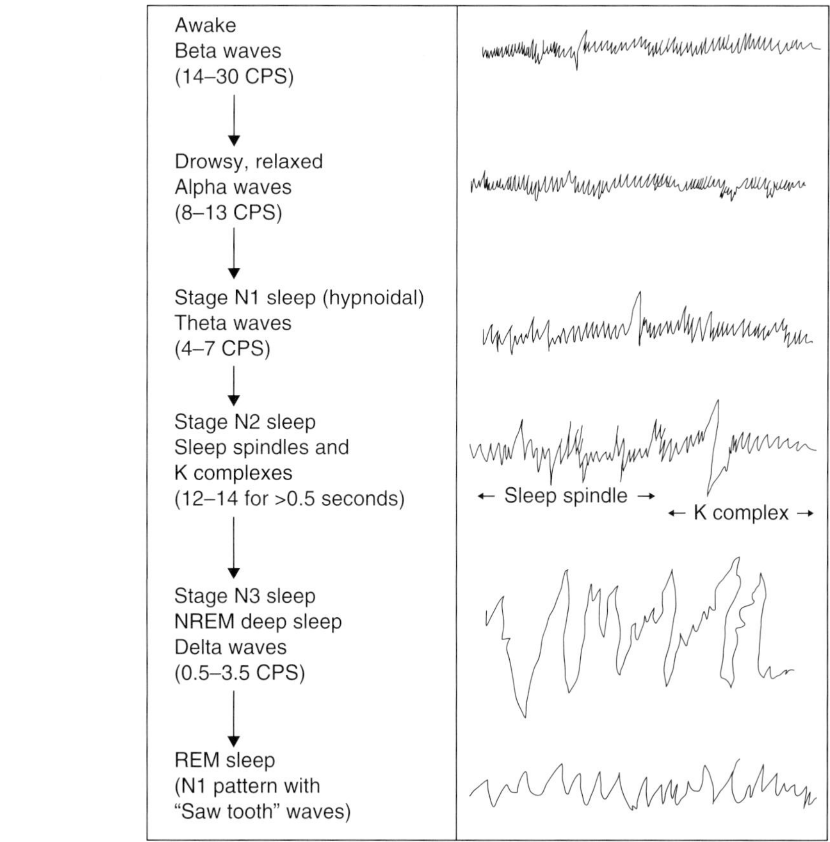

Figure 14.1 Brain wave activity during normal sleep.

Table 14.1 Differential diagnoses of excessive daytime sleepiness (EDS)/ hypersomnia.

- Upper airways resistance syndrome (UARS)
- Obstructive sleep apnoea/hypopnoea syndrome (OSAHS)
- Narcolepsy
- Periodic limb movement disorder (PLMD)/ Restless leg syndrome
- REM behaviour disorder (RBD)/parasomnia
- Idiopathic hypersomnia (IH)
- Nocturnal hypoventilation
- Insomnia
- Chronic sleep insufficiency
- Depression

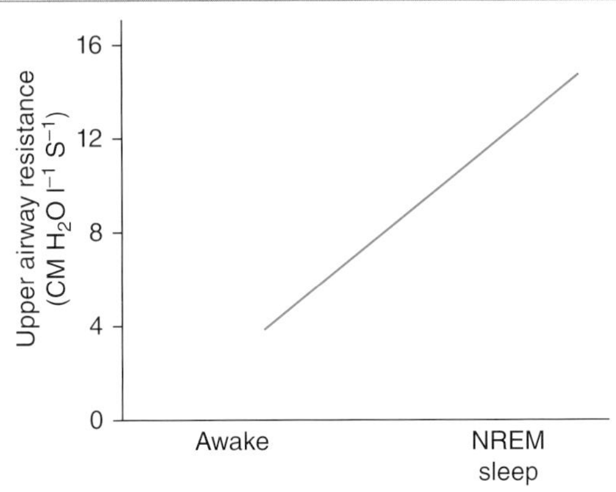

Figure 14.2 Increase in upper airway resistance during sleep.

Snoring

Snoring is a common symptom which can cause significant disruption to the sleep of the individual and to their bed partner. It can be a cause of excessive daytime sleepiness (EDS). Snoring can occur without any pathology when it is called "simple", due to upper airways resistance syndrome (UARS), or obstructive sleep apnoea/hypopnoea syndrome (OSAHS).

Simple snoring

Snoring is the noise made by vibration of the soft tissues in the oropharynx as the individual attempts to inhale air into the lungs against an obstruction. Simple snoring is a common condition which is more prevalent in men because they tend to have more fat deposition around their necks. It increases in prevalence with increasing weight and age. Snoring can be exacerbated by sleeping in the supine position, by taking sedatives and drinking alcohol. Snorers often breathe through their mouth and complain of a dry mouth. When severe, snoring can disturb the individual and their bed partner, and can result in disharmony. It can also cause sleep fragmentation and excessive daytime sleepiness.

Upper airways resistance syndrome (UARS)

Upper airways resistance increases during sleep, even in normal individuals, due to a reduction in the muscle tone of the upper airways and collapse of the upper airways (Figure 14.2). UARS, characterised by snoring and EDS, is at one end of the OSAHS spectrum, with severe OSA being at the other end. There is no accurate estimate of the prevalence of UARS in a population as these individuals do not usually report their symptoms to their doctor.

Oesophageal manometry and pneumotachographic airflow measurements show that while the negative inspiratory oesophageal pressure increases, the oronasal airflow decreases in UARS. Although these periods of upper airways resistance are not sufficient to cause an apnoea (complete cessation of breathing) or a desaturation of more than 4% in the oxygen level, they do result in brief EEG arousals which cause sleep fragmentation and daytime sleepiness. More than 10 EEG arousals/hour is also associated with an increase in diurnal diastolic blood pressure, possibly due to sympathetic activation and changes in intra-thoracic pressure.

UARS can result from any cause of upper airway obstruction, including enlarged tonsils, large nasal polyps, deviated nasal septum and craniofacial abnormalities, such as a low soft palate, and a long uvula. The male-to-female prevalence of UARS is similar, whereas OSAHS is commoner in men. Most individuals with UARS are non-obese and younger than the average patient with OSAHS. The average age of an individual with UARS is 37.5 years whereas the majority with OSAHS are over 50 years old.

Management of UARS

Management of UARS depends on the cause. If the obstruction can be dealt with by surgery, for example, septoplasty or tonsillectomy, this may improve symptoms. Craniofacial abnormalities

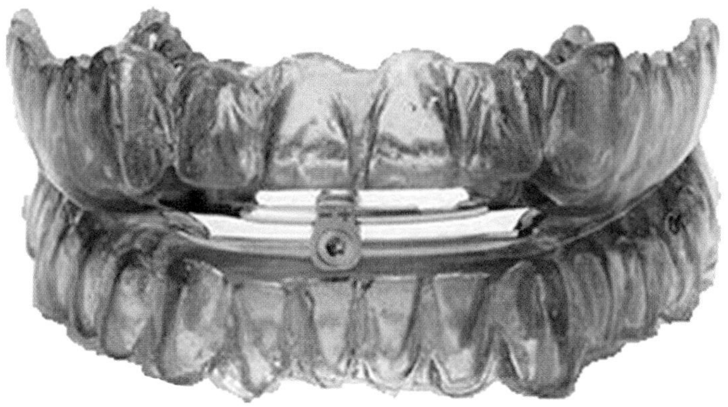

Figure 14.3 Mandibular advancement device (MAD).

are much harder to correct surgically. Patients should be advised to avoid alcohol and sedatives at night and to avoid sleeping in the supine position. Patients were told to sew a tennis ball in the back of their pyjama top to prevent them from rolling onto their back, and this advice is still given by many doctors. An intra-oral device, such as a mandibular advancement device (MAD), pulls the lower jaw forward and increases the space in the oropharynx (Figure 14.3). When no surgically correctable cause is identified and if a MAD is not helpful, symptomatic individuals may benefit from CPAP.

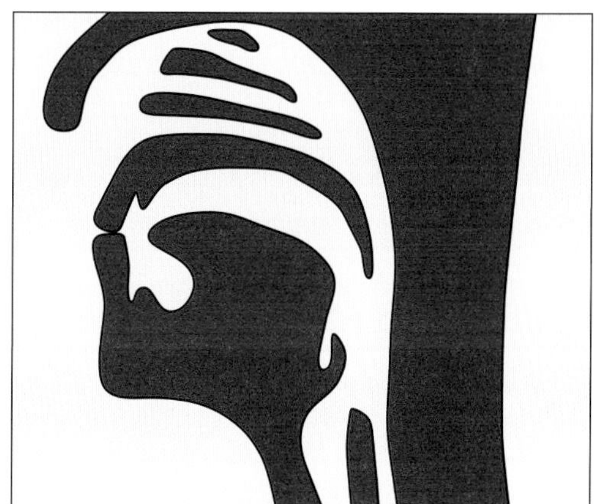

Figure 14.4 Normal upper airway.

Obstructive sleep apnoea/hypopnoea syndrome (OSAHS)

OSAHS is a common, chronic condition characterised by recurrent episodes of upper airway collapse during sleep resulting in hypoxia and sleep fragmentation (Figure 14.4, Figure 14.5). The diagnosis of OSAHS is made when the patient has symptoms of snoring and excessive daytime sleepiness, and a sleep study shows apnoeic episodes and desaturation of oxygen by at least 4% from baseline.

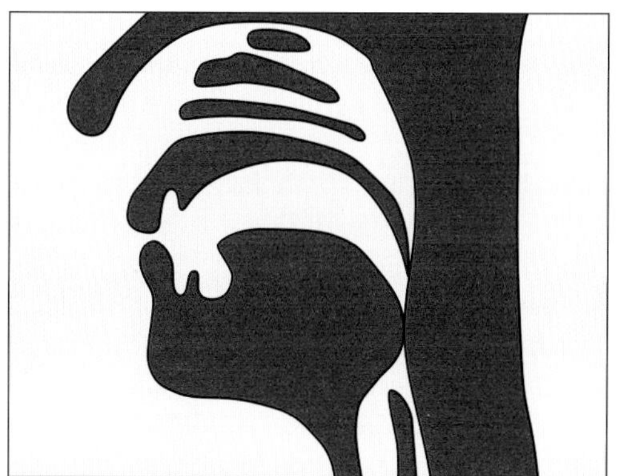

Figure 14.5 Narrowed upper airway in apnoea-hypopnoea syndrome.

OSAHS is an independent risk factor for developing systemic hypertension which could increase the risk of cardiovascular and cerebrovascular disease, although there is no direct evidence to suggest this. Retrospective data suggests that morbidity and mortality are greater in patients with an apnoea/hypopnoea index (AHI) of greater than 20/hour. Excessive sleepiness during the day is associated with an increase road traffic accidents. Table 14.2 contains the definitions of AHI from the SIGN Guidelines 2003.

Table 14.2 Definitions.

These definitions are arbitrary and exact cut-offs can vary between laboratories. The AHI is a continuous variable, like blood pressure, so separating normal from abnormal is difficult. The severity of symptoms can vary from night to night and can depend on exogenous factors, such as the amount of alcohol drunk. The severity of the apnoeic episodes measured does not always correlate with the severity of symptoms experienced by the patient.

- Apnoea: complete obstruction of airways for >10 sec
- Hypopnoea: >50% obstruction of airways for >10 sec
- Apnoea/Hypopnoea index (AHI) or Respiratory Disturbance Index (RDI): number of apnoeas and hypopnoeas/hour
- Mild OSA: AHI 5–14 h^{-1}
- Moderate OSA: AHI 15–30 h^{-1}
- Severe OSA: AHI > 30 h^{-1}

Source: adapted from SIGN guidelines (2003)

Epidemiology of OSAHS

OSAHS is a common condition affecting at least 3–7% of men and 2–5% of women in the general population. It is likely that many more individuals have a high AHI but are asymptomatic. Estimates of prevalence vary greatly between studies because of inconsistencies in the definitions and measurements used in different laboratories.

The prevalence of OSAHS is directly related to the prevalence of obesity in the population. Studies have shown a direct correlation between OSAHS and an increase in BMI, neck circumference, and waist circumference. Fat deposition in the parapharyngeal area causes narrowing of the upper airways and predisposes to airway collapse. In the Wisconsin Sleep Cohort Study it was found that individuals who had a 10% increase in weight had a 32% increase in the AHI and a sixfold increased risk of developing moderate to severe OSAHS compared to those who maintained a stable weight. Weight loss has been shown to improve the severity of OSAHS, and even completely eradicate it.

Several epidemiological studies have shown that the prevalence of OSAHS increases with age in both men and women, reaching a plateau after 60 years, where rates of 18% in men and 7% in women have been reported. This may be due to anatomical changes in the pharynx and soft palate, with increased deposition of fat in the parapharyngeal area.

The male-to-female ratio of OSAHS is 2–3:1 in epidemiological studies and 5–8:1 in clinic-based studies. This discrepancy may be partly because women are more likely to notice snoring in their male bed partners, whereas men under-report snoring in their female bed partners. Doctors too may be less likely to suspect OSAHS in women.

The reason for a male preponderance is mainly due to greater fat deposition around the neck and upper body compared to women which predisposes to airways narrowing and collapse. Hormonal factors are also implicated as the prevalence of OSAHS increases in women after the menopause, and hormone replacement therapy has been shown to reduce the prevalence of OSAHS in post-menopausal women. Exogenous androgen therapy can exacerbate the severity of OSAHS, and women with polycystic ovary syndrome have a higher rate of OSAHS. Women have a lower AHI in non-REM sleep and their apnoeic episodes are of shorter duration, with less severe oxygen desaturations than in men.

The prevalence of OSAHS is broadly similar in different ethnic groups, but the aetiology varies. Differences in craniofacial morphology may be relevant in the Asian and Oriental population, who tend to be less obese than the Caucasian populations of Europe and the USA. The greater prevalence of OSAHS in African Americans over 65 years of age may be due to an increase in the size of the tongue and soft palate. Care must be taken, however, when interpreting data regarding race and prevalence of OSAHS as socio-economic rather than genetic factors may be implicated.

OSAHS can occur within families, with first degree relatives of those affected having a greater risk of developing the condition. Several studies, including the Cleveland Family Study, have suggested that genetic factors, including inherited abnormalities affecting the control of breathing, may be implicated. However, confounding factors such as obesity and craniofacial or pharyngeal abnormalities within a family could also explain this. Further genetic studies are required to clarify the role of genes in the development of OSAHS.

The prevalence of OSAHS in children reaches a peak at around the age of 5 years and is estimated to be as high as 4% because of tonsillar and adenoid hypertrophy. Children who are sleep-deprived present with hyperactivity, loss of concentration, poor behaviour, and growth retardation. As children get older, their tonsils and adenoids atrophy, and the prevalence decreases. Tonsillectomy and/or adenoidectomy are possible, but rarely considered.

Pathophysiology of OSAHS

The patency of the upper airway is a dynamic process and reliant on a combination of anatomical features, neuromuscular activity, and whether the individual is awake or asleep. The upper airway is kept open when awake by activation of the pharyngeal dilator muscles and the rings of cartilage in the trachea. In response to negative intra-pharyngeal pressure, the tone of the main pharyngeal dilator muscle, the genioglossus, increases during inspiration and decreases during expiration. During sleep, particularly REM sleep, the muscle tone is reduced and is insufficient to keep the airway patent. In OSAHS there is also narrowing and vascular engorgement of the upper airway, causing collapse at multiple sites, with reduced or no airflow into the lungs despite continued respiratory effort Alcohol and sedatives cause relaxation of the upper airway dilator muscles, exacerbating the problem.

The reduction in airflow (hypopnoea) or cessation of airflow (apnoea) results in hypoxia which activates the respiratory centre, resulting in an arousal which is accompanied by an increase in pulse, an increase in blood pressure by about 50 mmHg and a surge in catecholamine release. The individual wakes up briefly to breathe, and there is an increase in inspiratory effort to overcome the obstruction, with the diaphragm and intercostal muscles working hard. This results in a breath being taken, often with a snort or grunt. This whole process can occur repeatedly throughout the night, up to 100 times every hour. The repeated arousals cause sleep fragmentation, resulting in poor quality, restless sleep, and excessive sleepiness during the day. Nocturia is associated with OSAHS due to an increase in atrial natriuretic peptide (ANP) levels.

Table 14.3 lists the presenting symptoms of OSAHS. Patients with OSAHS can present with any, or all, of these symptoms, which develop insidiously over many years. Occasionally, the patient may be asymptomatic despite proven OSA on a sleep study. Often it is the partner of the patient who reports loud, persistent, and disturbing snoring, in some cases prompting them to sleep in a separate room. The partner may also report that the patient stops breathing (witnessed apnoeic episodes), and then starts breathing accompanied by grunts and snorts. The patient could be disturbed by his/her own snoring which can wake them up from sleep. Even if an individual has no symptoms, those presenting with resistant hypertension and raised urinary catecholamines suggestive of sympathetic activation should also be investigated for OSAHS. Patients with metabolic syndrome and hypothyroidism are at increased risk of developing OSA.

Table 14.3 Presenting symptoms and signs of OSAHS.

- Snoring
- Apnoea (Greek word meaning 'without breath'), usually witnessed by a partner
- Restless/disturbed sleep
- Mouth breathing
- Dry mouth on waking
- Nocturnal choking
- Unrefreshed on waking
- Morning headache
- Nocturia
- Nocturnal sweating
- Excessive daytime sleepiness
- Reduced cognition, concentration, memory, and libido
- Irritability
- Change in mood
- Road traffic accidents

Table 14.4 lists the risk factor for, and clinical features of, OSAHS. As well as eliciting a history of snoring and the risk factors for OSAHS, it is essential to ascertain how sleepy the patient is using the Epworth Sleepiness Scale (ESS), which is a validated score that assesses the tendency to fall asleep under various situations (see Appendix 14.A). Ideally, the ESS should be completed by the patient, together with their partner, when they first present, as there is a tendency for the patient to underestimate the severity of their sleepiness. The baseline score is used to monitor improvement once treatment has been initiated.

- ESS < 11: normal
- ESS 11–14: mild sleepiness
- ESS 15–18: moderate sleepiness
- ESS > 18: severe sleepiness

Table 14.4 Risk factors for and clinical features of OSAHS.

Risk factor	History suggestive of	Features on clinical examination
Obesity	Increase in weight	BMI >30 (weight (kg)/height (M^2)
Large neck size	Large collar size	Neck size>17 inches (33 cm)
Retrognathia	Craniofacial abnormality	Maxillary and mandibular retroposition
Micrognathia	Craniofacial abnormality	Small mandible
Sedative drugs	Use of sedative drugs	None
Alcohol use at night	Alcohol intake at night	None
Enlarged tongue	Upper airway obstruction and snoring	Macroglossia
Low lying soft palate	Upper airway obstruction and snoring	Narrowed oropharynx
Long uvula	Upper airway obstruction and snoring	Long, oedematous uvula
Enlarged tonsils	Upper airway obstruction and snoring	Large tonsils
Enlarged adenoids	Upper airway obstruction and snoring	Large adenoids
Nasal pathology	Nasal trauma Nasal surgery	Broken nose Septal deviation Nasal polyps Reduced nasal inspiratory pressure
Asthma	Breathlessness, wheeze	Wheeze
Hypothyroidism	Weight gain Other symptoms of hypothyroidism	Features of hypothyroidism
Acromegaly	Increase in size of head, feet, and hands	Features of acromegaly
Marfan's syndrome	Marfan's syndrome	High arched palate Other Marfanoid features
Down's syndrome	Down's syndrome	Features consistent with Down's syndrome
Hypertension	Usually asymptomatic	Hypertension
Diabetes	May be asymptomatic	Hyperglycaemia on testing glucose
Musculoskeletal disorders	Nocturnal difficulty in breathing	Scoliosis Kyphosis
Neuromuscular Disease	Symptoms of neuromuscular disease	Features of neuromuscular disease
Polycystic Ovary Syndrome	Irregular menstrual cycle	Obesity Acne Hirsutism
Third Trimester of Pregnancy	Snoring and EDS during pregnancy	Pregnant Obese

Other causes of excessive sleepiness, such as narcolepsy, should be considered in patients who have a very high score of more than 18. Patients who are excessively sleepy should be strongly advised to stop driving immediately until investigations have been completed and appropriate treatment commenced. They should be advised to inform the DVLA.

Investigations for possible OSAHS

- Bloods: full blood count, urea, and electrolytes, fasting glucose, fasting lipids, thyroid function.
- ENT Investigations: nasendoscopy.
- Cardiac: blood pressure, ambulatory blood pressure monitoring, ECG, and echocardiogram.
- CXR if respiratory symptoms and/or hypoxia.
- Arterial blood gases if respiratory symptoms and/or hypoxia.
- Spirometry if respiratory symptoms and/or hypoxia.
- Overnight pulse oximetry.
- Limited sleep study.
- Full polysomnography (PSG).

Patients suspected of having severe OSA should have investigations and treatment without delay. Patients with co-morbid conditions, including ischaemic heart disease, arrhythmias, and COPD are at increased risk of fatal events during hypoxic episodes, so should be investigated urgently. Individuals who undertake dangerous tasks, work with machinery, or drive any vehicle (cars, Heavy Goods Vehicles (HGV), trains, buses), should be advised to stop work immediately and be referred for urgent investigations.

Overnight pulse oximetry may be sufficient to make a diagnosis of OSAHS in many patients. A drop of at least 4% or more of the oxygen saturation is considered a **desaturation** and the total number of desaturations per hour is counted. An increase in pulse rate may indicate an arousal and act as a surrogate marker of an apnoeic episode. However, oximetry alone may not reliably exclude OSAHS in a third of patients. False positive results can occur in those with respiratory disease and hypoxia at rest and those with Cheyne-Stokes breathing when there are oscillations in the oxygen saturation. Oximetry is also unreliable if tissue perfusion is poor, and can give false negative results in young, thin patients.

A **limited sleep study**, which can be done overnight in the patient's own home, is the most commonly used and cost-effective investigation for those suspected of having OSAHS. The patient is fitted with an oximeter to measure oxygen saturation, thoracic and abdominal belts to detect respiratory movements, oronasal airflow sensors or a thermistor and snore sensors which can measure the frequency and volume of snoring (Figure 14.6, Figure 14.7). This is cheaper than a full polysomnography (PSG) and more convenient for the patient.

Full polysomnography, including EEG monitoring to determine the stages of sleep, is not necessary in most patients suspected of having OSAHS (Figure 14.8, Figure 14.9). PSG is conducted in a sleep laboratory with trained sleep technicians, usually in a regional sleep centre, so is a time-consuming and expensive investigation. PSG should be reserved for patients with atypical features, those with neurological symptoms

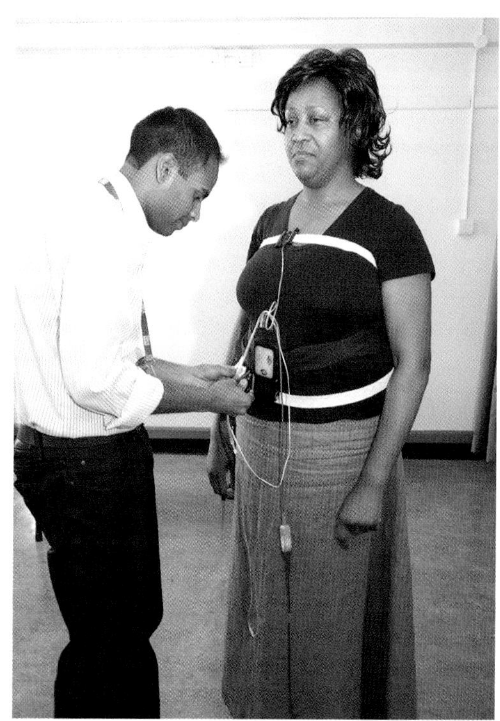

Figure 14.6 An individual being fitted with a home (limited) sleep study.

and when a limited sleep study is not diagnostic. The patient is fitted with an oximeter, thoracic and abdominal belts to detect chest and abdominal wall movements, oronasal airflow sensors, snore sensors, ECG to record heart rate, a blood pressure monitor, EEG to record the stages of sleep, EOG to detect rapid eye movement, and EMG to monitor limb movement (usually tibialis). Video recording can be used to correlate the patient's position and movement with apnoeas and arousals.

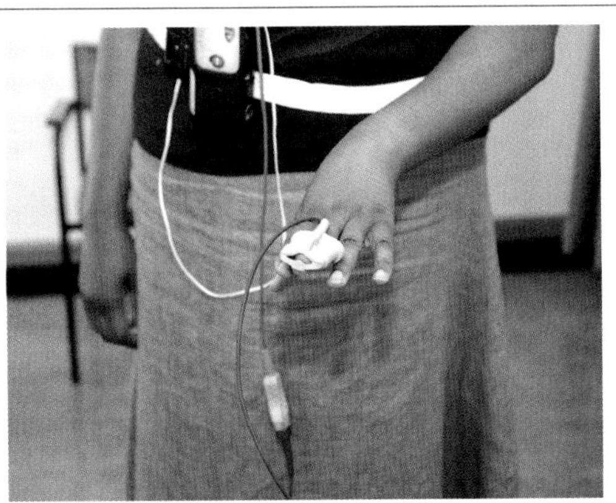

Figure 14.7 An oximeter being fitted for a home (limited) sleep study.

Diagnosis of OSA

A diagnosis of OSA is made when the AHI is greater than 10/hour in a patient who has symptoms suggestive of OSA as described in Table 14.2. Medical conditions, including hypothyroidism, diabetes, and hypertension should be actively excluded.

Consequences of OSA

OSAHS impairs cognition, mood, and quality of life. This can result in difficulty with work, social activities, and driving.

Initially, the link between OSAHS and systemic hypertension was thought to be due to confounding factors such as obesity and the metabolic syndrome. However, large epidemiological studies and controlled clinical trials have concluded that untreated OSAHS is an independent risk factor for developing systemic hypertension, with up to 60% of patients with OSAHS developing hypertension, often resistant to antihypertensive treatment. Patients with OSAHS were found to have a significantly higher

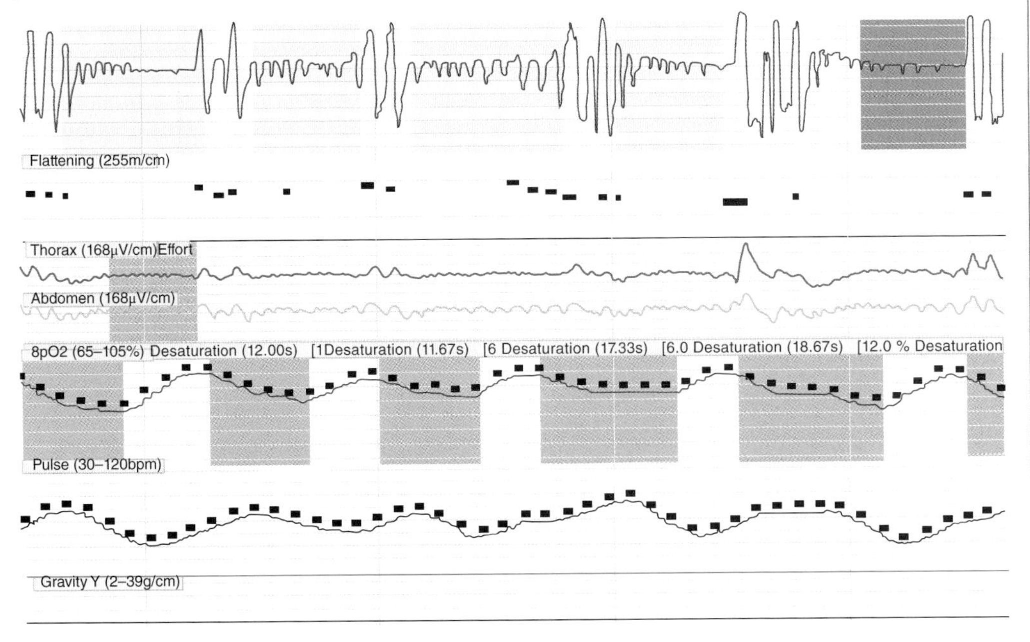

Figure 14.8 Home (limited) sleep study tracing showing obstructive sleep apnoea.

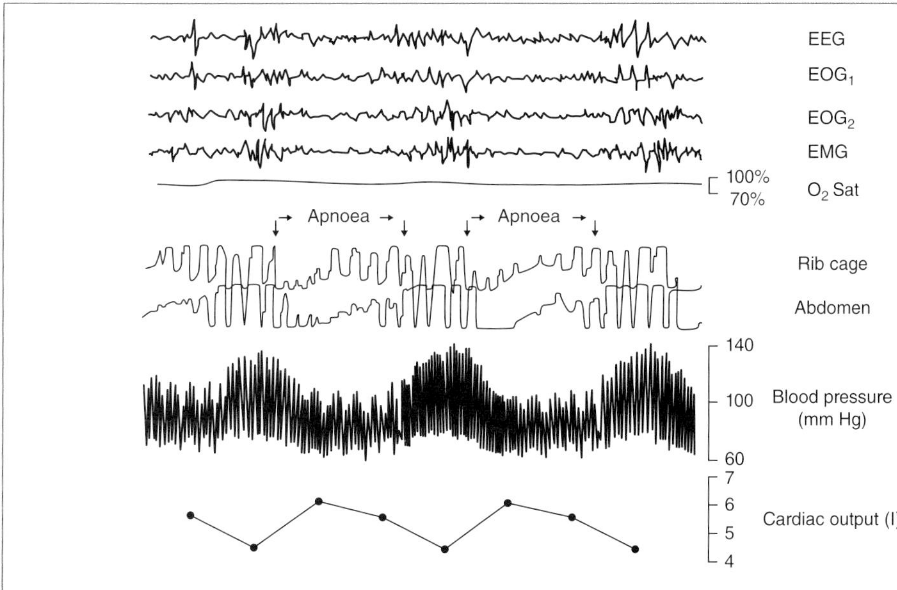

Figure 14.9 Full polysomnography tracing showing obstructive sleep apnoea.

blood pressure than matched controls, and treatment with CPAP resulted in a 5 mmHg reduction in blood pressure over a 24-hour period; this was most pronounced in patients with the most severe disease. That OSAHS alone results in an increased risk of cardiovascular and cerebrovascular morbidity and mortality has not been shown in any trial yet; a longer period of follow-up may be required.

It is postulated that recurrent episodes of hypoxaemia result in the formation of reactive oxygen species which damage the vascular endothelium. There is a reduction in nitric oxide levels and an increase in the levels of Endothelin-1, which results in vasoconstriction and an increase in peripheral vascular tone. There is a strong link between the metabolic syndrome (visceral obesity, insulin resistance, hypertension, and dyslipidaemia) and OSAHS, and apnoeic episodes may be associated with erratic glycaemic control. Individuals with OSAHS have reduced levels of growth hormone and testosterone and increased levels of cortisol, suggesting that the body is in a state of 'stress'. There is also a surge of catecholamine release with each arousal which may cause further damage to the vascular endothelium. It is thought that the high rates of sudden death during sleep associated with these conditions may be related to undiagnosed OSA.

Patients with COPD and OSAHS (called the Overlap Syndrome) have a high risk of nocturnal hypoxaemia, acute respiratory failure, pulmonary hypertension, and cor pulmonale.

Some obese patients with OSAHS will develop nocturnal hypoventilation and Type 2 Respiratory Failure which can be diagnosed with a full polysomnography and CO_2 measurements. These patients will require non-invasive ventilation (NIV) using BiPAP rather than CPAP. The causes and management of type 2 respiratory failure are discussed in Chapter 13.

OSAHS and driving

Driving when sleepy is extremely dangerous and can result in road traffic accidents. It is estimated that up to a quarter of all road traffic accidents occur due to people falling asleep at the wheel. Epidemiological studies have shown a high prevalence of OSAHS in truck drivers.

The doctor must inform the patient who has OSAHS that they should refrain from driving while excessively sleepy, that it is their duty to inform the DVLA and that it is a criminal offence leading to prosecution if they fall asleep at the wheel. The patient should also be told to inform their insurance company about their diagnosis.

The doctor should document the discussion in the notes and inform the patient's General Practitioner.

Individuals with OSAHS are legally required to inform the DVLA of a diagnosis of OSAHS. The DVLA will send them a questionnaire which they must complete, and their licence will be revoked until they can demonstrate that they are compliant with any treatment and that they are not excessively sleepy. Drivers holding Group 1 Licences (normal car licence) can drive when they are commenced on treatment for OSAHS and are no longer symptomatic. Group 2 Licence Holders (HGV, PSV = Public service vehicle and PCV = passenger carrying vehicle drivers) will be permitted to drive when it has been verified by a sleep specialist that they are using their CPAP for at least three hours each night, that they have a normal ESS and a normal sleep study when using CPAP.

Management of OSA

Patients who are symptomatic and who have moderate or severe OSAHS (AHI > 15 h^{-1}) are more likely to comply with advice and treatment.

Lifestyle changes

Patients who are overweight should be advised to reduce weight by modifying their diet and by exercise. Even a small weight loss can have significant benefits, with weight loss of 10% significantly decreasing the severity of obstructive events. Increasingly, patients who are morbidly obese are having bariatric surgery with significant improvement in the severity of their OSA. Patients should be advised to stop smoking and avoid sedatives, sleeping tablets, and alcohol consumption at night. Patients should also be advised to avoid sleeping in the supine position.

Surgery

Somnoplasty is a common procedure for snoring, but OSA must be excluded prior to surgery. Patients who have a deviated nasal septum, large nasal polyps, large tonsils, or adenoids may benefit from appropriate surgery. Uvulopalatopharyngoplasty (UPPP) and laser-assisted uvulopalatopharyngoplasty (LAUP) used to be common procedures, whereby parts of the soft palate, uvula, and pharyngeal walls were excised to increase the size of the airway and overcome the obstruction. The results of clinical trials on UPPP have not been favourable, and this procedure is now contra-indicated. UPPP was associated with an increase in peri-operative death, significant post-operative pain, and nasal regurgitation of food without a meaningful reduction in the number of apnoeas. In addition, patients who have had this procedure cannot use CPAP for OSAHS.

Rarely, in severe cases of OSAHS, when all other treatments have failed, tracheostomy can be considered.

Intra-oral devices

Mandibular advancement devices and tongue-retaining devices are used to increase the amount of space in the oropharynx.

Mandibular advancement device (MAD)

MAD is recommended for patients with mild OSAHS, UARS, and snoring. It holds the lower jaw forward, thereby increasing the space in the oropharynx. A moulded device can be made at home or a fixed device can be fitted by an orthodontist. Intra-oral devices are not recommended as first-line treatment for moderate or severe OSAHS as they have not been shown in cross-over studies to significantly reduce the number of apnoeas compared to CPAP. However, MADs have been shown to reduce snoring and sleepiness compared to placebo, so should be considered in patients with UARS, mild OSAHS and in those who are unable to tolerate CPAP. Side effects include hypersalivation, tooth pain, jaw pain and temperomandibular joint pain which usually improve over time.

Continuous positive airway pressure (CPAP)

CPAP is the treatment of choice for patients (adults) with moderate and severe OSAHS (AHI > 15 h^{-1}) but is not recommended for children. Randomised controlled trials using sham devices and Cochrane meta-analysis data have confirmed that compared to intra-oral devices and lifestyle changes alone, CPAP treatment is effective in reducing apnoeas, improving symptoms of sleepiness and improving quality of life in patients with moderate and severe OSAHS. The more severe the apnoeic episodes are, and the greater the ESS, the more likely the improvement in symptoms with

CPAP. The evidence is less clear for mild OSAHS (AHI < $14\,h^{-1}$), probably because of poor compliance in this group.

Regular use of CPAP for more than three hours each night for several months has been shown to reduce systemic blood pressure, with an average reduction of 4 mmHg in those with severe OSAHS compared to controls. It is inferred that this would lead to a reduction in cardiovascular and cerebrovascular risk.

CPAP treatment for those with OSAHS has been shown to improve sleepiness, driving simulator performance, steering accuracy, and reaction times. Meta-analysis of trial data and epidemiological data suggests that the use of CPAP is associated with a reduction in road traffic accidents by 83%.

A CPAP device consists of a unit that generates airflow and is connected to either a nasal or full-face mask via a tube (Figure 14.10, Figure 14.11). A pressure of about 5–15 cm H_2O is generated which splints the pharynx open by exerting positive airways pressure, thus preventing the airway from collapsing. A fixed CPAP device delivers air at a constant pressure throughout the night and the pressure required for each patient can be determined by an overnight titration study. Auto-titrating devices, which continually adjust the pressure delivered throughout the night, are more comfortable and better tolerated, but are more expensive. There is no evidence that their use results in a better outcome. A CPAP device costs £250–£500 and can last for five to seven years. A standard mask costs £100 and lasts for 6–12 months.

Claustrophobia, air leaks, and abdominal bloating are the main side effects of CPAP which stop the patient from using it. This can be reduced by ensuring that the mask fits properly and by using a chin support. Dry mouth, nasal congestion, and rhinitis can be reduced by humidification of the air that is breathed in. Damage to the skin, particularly on the bridge of the nose caused by a tightly fitting mask, can be prevented by using a nasal cushion. Epistaxis and paranasal sinusitis are rare complications.

Dedicated and experienced technicians who offer their support and expertise will improve compliance up to 95% for a 3–5 hours usage each night. CPAP machines record the hours of use which is essential when checking compliance, especially when the individual is intending to resume driving. Patients on CPAP should be regularly reviewed, their machines checked, and new masks fitted.

Patients with OSAHS should be carefully assessed prior to a general anaesthetic and regional anaesthesia recommended whenever possible. Sedative and opiate drugs should be avoided if possible. Patients should continue to use their CPAP machine post-operatively and should be monitored on HDU or ICU.

In patients who remain sleepy despite the use of CPAP, other causes of sleepiness, such as narcolepsy or periodic limb movement disorder, should be excluded. Modafanil, a stimulant working directly on the hypothalamus, can improve the symptoms of sleepiness in some patients, but should not be used as first line therapy for OSAHS.

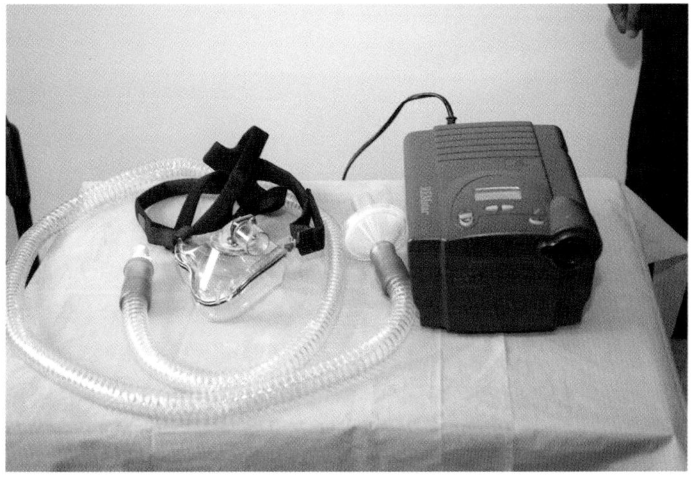

Figure 14.10 CPAP machine and circuit.

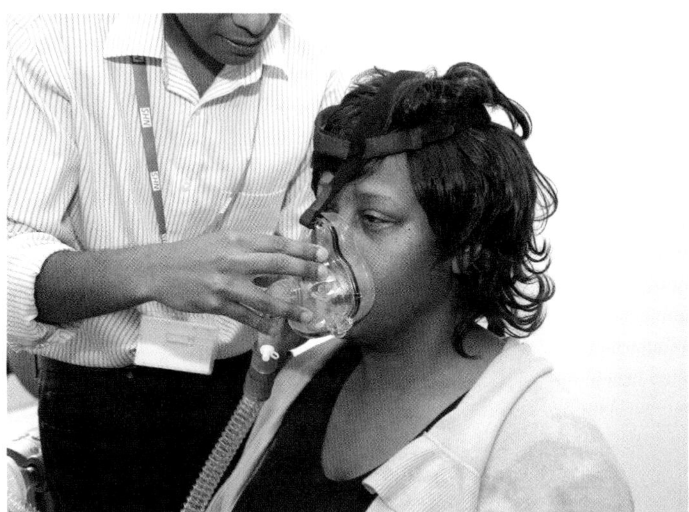

Figure 14.11 Individual having CPAP fitted.

Narcolepsy

Narcolepsy (meaning 'to be seized by somnolence'), is a serious sleep disorder which is usually insidious in onset, although occasionally it can develop more acutely over weeks or months. The incidence of narcolepsy is 1:2000, usually in early adolescence. Narcolepsy in children and older people is rare and often overlooked.

Pathophysiology

Primary narcolepsy results from a mutation in the hypocretin receptors in the hypothalamus of the brain. The hypocretin system regulates the sleep-wake cycle, maintaining wakefulness. Disorders result in excessive sleepiness. Secondary narcolepsy can result from a loss of the hypocretin-secreting neurones in the hypothalamus due to an autoimmune process (which is associated with HLA phenotype DQB1 0602), viral illness or head injury.

Clinical features

The main feature is EDS resulting in the irresistible need to fall asleep without notice. These episodes are often called 'sleep attacks', and short naps of 15 minutes are typically restoring. Cataplexy, which occurs in 65% of patients, is characterised by muscle paralysis for several seconds to a few minutes without loss of consciousness. Minor episodes may manifest as jerking of the face or head and slurring of speech. Episodes of cataplexy may be precipitated by strong emotions such as laughter, surprise, and anger. Other symptoms include parasomnias, sleep paralysis and hallucinations (visual, auditory, and tactile). As the hypothalamus is affected, appetite dysregulation with food cravings can occur, particularly in adolescent females, resulting in huge weight gain.

Investigations

A multiple sleep latency test (MSLT) is a standard measure of daytime sleepiness. It is used to make a diagnosis of narcolepsy and to monitor response to treatment. A normal MSLT score is 10–20 minutes, although it is dependent on how much sleep the individual has had the night before. Patients with narcolepsy will fall asleep within 8 minutes on a MSLT. Full polysomnography will show a reduced latency to REM sleep, with at least two sleep-onset REM episodes in a series of latency tests during the day. Hypocretin levels in cerebrospinal fluid (CSF) will be very low or undetectable, although this is not an investigation used routinely in clinical practice, but mainly used for experimental purposes.

Management

Lifestyle changes, such as planned short naps during the day and adjustment to the sleep cycle, may help. Employers and family members who appreciate the difficulty of this condition and are flexible can ensure that the individual continues to work and functions as normally as possible.

Modafinil, which stimulates the neurones in the hypothalamus, is the most effective drug for EDS. It is contraindicated if there are serious cardiovascular problems and can cause gastrointestinal upset and headaches. Stimulants, such as dexamfetamine and methylphenidate, can be helpful. Antidepressants, such as venlafaxine and clomipramine, are effective in cataplexy as they suppress REM sleep. Sodium oxybate is very effective, but expensive, and not yet recommended by NICE. Other drugs with less evidence of clinical benefit include melatonin and intravenous immunoglobulins if an autoimmune process is suspected.

Narcolepsy has a variable prognosis. Most patients improve to some extent with lifestyle modifications and medication. Some patients continue to be significantly affected so that they are unable to work or partake in social activities. Patients with narcolepsy must inform the DVLA and can only drive if their symptoms of sleepiness and cataplexy are effectively controlled.

Periodic limb movement disorder (PLMD)

PLMD is characterised by repetitive, involuntary, jerking movements of limbs which occur every 20–40 seconds and can last for many hours. Movement of the lower limbs is more common than that of the upper limbs. This can range from minor movements of feet or significant movements of all four limbs. PLMD occurs during the non-REM sleep stages, and so is more likely to occur during the first part of the night. Patients may not be aware of these movements which are noticed by their bed partner. These movements can cause sleep disruption and EDS. PLMD is commoner in patients suffering with Parkinson's disease and narcolepsy and associated with shift working, excessive stress, excessive caffeine intake, benzodiazepine withdrawal, and mental health disorders.

The incidence of PLMD is 4% and is commoner in elderly females. PLMD can be diagnosed with a history from a partner and by a PSG which demonstrates at least three episodes during the night, lasting from a few minutes to an hour, each with at least 30 movements followed by a partial arousal.

Treatment for PLMD includes anti-Parkinson medications, dopaminergic medication, anticonvulsants, benzodiazepines, and narcotics. Tri-cyclic antidepressants, alcohol, SSRIs, and caffeine should be avoided.

Restless leg syndrome (RLS)

Restless leg syndrome is characterised by an uncomfortable sensation in the legs which can occur when the patient is asleep or awake. When awake, the patient moves their legs voluntarily to relieve the sensation. Many of these patients (80%) will also have PLMD but the reverse is not true.

REM behaviour disorder (RBD)/parasomnia

RBD is a neurodegenerative disorder, mainly affecting elderly men. Idiopathic RBD is uncommon. Individuals with RBD act out their dreams, sometimes in a violent way, with potential for injuring themselves or their partner. During normal REM sleep the electrical activity, as measured by EEG, is the same as when awake, but there is muscle paralysis. In RBD, the distinction between REM sleep and the awake state is blurred. Episodes of RBD can occur up to four times during a night, especially in the morning hours, when REM sleep occurs more frequently. RBD results in sleep deprivation and is a cause of EDS. There may be a link between RBD and Parkinson's disease, Lewy body dementia, and multiple system atrophy. A diagnosis is usually made with a partner reporting nocturnal activity and with the use of PSG and a video camera. Clonazepam is the most effective medication for this condition. Antidepressants and melatonin can also help.

Idiopathic hypersomnia (IH)

Idiopathic hypersomnia is a diagnosis of exclusion. Other causes of excessive sleepiness, including the use of medication, alcohol, hypothyroidism, and depression need to be excluded. It is a chronic, debilitating condition characterised by excessive daytime sleepiness which develops insidiously over many years. The true prevalence of IH is unknown. It may be a disorder of the norepinephrine system of the brain or hypersensitivity to GABA. Decreased levels of histamine in CSF has been found in patients with IH.

The individual concerned may sleep up to 18 hours each day and still have difficulty waking up, with disorientation on waking. Unlike narcolepsy, the patient does not fall asleep suddenly, experience episodes of cataplexy, or find short naps refreshing. Anxiety, depression, and reduced appetite may occur. As the diagnosis is one of exclusion, it will require PSG, MSLT, measurement of hypocretin in CSF to exclude narcolepsy, and even a psychiatric review. Management includes stimulants, such as modafanil and amphetamines, although they are not as effective as they are in narcolepsy. Substances that act like histamine, GABA antagonists, clarithromycin, and hypocretin agonists may be suitable wake-promoting agents in the future.

Insomnia

Insomnia is a common cause of EDS. Stress, excessive caffeine, shift work, and jet lag are some causes of the causes. Chronic insomnia can be hard to cure. Management includes a detailed sleep diary, sleep hygiene advice, ensuring that the sleep environment is conducive to sleeping, and avoiding stimulants at night.

Chronic sleep insufficiency

There are many causes of chronic sleep insufficiency, including long hours at work, shift work and small children who might disrupt sleep. Management comprises of lifestyle modifications.

Central sleep apnoea (CSA)

CSA is much less common than OSAHS. It is due to an absent or reduced ventilatory drive but with no evidence of upper airways obstruction. The most common cause of CSA is due to damage to the brainstem from strokes, tumours, and conditions such as syringobulbia. Ondine's curse is a congenital form of CSA due to abnormal development of the neural crest. Cheyne-Stokes breathing, consisting of periods of apnoeas followed by hyperventilation, is associated with left ventricular failure (Figure 14.12). The prolonged circulation time means that the carotid body does not respond quickly to changes in ventilation.

Nocturnal hypoventilation

Nocturnal hypoventilation can be due to a variety of conditions, including neuromuscular and musculoskeletal diseases, which can result in mechanical ventilatory failure. Obesity is another common cause. The patient is usually able to maintain ventilation when awake but decompensates when asleep, resulting in type 2 respiratory failure (hypoxia and hypercapnoea). Causes and management of type 2 respiratory failure are discussed in Chapter 13.

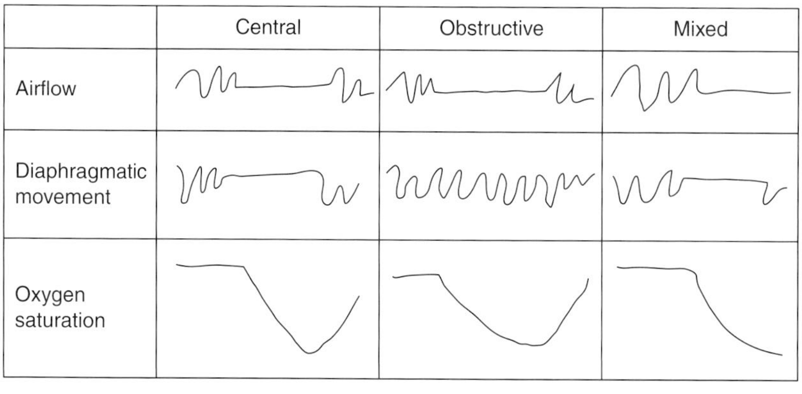

	Central	Obstructive	Mixed
Airflow			
Diaphragmatic movement			
Oxygen saturation			

Figure 14.12 Sleep tracing showing obstructive, central, and mixed apnoea.

SUMMARY OF LEARNING POINTS

- During REM sleep there is a reduction in ventilatory drive which adversely affects respiration.
- During REM sleep there is a reduction in muscle tone which can contribute to upper airway collapse and lead to airway obstruction.
- UARS is a common condition which can result in excessive daytime sleepiness and hypertension.
- UARS can be differentiated from OSAHS because there are no oxygen desturations.
- UARS can be treated with an intra-oral device, lifestyle modification, and CPAP if symptoms are severe.
- OSAHS is a common condition with a male preponderance, more common in the elderly and associated with obesity and the metabolic syndrome.
- The diagnosis of OSAHS can be made by a limited sleep study at home.
- Severe OSAHS is associated with hypertension.
- Patients who are excessively sleepy must be advised not to drive and to inform the DVLA until they have a diagnosis, treatment has been commenced and they are no longer sleepy.
- CPAP is the treatment of choice for moderate and severe OSAHS.
- CPAP results in a reduction in blood pressure in those with severe OSA.
- CPAP results in an improvement in sleepiness in those with severe OSA.
- CPAP results in a reduction in road traffic accidents in those who have OSA.
- Mild OSAHS can be treated with an intra-oral device and lifestyle modifications.
- Narcolepsy is a cause of excessive daytime sleepiness and can be diagnosed using a MSLT.
- Modafinil is the treatment of choice for narcolepsy.
- Other causes of excessive daytime sleepiness include periodic limb movement disorder, REM behaviour disorder, idiopathic hypersomnia, insomnia, and chronic sleep insufficiency.
- Central sleep apnoea can be distinguished from OSAHS because of the absence of ventilatory drive.
- CSA can occur due to neurological and cardiac causes.

MULTIPLE CHOICE QUESTIONS

14.1 During REM sleep the individual experiences which condition?

A Increase in respiratory rate
B Increase in libido
C Decrease in muscle tone
D Increased leg movement
E Decrease in eye movements

Answer: C

During REM sleep the individual has reduction in muscle tone and a reduction in ventilation and breathing associated with sleep paralysis.

14.2 UARS is NOT characterised by which of these conditions?

A Snoring
B Sleep fragmentation
C Hypertension
D Oxygen desaturation
E Exacerbation with alcohol

Answer: D

UARS results in snoring, sleep fragmentation, frequent arousals, and systemic hypertension. There is, however, no oxygen desaturation as occurs with OSAHS.

14.3 For which condition is Modafanil the treatment of choice?

A Central sleep apnoea
B Cheyne-Stokes breathing
C Narcolepsy
D Restless leg syndrome
E Upper airways resistance syndrome

Answer: C

Modafanil, which stimulates the hypothalamus, is indicated in the management of narcolepsy. It is not indicated in any of the other conditions.

14.4 What is the best treatment for moderately severe OSAHS?

A BiPAP
B CPAP
C Intra-oral device
D Modafanil
E UPPP

Answer: B

Several RCTs, Cochrane meta-analysis and NICE guidelines recommend CPAP as the treatment of choice for patients with moderate and severe OSAHS.

14.5 The most cost-effective investigation for patients suspected of having OSAHS is which of the following?

A Flow volume loop measurement
B Limited sleep study
C Nasendoscopy
D Overnight oximetry
E Polysomnography

Answer: B

A limited sleep study, done at the patient's home, is sufficient to make a diagnosis of OSAHS in most cases. PSG is rarely indicated and overnight oximetry has a lot of false positives and false negatives.

14.6 Randomised controlled trial evidence shows that treatment of severe OSA with CPAP does which of the following?

A Improves glycaemic control
B Improves systemic blood pressure
C Reduces all-cause mortality
D Reduces death from myocardial infarction
E Reduces the risk of stroke

Answer: B

There is RCT evidence that CPAP treatment results in a reduction of 4 mmHg in systemic blood pressure in patients with severe OSA. There is no evidence for the others, although it has been inferred that an improvement in blood pressure may result in reduction in cardiovascular and cerebrovascular events.

14.7 What is central sleep apnoea characterised by?

A Increase in thoracic movements
B Increase in abdominal movements
C Reduction in ventilatory drive
D Significant snoring
E Sleep fragmentation

Answer: C

Central sleep apnoea is caused by a reduction in, or absence of, ventilatory drive. The features of obstruction found with OSA are not present.

14.8 What is characteristic of Periodic Limb Movement Disorder (PLMD)?

A It affects the upper limbs
B It causes voluntary movements of the limbs
C It occurs in young men
D It occurs in non-REM sleep
E It occurs in REM sleep

Answer: D

PMLD occurs in non-REM sleep, is characterised by involuntary movement of the lower limbs, and occurs most commonly in elderly women.

14.9 How can narcolepsy be most reliably diagnosed?

A Hypocretin levels in CSF
B MRI of brain
C MSLT
D Overnight oximetry
E Home sleep study

Answer: C

The MSLT is used to make a diagnosis of narcolepsy. Hypocretin levels in CSF will only be low in Primary Narcolepsy and is still only available in a few centres. The other investigations will not be diagnostic.

14.10 Which of the following statements about REM behaviour disorder (RBD) is true?

A RBD occurs most frequently during non-REM sleep
B RBD occurs most frequently during REM sleep
C RBD occurs most often in adolescent men
D RBD results in muscle atonia
E RBD occurs soon after the patient goes to sleep

Answer: B

RBD occurs during REM sleep, so is more frequent in the early hours of the morning. It is more common in elderly men and the muscle paralysis that is usually seen in REM sleep is absent.

Appendix 14.A Epworth Sleepiness Scale (ESS)

How likely are you to doze off or fall asleep in the following situations in contrast to just feeling tired? This refers to your usual way of life in recent times. Even if you have not done some of these things, try to work out how they would have affected you.

Use the following scale to choose the most appropriate number for each situation.

1. would never doze
2. slight chance of dozing
3. moderate chance of dozing
4. high chance of dozing

Situation	Chance of dozing
Sitting and reading	
Watching TV	
Sitting inactive in a public place (e.g. theatre or meeting)	
As a passenger in a car for a hour without a break	
Lying down to rest in the afternoon when circumstances permit	
Sitting and talking to someone	
Sitting quietly after lunch without alcohol	
In a car, while stopped for a few minutes in traffic	
Total Score (maximum 24)	
ESS < 11: normal	
ESS 11–14: mild sleepiness	
ESS 15–18: moderate sleepiness	
ESS > 18: severe sleepiness	

FURTHER READING

American Academy of Sleep Medicine, European Sleep Research Society, Japanese Society of Sleep Research and Latin American Sleep Society (2001). *The International Classfication of Sleep Disorders, Revised: Diagnostic and Coding Manual.* Darien, IL: American Academy of Sleep Medicine.

Billiard, M. (2007). Diagnosis of narcolepsy and idiopathic hypersomnia. An update based on the international classification of sleep disorders, 2nd edition. *Sleep Medicine Reviews* 11 (5): 377–388.

Dean, D.A., Goldberger, A.L., Mueller, R. et al. (2016). Scaling up scientific discovery in sleep medicine: the National Sleep Research Resource. Sleep (5): 1151–1164.

Giles, T., Lasserson, T., Smith, B. et al. (2006). Continuous positive airways pressure for obstructive sleep apnoea in adults (review). *Cochrane Database of Systematic Reviews* 3: 4–6.

Johns, M.W. (1991). A new method for measuring daytime sleepiness: the Epworth sleepiness scale. *Sleep* 14 (6): 540–545.

National Institute for Health and Care Excellence (2008). Continuous positive airway pressure for the treatment of obstructive sleep apnoea / hypopnoea syndrome. National Institute for Health and Care Excellence Guideline, (March) 26. www.nice.org.uk/guidance/ta139/resources/continuous-positive-airway-pressure-for-the-treatment-of-obstructive-sleep-apnoeahypopnoea-syndrome-82598202209221.

Redline, S., Tishler, P.V., Tosteson, T.D. et al. (1995). The familial aggregation of obstructive sleep apnoea. *American Journal of Respiratory and Critical Care Medicine* 3 (Pt 1): 682–687.

Scottish Intercollegiate Guidelines Network (SIGN) (2003) Management of obstructive sleep apnoea/hypopnoea syndrome in adults: a national clinical guideline (73), (June), [online] Available at: papers2://publication/uuid/58D1FFC8-0C53-466F-8802-6785A074ED4E.

Sheerson, J.M. (2005). *Sleep Medicine: A Guide to Sleep and its Disorders.* Oxford: Blackwell Publishing Ltd.

Sleep Apnoea Trust Association (2016) Sleep Apnoea Trust, [online] Available at: http://www.sleep-apnoea-trust.org (accessed 13 March 2017).

Young, T. (2009). Rationale, design, and findings from the Wisconsin Sleep Cohort study: toward understanding the total societal burden of sleep-disordered breathing. *Sleep Medicine Clinics* 4 (1): 37–46.

Young, T., Finn, L., Peppard, P.E. et al. (2008). Sleep disordered breathing and mortality: eighteen-year follow-up of the Wisconsin Sleep Cohort. *Sleep* 31 (8): 1071–1078.

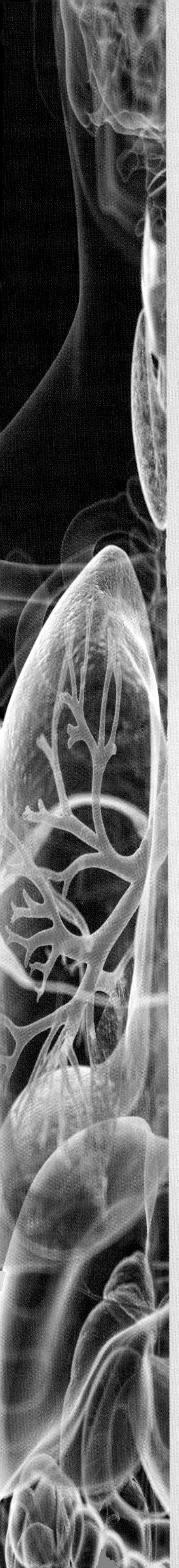

CHAPTER 15

Occupational, environmental, and recreational lung disease

Learning objectives

- To understand occupational, environmental, and recreational causes of lung disease
- To recognise the diagnosis and management of occupational asthma
- To understand the diagnosis and management of asbestosis
- To understand the diagnosis and management of other pneumoconiosis
- To understand the damage to lungs from inhalation of recreational drugs
- To appreciate the impact of air pollution on the lungs
- To appreciate the impact of the weather on the lungs

Essential Respiratory Medicine, First Edition. Shanthi Paramothayan.

Companion website: www.wiley.com/go/paramothayan/essential_respiratory_medicine

Abbreviations

ALI	acute lung injury
ARDS	adult respiratory distress syndrome
BAL	bronchoalveolar lavage
COPD	chronic obstructive pulmonary disease
CXR	chest X-ray
DAD	diffuse alveolar damage
DNA	deoxyribonucleic acid
DPLD	diffuse parenchymal lung disease
FDG-PET	fluoro-deoxyglucose positron emission tomography
FEV_1	forced expiratory volume in one second
FVC	forced vital capacity
HRCT	high-resolution computed tomography
IPF	idiopathic pulmonary fibrosis
LTOT	long term oxygen therapy
MCE	mucociliary escalator
NRT	nicotine replacement therapy
PEF	peak expiratory flow
RADS	reactive airways disease syndrome
THC	tetrahydrocannabinol
TLC	total lung capacity
TLCO	diffusing capacity to carbon monoxide
VC	vital capacity

Occupational, environmental, and recreational lung diseases

Many respiratory diseases occur after exposure to dust particles, smoke, fumes, chemical irritants, and biological agents arising from the environment, at work, in a social setting, or at home. Inhalation of smoke particles and irritant fumes can occur because of air pollution, contributed to by vehicle emissions and factory fumes. Individuals may be exposed to chemicals in their home or be exposed to organic particles when carrying out their hobbies. Individuals can be exposed to chemical and biological substances at work that cause lung damage, or allergens that can provoke asthma. A significant proportion of the population deliberately inhale drugs for recreational purposes and these can cause damage to the lungs. The consequences of inhalation will depend on the size, solubility, and toxicity of the particles inhaled, and the intensity and duration of exposure.

It is important to consider an occupational, environmental, or recreational cause for the patient's presentation, especially if the symptoms are new or unexplained. It is essential to take a detailed history of the patient's occupation, hobbies, and home environment. History taking is discussed in Chapter 5.

The commonest occupational lung disease is asthma. Individuals can also develop bronchitis, hypersensitivity pneumonitis (see Chapter 7), pneumoconiosis, malignancy (see Chapter 9) and acute lung injury (see Chapter 17) after exposure to a variety of substances.

Occupational lung disease

Occupational lung diseases have been a common cause of morbidity and mortality in the industrialised, urban population for decades. In the past 50 years, recognition of these conditions by employers and the government has resulted in the identification of risk factors, early detection of work-related illnesses, preventative measures at work, and strict health and safety regulations and legislation. For certain occupational lung diseases, the employee can seek compensation from the employer.

When considering an occupational lung disease, it is important to identify a temporal relationship between exposure to a substance and the development of symptoms. Other diseases that could be responsible for the symptoms need to be excluded. The accurate diagnosis and management of occupational lung diseases may be difficult for non-specialists. Most patients, particularly if they wish to get compensation for their illness, will be referred to a specialist in Occupational Lung Diseases.

Occupational asthma

Occupational asthma is the commonest occupational lung disease, with an incidence of 3000 cases each year. It is estimated that 10–15% of those with adult-onset asthma have an occupational cause. Occupational asthma can develop for the first time in an individual exposed to an irritant or sensitizer. Occupational exposure can also exacerbate symptoms in patients who have a known diagnosis of asthma (work-exacerbated asthma), and the estimated prevalence of this is 21%. A history of atopy or asthma has a poor positive predictive value for developing occupational asthma.

Occupational asthma, just like non-occupational asthma (see Chapter 6), is characterised by reversible and variable airflow obstruction. Exposure to a variety of substances at work can result in sensitization, resulting in inflammation of the airways and bronchospasm. Non-immunological agents can irritate the nose and upper airways, resulting in symptoms within minutes or hours of inhalation. The rapidity with which symptoms develop depends on the size of the substance; low molecular weight agents have a shorter latency period. A single exposure to highly soluble toxic gases, for example, sulphur dioxide, ammonia, or chlorine gas, can directly damage the upper airways, and cause reactive airways disease syndrome (RADS), the symptoms of which include persistent dry cough, dyspnoea, and wheeze. More severe or prolonged exposure can result in damage to the alveolar epithelial cells and the development of acute lung injury (ALI) and adult respiratory distress syndrome (ARDS). The long term consequence of this might be the development of bronchiolitis obliterans.

Exposure to immunologic stimuli will result in a period of sensitization and the development of symptoms at a later stage: this latent period may vary from a few weeks to several years. Further exposure to the same agent in a sensitised individual can result in an early (30 minutes) or late (12 hours) response.

Individuals with occupational asthma will develop symptoms of cough, wheeze, chest tightness, and breathlessness while at work, usually within several hours of being in that environment. Their symptoms will generally improve when they are away from the workplace, for example, at weekends or during holidays, and return when they go back to work. This temporal relationship between exposure and symptoms is important in making a diagnosis of occupational asthma. The agent that is likely to be causing the symptoms should be sought by careful evaluation of all the products that the individual is being exposed to. Prolonged and recurrent exposure to the agent could result in chronic asthma and irreversible lung damage, with the individual developing persistent symptoms even when they are away from the workplace.

It is important to remember that other conditions, such as COPD, hypersensitivity pneumonitis and non-occupational asthma will present with similar symptoms, and will need to be excluded when making a diagnosis of occupational asthma.

Individuals suspected of having an occupational cause for their asthma should have careful monitoring of their peak expiratory flow (PEF) and spirometry at work and when away from work. They may require bronchial hyper-responsiveness testing using histamine or methacholine in some cases. If these investigations are normal, then occupational asthma is unlikely. Additional investigations that may be useful include skin prick testing and measurement of immunoglobulin E RAST to specific allergens, as discussed in Chapter 6.

Once a diagnosis of occupational asthma has been confirmed, the most important thing is to reduce exposure to the agent provoking it. Ideally, this might mean removing the individual from the workplace altogether. If this is not possible, the employer will have to ensure that safety measures are in place to reduce exposure. This would include adequate ventilation, the wearing of protective masks, screening of other workers, and regular health checks.

Table 15.1 lists some common causes of occupational asthma. This list is not exhaustive. These agents can also result in exacerbation of COPD and other lung diseases.

Pneumoconiosis

Pneumoconiosis is lung fibrosis occurring as the result of inhalation of a variety of inorganic particles and mineral dusts at work. Asbestos, silica, and talc are fibrogenic, beryllium causes non-caseating granuloma, and iron, tin and barium are inert metals. In the last 50 years, recognition of the harmful effects of these dusts has led to strict regulations in the work-place and compensation for those affected, at least in developed countries.

As most of the pneumoconiosis have a characteristic radiological appearance, tissue biopsy is not usually required to make a diagnosis. HRCT has a higher sensitivity and specificity for classifying pneumoconiosis than CXR. FDG-PET may be helpful when lung malignancy is of concern (see Chapter 9).

The International Labour Organisation uses a standardised system for classifying the radiological abnormalities associated with pneumoconiosis which is used in research, for screening of workers and for determining disability claims.

Table 15.1 Common causes of occupational asthma.

Occupation	Agent
Healthcare workers	Latex
Car paint sprayers	Toluene di-isocyanate Acrylates Amines
Cleaners	Sodium hypochlorite in bleach Ammonia Trichloroethane Potassium hydroxide in oven and drain cleaners Sodium hydroxide in oven and drain cleaners
Hairdressers	Hair spray Solvent Persulfate salts
Carpenters	Wood dust
Painters and decorators	Paint and varnish solvents: turpentine, xylene, toluene, methanol, methylene, acetone, chlorine Toxic pigments: arsenic, cadmium, chromium, lead, mercury, acrylic emulsion
Baker	Flour
Photography	Hydroquinone, acetic acid, chromium, acetic acid-sulfur dioxide, formaldehyde
Electronic	Colophony from electronic soldering flux
Pharmaceutical	Antibiotics: penicillin Enzymes Glutaraldehyde
Plastic manufacture	Azodicarbonamide
Ceramics	Colours and glazes: barium carbonate, lead, chromium, uranium, cadmium, manganese
Gardeners	Malathion, dichlorvos, carbaryl and methoxychlor in pesticides
Farmers	Mushrooms

Source: Adapted from Goldman and Peters (1981:2831).

Asbestosis

Asbestos is a naturally occurring fibre composed of hydrated magnesium silicate. Prior to the recognition that inhalation of asbestos fibres was harmful, asbestos was widely used without any protective measures in a variety of industries, as listed in Box 15.1.

Since the early 1970s, strict regulations in developed countries have resulted in banning the use of asbestos, and the implementation of health and safety measures to reduce exposure in those who might be exposed to it. However, the long lag period between exposure and developing the disease means that patients exposed to asbestos many

Box 15.1 Occupations associated with asbestos exposure.

• Plumbers	• Construction workers	• Firefighters	• Mechanics	• Blacksmiths
• Builders	• Shipyard workers	• Carpenters	• Chemical plant workers	
• Roofers	• Cement plant workers	• Electricians	• Power plant workers	

decades ago are still presenting with asbestosis and mesothelioma. Therefore, it is important to take a full occupational history. In less developed countries, asbestos, which is a cheap material, is still widely used without any regulation.

Asbestos occurs in natural sources, such as rocks, so those living in certain geographical regions are exposed to low levels. Those living or working in a building which contains asbestos, for example, a house or school, are also exposed. Those who breathe in asbestos fibres from the workclothes of partners are also at risk. This type of exposure increases the risk of mesothelioma but does not increase the risk of asbestosis.

Asbestos comes in two main forms: serpentine and amphibole. Chrysotile, or white asbestos, is serpentine and accounts for most of the asbestos used commercially. Chrysotile is composed of curly fibres, 2 cm long and 1–2 μm wide. These fibres do not penetrate the lung tissue as much as crocidolite and are therefore less toxic. Crocidolite, blue asbestos, is composed of stiff amphibole fibres, 50 μm long and 102 μm wide. These shorter fibres penetrate the lung tissue, are not easily broken down and result in damage to the lung tissue. Amosite (brown asbestos) and tremolite are also amphiboles but are less prevalent.

Asbestos fibres, which contain iron molecules, have a direct toxic effect on pulmonary parenchymal cells. Alveolar macrophages, neutrophils, lymphocytes, and eosinophils accumulate around the fibres and release proteases, cytokines, reactive oxygen species, and free radicals which damage DNA causing genetic mutations and malignancy. These inflammatory cells also release cytokines that cause fibroblast proliferation and collagen formation. Inhaled asbestos fibres are deposited in the respiratory bronchioles and at the bifurcation of alveolar ducts. Some of the asbestos fibres are removed by mucociliary clearance mechanisms. The remaining fibres are removed by alveolar macrophages and type 1 alveolar cells.

Inhalation of asbestos fibres can cause several types of damage to the lungs. Pleural disease and mesothelioma are discussed in Chapter 10 and bronchogenic carcinoma is discussed in Chapter 9. Asbestosis, which is pulmonary fibrosis resulting from inhalation of asbestos fibres, is a slowly progressive, irreversible disease resulting in respiratory failure and death. The lag period between exposure and development of asbestosis is 10–25 years, which is less than the lag period for developing mesothelioma. Heavy and more intense exposure to asbestos fibres will result in development of fibrosis in a shorter period.

The clinical and radiological presentation is identical to that of other Diffuse Parenchymal Lung Diseases (DPLDs), particularly idiopathic pulmonary fibrosis (IPF), which is discussed in Chapter 7. Patients with asbestosis will have bibasal, fine crackles and a third will have finger clubbing. They will become hypoxaemic and, in the late stages, develop cor pulmonale. Pulmonary function tests will show a restrictive picture, with reduced lung volumes (VC and TLC) and reduced diffusing capacity (TLCO), which are the most sensitive measures.

CXR may appear normal in the early stages but will progress to show bilateral, basal, reticulonodular shadowing (Figure 15.1). With progressive disease, these changes will involve the mid and upper zones, and with advanced disease there will be honeycombing. HRCT is more sensitive than CXR at detecting early changes and will show sub-pleural linear densities, peribronchiolar, intralobular, and interlobular septal fibrosis. The presence of benign pleural plaques on the chest X-ray is pathognomonic of asbestos exposure (Figure 15.2).Images of pleural plaques are shown in Chapter 10.

If the history of asbestos exposure is clear, and the clinical and radiological features are typical of

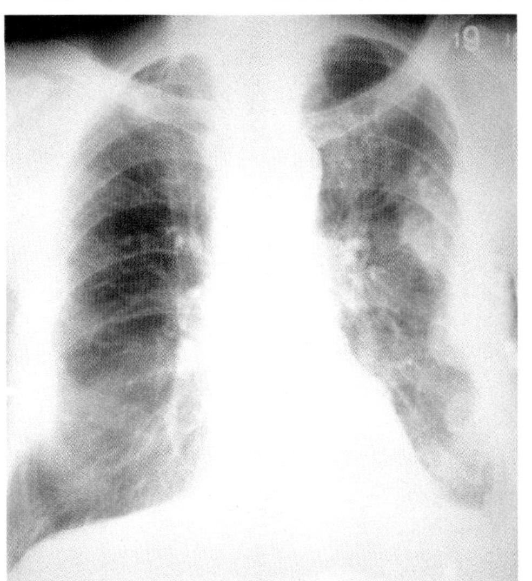

Figure 15.1 Chest X-ray of asbestosis and mesothelioma.

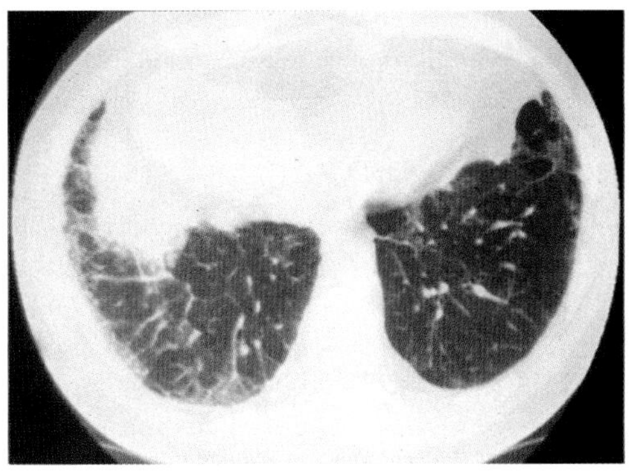

Figure 15.2 CT thorax of asbestosis.

asbestosis, a histological diagnosis is not required. A bronchoalveolar lavage (BAL) and lung biopsy will be required if there is uncertainty about the diagnosis or if concurrent infection is suspected. Lung biopsy will reveal asbestos bodies which are transparent asbestos fibres coated with iron and protein. The presence of asbestos fibres and asbestos bodies in sputum, a BAL and lung biopsy only indicates asbestos exposure. Patients with asbestosis will have 10–20 times more asbestos fibres than found in normal lung, with more than 1000 asbestos bodies g^{-1} of lung tissue, which correlates to more than one asbestos body ml^{-1} of BAL fluid. These 'ferruginous bodies', as they are also called, can also be found in individuals exposed to glass, talc, iron, and carbon.

There is no specific treatment for individuals who develop asbestosis. Management is symptomatic and supportive, with long term oxygen therapy (LTOT) and ambulatory oxygen when patients develop respiratory failure. Smoking cessation should be strongly encouraged as smoking is an additional risk factor for developing mesothelioma and asbestosis.

Individuals who develop asbestosis are eligible for compensation, as are those who develop malignant mesothelioma. This is discussed in Appendix 2 of Chapter 10.

Coal worker's pneumoconiosis

Coal worker's pneumoconiosis, which results from the inhalation of carbon or coal dust, was a significant problem in the early part of the twentieth century among coal miners, many of whom died from respiratory failure. The risk of developing lung fibrosis is directly related to the amount of exposure to coal dust. Coal dust is taken up by alveolar macrophages in the lungs and cleared by the mucociliary escalator and by lymphatic drainage. If these systems are overwhelmed by the amount of dust inhaled, then the macrophages within the respiratory bronchioles ingest the dust and die, releasing cytokines which induce fibrosis.

In **simple coal worker's pneumoconiosis**, there is accumulation of small, < 4 mm particles throughout the lung parenchyma, particularly in the upper lobes, giving a mottled appearance on CXR. These particles contain coal dust, dust-laden macrophages, and fibroblasts. The individual is not usually symptomatic, despite the abnormal CXR, unless they are concurrent smokers; in smokers, focal emphysema is often present.

Progressive massive fibrosis (PMF) is a serious condition with significant morbidity and mortality. It results in severe breathlessness, and can progress to respiratory failure (Figure 15.3). The CXR will show large (> 1 cm) fibrotic masses in the upper zones of the lung fields composed of collagen and coal dust. These masses may cavitate, resulting in the patient coughing up black sputum, which is called **melanoptysis**. Lung function tests will demonstrate reduced lung volumes, decreased diffusing capacity, and irreversible airflow obstruction.

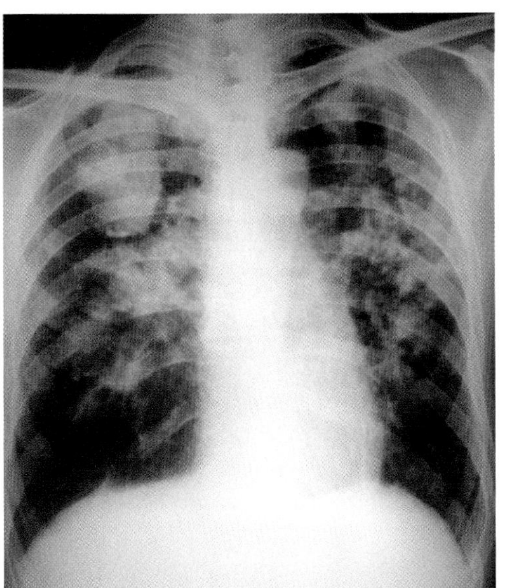

Figure 15.3 CXR showing progressive massive fibrosis.

Box 15.2 Industries with exposure to silica.

- Mining for: gold, tin, iron, copper, nickel, silver, coal, tungsten, and uranium
- Tunnelling through rock with high silica content
- Quarrying
- Stone cutting
- Sandblasting
- Foundry work
- Pottery

Caplan's syndrome is a pneumoconiosis which occurs in coal miners with rheumatoid arthritis. Less commonly, it can occur after exposure to asbestos and silica. Patients develop multiple nodules, 0.5–2 cm in size, and may have symptoms of breathlessness and cough. Patients may also develop subcutaneous rheumatoid nodules.

Coal miners who develop respiratory disease because of their occupation are eligible for compensation from the Department of Social Security if they have worked for more than 20 years and have abnormal lung function. With fewer people working in the coal industry and the introduction of health and safety measures at work (better ventilation in coal mines and the wearing of protective masks), fewer deaths are associated with this industry these days.

Silicosis

Inhalation of free silica (silicon dioxide) results in lung injury. Box 15.2 lists industries that are associated with silica exposure. As with other pneumoconiosis, stringent health and safety measures in the UK have reduced the incidence of silicosis, although it remains a problem worldwide.

Individuals who have inhaled silica may be asymptomatic, even when they have CXR changes.

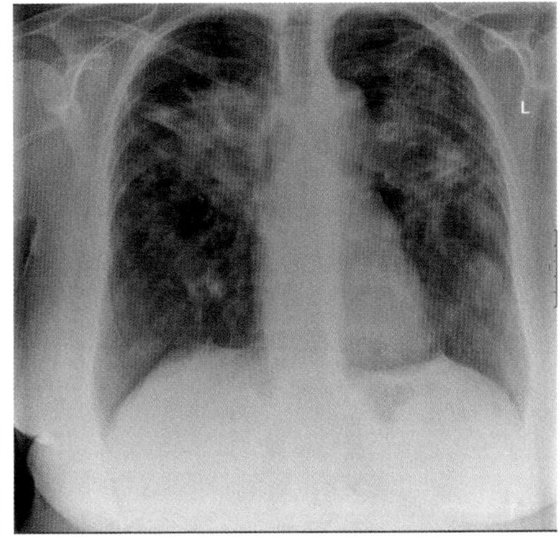

Figure 15.4 CXR showing silicosis and progressive massive fibrosis.

Significant exposure results in symptoms of chronic productive cough and breathlessness, progressively worsening to respiratory failure. Unlike asbestosis, finger clubbing and crackles do not occur.

In the early stages, the CXR typically shows eggshell calcification of the hilar lymph nodes and upper zone nodular fibrosis, with pleural thickening in some cases (Figure 15.4, Figure 15.5). With advanced disease, there will be extensive fibrosis, mainly in the upper zones. Pulmonary function tests will be consistent with a restrictive process, with reduction in VC, TLC and TLCO. Histology of the silicotic nodules characteristically reveals dust, bi-refringent quartz crystals, and macrophages surrounded by concentric layers of collagen. Silica is highly toxic to macrophages and is fibrogenic. Silicosis therefore predisposes to

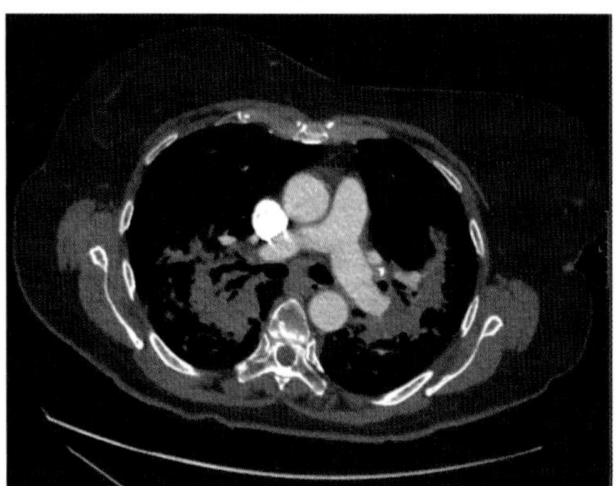

Figure 15.5 CT thorax showing silicosis and progressive massive fibrosis.

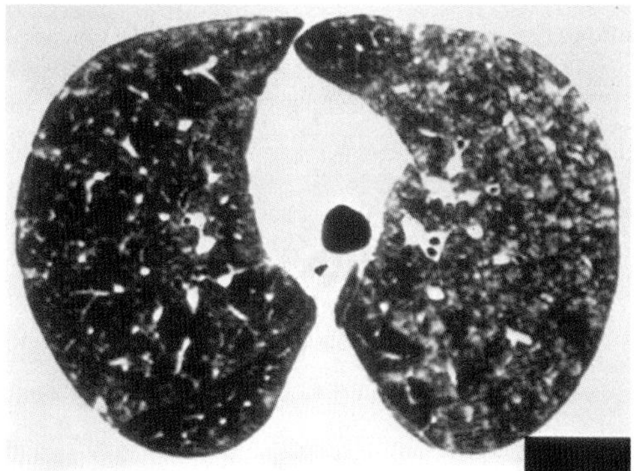

Figure 15.6 CT thorax showing changes associated with hard metal sensitivity.

mycobacterium tuberculosis infection and an increased risk of lung cancer.

Management of silicosis is the immediate removal of exposure, smoking cessation in smokers and symptomatic treatment. LTOT may be required in end-stage disease.

Siderosis

Individuals working in the iron and steel industry, especially those welding metals, may inhale iron oxide. These individuals are usually asymptomatic, with normal lung function, but CXR may have a characteristic mottled appearance because of the high radio-density of iron. Exposure to antimony, tin and other metals can result in similar radiological changes (Figure 15.6).

Byssinosis

Byssinosis develops due to chronic inhalation of raw cotton, hemp, or flax. This can cause bronchoconstriction with symptoms of breathlessness, cough, chest tightness, wheeze, and fever. Symptoms develop within hours of starting work, but gradually improve over the next few days. The CXR is usually normal, but with regular exposure, pulmonary function tests will show airflow limitation.

Berylliosis

Beryllium is a lightweight metal used in the dental, computer, and aerospace industries. It has a latency period of 3–30 years and affects 5–20% of exposed workers. Beryllium causes non-caseating granuloma, almost identical to that seen in sarcoidosis. The CXR shows multiple, small, calcified nodules in the upper lobes which may coalesce causing parenchymal distortion, volume loss and bullae formation, with an increased risk of pneumothorax. Mediastinal and hilar lymph node enlargement is common. As with sarcoidosis (discussed in Chapter 7), HRCT shows nodular beading along bronchovascular bundles in a peri-lymphatic distribution and ground glass opacities. Beryllium produces a specific immune response, which can be used to differentiate berylliosis from sarcoidosis.

Hypersensitivity pneumonitis

Individuals exposed to organic dusts, for example, from avian droppings or mouldy hay, may develop hypersensitivity pneumonitis, also called extrinsic allergic alveolitis. This is discussed in Chapter 7.

Recreational drugs and the lungs

Inhalation of substances for recreational purposes is widespread. Cigarette, cigar, and pipe smoking is legal, although recent legislation has restricted the places where these can be smoked. Many young people sniff glue and solvents as these are cheap and easily obtainable. There were 1700 deaths from inhaling solvent and sniffing glue and paint thinners between 1983 and 2000. Cannabis smoking is common, especially in young people. Inhalation of crack cocaine, amphetamines and heroin is carried out by 2% of the population. Insufflation of poppers, amyl nitrites, and toluene (fine spray inhaled quickly) can damage the lungs. The use of aerosol propellant gases with a plastic bag held over the mouth has a high risk of hypoxia, aspiration, suffocation, and respiratory arrest.

Lungs have a large surface area and can absorb large quantities of inhaled drugs within seconds. These drugs are carried swiftly in the bloodstream to the brain, having immediate effects. Rapid inhalation of powders and solvents can result in pneumonitis, bronchitis, and pneumonia. Crack cocaine and heroin, which are snorted through the nostrils, can cause epistaxis, and destroy the nasal cartilage.

Smoking

Smoking tobacco products is the single, greatest preventable cause of death in the UK, responsible for 120 000 deaths every year. Worldwide, approximately two billion people smoke, and smoking is responsible for five million deaths each year. In the UK, 17.7% of men and 15.8% of women smoke. Children whose parents smoke, and who are more socially deprived, tend to take up smoking. The pressure to smoke is compounded by peers and tobacco advertising. Cigarette smoking increases the risk of lung cancer, bladder cancer, renal cell cancer, COPD, interstitial lung disease, ischaemic heart disease, peripheral vascular disease, stroke, and respiratory infections. Smoking during pregnancy results in foetal growth retardation.

Smoking cigarettes is the main risk factor for developing lung cancer. Cigarette smoke contains a variety of carcinogens which cause genetic mutations, thus increasing the risk of lung cancer. The link between smoking and lung cancer was first considered in 1912 and clearly established in 1950 by Richard Doll. Passive smoking, which is inhaling 'second-hand smoke', also increases the risk of lung cancer. Smoking cessation decreases the risk of lung cancer within the first five years after cessation, but remains higher than in a never smoker. Individuals who stop smoking gain 6–10 years of life. Cigar smoking is associated with an increased risk of lung cancer, with a relative risk of 2.1. Pipe smoking also increases the risk of lung cancer with a relative risk of five. Lung cancer is discussed in Chapter 9.

Tobacco smoke contains carbon monoxide, which has a great affinity for haemoglobin, thus displacing oxygen to form carboxyhaemoglobin. Smokers have CO levels of 15% compared to non-smokers who have levels of <3%. Cigarette smoke destroys the cilia lining the respiratory epithelium and impairs the function of the mucociliary escalator. It also causes hyperplasia of the goblet cells, resulting in an increase in the amount of mucus production, one of the key symptoms in patients with COPD. The diagnosis and management of obstructive airways disease is discussed in Chapter 6. Exposure to cigarette smoke can irritate the airways and cause exacerbation of asthma. Children exposed to cigarette smoke have an increased risk of developing asthma.

The main reason people continue to smoke cigarettes, even when they know of its detrimental effects, is because nicotine, one of the key components of tobacco, binds to the nicotinic acetylcholine receptors in the brain, resulting in the release of a variety of neurotransmitters, including dopamine, serotonin, β-endorphins, vasopressin, and noradrenaline. These neurotransmitters increase the sensation of pleasure, reduce anxiety, and suppress appetite, among other things. Nicotine leads to dependence, therefore smoking cessation results in severe physical and psychological withdrawal symptoms.

All healthcare professionals should advise and assist smokers to stop smoking by offering them pharmacological products and by offering them counselling and support. Box 15.3 lists the approach for counselling for smoking cessation. It has been shown that a simple counselling session results in a one year quit rate of 1–3%, whereas more intense counselling, including group counselling, can improve this up to 20%, especially when nicotine replacement therapy (NRT), Bupropion or Varenicline are prescribed. E-cigarettes are also now being use by many smokers to help them quit. The pharmacological agents available for smoking cessation is discussed in Chapter 3.

Box 15.3 Counselling for smoking cessation.

- **Ask** how many cigarettes the individual smokes every day and calculate pack years
- **Assess** the risk of smoking
- **Advise** how to stop smoking and refer to the smoking cessation counsellor
- **Assist** with pharmacological and behavioural therapy
- **Arrange** follow-up

Cocaine

Cocaine, an alkaloid, is a commonly used illegal drug. It is derived from the leaves of Erythroxylon coca, found mainly in Central and South America. Cocaine stabilises cell membranes and has local anaesthetic properties. Cocaine interferes with the re-uptake of catecholamines and serotonin in the brain, resulting in stimulation and a sensation of euphoria. Due to its potent sympathomimetic effects, cocaine also causes cardiovascular complications.

Cocaine hydrochloride, a white powder, can be snorted or injected intravenously. Crack cocaine, which is formed by boiling cocaine with baking soda and water and then extracted with alcohol or ether, can be smoked (free-basing). Crack cocaine is often mixed with either marijuana or tobacco and smoked. Cocaine is quickly absorbed into the pulmonary circulation and reaches the central nervous system within a few seconds. It has a half-life of 60–90 minutes in blood.

Crack cocaine has acute pulmonary toxicity by a variety of mechanisms. Thermal injury and cellular toxicity can result in diffuse alveolar damage (DAD), hyaline membrane formation, acute alveolitis, and pulmonary oedema within hours of inhalation. Acute eosinophilic pneumonia can occur within days of inhalation. Patients present with severe dyspnoea, pleuritic chest pain, fever, haemoptysis, and cough. Occasionally, patients may cough up black sputum, called melanoptysis. CXR and HRCT will show ground-glass changes. Those inhaling crack cocaine often use the Valsalva manoeuvre which can result in life-threatening pneumothorax, pneumopericardium, and pneumomediastinum.

Management of 'acute crack lung', which can progress to acute lung injury (ALI) and adult respiratory distress syndrome (ARDS), is supportive and includes supplemental oxygen, non-invasive ventilation, or intubation and ventilation. Bronchodilators and antibiotics may be required. Steroids are only indicated when there is an acute eosinophilic picture. ALI and ARDS are discussed in Chapter 17.

Chronic cocaine use can result in bronchiectasis, foreign body granulomatosis, bronchiolitis obliterans and recurrent alveolar haemorrhage with haemosiderosis. CXR and HRCT will show ground-glass or consolidative changes. Vasospasm can result in ventilation-perfusion mismatch which can progress to pulmonary hypertension, and which can be confused with acute pulmonary embolism. Those who smoke cocaine and cigarettes together have a higher risk of developing bullous emphysema.

Cannabis

Cannabis (marijuana) is used by many as a recreational drug. It is also reported to have benefit in relieving the pain of multiple sclerosis and in certain types of epilepsy. Cannabis is a Class B drug (under the Misuse of Drugs Act, 1971) and individuals can be sent to prison for five years for possessing cannabis, and up to 14 years for supplying it.

Marijuana is made from the Cannabis sativa hemp plant. It can be smoked after being rolled into joints, smoked in pipes, in bongs (water pipes), or in blunts, which are hollowed out cigars filled with a mixture of tobacco and marijuana. It can also be ground into hash and eaten as hash cakes or cookies.

Cannabis smoking is almost as prevalent as cigarette smoking in the young; 20% of the population are estimated to have used cannabis at least once. Cannabis is addictive, with one in six regular users becoming dependent.

Cannabis contains a chemical called delta-9-tetrahydrocannabinol (THC) which stimulates the secretion of dopamine in the brain, causing feelings of euphoria. The concentration of THC in cannabis joints varies considerably from 2.3% to 8%. Cannabis contains 33 carcinogens and tar, which is deposited in the lungs. As cannabis joints are unfiltered, more tar is deposited than with cigarette smoke and deposited more deeply into the lungs. Inhaling cannabis also results in an increase in the concentration of carbon monoxide in the blood.

The average cannabis user will smoke it two to three times a month, therefore is much less exposed to toxic substances than a tobacco smoker who usually smokes daily. Cannabis irritates the lungs, resulting in a productive cough, chest tightness, bronchospasm, and wheezing. These individuals may be predisposed to chest infections. Heavier and regular use of cannabis will result in a decline in pulmonary function. Studies have not found an increased risk of lung cancer with cannabis use alone, but it is difficult to find the evidence as most heavy cannabis smokers also smoke cigarettes.

Users of cannabis often inhale deeply and breath-hold, with an increased risk of pneumothorax or a pneumomediastinum and will present with sharp, pleuritic chest pain and breathlessness. Cannabis is associated with an increased risk of psychotic symptoms, increase in the risk of road traffic accidents, and foetal growth retardation if smoked by a pregnant woman.

The environment and the lungs

Pollution

Air pollution has been shown to increase morbidity and mortality by increasing the risk of cardiovascular and respiratory illnesses. Air pollution also adversely affects lung development in children.

Individuals living in urban areas with high amounts of road traffic may be more susceptible to lung diseases. Exposure to traffic fumes containing high concentrations of particulate matter, including carbon, sulphite, and carbon monoxide can cause respiratory symptoms, especially in individuals with underlying lung disease. An increase in the amount of carbon particles in lung macrophages correlates with a reduction in lung function. A reduction in the number of fine particles in the atmosphere results in increased life expectancy. Reducing diesel in cars may reduce the risk of pollution-related respiratory disease. Environmentalists are calling for the use of electric cars and for stricter regulations on traffic fumes in urban areas.

Toxic substances

Toxic drugs in the environment may predispose to the development of malignancies, including lung cancer. These agents act synergistically with tobacco smoke to increase the risk of lung cancer. Box 15.4 lists some of the agents which have been implicated.

Radon is a gaseous decay product of Uranium-238 and radium-226 which is found in soil, rock, and groundwater. Radon emits alpha particles, which damage the respiratory epithelium. Radiotherapy used to treat malignancies can also increase the risk of primary lung cancer. Patients who have had radiotherapy for breast cancer have a relative risk of 3–4 of developing lung cancer, and those who have had radiotherapy for Hodgkin's lymphoma have a relative risk of 3–7 of developing lung cancer. Exposure to particulate matter in polluted air increases the risk of lung cancer, as does inhalation of smoke from indoor wood and coal burning fires.

Box 15.4 Environmental agents associated with malignancies.

• Air pollution	• Asbestos	• Chromium
• Formaldehyde	• Hard metal dust	• Ionising radiation
• Polycyclic aromatic hydrocarbons	• Vinyl chloride	• Nickel
• Bis-chloromethyl ether	• Arsenic	• Radon

Inhaled allergens and irritants

Inhaled allergens and respiratory irritants, both indoor and outdoor, can trigger an acute exacerbation of asthma and COPD. Box 15.5 lists some common environmental allergens.

Fumes from unvented fireplaces, gas stoves, heaters, chlorine-based cleaning products, and volatile organic compounds, including formaldehyde, can cause bronchoconstriction, wheezing, and dyspnoea. Individuals with asthma can develop symptoms of cough, wheezing and breathlessness when exposed to aerosol sprays, including air fresheners and perfumes.

Weather

Changes in temperature and weather are associated with asthma and COPD exacerbations. Inhalation of cold, dry air can result in bronchoconstriction, possibly due to loss of water from the airways. Breathing hot, humid air can cause bronchoconstriction secondary to vagal mechanisms.

Thunderstorms result in increased concentrations of pollen debris which can cause an allergic exacerbation of asthma, as can an increase in the level of ozone on hot, sunny days. Damp weather results in increased levels of dust mites, moulds, and carbon dioxide levels, resulting in bronchoconstriction. Desert dust, containing particles of crystalline silica, can be blown across continents during storms, causes respiratory symptoms and an increase in hospitalisation with acute exacerbation of asthma and COPD. Weather forecasts now warn patients with respiratory disease about high pollen count and thunderstorms, and this may help to reduce the risk of exacerbations.

Box 15.5 Common indoor and outdoor allergens and irritants.

	Indoor	Outdoor
Allergens	House dust mite Mould	Grass pollen Tree pollen Mould
Irritants	Tobacco smoke Perfume Aerosol spray Fumes from gas stoves Chlorine-based cleaning products Paint sprays Formaldehydes	Cold, dry air Sulfite NO_2 Ozone Carbon particles Desert dust (crystalline silica)

SUMMARY OF LEARNING POINTS

- Occupational lung diseases are a common cause of morbidity and mortality.
- A comprehensive history of ALL the jobs the individual has done is required.
- Occupational asthma is the commonest occupational lung disease, affecting 3000 new individuals each year.
- To make a diagnosis of occupational asthma, a temporal association between exposure to an agent and the development of new symptoms needs to be established.
- Individuals with occupational lung disease develop symptoms of cough, dyspnoea, and wheeze while at work or soon afterwards, with symptoms improving at weekends or during holidays.
- Management of occupational asthma includes removal from the workplace or measures to reduce exposure to the allergen, such as wearing a mask.
- Pneumoconioses are restrictive lung disorders that result from the inhalation of inorganic dust particles.
- Pneumoconiosis can progress to severe pulmonary fibrosis and respiratory failure in some cases.
- Asbestosis is associated with the inhalation of Crocidolite, or blue asbestos fibres, and has a lag period of 10–20 years.
- Asbestosis increases the risk of lung cancer.
- Silicosis, caused by exposure to silica, can also result in the development of silicotic nodules, pulmonary fibrosis, increased risk of pulmonary tuberculosis, and lung cancer.
- Smoking tobacco is the single, greatest preventable cause of pulmonary disease worldwide.
- Tobacco is addictive, with smokers getting withdrawal symptoms on cessation.
- Healthcare professionals should advise smokers about cessation, prescribe pharmacological therapy, and refer for counselling.
- Smoking causes malignancies, COPD, peripheral vascular disease, ischaemic heart disease, and stroke.
- Cannabis can cause significant damage to the lungs, with reduction in lung function and an increased risk of pneumothorax.
- Inhaling crack cocaine can result in thermal injury, risk of pneumothorax and acute lung injury.
- Particulate matter, particularly carbon particles in the atmosphere, can result in reduction in lung function and increased mortality.
- Many environmental agents increase the risk of malignancies: radon, chromium, nickel, and hard metal dust.
- The temperature and weather patterns can result in exacerbations of lung disease.

MULTIPLE CHOICE QUESTIONS

15.1 Which of the following has NOT been shown to be strongly associated with cannabis inhalation?

A Chest infection
B Cough
C Euphoria
D Lung cancer
E Pneumothorax

Answer: D

Inhaling cannabis causes cough, chest infections, euphoria and, if inhaled deeply with breath-holding (Valsalva manoeuvre), can result in a pneumothorax and a pneumopericardium. Although cannabis contains several carcinogens, there is no clear evidence that it causes lung cancer. Studies are made difficult by the fact that most heavy users of cannabis also smoke cigarettes and are young.

15.2 Which of the following is NOT associated with crack cocaine use?

A Bronchiolitis obliterans
B Diffuse alveolar damage
C Eosinophilic pneumonia
D Pneumothorax
E Sarcoidosis

Answer: E

Snorting cocaine or smoking crack cocaine can cause acute and chronic lung injury. It can result in all the above conditions as well as alveolar haemorrhage, haemosiderosis and foreign body granulomatosis. However, cocaine abuse is not associated with sarcoidosis.

15.3 Which of the following statements about occupational asthma is true?

A The latency period for developing asthma is longer with low molecular weight agents
B Symptoms of asthma always improve when the individual is away from work
C A history of atopy is accurate at predicting the likelihood of developing occupational asthma
D Occupational asthma is an extremely rare diagnosis
E If spirometry, peak expiratory flow monitoring, and bronchial hyper-responsiveness tests are normal then occupational asthma is unlikely

Answer: E

The latency period for developing occupational asthma is longer with high molecular weight agents. Individuals exposed over a long period of time may develop chronic asthma and become symptomatic even when away from work. A history of atopy is not good at predicting the risk of developing occupational asthma. Occupational asthma is the commonest occupational lung disease, accounting for 10–15% of adult-onset asthma.

15.4 Which of the following statements about asbestosis is true?

A Chrysotile is more likely to cause asbestosis than crocidolite
B Chest X-ray may be normal in up to 30% of patients with asbestosis
C Corticosteroid treatment is effective in asbestosis
D FEV_1/FVC ratio will be reduced in asbestosis
E Pulmonary fibrosis develops 30–40 years after exposure to asbestos

Answer: B

Crocidolite, blue asbestos, is more likely to cause asbestosis and malignant mesothelioma as it is composed of short fibres which are cleared less easily from the lungs and are more toxic. Asbestosis results in a restrictive lung process, with an increase in the FEV_1/FVC ratio, reduced VC, TLC and TLCO. Pulmonary fibrosis (asbestosis) develops 10–20 years after exposure to asbestos, unlike mesothelioma which develops 30–40 years after exposure. The CXR may appear normal in the early stages in approximately a third of patients.

15.5 Which of the following radiological features is most likely to be found in someone who works quarrying sandstone?

A Ground-glass opacification
B Eggshell calcification of hilar lymph nodes
C Massive fibrotic nodules
D Mottled micronodules
E Reticulonodular opacities at the lung bases

Answer: B

Working with sandstone increases the risk of silicosis, which typically presents with eggshell calcification of the hilar lymph nodes. Ground-glass opacification is non-specific, usually associated with non-specific interstitial pneumonia. Massive fibrotic nodules are seen in coal worker's pneumoconiosis and reticulonodular opacities at the bases can be seen in idiopathic pulmonary fibrosis.

15.6 Which of the following statements about occupational asthma is NOT true?

A Occupational asthma can occur after one exposure
B Occupational asthma can only occur in someone with known asthma
C Occupational asthma can occur after exposure to a variety of substances
D Occupational asthma is the commonest occupational lung disease
E Occupational asthma will improve if the individual is removed from the workplace

Answer: B

Occupational asthma can occur for the first time after exposure to an allergen in the workplace. All the other statements are true.

15.7 Non-caseating granulomas are associated with inhalation of which substance?

A Beryllium
B Cadmium
C Iron
D Nickel
E Silica

Answer: A

Berylliosis presents with non-caseating granuloma which is like that in sarcoidosis. Individuals who worked with fluorescent lights and work with dental material and in the computer and aerospace industry may be exposed.

15.8 Patients with which one of the following conditions are NOT eligible for compensation?

A Asbestosis
B Benign pleural plaque
C Occupational asthma
D Progressive massive fibrosis
E Silicosis

Answer: B

The development of benign pleural plaque indicates exposure to asbestos, but the individual is asymptomatic and does not progress to either asbestosis or malignant mesothelioma. All the other conditions are eligible for compensation.

15.9 Which of the following is NOT associated with an increased risk of lung cancer?

A Asbestosis
B Massive pulmonary fibrosis
C Passive smoking
D Siderosis
E Silicosis

Answer: D

Siderosis is the result of inhalation of iron. Although there are chest X ray changes, the individual is asymptomatic, with no increased risk of lung cancer.

15.10 Which of the following features of a particle does not determine its risk of deposition in the lungs?

A Molecular weight of particle
B Origin of particle
C Shape of particle
D Size of particle
E Solubility of particle

Answer: B

The origin or source of the particle (inorganic dust, organic material) does not influence deposition in the lungs. All the other factors do influence deposition.

FURTHER READING

American Thoracic Society, Guidotti, T.L., Miller, A. et al. (2004). Diagnosis and initial management of nonmalignant diseases related to asbestos. *American Journal of Respiratory and Critical Care Medicine* 170 (6): 691–715.

Barne, C., Alexis, N.E., Bernstein, J.A. et al. (2013). Climate change and our environment: the effect on respiratory and allergic disease. *The Journal of Allergy and Clinical Immunology in Practice* 1 (2): 137–141.

Borgelt, L.M., Franson, K.L., Nussbaum, A.M., and Wang, G.S. (2013). The pharmacologic and clinical effects of medical cannabis. *Pharmacotherapy* 33 (2): 195–209.

Brambilla, E., Travis, W.D., Brennan, P. et al. (2009) Lung cancer. In World Cancer Report 2014, WHO, Lyon, pp. 350–361, [online]. Available at: http://publications.iarc.fr/Non-Series-Publications/World-Cancer-Reports/World-Cancer-Report-2014 (accessed 16 March 2017).

British Lung Foundation (2017). Asbestos and mesothelioma, [online] Available at: www.blf.org.uk/support-for-you/mesothelioma/what-is-it.

Canova, C., Heinrich, J., Anto, J.M. et al. (2013). The influence of sensitisation to pollens and moulds on seasonal variations in asthma attacks. *European Respiratory Journal* 42 (4): 935–945.

Copas, J.B. and Shi, J.Q. (2000). Reanalysis of epidemiological evidence on lung cancer and passive smoking. *BMJ (Clinical research ed.)* 320 (7232): 417–418.

D'Amato, G., Liccardi, G., and Frenguelli, G. (2007). Thunderstorm-asthma and pollen allergy. *Allergy: European Journal of Allergy and Clinical Immunology* 62 (1): 11–16.

Devlin, R.J. and Henry, J.A. (2008). Clinical review: major consequences of illicit drug consumption. *Critical Care* 12 (1): 202.

Doll, R. and Hill, A.B. (1950). Smoking and carcinoma of the lung; preliminary report. *British Medical Journal* 2 (4682): 739–748.

Eggleston, P.A. and Bush, R.K. (2001). Environmental allergen avoidance: an overview. *The Journal of Allergy and Clinical Immunology* 107 (3 Suppl): S403–S405.

Ernst, A. and Zibrak, J.D. (1998). Carbon monoxide poisoning. *New England Journal of Medicine* 339 (22): 1603–1608.

Fishwick, D., Barber, C.M., Bradshaw, L.M. et al. (2008). Standards of care for occupational asthma. *Thorax* 63 (3): 240–250.

Goldman, R.H. and Peters, J.M. (1981). The occupational and environmental health history. *JAMA* 246 (24): 2831–2836.

Haponik, E.F., Crapo, R.O., Herndon, D.N. et al. (1988). Smoke inhalation. *The American Review of Respiratory Disease* 138 (4): 1060–1063.

Mapp, C.E., Boschetto, P., Maestrelli, P., and Fabbri, L.M. (2005). Occupational asthma. *American Journal of Respiratory and Critical Care Medicine* 172 (3): 280–305.

Mehra, R., Moore, B.A., Crothers, K. et al. (2006). The association between marijuana smoking and lung cancer: a systematic review. *Archive of Internal Medicine* 166 (13): 1359–1367.

National Institute for Occupational Safety and Health (NIOSH) (2010) A story of impact: NIOSH research methods demonstrate that breathing nanoparticles may result in damaging health effects, DHHS (NIOSH) Publication Number 2010–158, [online] Available at: https://www.cdc.gov/niosh/docs/2010-158.

Nicholson, P.J., Cullinan, P., Taylor, A.J. et al. (2005). Evidence based guidelines for the prevention, identification, and management of occupational asthma. *Occupational and Environmental Medicine* 62 (5): 290–299.

Oasys Research Group part of the Midland Thoracic Society (2017). Agents that cause Occupational Asthma, Oasys Website, [online] Available at: http://www.occupationalasthma.com/occupational_asthma_causative_agents.aspx (accessed 13 March 2017).

Oasys Research Group, part of the Midland Thoracic Society (2017). Occupational asthma causative agents/sensitizers, [online] Available at: http://www.occupationalasthma.com/occupational_asthma_causative_agents.aspx (accessed 13 March 2017).

Pope, C.A. III, Ezzati, M., and Dockery, D.W. (2009). Fine-particulate air pollution and life expectancy in the United States. *New England Journal of Medicine* 360 (4): 376–386.

Sigsgaard, T., Nowak, D., Annesi-Maesano, I. et al. (2010). ERS position paper: work-related respiratory diseases in the EU. *European Respiratory Journal* 35 (2): 234–238.

Voelker, R. (2012). Asthma forecast: why heat, humidity trigger symptoms. *JAMA* 308 (1): 20.

Wagner, G.R. (1997). Asbestosis and silicosis. *Lancet.* 349 (9061): 1311–1315.

Zimmerman, J.L. (2012). Cocaine intoxication. *Critical Care Clinics* 28 (4): 517–526.

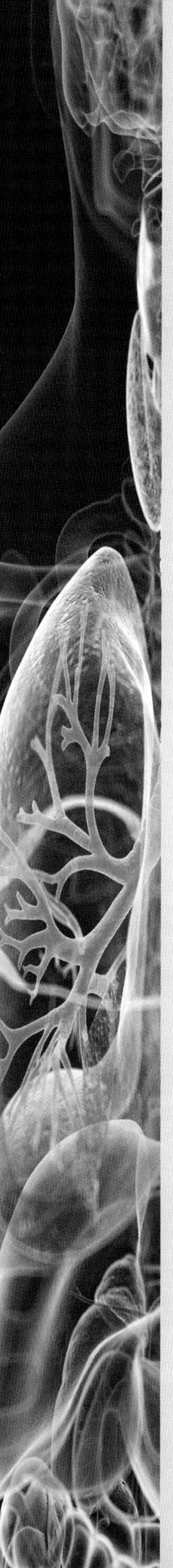

CHAPTER 16 Disorders of the mediastinum

Learning objectives

- To understand the basic anatomy of the mediastinum
- To understand the diagnostic pathway for patients presenting with a mediastinal mass
- To understand the differential diagnosis and management of a mass in the anterior mediastinum
- To understand the differential diagnosis and management of a mass in the middle mediastinum
- To understand the differential diagnosis of mediastinal lymphadenopathy
- To understand the differential diagnosis and management of a mass in the posterior mediastinum
- To understand the aetiology and management of acute and chronic mediastinitis
- To understand the aetiology and management of a pneumomediastinum

Essential Respiratory Medicine, First Edition. Shanthi Paramothayan.

Companion website: www.wiley.com/go/paramothayan/essential_respiratory_medicine

Abbreviations

AFP	alpha-feta protein
β-hcg	β-human chorionic gonadotrophin
CXR	chest X-ray
CT	computed tomography
FNA	fine needle aspiration
LDH	lactate dehydrogenase
MEN	multiple endocrine neoplasia
MG	myasthenia gravis
MRI	magnetic resonance imaging
PA	postero-anterior
PET-CT	positron emission tomography with computed tomography
SVCO	superior vena cava obstruction
VATS	video assisted thoracoscopic surgery
WHO	World Health Organisation

Anatomy of the mediastinum

The anatomy and physiology of the lungs are discussed in Chapter 2. The mediastinum is the central part of the thorax with the lungs on either side, the thoracic inlet above, the vertebral bodies behind, and the diaphragm below. The mediastinum contains the heart, trachea, oesophagus, thoracic duct, thymus, lymph nodes, aorta, pulmonary arteries, pulmonary veins, azygous vein, superior vena cava, inferior vena cava, phrenic nerves, sympathetic chain and parasympathetic chain. These structures are held together by connective tissue and fatty tissue. The mediastinum is divided into three areas: the anterior (or antero-superior), the middle and the posterior (Table 16.1). These are not anatomical divisions as there are no tissue planes separating them, but are arbitrary radiological divisions used to facilitate the classification of masses within the mediastinum.

Diagnosis of a mediastinal mass

Some 75% of mediastinal masses are benign, and more likely to be so in an adult. Thymomas, thyroid masses, lymph nodes, and benign cysts are the commonest mediastinal masses in adults. In children, over 80% of masses are neurogenic tumours, germ cell tumours, or foregut cysts.

A slow-growing, benign, mediastinal mass may be asymptomatic and found incidentally on a chest X-ray. As the mass enlarges, it can cause symptoms of cough, chest pain, and breathlessness. If the mass compresses adjacent structures, such as the trachea, oesophagus, or superior vena cava, it can cause stridor, dysphagia, and superior vena cava obstruction (SVCO). The patient may also develop systemic symptoms, depending on the mass.

History and examination

The patient should be asked about symptoms of fatigue, night sweats, fevers, and weight loss. Examination should look for lymphadenopathy, signs of ptosis, ophthalmoplegia and inability to maintain upward gaze suggestive of myasthenia gravis (MG) (Box 16.1). The testes should be examined in men.

Table 16.1 Structures in the mediastinum.

Anterior mediastinum	Middle mediastinum	Posterior mediastinum
Thymus	Tracheal bifurcation	Sympathetic ganglia
Lymph nodes	Oesophagus	Spinal nerve roots
Thyroid	Lymph nodes	Lymph nodes
Ascending aorta	Part of azygous vein	Parasympathetic chain
Pulmonary artery	Inferior vena cava	Oesophagus
Phrenic nerves	Posterior heart	Thoracic duct
	Lower half of superior vena cava	Descending thoracic aorta
	Aortic arch	Vertebrae
	Pulmonary artery	
	Pulmonary vein	

Box 16.1 Investigations of a mediastinal mass.

- Chest X-ray (CXR): postero-anterior (PA) and lateral
- CT thorax, abdomen and pelvis with contrast
- MRI scan
- PET-CT scan
- Other scans as indicated: barium swallow, angiography, sestamibi parathyroid scintigraphy, radioiodine uptake scan
- Tumour markers as indicated
- CT-guided percutaneous fine-needle aspiration (FNA) or biopsy

Box 16.2 Tumour markers.

Alpha-fetoprotein (AFP) levels are elevated in some germ cell tumours

β-human chorionic gonadotrophin (β-hcg) levels are elevated in germ cell tumours

Acetylcholine receptor antibody levels are elevated in thymoma associated with myasthenia gravis

Lactate dehydrogenase (LDH) levels are elevated in several conditions, including lymphoma

Chest X-ray: PA and lateral

It should be possible, with a combination of a PA and lateral chest X-ray, to determine whether the mass is in the mediastinum, and then to locate it within the anterior, middle, or posterior compartments. A spiculated or nodular mass is likely to be within the lung and may contain air bronchograms, whereas a mediastinal mass will have a broad base, a smooth edge and will not contain air bronchograms. The right superior mediastinal border is formed of the right brachiocephalic vein and the superior vena cava, and is usually straight and vertical. A mediastinal mass will cause widening of the upper mediastinum, and the right superior mediastinal border will become distorted and indistinct. The left mediastinal border is formed of the left carotid artery, left subclavian artery, left brachiocephalic vein, and left jugular vein. When there is a mediastinal mass on the left side, the aortic knuckle may be poorly defined.

On the lateral CXR, the anterior and middle compartments can be divided by an imaginary line anterior to the trachea and posterior to the inferior vena cava. The middle and posterior compartments can be divided by an imaginary line passing 1 cm posterior to the anterior border of the vertebral bodies. A two-dimensional CXR will not, however, give sufficient detail about the structure or location of the mass and a CT scan with contrast is required for that.

CT thorax with contrast is essential to determine the exact anatomical structure and position of the mass and any possible invasion into surrounding tissues. The radiologist will consider whether the mass contains predominantly fat, fluid, or solid components, and whether it enhances after intravenous contrast. As different types of lesions have specific radiological characteristics, it may be possible to make a clear diagnosis without histology, for example, with a thymoma. Fluid-containing lesions are usually cysts or necrotic lymph nodes. Solid components increase the likelihood of the lesion being malignant. Fat-containing lesions are usually benign, and include teratomas and lipomas.

An **MRI scan** will be required to assess a posterior mediastinal mass to see if there is any tumour extension into the spinal canal, and is essential prior to surgery. **Angiography** is recommended prior to any invasive procedure if a vascular lesion is suspected. **PET-CT** may be helpful if a malignant mass is suspected, and may be required prior to surgery.

Tumour markers (Box 16.2) can be helpful in narrowing the differential diagnosis of a mediastinal mass and in monitoring response to treatment.

Anterior mediastinal mass

The anterior mediastinum is behind the sternum and in front of the pericardium (Figure 16.1, Figure 16.2, Figure 16.3). On a CXR, the hilum overlay sign (one can see the hilar vessels through the mass), displacement of the anterior junction line, obliteration of the retrosternal space and a hazy cardio-phrenic angle suggest an anterior mediastinal mass (Box 16.3).

Thymoma is a tumour of epithelial cells arising in the thymus. It is commonest in men over 50 years and rare in patients younger than 20 years. It is associated with myasthenia gravis in 30–40%

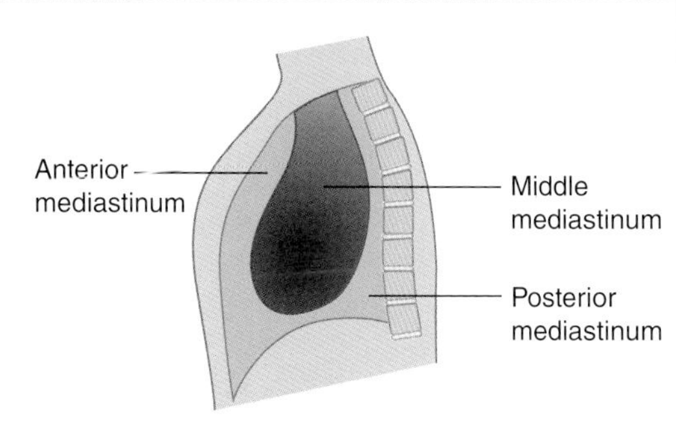

Figure 16.1 Outline of the mediastinum.

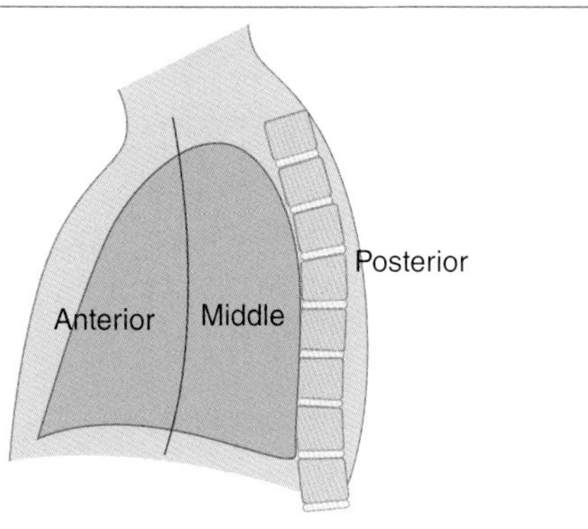

Figure 16.2 Compartments of the mediastinum on a lateral CXR.

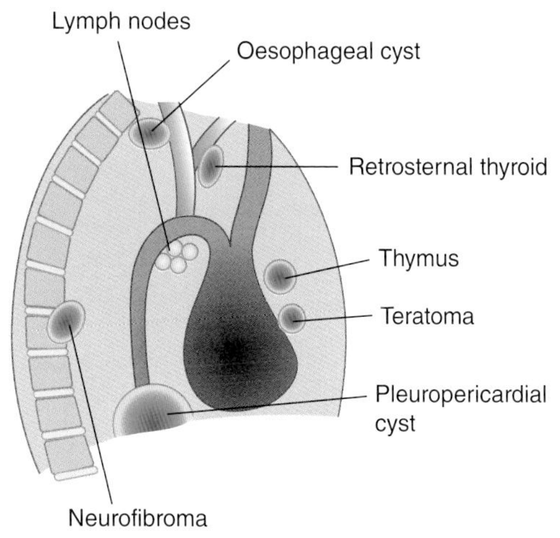

Figure 16.3 Common mediastinal masses in the anterior, middle, and posterior mediastinum.

Box 16.3 Differential diagnosis of anterior medistinal mass.

- The common mnemonic used for an anterior mediastinal mass is 'the Four T's': thymus, teratoma (germ cell tumour), thyroid and terrible lymphoma
- Thymoma
- Thymic cyst
- Thymic carcinoid
- Germ cell tumour (includes teratoma/ dermoid cyst)
- Lymphoma
- Thyroid goitre
- Parathyroid adenoma
- Ascending aortic aneurysm
- Pleuropericardial cyst
- Pericardial fat pad
- Morgagni anterior diaphragmatic hernia (congenital)

of cases, and 20% of patients presenting with myasthenia gravis (MG) are found to have a thymoma. Patients with MG have positive acetylcholine receptor autoantibodies which bind to acetylcholine receptors at the post-synaptic motor endplate causing nerve fatigue. Patients with thymoma and MG complain of pain, dyspnoea, dysphagia, and muscle weakness with repeated contraction, and the inability to maintain an upward gaze.

Thymomas contained within the thymic capsule tend to be relatively benign. If a thymoma is suspected radiologically, the case should be discussed with a thoracic surgeon and oncologist at the lung multidisciplinary meeting prior to a fine needle aspiration of the mass.

The treatment is with thymectomy, usually through a median sternotomy scar. A VATS procedure may be possible for small thymomas. A transcervical thymectomy may also be indicated in patients with myasthenia gravis without a thymoma as this can improve symptoms in many and result in complete remission in 30–40% of cases. Best results are obtained in younger patients with detectable acetylcholine receptor antibodies who present with early disease. Symptoms of myasthenia gravis should also be treated with pyridostigmine and with immunosuppressants, such as prednisolone or azathioprine.

Malignant thymomas extend outside the capsule and spread by 'seeding', invading local structures and spreading to the pleural space (Figure 16.4, Figure 16.5). The most widely used staging system for thymoma is the Masaoka system, which is based on the degree of capsular invasion (Table 16.2). The WHO system, which is based on the microscopic appearance of the cells, has subtypes A, B and C. Type C tumours are thymic carcinomas, which have the worst prognosis.

Thymic cysts can be congenital or acquired secondary to inflammation. They are asymptomatic unless large and cause symptoms of compression, in which case they should be excised. Thymic lipoma and thymic hyperplasia can also appear as an anterior mediastinal mass. **Thymic carcinoids** can behave aggressively, with local invasion and distant metastases. These tumours are not associated with myasthenia gravis but may be associated with Cushing's syndrome. Treatment is with surgery, chemotherapy, and octreotide.

Germ cell tumours are a diverse group of benign and malignant tumours which account for 10–15% of anterior mediastinal neoplasms in adults. They result from a failure of immature germ cells to migrate during embryogenesis, with the mediastinum being the commonest extragonadal site. Benign, mature **cystic teratomas (dermoid cysts)** are the commonest germ cell tumours in adults, accounting for 60–70% of cases, and occurring in the third decade. These well-differentiated tumours contain fat, skin, hair, eyes, nails, sweat glands, cartilage, and teeth. They usually

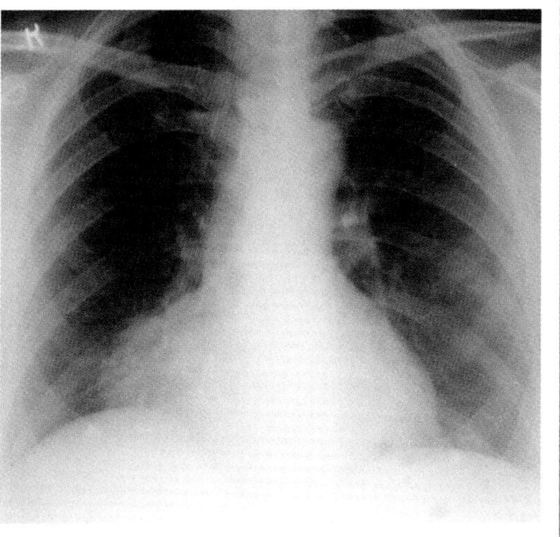

Figure 16.4 CXR of thymoma.

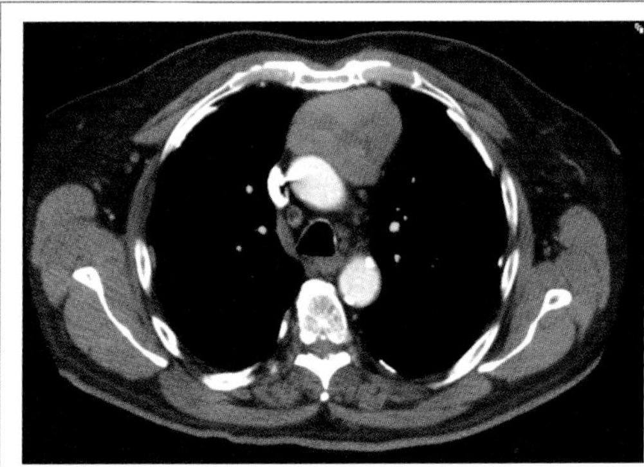

Figure 16.5 CT thorax showing thymoma.

Table 16.2 Masaoka system.

Stage	Extent of tumour invasion	Management	Cure rates (%)
1	No tumour invasion into capsule	Thymectomy	90–95
11	Tumour invasion into the fatty tissue around thymus and microscopic capsular invasion	Thymectomy + radiotherapy	85–90
111	Tumour invasion into surrounding organs	Chemotherapy or chemo-radiation followed by thymectomy	50–70
1VA	Tumour extension to the pleura and pericardium	Chemo-radiation + thymectomy in some cases	20–50
1VB	Spread to lymph nodes +/or distant metastases by haematogenous spread	Chemo-radiation + thymectomy in some cases	20

present with symptoms of compression and rarely with expectoration of hair (trichoptysis), sebum or fluid from a connection that forms between the tumour and the airways. Tumour markers are negative with a teratoma. CXR and CT thorax will reveal a well-circumscribed, multi-loculated, cystic mass with a fat-fluid level and calcification. Teeth and hair may be present. The prognosis is excellent with surgery.

The majority of malignant mediastinal germ cell tumours occur in men who will be symptomatic. Serum levels of β-hcg and/or AFP will be elevated in 80–85% of cases. **Seminomas** account for about half of malignant germ-cell tumours and affect men in their twenties and thirties. The CXR will depict a large, lobulated, well-defined anterior mediastinal mass. Local invasion of mediastinal structures is uncommon, although lymph node, lung, and bone metastases can occur. Treatment is with radiotherapy, chemotherapy and surgery, and the prognosis has improved significantly in the past decade. Measurement of tumour markers can be helpful in monitoring the disease.

Other malignant germ cell tumours affecting young men include choriocarcinoma, embryonal cell carcinoma, endodermal sinus tumour, and mixed germ-cell tumour. These too may secrete AFP and β-hcg. Some 20% of these men have Klinefelter's syndrome, and the tumour may also be associated with haematological malignancies. These lesions appear as a large, irregular, heterogeneous mass with central necrosis, haemorrhage, and cyst formation. Invasion of adjacent structures with pleural and pericardial effusions can occur. Distant metastases occur at an advanced stage. Treatment is with chemotherapy and surgery, and the five-year survival rate is 50%.

Lymphomas can arise from lymph nodes in the anterior or middle mediastinum. B-cell Hodgkin's lymphoma is the commonest type of lymphoma. Patients may present with B symptoms (fever, night sweats, and weight loss), and LDH levels may be elevated significantly. A surgical biopsy is recommended to confirm the histological diagnosis. The patient should be referred urgently to the haemo-oncologist for chemotherapy and further management.

A large, retrosternal **thyroid goitre** can appear as an antero-superior mediastinal mass. Patients are usually euthyroid, but may experience symptoms of dyspnoea and dysphagia because of compression of the trachea and oesophagus. The CXR and CT thorax may show tracheal deviation (Figure 16.6). The contrast CT scan may reveal enhancement of an encapsulated mass with haemorrhagic and cystic changes, and possible calcification. Further imaging with radioactive iodine (^{123}I or ^{131}I) scan and a thyroid ultrasound will be required, as well as thyroid function tests and measurement of thyroid antibodies. Surgery should be considered if the patient is symptomatic.

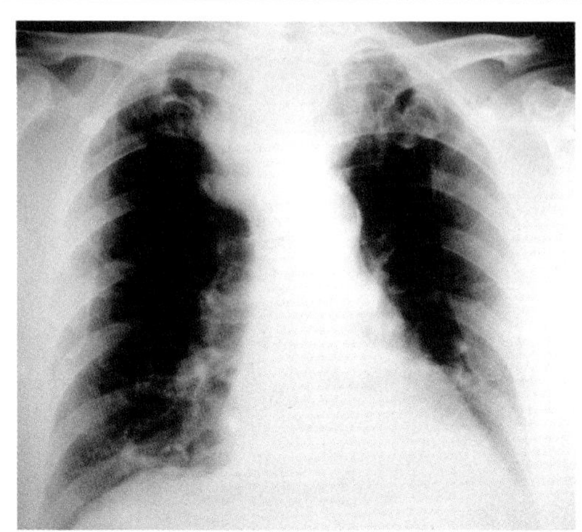

Figure 16.6 CXR showing retrosternal thyroid.

Parathyroid adenomas occur in elderly women and should be considered in those who have persistent hyperparathyroidism and hypercalcaemia despite parathyroidectomy. These benign functioning ectopic adenomas occur in the anterior mediastinum near the thymus. They may be too small to be detected on a CXR. A contrast CT thorax will show an encapsulated mass and there will be increased uptake with ^{99m}Tc sestamibi scintigraphy. Management is with surgical excision.

Middle mediastinal mass

The middle mediastinum is the area between the anterior and posterior mediastinum. A middle mediastinal mass may appear in the aorto-pulmonary window with widened paratracheal stripes, displacement of the azygo-oesophageal recess on the right, and a pseudoparavertebral line on the left (Box 16.4).

The commonest mass in the middle mediastinum is due to lymph node enlargement (Figure 16.7), which can be due to a variety of aetiologies (Box 16.5).

Box 16.4 Differential diagnosis for middle mediastinal mass.

- Lymphadenopathy
- Foregut duplication cysts: bronchogenic cyst, oesophageal duplication cyst
- Pericardial cyst
- Vascular anomalies: aortic arch anomalies
- Foramen of Morgagni diaphragmatic hernia

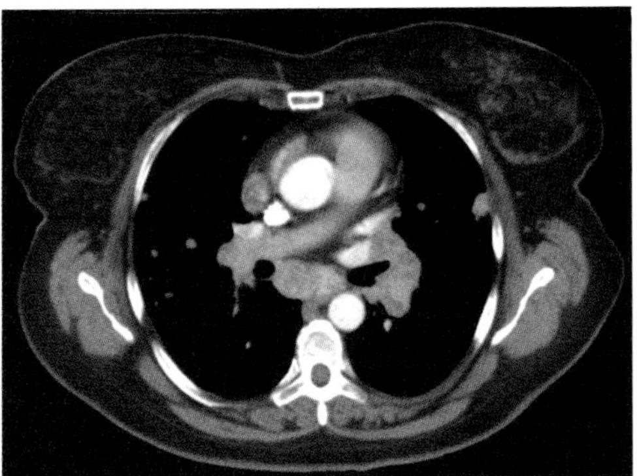

Figure 16.7 CT thorax with contrast showing lymphadenopathy.

Box 16.5 Causes of lymphadenopathy in mediastinum.

- Infectious granulomatous disease: mycobacterium tuberculosis, histoplasmosis, coccidiodomycosis
- Non-infectious granulomatous disease: sarcoidosis, silicosis
- Lymphoma: Hodgkin's lymphoma or non-Hodgkin's lymphoma
- Metastases to lymph node from lung, breast, renal cell carcinoma, gastrointestinal malignancy, mesothelioma, and prostate
- Reactive hyperplasia from viral or bacterial infection
- Amyloidosis
- Castleman's disease (giant lymph node hyperplasia)
- Drugs: phenytoin, methotrexate

Sarcoidosis commonly presents with symmetrical, bilateral, hilar lymphadenopathy. The other conditions listed can present with asymmetric lymph node enlargement. Calcification of lymph nodes can occur with tuberculosis and histoplasmosis. Silicosis is associated with 'eggshell calcification'.

Foregut duplication cysts account for 20% of mediastinal masses and are commoner in children. They are usually asymptomatic when small, but may cause symptoms of compression if they enlarge. Diagnosis can be made from characteristic radiological features, although biopsy or percutaneous CT-guided FNA may be necessary.

Some 50–60% of these are **bronchogenic cysts** which are the result of abnormal budding of the ventral foregut in embryogenesis. They can occur in adults of all ages and equally in men and women. They are asymptomatic unless they become infected or bleed. These occur most commonly in the subcarinal and paratracheal regions, although some can occur in the pulmonary parenchyma. CXR will show a well-circumscribed, spherical, homogeneous mass with fluid and calcification. There will be no enhancement with contrast on a CT scan. Bronchogenic cysts are lined with pseudostratified, columnar, ciliated respiratory epithelium and can contain fluid, mucus, milky fluid with calcium, blood, or purulent material. This material can be analysed from a FNA.

Oesophageal duplication cysts and neuroenteric cysts are commoner in children and originate from the dorsal foregut. They account for 10–15% of all cysts. Oesophageal cysts are located close to the distal oesophagus on the right, are lined by squamous or enteric epithelium and can contain gastric mucosa or pancreatic tissue. Neuroenteric cysts may also occur in the posterior mediastinum and contain neural tissue. These may be associated with spina bifida and other vertebral abnormalities.

Foregut duplication cysts should be followed up clinically and radiologically. Surgery should be considered if symptoms develop.

Pericardial cysts (also called spring water or clear water cysts) are rare, usually asymptomatic, and found incidentally in middle-aged adults. They appear as well-circumscribed, fluid-containing lesions abutting the heart, diaphragm, and the anterior chest wall, typically in the right cardiophrenic angle. The cyst does not enhance on a contrast CT scan. Management is conservative unless symptoms arise (Figure 16.8).

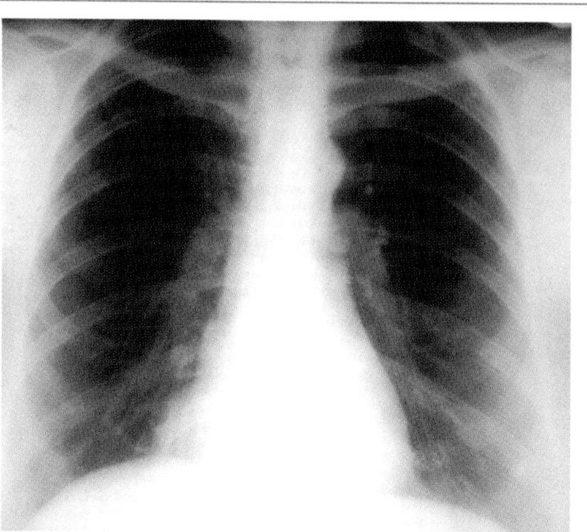

Figure 16.8 CXR showing a pericardial cyst.

Box 16.6 Differential diagnosis of posterior mediastinal mass.

- Neurogenic tumour
- Lipoma
- Descending aortic aneurysm
- Bochdalek posterior diaphragmatic hernia (congenital)
- Foregut duplication cyst
- Lateral thoracic meningocele

Vascular anomalies originate from the arterial or venous parts of the systemic or pulmonary circulation and account for 10% of all mediastinal masses. It is advisable to confirm that the lesion is vascular with angiography prior to any attempt at a biopsy to avoid catastrophic consequences.

Diaphragmatic hernias are common and can be due to congenital defects in the diaphragm. A foramen of Morgagni diaphragmatic hernia appears as a mass in the right cardiophrenic angle. CT thorax, combined with barium studies, can usually confirm the diagnosis.

Posterior mediastinal mass

The posterior mediastinum is the area behind the pericardium and in front of the vertebral bodies (see Figures 16.1–16.3). On a CXR, the mass extends above the superior clavicle (cervicothoracic sign) with widening of the paravertebral stripes (Box 16.6).

Most **neurogenic tumours** (90%) occur in the posterior mediastinum and account for 75% of primary, posterior mediastinal neoplasms. They constitute 15–20% of posterior mediastinal masses in adults, most of which are benign. They make up 40% of posterior mediastinal tumours in children, and 50% will be malignant. Neurogenic tumours can be divided into peripheral nerve sheath tumours, sympathetic ganglia tumours and paragangliomas.

Peripheral nerve sheath tumours include **neurofibromas** and schwannomas which are the commonest cause of a posterior mediastinal mass, and are usually benign in adults. Neurofibromas are slow-growing and arise from a posterior spinal nerve root and can involve any nerve in the thorax. They occur equally in men and women in their twenties and thirties and are asymptomatic when small. In 10% of cases, neurofibromas are multiple. 30–45% of neurofibromas occur in individuals with neurofibromatosis (von Recklinghausen's disease), who are at increased risk of malignant transformation of a pre-existing neurofibroma. If a neurofibroma increases in size, it can cause pain, pressure in the back, with erosion of ribs, vertebral bodies and neural foramina, and, in rare cases, results in spinal cord compression. If the neuroma is large enough to cause symptoms, surgery should be conducted after an MRI scan to ensure that there is no intraspinal extension. Symptoms of pain and a rapidly enlarging mass should alert the clinician to the possibility of a malignant transformation.

A neurofibroma appears as a round or lobulated, paravertebral, posterior, mediastinal mass, spanning one or two vertebral bodies. As it increases in size, it can appear as a dumb-bell structure straddling the intervertebral foramen. A CT scan demonstrates a heterogeneous mass which may contain calcification and low areas of attenuation.

Malignant tumours of the nerve sheath/neurosarcomas are a rare group of spindle cell sarcomas occurring equally in men and women in their twenties to their forties. Some 50% occur in patients with neurofibromatosis (Figure 16.9, Figure 16.10). They can invade locally and metastasize.

Sympathetic chain ganglia tumours include neuroblastomas, which occur in young children, and are the commonest neurogenic tumour in this age group. Ganglioneuromas and ganglioneuroblastomas occurs in older children. These are rare

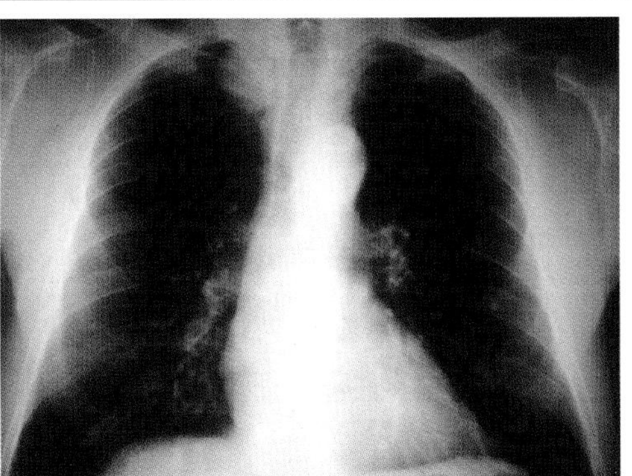

Figure 16.9 CXR showing a neurofibroma.

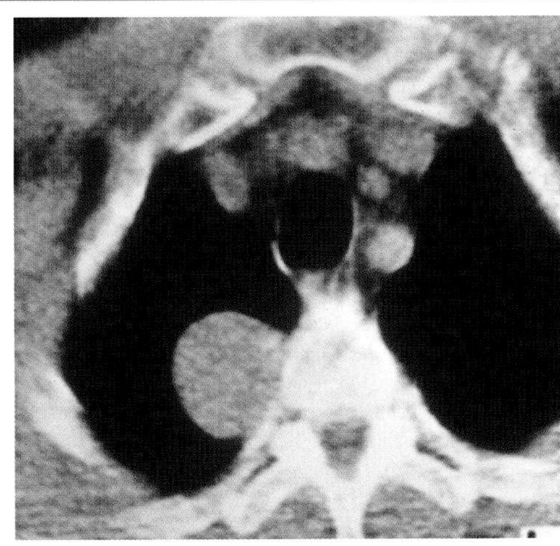

Figure 16.10 CT thorax showing a neurofibroma.

in adults. Some 50% arise from adrenal glands, with one-third in the mediastinum, the most common extra-abdominal location. Treatment is with surgery and chemotherapy.

Paragangliomas are rare neuroendocrine tumours that occur in men in the third and fourth decade; 75% of these occur sporadically, but 25% are hereditary and may be associated with a mutation of the gene for succinate dehydrogenase, or be part of Type 2a or 2b multiple endocrine neoplasia (MEN) syndrome. Paragangliomas usually arise from the adrenal gland, but 10% are extra-adrenal, occurring in the head, neck, thorax, or abdomen. Less than 2% of these are intra-thoracic, but these are more likely to be malignant. Only 3% are malignant and spread to distant sites; 1–3% of tumours secrete catecholamines and the clinical presentation is like that of a phaeochromocytoma. Management is surgical resection.

Lateral thoracic meningocele is a rare lesion that consists of redundant meninges.

Other mediastinal conditions

Conditions such as mediastinitis, haematoma, vascular lesions, and malignancies are can occur in any part of the mediastinum.

Mediastinitis can be caused by infection or inflammation (Box 16.7).

Acute mediastinitis can be secondary to bacterial infection or iatrogenic secondary to endoscopic surgical procedures. It is usually rapidly progressive and often fatal. Patients with acute mediastinitis are systemically unwell and present with fever,

Box 16.7 Causes of acute mediastinitis.

- Oesophageal rupture
- Tracheo-bronchial perforation
- Penetrating chest injury
- Post-operative sternal wound infection
- Oro-pharyngeal infection
- Paravertebral abscess
- Vertebral abscess
- Radiotherapy
- Anthrax
- Malignancy

rigors, chest wall tenderness, dyspnoea, and dysphagia. A CT thorax may show mediastinal widening, emphysema, pneumomediastinum, mediastinal air-fluid level, and pleural effusions. Treatment is that of the underlying cause and includes surgical drainage, debridement, and intravenous antibiotics.

Chronic (fibrosing) mediastinitis results from long-standing inflammation and the formation of dense fibrous tissue in the carinal, paratracheal, and hilar regions (Box 16.8). This results in significant compression of the mediastinal structures, causing dysphagia, breathlessness, and superior vena cava obstruction. CXR, contrast CT thorax, MRI scan, perfusion scintigraphy and biopsy may be required to exclude

Box 16.8 Causes of chronic mediastinitis (fibrosing mediastinitis).

- *Mycobacterium tuberculosis*
- *Histoplasmosis*
- Sarcoidosis
- Silicosis
- Autoimmune disease: retroperitoneal fibrosis, Riedel's thyroiditis, systemic lupus erythematosus, rheumatoid arthritis, sclerosing cholangitis
- Drugs: methysergide, practolol
- Mediastinal haematoma
- Radiation therapy

malignancy and infection, and to make the diagnosis. Unfortunately, no effective treatment is available, although surgery may relieve symptoms of compression.

Pneumomediastinum can result from rupture of the airways, causing air to track into the pulmonary interstitium and the soft tissues of the neck. It can be the caused by penetrating injury, for example, gunshot wounds, or oesophageal or tracheobronchial perforation. A pneumomediastinum can occur secondary to violent vomiting, acute airway obstruction (for example, in acute asthma) or severe coughing. Increased alveolar pressure from the Valsalva manoeuvre, the Heimlich manoeuvre, and mechanical ventilation can also result in a pneumomediastinum, as can iatrogenic causes such as mediastinal surgery, mediastinoscopy, tonsillectomy, or thyroidectomy. Pneumomediastinum can also be secondary to cervical emphysema or pneumoperitoneum that tracks into the mediastinum, often secondary to infection with gas-forming organisms. Patients with abnormal lungs are at greater risk.

The clinical symptoms include pleuritic chest pain, neck pain, dyspnoea, and dysphagia. Clinical signs include subcutaneous emphysema with crepitations in the neck and Hammans sign, which is a mediastinal crunch on auscultation. A CXR will show air outlining the mediastinal structures, and a lateral chest X-ray will reveal retrosternal air which will not move with a change in position (Figure 16.11, Figure 16.12).

There is a risk of developing a tension pneumothorax or a tension pneumopericardium, as well as mediastinitis. The prognosis depends on the underlying cause, but a pneumomediastinum usually resolves within a week.

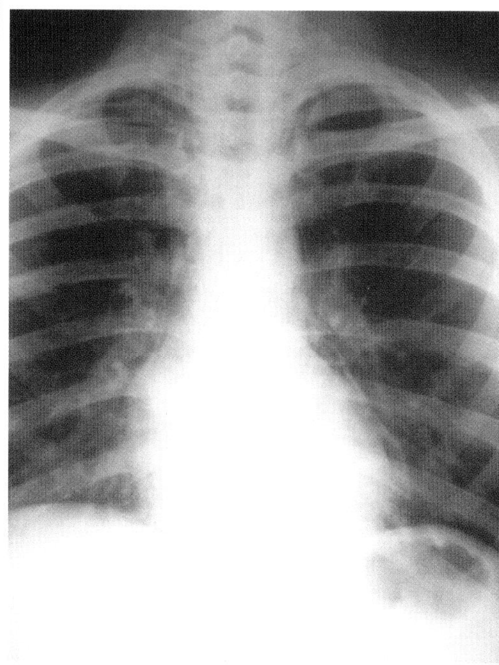

Figure 16.11 CXR showing a pneumomediastinum.

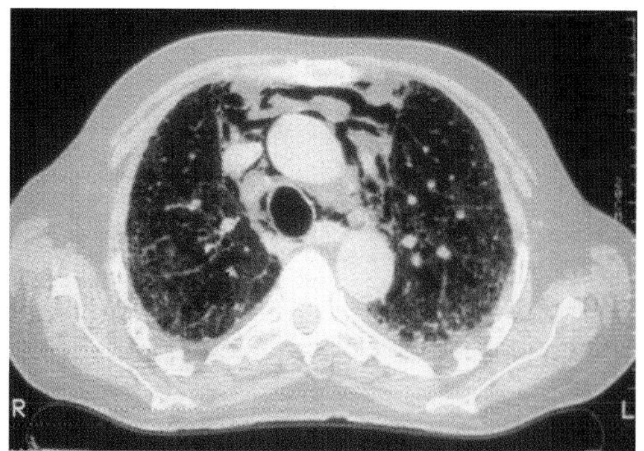

Figure 16.12 CT thorax showing a pneumomediastinum.

SUMMARY OF LEARNING POINTS

- The mediastinum is an area in the thorax between the lungs, vertebral bodies, thoracic inlet, and diaphragm.
- The mediastinum can be artificially separated into the anterior, middle, and posterior mediastinum.
- A contrast CT scan is necessary to understand the structure and exact location of a mediastinal mass.
- Masses in the mediastinum are often asymptomatic when small, causing symptoms of compression when they enlarge.
- The differential diagnoses of mediastinal masses varies in adults and children.
- Children are more likely to have a posterior mediastinal mass which is more likely to be malignant.
- Common causes of an anterior mediastinal mass in adults include thymoma, thyroid mass, teratoma (germ cell tumour), and lymphadenopathy.
- A thymoma is usually benign but may be associated with myasthenia gravis.
- Surgical resection of a thymoma is usually curative and relieves the symptoms of myasthenia gravis in a significant proportion of patients.
- Thymectomy may improve the symptoms of myasthenia gravis even in those without a thymoma.
- The majority of germ cell tumours in adults (teratomas) are benign.
- Seminomas are the commonest germ cell tumours in men and may secrete AFP and β-hcg.
- There are several causes of mediastinal lymphadenopathy, including infections, malignancies, sarcoidosis, and drugs.
- Bronchogenic cysts are developmental anomalies which are benign.
- Neurogenic tumours are the commonest cause of a posterior mediastinal mass.
- Neurofibromas are usually benign, but can become malignant in individuals with neurofibromatosis.
- Acute mediastinitis is a serious condition caused by infection and inflammation of the mediastinum, often secondary to trauma or procedures.
- Chronic (fibrosing) mediastinitis occurs from long-standing infection or inflammation, resulting in the formation of fibrous tissue.
- Chronic fibrosis can compress mediastinal structures and cause dysphagia and SVCO. There is no effective treatment for this.
- Pneumomediastinum can occur after penetrating chest injury, endoscopic procedures, barotrauma, or due to gas-forming bacteria from the peritoneum.

MULTIPLE CHOICE QUESTIONS

16.1 Which of the following statements about the mediastinum is true?

A The anterior mediastinum lies behind the pericardium
B The oesophagus lies within the anterior mediastinum
C The thymus is within the anterior mediastinum
D The middle mediastinum contains the sympathetic ganglia
E The posterior mediastinum contains the ascending aorta

Answer: C

The thymus lies in the anterior mediastinum, which is in front of the pericardium and behind the sternum. The oesophagus runs through the middle and posterior mediastinum. The ascending aorta is in the anterior mediastinum, while the posterior mediastinum contains the descending aorta and the sympathetic ganglia.

16.2 Which statement is true of most mediastinal masses?

A In adults they are malignant
B In children they are duplication cysts
C They have a poor prognosis

D In children they are congenital
E They secrete hormones

Answer: D

Overall, most mediastinal masses are benign, although they are more likely to be malignant in children. The commonest mediastinal tumours in children are neurogenic tumours. Only some germ-cell tumours and paragangliomas secrete hormones.

16.3 Which statement is true of a thymoma?
A It occurs most commonly in young women
B It can be associated with myasthenia gravis in 90% of cases
C It usually metastasises early
D It often transforms to a malignant thymoma
E It has a good prognosis

Answer: E

Thymomas are common in middle-aged men and are associated with myasthenia gravis in 30–40% of cases. They are usually benign and spread to local structures by breaching the capsule and seeding. Thymomas have a good prognosis if detected early. They do not commonly transform to a malignant thymoma.

16.4 Which of the following statements about germ cell tumours is true?
A Teratomas are the commonest germ cell tumour in adults
B Germ cell tumours account for 50% of anterior mediastinal masses
C Seminomas occur in elderly men
D Teratomas metastasise to the lungs and the heart
E The five-year survival with seminoma is less than 10%

Answer: A

Teratomas (dermoid cysts) are the commonest germ cell tumours in adults and are benign. Germ cell tumours account for 10–15% of anterior mediastinal masses in adults, most commonly in young men. Advances in treatment have resulted in significant improvement in survival.

16.5 What is the commonest cause of a middle mediastinal mass in an adult?
A Bronchogenic cyst
B Retrosternal thyroid
C Lymphadenopathy
D Pericardial cyst
E Diaphragmatic hernia

Answer: C

Lymphadenopathy (various causes) is the commonest middle mediastinal mass in an adult.

16.6 Which statement is true of bronchogenic cysts acquired secondary to infection?
A They can contain blood and mucus
B They are much commoner in women than in men
C They are lined with lung parenchymal cells
D They enhance with contrast CT scan
E They are associated with Neurofibromatosis

Answer: A

Bronchogenic cysts are development anomalies which occur equally in men and women. They are lined with pseudostratified, columnar, ciliated respiratory epithelium and can contain fluid, blood, and mucus. They do not enhance with contrast.

16.7 Which statement is true of posterior mediastinal masses?
A They are commoner in children than adults
B They are more likely to be malignant in adults
C They commonly present with spinal cord compression
D They usually secrete catecholamines
E They cause narrowing of the paravertebral stripe on a chest X-ray

Answer: A

The commonest posterior mediastinal masses are neurogenic tumours which are more common in children, and more likely to be malignant in children. They rarely cause spinal cord compression and only a small percentage of paragangliomas secrete catecholamines. On a chest X-ray there is widening of the paravertebral stripes.

16.8 Which of the following statements about neurogenic tumour is true?

A Neurogenic tumours grow rapidly
B They arise from the sympathetic ganglia
C They can occur in von Recklinghausen's disease
D They may secrete catecholamines
E They may be part of MEN Type 2a

Answer: C

Neurogenic tumours are slow-growing tumours that arise from peripheral nerves or nerve sheaths. Some 30% of individuals with neurofibroma have neurofibromatosis (von Recklinghausen's disease) and present with multiple neurofibromas. Paragangliomas are associated with MEN Types 2a and 2b and secrete catecholamines.

16.9 Which of the following statements is true of chronic mediastinitis?

A It can present with superior vena cava obstruction
B It can be treated effectively with intravenous steroids
C It can be caused by oesophageal rupture
D It can be treated with immunosuppression
E It can improve with cessation of the drug causing it

Answer: A

Chronic fibrosing mediastinitis results from long-standing inflammation secondary to infection, drugs, sarcoidosis, or autoimmune disease. When advanced, the fibrosis can cause compression of organs, including SVCO. There is no effective treatment for this.

16.10 Which statement is true of pneumomediastinum?

A It has a mortality rate of 80%
B It can be caused by the Valsalva manoeuvre
C It can be managed with a small chest drain
D It can improve with hyperbaric oxygen
E It always requires thoracic surgery

Answer: B

A pneumomediastinum can occur from trauma or alveolar over-distension and usually has a reasonable prognosis, resolving within seven days. This does, however, depend on the underlying cause. Chest drain, surgery or hyperbaric oxygen are not indicated.

FURTHER READING

Armstrong, P., Wilson, A., Dee, P., and Hansell, D. (1995). *Imaging of Diseases of the Chest*, 2nde. St. Louis, MO: Mosby.

Hill, N.S. (1999). Noninvasive mechanical ventilation. In: *Comprehensive Respiratory Medicine* (ed. R.R. Albert, S.C. Spiro and J.R. Jett), 12.1–12.10. London: Mosby.

Strollo, D.C., Rosado de Christenson, M.L., and Jett, J.R. (1997). Primary mediastinal tumors. Part 1: tumors of the anterior mediastinum. *Chest* 112 (2): 511–522.

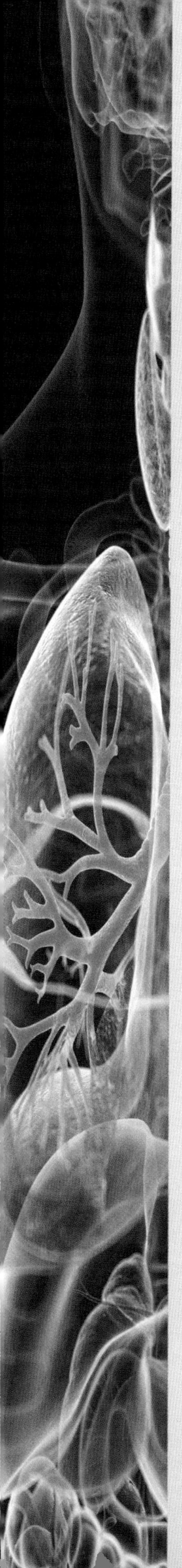

CHAPTER 17
Acute lung injury and acute respiratory distress syndrome

Learning objectives

- To understand some of the common causes of acute lung injury
- To understand the aetiology and pathogenesis of ARDS
- To understand the clinical features and diagnosis of ARDS
- To understand the prognosis and outcome of ARDS
- To appreciate the management of ARDS
- To appreciate the aetiology, presentation, and management of TRALI
- To appreciate the management of acute chest syndrome in sickle cell disease
- To understand the management of smoke inhalation
- To recognise the presentation and management of carbon monoxide poisoning
- To learn the physiological effects of drowning
- To understand the physiological consequences of deep sea diving
- To understand the presentation and management of acute altitude sickness

Essential Respiratory Medicine, First Edition. Shanthi Paramothayan.

Companion website: www.wiley.com/go/paramothayan/essential_respiratory_medicine

Abbreviations

ABG	arterial blood gas
ACS	acute chest syndrome
ALI	acute lung injury
APACHE 11	Acute Physiology and Chronic Health Evaluation
ARDS	acute respiratory distress syndrome
CO	carbon monoxide
COHB	carboxyhaemoglobin
COP	cryptogenic organising pneumonia
COPD	chronic obstructive pulmonary disease
CPAP	continuous positive airways pressure
CVP	central venous pressure
CXR	chest X-ray
ECG	electrocardiogram
ECMO	extra corporeal membrane oxygenation
FiO2	inspired oxygen concentration
GCS	Glasgow Coma Scale
HACE	high altitude cerebral oedema
HAPE	high altitude pulmonary oedema
HB	haemoglobin
HBO	hyperbaric oxygen
HBSS	homozygous sickle cell disease
HLA	human leukocyte antigen
HRCT	high-resolution computed tomography
ICU	intensive care unit
IL-1	interleukin 1
IL-6	interleukin 6
LVF	left ventricular failure
NIV	non-invasive ventilation
NO	nitric oxide
PCO_2	partial pressure of carbon dioxide
PEEP	positive end-expiratory pressure
PIP	peak inspiratory pressure
PO_2	partial pressure of oxygen
TNF-α	tumour necrosis factor alpha
TRALI	transfusion-related acute lung injury
TPN	total parenteral nutrition
V/Q	ventilation perfusion

Acute lung injury (ALI) and acute respiratory distress syndrome (ARDS)

Acute lung injury (ALI) can occur due to direct insult to the lungs or secondary to a systemic inflammatory response. ALI, which can develop over hours to days, causes a diffuse, inflammatory lung injury. ALI can progress to acute respiratory distress syndrome (ARDS) over a period of days. ALI progressing to ARDS has significant morbidity and mortality. Box 17.1 lists common causes of ALI and ARDS.

Box 17.1 Aetiology of ALI and ARDS.

Direct causes	Indirect causes
Lung infection: pneumonia	Anaphylaxis
Pulmonary trauma causing contusion	Eclampsia
Near drowning	Sepsis
Inhalation of toxic gases: ammonia, chlorine, phosgene	Hypotensive shock
Smoke inhalation	Drugs: salicylates, barbiturates
Aspiration of gastric contents (pH < 2)	Bowel infarction
Oxygen toxicity (FiO_2 > 0.8)	Burns
Amniotic fluid embolism	Haemorrhage
Fat embolism	Multiple blood transfusion
	Post cardiac arrest
	Pancreatitis
	Disseminated intravascular coagulopathy (DIC)

Diagnosis of ALI and ARDS

Patients with ALI and ARDS develop acute respiratory failure refractory to supplemental oxygen. They present with severe breathlessness, fever, cyanosis, tachycardia, and hypotension. As the condition worsens, patients display symptoms and signs of multi-organ failure, which includes delirium, crackles in the lungs, haemodynamic compromise, and renal failure. Serial arterial blood

Box 17.2 International criteria for diagnosis of ARDS: Berlin definition.

- Respiratory symptoms within a week of a known clinical insult
- Severe hypoxaemia ($PaO_2/FiO_2 < 200$)
- Bilateral diffuse parenchymal infiltrates on CXR
- Pulmonary artery occlusion pressure < 18 mmHg to exclude fluid overload

gas sampling will demonstrate worsening hypoxaemia and a metabolic acidosis. A chest-X-ray (CXR) typically shows bilateral pulmonary infiltrates.

Intubated patients with ARDS develop high peak and plateau airway pressures and increased amounts of frothy, exudative fluid from the lungs with a high neutrophil count. As this is not due to left ventricular failure (LVF), the pulmonary capillary wedge pressure will not be increased.

The differential diagnoses of ARDS includes respiratory infection, pulmonary oedema, pulmonary haemorrhage, acute exacerbation of interstitial lung disease, cryptogenic organising pneumonia (COP), acute eosinophilic pneumonia, acute interstitial pneumonia (Hamman-Rich syndrome), and disseminated malignancy. The diagnosis of ARDS is, therefore, made after excluding the above conditions.

Microbiological analysis of bronchoalveolar lavage fluid can point to an infective aetiology and a differential cell count can be helpful in determining the underlying cause. For example, a raised eosinophil count in the fluid may suggest acute eosinophilic pneumonia, while in COP there is a mixed pattern of increased lymphocytes, neutrophils, and eosinophils with a reduction in the number of macrophages. Patients who develop acute respiratory failure secondary to pulmonary haemorrhage will produce blood-stained secretions, with haemosiderin-laden macrophages in the lavage fluid, and may drop their haemoglobin (HB) if the haemorrhage is severe. Plasma brain natriuretic peptide level (BNP) < 100 $pg\,ml^{-1}$, a normal echocardiogram and a pulmonary capillary wedge pressure of <18 mmHg will exclude pulmonary oedema secondary to cardiac dysfunction.

If the aetiology of ARDS is not clear, then a surgical lung biopsy is recommended. This has a complication rate of 39%, but a relatively low mortality rate, and a specific diagnosis resulting in a change in management is made in 60% of cases. Box 17.2 lists the internationally agreed criteria for the diagnosis of ARDS.

The severity of ARDS depends on the level of hypoxaemia and is measured in a ventilated patient with a positive end-expiratory pressure (PEEP) of greater than 5 cm H_2O.

- **Mild ARDS:** $PaO_2/FiO_2 < 300$ mmHg > 200 mmHg on a ventilator setting that include PEEP >5 cm H_2O.
- **Moderate ARDS:** $PaO_2/FiO_2 < 200$ mmHg > 100 mmHg on a ventilator setting that include PEEP >5 cm H_2O.
- **Severe ARDS:** $PaO_2/FiO_2 < 100$ mmHg on a ventilator setting that include PEEP >5 cm H_2O.

To measure the PaO_2/FiO_2 ratio, the PaO_2 is measured in mmHg and the FiO_2 is expressed as a decimal between 0.21 and 1.

Incidence and mortality of ALI and ARDS

The incidence of ARDS is 2–8 cases/100 000 population per year. ALI is more common but is often not recognised. The overall mortality for ARDS is about 50%, but depends on the underlying cause and is greater in patients over the age of 60. For example, mortality may be 35% for ARDS secondary to trauma, 50% when sepsis is the cause and 80% for aspiration pneumonia. Death is usually secondary to multi-organ failure caused by tissue hypoxia. Survivors often develop chronic pulmonary fibrosis and impaired lung function, although those with ALI who are managed optimally can recover completely, with normal lung function.

Pathogenesis of ALI and ARDS

Insult to the lungs from a direct or indirect aetiology results in an acute inflammatory process. The initial acute inflammatory phase, which causes diffuse alveolar damage, lasts for 3–10 days, and causes widespread endothelial damage and the release of inflammatory cytokines, including IL-1, IL-6, and TNF-α. These cytokines activate neutrophils and monocytes which adhere to the endothelium and the alveolar epithelium and release proteolytic enzymes. These enzymes damage the alveolar-capillary membrane, resulting in loss of surfactant, increased alveolar-capillary permeability, alveolar collapse, and pulmonary oedema. The reduction in functioning alveoli causes ventilation/perfusion mismatch, worsening hypoxaemia, and respiratory failure. The alveolar arterial (A-a) gradient is widened.

After the acute inflammatory phase, as ALI progresses to ARDS, there is pulmonary fibrosis with hyaline membrane formation. The lungs become stiffer, with reduced compliance and increased dead space. Microthrombi can form in the pulmonary capillaries and progress to DIC, causing pulmonary vasoconstriction and pulmonary hypertension. Reduced tissue perfusion results in multi-organ failure. Secondary respiratory and systemic infections can occur.

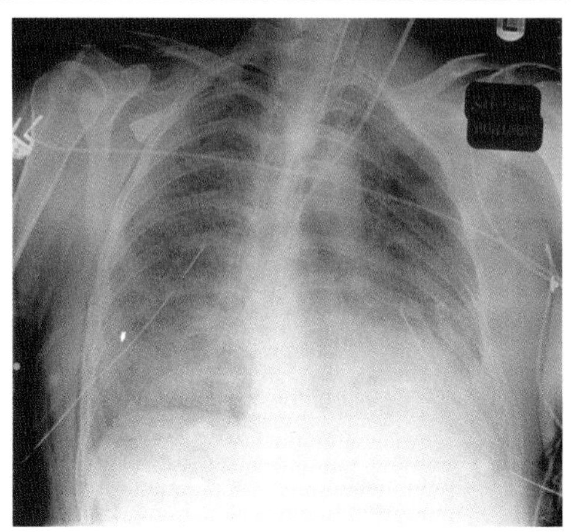

Figure 17.1 Chest X-ray showing ARDS.

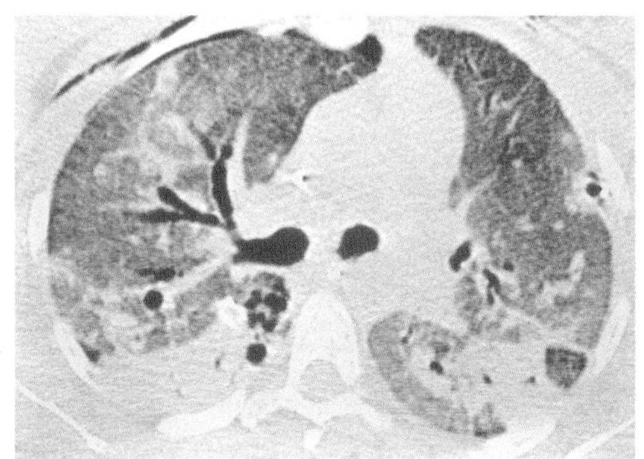

Figure 17.2 High resolution CT scan showing ARDS.

Investigations in patients suspected of ALI and ARDS

Early recognition of patients at risk of developing ALI is essential. Careful clinical monitoring on the high dependency unit (HDU) or intensive care unit (ICU) is recommended to pick up signs of deterioration, which may be subtle in the early stages. Serial arterial blood gas measurements through an arterial line, the measurement of central venous pressure and left atrial pressure will distinguish between pulmonary oedema secondary to left ventricular failure and ARDS. Careful assessment for signs of sepsis, including blood and urine cultures, as well as bronchial lavage, may be indicated. Chest X-ray and high-resolution CT thorax (HRCT) initially show widespread diffuse or patchy infiltrates with evidence of airspace consolidation, particularly in the dependent areas of the lung (Figure 17.1, Figure 17.2). Once ARDS is established, coarse, reticular changes, consistent with pulmonary fibrosis, develop.

Management of ALI and ARDS

Patients with ALI and ARDS are extremely unwell and should be managed in the ICU. Management consists of treating the underlying cause, treating secondary sepsis aggressively, appropriate fluid resuscitation, and oxygenation to reduce the risk of multi-organ failure. It is essential to avoid excessive intravenous fluid administration and to aim for a central venous pressure (CVP) of <4 mmHg. A combination of diuretics, systemic vasodilators, inotropes, and vasoconstrictors may be required to obtain adequate cardiac output and perfusion pressures at low left-atrial filling pressures.

General supportive care includes optimal nursing care, daily chest physiotherapy to clear secretions, nutritional support with total parenteral nutrition (TPN) to reduce hypoalbuminaemia, avoidance of pressure ulcers, prophylaxis against the development of venous thromboembolism, proton pump inhibitor to prevent gastrointestinal stress ulcers, and correction of anaemia. There is some evidence that medication to reduce body temperature will reduce the catabolic state which can worsen tissue hypoxia and contribute to multi-organ failure. Deep sedation and neuromuscular blockade are used to treat agitated delirium. This can help to optimise mechanical ventilation by reducing asynchrony with the ventilator and may improve survival in patients with severe ARDS.

Nosocomial infection in patients who are intubated and ventilated is a common cause of morbidity and mortality. This can be difficult to distinguish from ARDS, so if any doubt exists, patients should receive broad spectrum intravenous antibiotics.

Principles of mechanical ventilation in ARDS

In the initial stages of ALI, high inspired oxygen concentrations can be delivered using CPAP. However, as the condition deteriorates, patients will require mechanical ventilation. As lung compliance decreases secondary to pulmonary fibrosis and consolidation, high peak inspiratory pressures (PIP) and high positive end-expiratory pressures (PEEP) of >10 cm H_20 may be required to achieve normal tidal volumes.

The high pressures used in mechanical ventilation can result in ventilator-induced barotrauma to the normal alveoli, which are easier to inflate. Repeated alveolar collapse and re-expansion result in atelectasis and damage to the normal alveoli, exacerbating the ventilation-perfusion (V-Q) mismatch. Complications of mechanical ventilation include pneumothoraces and the formation of lung cysts. High oxygen concentrations can result in oxygen toxicity. Ventilator-induced barotrauma is associated with a poor outcome in ARDS.

Ventilating at low tidal volumes and keeping the plateau airway pressure to less than 30 cm H_2O reduces alveolar over-distension, recruits collapsed alveoli, is associated with fewer complications, and improves mortality in patients with ARDS. Patients with moderately severe or severe ARDS ($PaO_2/FiO_2 < 200$ mmHg) (26.6 kPA) may require a high PEEP. Permissive hypercapnia, resulting from low tidal volume ventilation, is well tolerated. Nursing the patient in a prone position ensures that blood flow is greatest in areas of the dependent lung and improves the VQ mismatch.

Extra-corporeal membrane oxygenation (ECMO) in a specialist centre may be necessary if the usual ventilatory methods fail, although improved survival has not been proven in adults.

Other therapies for ARDS

Inhaled nitric oxide (NO) increases capillary blood flow to the ventilated alveoli and reduces the VQ mismatch, but has not been shown to reduce mortality. Inhaled prostacyclin and prostaglandin E1 have improved physiological parameters in trials but have not been shown to improve survival. There is some debate as to whether corticosteroids given in the initial 7–10-day period reduce the risk of developing pulmonary fibrosis and influence the long term prognosis of patients with ARDS. Corticosteroids are contra-indicated in the latter stages of the condition.

There is currently limited evidence for the use of exogenous surfactant or antioxidant therapy. β-2 agonists, N-acetylcysteine, and ibuprofen have not been shown to be beneficial. Trials looking at human mesenchymal stem cells and recombinant human activated protein C are currently underway.

Morbidity and mortality in ARDS

Patients with ARDS die from the underlying cause of the ARDS and secondary complications, particularly nosocomial infection, rather than from respiratory failure. Survivors can take several months to improve. Many are left with persistent cognitive impairment resulting from hypoxic brain injury, myopathy, renal impairment, pulmonary fibrosis, and pulmonary hypertension.

Transfusion-Related Acute Lung Injury (TRALI)

Transfusion-related acute lung injury (TRALI), an important cause of transfusion-related death, can occur within a few hours of the transfusion of any blood product, although most cases are related to red blood cell transfusion. TRALI occurs when the donor plasma has antibodies to human leukocyte and human neutrophil antigens, and this is more likely to occur when plasma or blood products from a multiparous female donor are used. The recipient neutrophils are sensitised by the underlying clinical condition and are then activated by the anti-leukocyte antibodies.

The true incidence of TRALI is unknown, but is estimated to occur in 0.04–0.1% of transfused patients and in up to 8% of critically ill patients, which equates to 1:5000 transfused blood components. TRALI is more likely to occur in patients who have a high APACHE 11 score, and particularly prevalent in patients who have had surgery, those with sepsis, those who have received a large transfusion, and in alcoholics.

Patients developing TRALI become breathless and severely hypoxic during or immediately after transfusion of a blood product. When TRALI is suspected, the transfusion should be stopped immediately and the transfusion service should be notified. Supportive treatment includes oxygenation and appropriate ventilatory support using lung protective strategies. Mortality depends on the patient's underlying illness and can be up to 60%. Patients who survive usually make a complete recovery. The incidence of TRALI has decreased with the use of plasma products primarily from male donors, female donors without prior pregnancy or those who test negative for HLA antibodies.

Acute chest syndrome with sickle cell disease

Acute chest syndrome (ACS) developing during a sickle cell crisis is the most common cause of death in adults with homozygous sickle cell disease (HBSS). Approximately 50% of patients with HBSS will have an episode of ACS, the majority associated with a vaso-occlusive pain crisis. Patients with other phenotypes of sickle cell disease are at a lower risk of ACS.

Most episodes of ACS are secondary to bone marrow ischaemia and necrosis, causing fat emboli and bone marrow to enter into the venous circulation, which mainly affects the lungs and the central nervous system. The fat emboli mechanically obstruct the blood vessels, but also release free fatty acids which cause inflammation and tissue injury. Additionally, there is accumulation of microthrombi in the pulmonary vessels.

A diagnosis of fat emboli can be difficult to make. Clinical signs include a petechial rash and lipaemia retinalis. Induced sputum or bronchial lavage will show fat-laden alveolar macrophages. Bone marrow necrosis and fat emboli can also result in liver and kidney failure.

ACS presents with high fever, severe chest pain, dyspnoea, hypoxia, and new radiological changes on chest X-ray. The differential diagnoses includes pulmonary embolus and pneumonia. Supportive management includes supplemental oxygen, analgesia, intravenous fluids, thromboprophylaxis, antibiotics, bronchodilators, and incentive spirometry to reduce pulmonary atelectasis. Exchange blood transfusion is usually carried out to achieve a haemoglobin S% of 30%. Patients who have more than two episodes of ACS are usually commenced on hydroxyurea and a chronic transfusion programme to keep the HB S level < 50%. Haematopoietic cell transplantation could also be considered for those with recurrent episodes of ACS.

There is some evidence that repeated episodes of ACS predispose to the development of interstitial pulmonary disease, historically known as chronic sickle cell lung disease. This can progress to pulmonary hypertension and respiratory failure. There is little evidence that ACS directly causes pulmonary hypertension.

Smoke inhalation

Fire kills because of smoke inhalation and severe airway burns. Inhaled toxins, such as chlorine, phosgen, and sulphur dioxide, can cause erythema, oedema, and ulceration of the airways. It should be presumed that all patients with smoke inhalation have been exposed to CO and cyanide, which is formed from the burning of common household compounds, such as nylon, wool, and cotton. Cyanide can kill rapidly by inhibiting aerobic metabolism.

Patients who present with suspected smoke inhalation need a thorough assessment of their airway. Clinical features of concern include tachypnoea, erythema, burns to the face and neck and blistering of the oropharynx found at laryngoscopy. Symptoms of cough and wheeze will occur within seconds and respiratory distress will occur within 12–36 hours of exposure.

Patients should have serial arterial blood gas measurements of oxyhaemoglobin level and measurement of carboxyhaemoglobin, methaemoglobin, and lactate levels. A toxicology screen should be sent and a CXR obtained, although it is a poor indicator of lung injury. Patients with an unexplained lactic acidosis and a low $PaCO_2$ may have cyanide poisoning.

Patients should be given 100% inspired oxygen to reverse the tissue hypoxia and displace the CO and cyanide bound to proteins. The treatment for cyanide poisoning is with sodium thiosulfate and hydroxocobalamin. Nebulised bronchodilators and prophylactic antibiotics are usually prescribed and the patient must be continuously monitored. Patients who suffer with smoke inhalation can develop secondary airway obstruction due to oedema and secretions, develop secondary infections, and can progress to ARDS over days. Patients who develop stridor with worsening airway oedema are at risk of respiratory and cardiac arrest and should be intubated and ventilated.

Carbon monoxide poisoning

Carbon monoxide (CO) poisoning is common, often undiagnosed, and potentially fatal. It should be considered in all patients presenting with smoke inhalation but is also commoner in the winter months as it often occurs with faulty boilers and poorly ventilated fuel-burning devices. CO has an affinity for haemoglobin 240 times greater than oxygen, diffuses rapidly across the capillary membrane of the lungs and binds to haemoglobin, forming carboxyhaemoglobin (COHB). CO reduces the amount of oxygen transported to tissues for glycolysis.

Patients with CO poisoning present with non-specific symptoms, including headaches, confusion, nausea, dizziness, and general malaise: the symptoms are often mistakenly thought to have a viral aetiology. Patients are noted to have "cherry red" lips. When severe, patients may present with seizures and a reduced Glasgow Coma Scale (GCS).

Doctors should have a high index of suspicion and should take a detailed social history. A neurological examination is essential and evidence of end-organ damage, which includes cardiac ischaemia, should be sought. Pulse oximetry and blood gas measurements will be normal as these cannot distinguish between oxyhaemoglobin and carboxyhaemoglobin (COHB). COHB measurements can be obtained from a blood gas sample using co-oximetry. Non-smokers have CO levels < 3% while smokers may have levels up to 15%.

Patients with CO poisoning require continuous monitoring on a HDU or ICU. Management is with 100% inspired oxygen using a non-breathing face mask. The guidelines recommend hyperbaric oxygen therapy (HBO) if the CO level is >25%, if the CO level is >20% in a pregnant woman, if there is a severe metabolic acidosis with a pH < 7.1, or if there is evidence of cardiac ischaemia on ECG. There is some evidence that hyperbaric oxygen reduces the severity of cognitive defects. Patients who have a reduced GCS should be intubated and ventilated. The local council and fire departments should be alerted to seal off the premises to prevent harm to others.

Airway trauma

Direct trauma to the airway can occur secondary to any injury to the head, neck, oropharynx, or upper chest. Causes include blunt or penetrating injuries, burns, smoke inhalation, and ingestion of caustic substances. These injuries can result in immediate or delayed airways obstruction. The clinician needs to assess the patient and the airway for signs of obstruction and the likelihood of deterioration. Continuous pulse oximetry monitoring is essential. If oedema or a haematoma are likely to develop, then it is advisable to intubate the patient.

Near-drowning

Drowning, either in freshwater (90%) or sea water (10%), is a common cause of death worldwide, especially in children. Individuals submerged in water breath-hold until they exceed the breaking point. Aspiration of water occurs in 85% of cases before laryngospasm and bronchospasm set in. Drowning causes a loss of surfactant in the lung, resulting in atelectasis, and exudative fluid pours into the alveoli. This is exacerbated by the vasoconstriction that occurs in the pulmonary vessels secondary to hypoxia. If the individual is not removed from the water, there is worsening hypoxaemia, hypercapnoea, acidosis, and cardiac arrest.

Management is with immediate basic life support, oxygen, and treatment of any hypothermia, Prolonged resuscitation is recommended, especially in children and in those with hypothermia. Unconscious patients will need to be intubated and mechanically ventilated using high PEEP. Those who are conscious and appear to have recovered should be monitored carefully for at least six hours as pulmonary oedema can occur up to four hours after the event.

Deep sea diving

Diving to depths greater than 30 m (98 ft) has significant physiological effects on gas exchange. Divers breathe a mixture of gases, including Heliox. The greater density of gas results in increased airway resistance which increases the work of breathing. There is also a reduction in the maximum breathing capacity and a reduction in pulmonary compliance.

In addition, there is an increase in the dead space in the lungs which results in hypoventilation and hypercapnoea. Oxygen exchange in the alveoli is compromised when the gas density exceeds 25 $g l^{-1}$. Decompression stops during the dive are required to minimise this risk. There is also a risk of oxygen toxicity.

Asymptomatic lung rupture can occur in normal individuals, even at sea level, with everyday manoeuvres such as coughing, sneezing, and breath-holding. These are usually small and have no significant adverse effects. When a diver ascends, the volume of air in the lungs expands according to Boyle's Law. This can cause pulmonary barotrauma which can result in air embolism which then escapes into the arterial circulation. Divers often do "skip breathing" when they inhale, then pause, then exhale and this may predispose to lung rupture as the lungs are stretched to their elastic limit. There is a risk of developing a tension pneumothorax on ascent secondary to pulmonary barotrauma.

Individuals at risk of a pneumothorax, for example, those with chronic lung disease, are advised against deep sea diving. A fit and healthy young adult who has had a spontaneous pneumothorax should be safe to dive if they have had bilateral pleurectomies, have not had a pneumothorax for five years and if a CT thorax and lung function with flow volume loops are normal, as the risk of barotrauma is not significantly greater than that for the general population. An individual who has suffered a traumatic or iatrogenic pneumothorax, for example, after non-invasive ventilation, should be safe to dive so long as there has been complete resolution as assessed by CT thorax and full lung function tests. Pneumothorax is discussed in Chapter 10.

Nitrogen narcosis initially causes a feeling of euphoria which can rapidly progress to decreased consciousness and coma. A rapid ascent can result in decompression sickness or "the bends" when nitrogen dissolved in the blood and tissues forms bubbles and causes dysbaric osteonecrosis of bones, especially in the humerus and femur.

Acute altitude sickness

Acute altitude or mountain sickness is caused by rapid ascent to altitudes above 2400 m (8000 ft). Although the percentage of oxygen at high altitudes remains at 21%, the partial pressure of oxygen decreases, so climbers become progressively more hypoxaemic. Early flu-like symptoms, which include headaches, dizziness, fatigue, abdominal cramps, nausea, and vomiting, occur approximately eight hours after ascent. The symptoms usually resolve after two days of acclimatisation. Nosebleeds and insomnia are also common symptoms.

Ascent to over 3500 m (11 500 ft) without acclimatisation can result in high altitude pulmonary oedema (HAPE) and high altitude cerebral oedema (HACE), which can be fatal. Climbers with HAPE present with severe breathlessness at rest, fever, and a cough which is initially, dry but then productive of pink, frothy sputum. It is postulated to occur due to pulmonary vasoconstriction secondary to ventilation/perfusion (VQ) mismatch. HACE, which may develop secondary to vasodilation of cerebral blood vessels, presents with severe headaches, neurological symptoms, and can progress to coma and death. Factors which determine the development of HAPE and HACE include rate of ascent, the altitude reached, and an individual's susceptibility.

Acute mountain sickness, HAPE, and HACE can be prevented by ascending slowly, not undertaking strenuous physical activities for 24 hours and avoiding alcohol which can exacerbate the dehydration that occurs at high altitudes due to loss of water vapour. Management of acute mountain sickness includes immediate descent as well as supplemental oxygen, which can be given by a Gamow bag. Acetazolamide, given at 125 mg twice a day, relieves symptoms and improves oxygenation by stimulating the respiratory centre to increase the respiratory rate. Dexamethasone can be beneficial in the short term for HACE, but moving the patient to a lower altitude is essential.

Chronic mountain sickness (Monge's disease) occurs in people living at altitudes above 3000 m (10 000 ft), especially in the Andes in South America. It is linked to expression of genes ANP32D and SENP1. Chronic hypoxaemia causes an increase in erythropoiesis, resulting in polycythaemia (HB > 200 $g l^{-1}$ and haematocrit >65%), hyperviscosity and VQ mismatch. It can progress to pulmonary hypertension and cor pulmonale which may warrant urgent venesection. Descent to a lower altitude improves symptoms and reverses early physiological changes.

SUMMARY OF LEARNING POINTS

- ALI can result from direct or indirect insult to the lungs.
- ALI can progress to ARDS over several days with significant mortality.
- Clinical signs of ARDS include tachypnoea, tachycardia, and worsening hypoxaemia.
- The main differential diagnosis of ARDS is cardiogenic pulmonary oedema.
- Management of ARDS includes early recognition, treatment of the underlying cause, adequate oxygenation, and supportive treatment.
- Mechanical ventilation using lung-protective strategies has been shown to improve survival in ARDS.
- TRALI is a cause of ARDS which occurs after transfusion of blood products.
- Sickle cell lung crisis is a significant cause of morbidity and mortality in patients with HBSS.
- A lung crisis and ARDS can occur secondary to fat and bone marrow embolism in patients with HBSS.
- Individuals with smoke inhalation must have careful assessment of their upper airway and should be continuously monitored.
- Individuals with smoke inhalation must be presumed to have CO and cyanide exposure which need to be treated.
- Survivors of near-drowning need to be monitored for several hours as pulmonary oedema can occur four hours after the event.
- Deep sea diving results in significant physiological changes in gas exchange and is associated with an increased risk of pneumothorax.
- The risk of pneumothorax when diving is high in patients with chronic lung disease.
- An individual with a spontaneous, primary pneumothorax does not have a greater risk of developing a further pneumothorax when diving if they have had definitive surgery and their CT thorax and lung function are normal.
- Acute altitude sickness occurs over 2400 m in individuals who attempt a rapid ascent without acclimatisation.
- In severe cases, individuals can develop high altitude pulmonary oedema and or high altitude cerebral oedema, both of which can be fatal.
- Treatment of HAPE and HACE includes descent, oxygen therapy, dexamethasone, and acetazolamide.
- Chronic altitude sickness (Monge's disease) is associated with polycythaemia, hyperviscosity of blood, and can progress to cor pulmonale. Management is with descent and venesection.

MULTIPLE CHOICE QUESTIONS

17.1 Which of the following conditions is not a cause of ARDS?

A Blood transfusion
B Bowel obstruction
C COPD
D Near-drowning
E Sickle cell crisis

Answer: C

There is no association between COPD and ARDS.

17.2 Which of the following features makes ARDS unlikely?

A Bilateral infiltrates on chest X-ray
B Hypotension
C Increased pulmonary capillary wedge pressure
D Metabolic acidosis
E Reduced urine output

Answer: C

Increased pulmonary capillary wedge pressure suggests left ventricular failure which may result in pulmonary oedema, one of the main differential diagnoses. All the others are features of ARDS.

17.3 Which of the following investigations will NOT be helpful in identifying the aetiology of ARDS?

A Blood cultures
B Bronchoalveolar lavage
C Echocardiogram
D Open lung biopsy
E Serial ABG measurement

Answer: E

Serial ABG measurements will merely show worsening hypoxaemia but will not identify the cause of the ARDS. All the other investigations may give a clue as to the aetiology.

17.4 Which of the following strategies of mechanical ventilation have been shown to be beneficial?

A Ensuring that the PCO_2< 3 kPa
B Keeping plateau airway pressure <30 cm H_2O
C Nursing the patient on their side
D Ventilating at high volumes
E Ventilating at high pressures

Answer: B

To prevent barotrauma to normal alveoli, it is recommended that patients are ventilated using low tidal volumes and keeping the plateau pressure <30 cm H_2O. Hypercapnoea often develops but does not have a significantly harmful effect. Nursing the patient in a prone position improves VQ mismatch.

17.5 Which of the following treatments for ARDS has been shown to improve survival?

A Corticosteroids given at 14 days
B ECMO
C NO
D Surfactant
E Ventilating at low tidal volumes

Answer: E

Ventilating at low tidal volumes reduces barotrauma and therefore improves survival in patients with ARDS. NO, a vasodilator, increases capillary blood flow and reduces VQ mismatch but has not yet been shown to improve survival. There is limited trial benefit for the use of corticosteroids given after 14 days, ECMO, and exogenous surfactant.

17.6 What should the doctor do with patients presenting with smoke inhalation?

A Be discharged home if the initial arterial blood gas is satisfactory
B Be discharged home if the initial chest X-ray is normal
C Be intubated and ventilated on ICU
D Have methaemoglobin concentration measured
E Receive hyperbaric oxygen

Answer: D

Patients are at risk of developing complications 12–36 hours after smoke inhalation. This includes airway obstruction, secondary infection, and progression to ARDS. These patients should have serial ABG measurements and be continuously monitored. Methaemoglobin level should be measured.

17.7 When is TRALI more likely to occur?

A In a patient with a low APACHE 11 score
B In a patient with O negative blood
C Several days after a blood transfusion
D When the donor is male
E When the patient receives a large blood transfusion

Answer: E

TRALI is associated with large blood transfusions, especially in severely ill patients with a high APACHE 11 score. It occurs during or soon after the transfusion and is more common when the donor is a multiparous woman as the blood will contain antibodies to human leukocyte and human neutrophil antigens.

17.8 How can a diagnosis of CO poisoning initially be made?

A Arterial blood gas measurement
B Changes on chest X-ray
C Measurement of carboxyhaemoglobin level
D Pulse oximetry
E Toxicology screen

Answer: C

Measurement of carboxyhaemoglobin level is required in any patients presenting with smoke inhalation or symptoms suggestive of CO poisoning. There needs to be a high index of suspicion. Pulse oximetry and arterial blood gas measurements will be normal.

17.9 Patients with CO poisoning should be given hyperbaric oxygen if

A The CO level is >10%
B The woman is pregnant
C The patient is in a coma
D There are ischaemic changes on ECG
E The $PaCO_2 > 6\,kPa$

Answer: D

The indications for HBO include a CO level of >25%, a level > 20% in a pregnant woman and if there is evidence of end organ damage, which includes cardiac ischaemia and neurological symptoms. Patients with a reduced GCS should be intubated and ventilated without delay.

17.10 A young man, who had a spontaneous, unilateral pneumothorax six years earlier, asks if he can go scuba diving. What should he be advised?

A Diving is contraindicated
B Diving is safe after five years
C Diving is safe if CT scan if normal
D Diving is safe if lung function is normal
E Diving is safe if he had bilateral pleurectomies and CT scan and lung function are normal

Answer: E

The current advice is that a patient with a spontaneous primary pneumothorax does not have a risk of a pneumothorax greater than the general population when diving if he/she has had bilateral pleurectomies and the CT scan and full lung function test are normal.

FURTHER READING

Artigas, A., Bernard, G.R., Carlet, J. et al. (1998). The American-European consensus conference on ARDS, part 2: Ventilatory, pharmacologic, supportive therapy, study design strategies, and issues related to recovery and remodeling. Acute respiratory distress syndrome. *American Journal of Respiratory and Critical Care Medicine* 157 (4 Pt 1): 1332–1347.

Chastre, J., Trouillet, J.L., Vuagnat, A. et al. (1998). Nosocomial pneumonia in patients with acute respiratory distress syndrome. *American Journal of Respiratory and Critical Care Medicine* 157 (4 Pt 1): 1165–1172.

Ernst, A. and Zibrak, J.D. (1998). Carbon monoxide poisoning. *New England Journal of Medicine* 339 (22): 1603–1608.

Hackett, P.H. and Roach, R.C. (2001). High-altitude illness. *New England Journal of Medicine* 345 (2): 107–114.

Haponik, E.F., Crapo, R.O., Herndon, D.N. et al. (1988). Smoke inhalation. *The American Review of Respiratory Disease* 138 (4): 1060–1063.

Hudson, L.D., Milberg, J.A., Anardi, D., and Maunder, R.J. (1995). Clinical risks for development of the acute respiratory distress syndrome. *American Journal of Respiratory and Critical Care Medicine* 151 (2 Pt 1): 293–301.

Leitch, D.R. and Green, R.D. (1986). Pulmonary barotrauma in divers and the treatment of cerebral arterial gas embolism. *Aviation, Space, and Environmental Medicine* 57 (10 Pt 1): 931–938.

Neff, T.A., Stocker, R., Frey, H.-R. et al. (2003). Long-term assessment of lung function in survivors of severe ARDS. *Chest* 123 (3): 845–853.

Ranieri, V.M., Rubenfeld, G.D., Thompson, B.T. et al. (2012). Acute respiratory distress syndrome: the Berlin definition. *JAMA* 307 (23): 2526–2533.

Toy, P., Popovsky, M.A., Abraham, E. et al. (2005). Transfusion-related acute lung injury: definition and review. *Critical Care Medicine* 33 (4): 721–726.

Vichinsky, E.P., Neumayr, L.D., Earles, A.N. et al. (2000). Causes and outcomes of the acute chest syndrome in sickle cell disease. National Acute Chest Syndrome Study Group. *The New England Journal of Medicine* 342 (25): 1855–1865.

Index

Page numbers in **bold** indicate boxes and those in *italic* indicate tables.

Essential Respiratory Medicine, First Edition. Shanthi Paramothayan.

Companion website: www.wiley.com/go/paramothayan/essential_respiratory_medicine